PEDIATRICS, CHILD AND ADOLESCENT HEALTH

CHILD AND ADOLESCENT HEALTH YEARBOOK 2013

PEDIATRICS, CHILD AND ADOLESCENT HEALTH

SERIES EDITOR - JOAV MERRICK

NATIONAL INSTITUTE OF CHILD HEALTH AND HUMAN DEVELOPMENT, MINISTRY OF SOCIAL AFFAIRS, JERUSALEM

Child and Adolescent Health Yearbook 2011
Joav Merrick (Editor)
2012. ISBN: 978-1-61942-782-2 (Hardcover)
2012. ISBN: 978-1-61942-783-9 (e-book)

Child and Adolescent Health Yearbook 2012
Joav Merrick (Editor)
2012. ISBN: 978-1-61942-788-4 (Hardcover)
2012. ISBN: 978-1-61942-789-1 (e-book)

Child and Adolescent Health Yearbook 2013
Joav Merrick (Editor)
2014. ISBN: 978-1-63117-658-6 (Hardcover)

Child Health and Human Development Yearbook 2011
Joav Merrick (Editor)
2012. ISBN: 978-1-61942-969-7 (Hardcover)
2012. ISBN: 978-1-61942-970-3 (e-book)

Child Health and Human Development Yearbook 2012
Joav Merrick (Editor)
2012. ISBN: 978-1-61942-978-9 (Hardcover)
2012. ISBN: 978-1-61942-979-6 (e-book)

Developmental Issues in Chinese Adolescents
Daniel T. L. Shek, Rachel C. F. Sun and Joav Merrick (Editors)
2012. ISBN: 978-1-62081-262-4 (Hardcover)
2012. ISBN: 978-1-62081-270-9 (e-book)

Positive Youth Development: A New School Curriculum to Tackle Adolescent Developmental Issues
Hing Keung Ma, Daniel T. L. Shek and Joav Merrick (Editors)
2012. ISBN: 978-1-62081-384-3 (Hardcover)
2012. ISBN: 978-1-62081-385-0 (e-book)

Positive Youth Development: Theory, Research and Application
Daniel T. L. Shek, Rachel C. F. Sun and Joav Merrick (Editors)
2012. ISBN: 978-1-62081-305-8 (Hardcover)
2012. ISBN: 978-1-62081-347-8 (e-book)

Transition from Pediatric to Adult Medical Care
David Wood, John G. Reiss, Maria E. Ferris, Linda R. Edwards and Joav Merrick (Editors)
2012. ISBN: 978-1-62081-409-3 (Hardcover)
2012. ISBN: 978-1-62081-412-3 (e-book)

Tropical Pediatrics: A Public Health Concern of International Proportions
Richard R. Roach, Donald E. Greydanus, Dilip R. Patel, Douglas N. Homnick and Joav Merrick (Editors)
2012. ISBN: 978-1-61942-831-7 (Hardcover)
2012. ISBN: 978-1-61942-840-9 (e-book)

Understanding Autism Spectrum Disorder: Current Research Aspects
Ditza A. Zachor and Joav Merrick (Editors)
2012. ISBN: 978-1-62081-353-9 (Hardcover)
2012. ISBN: 978-1-62081-390-4 (e-book)

Child Health and Human Development: Social, Economic and Environmental Factors
I. Leslie Rubin and Joav Merrick (Editors)
2013. 978-1-62948-166-1 (Hardcover)

Guidelines for the Healthy Integration of the Ill Child in the Educational System: Experience from Israel
Yosefa Isenberg
2013. ISBN: 978-1-62808-350-7 (Hardcover)

Chinese Adolescent Development: Economic Disadvantages, Parents and Intrapersonal Development
Daniel TL Shek, Rachel CF Sun and Joav Merrick (Editors)
2013. ISBN: 978-1-62618-622-4 (Hardcover)

University and College Students: Health and Development Issues for the Leaders of Tomorrow
Daniel TL Shek, Rachel CF Sun and Joav Merrick (Editors)
2013. ISBN: 978-1-62618-586-9 (Hardcover)

Adolescence and Behavior Issues in a Chinese Context
Daniel TL Shek, Rachel CF Sun and Joav Merrick (Editors)
2013. ISBN: 978-1-62618-614-9 (Hardcover)

Advances in Preterm Infant Research
Jing Sun, Nicholas Buys and Joav Merrick (Editors)
2013. ISBN: 978-1-62618-696-5 (Hardcover)

Internet Addiction: A Public Health Concern in Adolescence
Artemis Tsitsika, Mari Janikian, Donald E. Greydanus, Hatim A. Omar Joav Merrick (Editors)
2013. ISBN: 978-1-62618-925-6 (Hardcover)

Promotion of Holistic Development of Young People in Hong Kong
Daniel TL Shek, Tak Yan Lee and Joav Merrick (Editors)
2013. ISBN: 978-1-62808-019-3 (Hardcover)

Human Developmental Research: Experience from Research in Hong Kong
Daniel TL Shek, Cecilia Ma, Yu Lu and Joav Merrick (Editors)
2013. ISBN: 978-1-62808-166-4 (Hardcover)

Chronic Disease and Disability in Childhood
Joav Merrick (Editor)
2013. ISBN: 978-1-62808-865-6 (Hardcover)

Break the Cycle of Environmental Health Disparities: Maternal and Child Health Aspects
I. Leslie Rubin and Joav Merrick (Editors)
2013. ISBN: 978-1-62948-107-4 (Hardcover)

Environmental Health Disparities in Children: Asthma, Obesity and Food
I. Leslie Rubin and Joav Merrick (Editors)
2013. ISBN: 978-1-62948-122-7 (Hardcover)

Environmental Health: Home, School and Community
I. Leslie Rubin and Joav Merrick (Editors)
2013. ISBN: 978-1-62948-155-5 (Hardcover)

Children, Violence and Bullying: International Perspectives
Joav Merrick, Isack Kandel and Hatim A. Omar (Editors)
2013. ISBN: 978-1-62948-342-9 (Hardcover)

Playing with Fire: Children, Adolescents and Firesetting
Hatim A. Omar, Carrie Howell Bowling and Joav Merrick (Editors)
2013. ISBN: 978-1-62948-471-6 (Hardcover)

School, Adolescence and Health Issues
Joav Merrick, Ariel Tenenbaum and Hatim A. Omar (Editors)
2014. ISBN: 978-1-62948-702-1 (Hardcover)

Adolescence and Sexuality: International Perspectives
Joav Merrick, Ariel Tenenbaum and Hatim A. Omar (Editors)
2014. ISBN: 978-1-62948-711-3 (Hardcover)

Adoption: The Search for a New Parenthood
Gary Diamond and Eva Arbel
2014. ISBN: 978-1-63117-710-1 (Hardcover)

PEDIATRICS, CHILD AND ADOLESCENT HEALTH

CHILD AND ADOLESCENT HEALTH YEARBOOK 2013

JOAV MERRICK
EDITOR

NOVA BIOMEDICAL
New York

For permission to use material from this book please contact us:
Telephone 631-231-7269; Fax 631-231-8175
Web Site: http://www.novapublishers.com

Library of Congress Cataloging-in-Publication Data

ISBN 978-1-63117-658-6

Published by Nova Science Publishers, Inc. † New York

CONTENTS

In: Child and Adolescent Health Yearbook 2013
Editor: Joav Merrick
ISBN: 978-1-63117-658-6

INTRODUCTION

Donald E Greydanus*, MD, Dr HC (ATHENS)[1] and Joav Merrick, MD, MMedSc, DMSc[2,3,4,5]

[1]Department Pediatrics and Adolescent Medicine Western Michigan University School of Medicine, Kalamazoo, Michigan, US
[2]National Institute of Child Health and Human Development, Jerusalem
[3]Division of Pediatrics, Hadassah Hebrew University Medical Center, Mt Scopus Campus, Jerusalem,
[4]Office of the Medical Director, Health Services, Division for Intellectual and Developmental Disabilities, Ministry of Social Affairs and Social Services, Jerusalem, Israel
[5]Kentucky Children's Hospital, University of Kentucky, Lexington, Kentucky, United States of America

"All of us pass through different phases like childhood, adolescence, adulthood, parenthood, others. In each phase, we experience certain difficult periods and come out with wonderful discoveries. With some insight into our lives, we can definitely say that 'teen years" or "adolescence" is one of the most challenging periods!" (1)

The term, adolescence, can be traced to the 15th century and is based on Latin etymology; adolescere refers to "growing into maturity." The current term, adolescence, identifies a critical period of human life that allows sufficient maturity for the human being to leave childhood dependency and pass through a dramatic period of immense physiological, psychological, and sociological consequences. The adolescent must accept the failures and successes of childhood with the initiation of puberty and in the end, starts his or her adult life as central nervous system maturity occurs. The tremendous peaks of growth and development are only exceeded by those seen in utero and in early childhood.

* *Correspondence:* Donald E Greydanus, MD, Dr. HC (ATHENS), Professor and Chair, Department of Pediatric and Adolescent Medicine, Western Michigan University School of Medicine, 1000 Oakland Drive, D48G, Kalamazoo, MI 49008-1284, United States. E-mail: Donald.greydanus@med.wmich.edu

Fascination with this period of development has been intense since the emergence of Homo sapiens sapiens over 60,000 years ago (2). Some of this fascination has been horror at the impulsive and sometimes confusing behavior of adolescents---as suggested in this classic quote of the Greek poet, Hesiod, in the 8th century BC (3):

> *"I see no hope for the future of our people if they are dependent on the frivolous youth of today, for certainly all youth are reckless beyond words... When I was a boy, we were exceedingly wise and impatient of restraint" (3)*

Research into issues of adolescence did not occur in earnest until over two millennia after the conclusions of Hesiod. This research was stimulated by the first PhD of psychology in America, G Stanley Hall (1844-1924), who wrote the inaugural classic work "Adolescence: Its psychology and its relationship to physiology". This two volume work details his observations and research on adolescence and led to the classic term "Sturm und Drang" (storm and tempest), that presented this period as a turbulent time in human life (4). Some of Professor Hall's conclusions were based on work done in the physiology laboratory of HP Bowditch, the researcher whose brilliant work on growth in 1877 (5) resulted in the classic opus ("Growth at adolescence") of James M Tanner (1920-2010) in England that was published in 1955 and 1962 (6).

Research on adolescence, overdue for thousands of years, lead to clinical interest in adolescents with the first medical clinic in the United States at Stanford University (Palo Alto, California) (7). Work in college health lead to interest in young adolescents that was launched by the physician James Rosswell Gallagher (1903-1995), who established the first clinic for teenagers in Boston in 1951 (7). Gallagher is particularly important, because he recorded his observations in a textbook on the medical care of teenagers that had three editions: 1960, 1966, and 1976 (8). This "father of adolescent medicine" suggested that the views of youth should outweigh the views of parents. In the preface to his first edition, he noted:

> *"Adolescents are different, and it is clearly desirable to think about them in different terms than one does of a little child or an adult. So, too, is the doctor's relationship to these patients different; no longer is it the parent who tells all the story, and now the patient requires very considerable evidence of his doctor's interest in him. How to talk to these young people (or better how to get them to talk to you!), how to deal with them effectively, how to utilize for their own good their tendency to accept advice from and to imitate and to talk freely to other adults than their parents—these we have considered to be important topics."* (8)

The baton of Gallagher was beautifully picked up by Adele Dellenbaugh Hofmann (1926-2001), professor of pediatrics at New York University who published her classic text "Adolescent medicine" in 1983 (9). As noted with the work of Gallagher, Hofmann's textbook went on to three formal editions: 1983, 1989, and 1997, She died in 2001 after influencing countless numbers of clinicians and scholars in the field of Ephebiatrics that continue now into the 21st century.

In this yearbook you will find the guiding work of these former masters of adolescent medicine (Ephebiatrics; Greek: Ephebos: youth) as we explore important concepts of medical disorders in the adolescents. Concepts of cardiology are considered that include dyslipidemias and their management (10). Treatment concepts of statins are reviewed and illustrate the complexities of evidence-based medicine. Statins have been available since the 1980s based on work from the 1970s and yet their use in healthy youth without risk of heart disease remains controversial. Recent data suggest that placing such individuals on statins over many years can increase the risk for diabetes mellitus in some females (11). Thus, clinicians must weigh the risks of such therapy with an examination of the actual benefits of pharmacology in this situation and with the heightened pressure for better living through chemistry in our society.

Pulmonary disorders in youth, particularly asthma and cystic fibrosis---the former often treated by primary care clinicians and the latter by specialists, is also presented. National and international guidelines for asthma care are available in classic articles (12,13). However, recent research suggests that clinicians do not follow these guidelines leading to reduced and lowered health care for this population (14,15). How can this be? After we finally are focusing on the healthcare of children and adolescents, how can we not optimize their health for the benefit of current and future society?

Interest musculoskeletal problems probably started with Homo sapiens' love of sports and competition dating to and before the ancient Olympic Games (776 BC to 393 AD) (16). Sports injuries, musculoskeletal disorders and rheumatologic conditions in youth (17-19) are also part of this developmental period. Though often relegated to orthopedic specialists and rheumatologists, such disorders must be understood by primary care clinicians as well. The interest in sports play brings many youth to clinicians both for injury management and also for improved sports play (17,18). Prevention of sports doping is important, as youth try a wide variety of chemicals in hopes of achieving success in sports and peer recognition (20). Indeed, the practice of adolescent medicine always involves principles of preventive medicine and teaching these vulnerable patients how to prevent health hazards in a dangerous, often unforgiving world.

Rheumatoid diseases include a variety of common and rare conditions often bewildering to both teen patients and clinicians alike. This issue offers a primer in these disorders, particularly the classic autoimmune diseases, JIA (juvenile idiopathic arthritis) and SLE (systemic lupus erythematosus). The pharmacologic management is also complex with have many potentially serious adverse effects. An individualized approach is suggested under the guidance of a rheumatologic expert. Implications for both the adolescent and the primary care clinicians are immense and ever-changing---hence, the challenge of adolescent medicine practice in the 21st century.

Perhaps even more challenging to clinicians are disorders that are usually diagnosed in the newborn or infancy stage and yet may not be seen until the adolescent or young adult years. Thus, we also discuss metabolic disorders (inborn errors of metabolism) in adolescents (21). Inborn errors of metabolism were first identified by Garrod in his classic 1902 Lancet article on alkaptonuria (22). We are now cognizant of hundreds of these complicated disorders that involve abnormalities in metabolic or biochemical pathways that are vital for healthy human existence. They are due to total or partial deficiency of various enzymes that may also lead to mental subnormality (23). This publication considers those that are seen in the adolescent age period and includes adrenoleukodystrophy, glycogen storage diseases, lyososomal storage diseases, and urea cycle disorders.

We conclude this symposium on medical disorders in adolescents with a discussion of one of the most physiologically complex organs of Homo sapiens, the kidney (24,25). Evolved over millions of years to allow for life both ancient and modern, normal renal function is vital for normal growth and health in all teenagers. A variety of conditions are considered including urinary tract infections, hematuria, proteinuria, and glomerulonephritis. We examine nephrotic syndrome, minimal changes disease (MCD), collapsing focal segmental glomerulosclerosis, IgA nephropathy, post-streptococcal glomerulonephritis, Henoch-Schönlein Purpura (HSP) Nephritis, hemolytic-uremic syndrome, lupus nephritis, and others. These conditions can have profound effects on both the medical and psychological health of youth.

Much has been learned about medical disorders of adolescents over the thousands of years of human existence, especially over the past few decades. This journal issue celebrates this knowledge in the best traditions of such giants in medicine as Hall, Gallagher, and Hofmann. There are many challenges and conundrums in our quest to improve the health of our youth. If we apply these known principles now in the early part of the 2nd decade of this current century, the result will be healthier adolescents with great benefit to themselves and the world as the 21st century inevitably unfolds into the next.

> *"I am full of hope, and even while I speak in some distress. My hope is that tomorrow's child will speak of great progress!"* (26)

REFERENCES

[1] Nair MKC. Adolescence and family life education. Bangalore, India: Standard Press, 2002.

[2] Magner LN. A History of the life sciences, 3rd ed. New York: Marcel Dekker, 2002.

[3] Greydanus DE. Adolescent sexuality: An overview and perspective. Pediatr Ann 1982;11:714-26.

[4] Stanley Hall G. Adolescence: Its psychology and its relationship to physiology, anthropology, sociology, sex, crime, religion, and education. New York: D Appleton, 1904.

[5] Bowditch HP. Growth of children. Boston: AJ Wright State Printer, 1877.

[6] Tanner JM. Growth at adolescence. Oxford: Blackwell Scientific, 1955; 1962.

[7] Gallagher JR. The origins, development, and goals of adolescent medicine. J Adolesc Health Care 1982;3:57-63.

[8] Gallagher JR. Medical care of the adolescent, 1st ed. New York: Appleton Century Crofts, 1960.

[9] Hofmann AD. Adolescent medicine. Menlo Park, CA: Addison Wesley, 1983.

[10] Third Report of the National Cholesterol Education Program (NCEP) Expert Panel on Detection, Evaluation, and Treatment of High Blood Cholesterol in Adults (Adult Treatment Panel III) final report. Circulation 2002;106(25):3143-421.

[11] Culver Al, Ockene IS, Balasubramanian R, Olendzki BC, Sepavich DM, Wactawski-Wende J et al. Statin use and risk of diabetes mellitus in postmenopausal women in The Women's Health Initiative. Arch Int Med 2012;172(2):144-52.

[12] Global Initiative for Asthma (GINA). Global strategy for asthma management and prevention: NHLBI/WHO Workshop Report. Bethesda, MD: National Institutes Health, National Heart Lung Blood Institute, 02-3659, 2002.

[13] National Asthma Education and Prevention Program. Expert panel report III: Guidelines for the diagnosis and management of asthma. Bethesda, MD: National Heart Lung Blood Institute, 08-4051, 2007.

[14] Finkelstein JA, Lozano P, Shulruff R, Inui TS, Soumerai SB, Ng M, Weiss KB. Self-reported physician practices for children with asthma: are national guidelines followed? Pediatrics 2000;106(4 Suppl):886-96.

[15] Cabana MD, Rand CS, Powe NR, Wu AW, Wilson MH, Abboud PAC, et al. Why don't physicians follow clinical practice guidelines? JAMA 1999;282:1458-65.

[16] Patel DR, Greydanus DE, Baker RJ. Pediatric practice: Sports medicine. New York: McGraw Hill, 2008.

[17] Patel DR, Greydanus DE, Omar HA, Merrick J, eds. Adolescence and sports. New York: Nova Science, 2010.

[18] Greydanus DE, Patel DR. Musculoskeletal disorders. State of the Art Rev Adolesc Med 2007;18(1).

[19] Moore MD. Rheumatic diseases. In: Greydanus DE, Patel DR, Pratt HD, eds. Essential adolescent medicine. New York: McGraw-Hill, 2006:201-34.

[20] Greydanus DE, Patel DR. Sports doping in the adolescent—the Faustian conundrum of hors de combat. Pediatr Clin North Am 2010;57(3):729-50.

[21] Kamboj MK. Inborn errors of metabolism. In: Patel DR, Greydanus DE, Omar HA, Merrick J, eds. Neurodevelopmental disabilities: Clinical care for children and young adults. New York: Springer, 2011:53-67.

[22] Garrod AE. The incidence of alkaptonuria: a study in chemical individuality. Lancet 1902;2:1616-20.

[23] Greydanus DE, Pratt HD. Syndromes and disorders associated with mental retardation. Indian J Pediatr 2005;72(10):859-64.

[24] Greydanus DE, Torres AD, Wan JH. Genitorurinary and renal disorders. In: Greydanus DE, Patel DR, Pratt HD, eds. Essential adolescent medicine. New York: McGraw-Hill, 2006;329-70.

[25] Sherwinter J, Foulds M, Greydanus DE. Nephrologic disorders in adolescents. Adolesc Med Clin 2005;16(1):1-247.

[26] WHO, UNICEF. A Healthy Start in Life. Report on the Global Consultation on Child and Adolescent Health and Development. March 12-13, 2002. Stockholm, Sweden. Geneva: WHO, 2002.

SECTION ONE – HEALTH ASPECTS OF ADOLESCENCE

In: Child and Adolescent Health Yearbook 2013
Editor: Joav Merrick
ISBN: 978-1-63117-658-6

Chapter 1

CARDIOLOGY IN CHILDHOOD AND ADOLESCENCE

James Loker, MD*
Bronson Pediatric Cardiology, Bronson Methodist Hospital,
Kalamazoo, Michigan, United States of America

ABSTRACT

This paper provides information regarding dyslipidemias that includes concepts of lipid metabolism, familial hypercholesterolemias, and secondary hyperlipidemias. Management of dyslipidemias is considered that focus on the role of statins as the mainstay of drug treatment for these disorders. Also reviewed are anticoagulants (i.e., warfarin, ximelegatran, rivaroxaban, others) and then medication used for syncope. Finally, this discussion considers the potential impact of stimulant medications on the cardiac system in those with heart disease and ADHD. Medications have an important role in the management of youth with cardiac disorders. The application of these pharmacologic agents will improve the lives of these youth and the future adults that will emerge.

Keywords: Cardiology, child, adolescent

INTRODUCTION

Pediatric cardiology can claim many recent advances. New surgical techniques, improvements in perfusion, and postoperative care have dramatically increased the survival rates for congenital heart surgery. Progress in catheter interventions, stents, and occluding devices has significantly improved morbidity by the need for surgery in many cases. Genetic analysis has not only helped confirm suspected diagnoses, but can screen other family members and help determine prognosis and treatment. New medications capitalize on a better understanding of the pathophysiology of cardiac diseases. All of these factors have improved

* Correspondence: James Loker MD, Bronson Pediatric Cardiology, Bronson Methodist Hospital, 601 John St. Suite M-351, Kalamazoo, Michigan 49007 United States. E-mail: lokerj@bronsonhg.org

survival so that currently there are more adults living with congenital heart disease than children. Adolescents with heart disease struggle to understand their condition, while starting the transition from the pediatric caregivers they have trusted for many years to adult specialists and specialty clinics.

Almost all of the cardiac medications used in pediatrics today are administered off-label (1). This increases the risk associated with treatment, as dosages are extrapolated for pediatric use. Unique features of the very young include a higher water- to-weight ratio and reduced intravascular space, which can dramatically affect pharmacokinetics. In addition, many medications do not come in liquid form. Dosing errors are the most common mistake made in prescribing medication, particularly in infants less than 1 year old (2). Cutting or crushing tablets, or making suspensions may increase the risk of dosage error and alter the bioavailability of the medication. Formulated suspensions frequently have a short shelf-life. Even in adolescents, the smallest available dosage is not always low enough.

Caution is therefore urged in using any medications, especially cardiovascular medications. This discussion has derived dosages from several sources, and readers are encouraged to evaluate these and become acquainted with any medication that is prescribed. This article only addresses the medications suitable for outpatient use. Intravenous medications and those requiring inpatient monitoring during initiation will not be discussed.

Dyslipidemias

Dyslipidemia can be broadly classified as primary, due to an underlying genetic abnormality with lipid metabolism, or secondary, due to obesity, diabetes, kidney or liver disease, hypothyroidism, or other conditions. The primary dyslipidemias are associated with overproduction and/or impaired removal of lipoprotein (see table 1). The impaired removal can result from an abnormality in either the lipoprotein itself or in the lipoprotein receptor. Secondary dyslipidemias are associated with dysregulation of key enzymes in the metabolic pathway, particularly lipoprotein lipase (LPL).

Numerous studies have documented the atherosclerotic changes that can occur in childhood, and have been the driving force behind increased efforts to screen and treat pediatric hyperlipidemias. Autopsy studies have shown that antemortem low-density lipoprotein (LDL) and total cholesterol are highly associated with aortic fatty streaks in people 7 to 24 years old (3). Berenson et al. reported that serum concentrations of total cholesterol, triglycerides, LDL, and high-density lipoprotein (HDL) were strongly associated with the extent of lesions in the aorta and coronary arteries at autopsy in young persons who died from trauma (4). The Pathobiological Determinants of Atherosclerosis in Youth (PDAY) study demonstrated raised fatty streaks, and accumulation of lipid-filled macrophages within the intima of the artery in 10% of coronary arteries and 30% of aortas in individuals 15 to 34 years of age (5).

Lipid metabolism

A brief introduction to lipid metabolism will help explain the mechanisms of atherosclerosis and how interventions can help. Lipoprotein particles are classified by their density on ultracentrifugation or their electrophoretic patterns (6). Triglycerides are the storage form of lipids, found mostly in adipose tissue but also in liver, heart, and muscle. Triglycerides originate from the dietary ingestion of fat and are secreted into lymph as chylomicrons. They can also be synthesized from carbohydrate and fatty acids in liver and secreted as very low density lipoprotein (VLDL), and end-product that can be hydrolyzed by LDL. Once the hydrolyzed particles enter the cell, they can be re-esterified into triglycerides. Lipolysis and free fatty acid (FFA) oxidation remove triglycerides from tissue. In the liver, VLDL secretion is increased by insulin, glucocorticoids, and ethanol, and decreased by glucagon.

Cholesterol is a key component of cell membranes, steroidogenesis, and bile acid formation. Cholesterol can be absorbed in the diet or synthesized in most tissues. The rate-limiting step is the conversion of HMG CoA to mevalonate by HMG CoA reductase. This enzymatic step is targeted by the statins.

Table 1. Lipoproteins

Lipoprotein Particle	Size	Origin and Function	Composition	Predominant Protein in Shell
Chylomicrons	Large lipids, low density, will float on plasma	Small intestine	Triglycerides Cholesterol (2%-4%)	Apolipoprotein B (Apo B)
Very low density lipoprotein (VLDL)	Smaller than chylomicron but may also float	Liver from triglycerides	Triglycerides Cholesterol (10%-15%)	Apo B 100
Intermediate density lipoprotein (IDL)		Intermediate in metabolism from VLDL to LDL	Cholesterol 20%-35% Protein shell 5%-40%	Apo B 100
Low density lipoprotein (LDL)	Derived from metabolism of VLDL as it shrinks	Functions to transport cholesterol	Cholesterol 35%-45% Surface protein 20%-30%	Apo B 100
High density lipoprotein (HDL)	Synthesized in liver and small intestine with complex metabolism	Functions in reverse cholesterol transport and is anti-atherogenic	Cholesterol 10%-20%	Apo A-l and Apo A-II

Table 2. Frederickson classification of Dyslipidemias

Phenotype	Major Lipid Increased	Frequency
I	Triglyceride	Very rare
IIA	LDL	Common
IIB	LDL triglyceride	Common
III	Total cholesterol, triglyceride	Rare
IV	Triglyceride	Common
V	Triglyceride	Uncommon

Internalized cholesterol inhibits cholesterol synthesis by decreasing HMG CoA and also limits further cholesterol uptake by down regulating the LDL receptor. Esterification by lecithin cholesterol acyl transferase (LCAT), and shuttling of cholesterol esters by cholesterol esterase transfer protein (CETP) moves cholesterol from HDL to VLDL to the LDL molecule.

Enzymes and cellular receptors associated with lipid metabolism

Lipoprotein lipase is present on the endothelium of vessels, mostly in fat and muscle, where it hydrolyzes triglycerides in chylomicrons and VLDL to release free fatty acids (FFA). The activity of this enzyme is regulated by insulin and is diminished in poorly controlled diabetes, causing elevation of LDL levels. Hepatic lipase (HLA) facilitates the lipolysis of VLDL and intermediate density lipoprotein (IDL) in hepatic endothelial cells, and hydrolyzes phospholipids and triglycerides in HDL. Its activity is modulated by sex steroid in which androgens increase and estrogens decrease its activity.

The LDL receptor (LDLR) is the key mediator of entry of cholesterol, as well as VLDL/LDL particles, into cells. The gene for this receptor is coded on chromosome 19, and defects in this receptor are responsible for familial hypercholesterolemia. The dyslipidemias are broadly grouped phenotypically by the lipid abnormality in the Fredrickson classification (see table 2). Research continues into the genetic basis of protein and receptor abnormalities. Genetic research has opened up new ways to treat the underlying disorder and may help establish more accurate prognoses (6).

Familial hypercholesterolemias

Familial chylomicronemia (type I) is characterized by chylomicrons and high triglycerides due to congenital deficiency of LPL or Apo C-II, which is required to remove triglycerides from chylomicrons. Symptoms include pancreatitis in children or young adults, eruptive xanthomas, and an enlarged liver and spleen but no coronary artery disease (CAD). The condition is very rare, occurring in 1 of 1 million individuals. Triglyceride levels are generally over 2,000 mg/dL. Secondary hypertriglyceridemia can be seen in patients with severe diabetic ketoacidosis and taking estrogen therapy.

Familial hypercholesterolemia FH (type IIA) occurs in 1 of 500 individuals as an autosomal dominant condition. It is due to abnormal LDL receptors, with over 150 mutations known. Type IIA FH includes a triad of hyperlipidemia, xanthoma, and premature CAD. Individuals heterozygous for this condition typically have LDL levels greater than 250 mg/dL. Diagnosis is based on LDL higher than 250 mg/dL, with a family history of premature CAD. Average life expectancy of heterozygous males with familial hypercholesterolemia is 45 years. Individuals homozygous for FH have total cholesterol levels exceeding 600 mg/dL, and can have a myocardial infarction by 3 years of age. Fortunately, this form of FH is very rare, occurring in only 1 of 1 million individuals.

Familial combined hyperlipidemia (type IIB) is also autosomal dominant trait with several genetic loci being implicated. It is seen in 1 in 300 individuals, although there may be significant overlap with secondary dyslipidemias, including metabolic syndrome. Type IIB FH appears to be more complex than FH and consensus diagnostic criteria are lacking, which makes diagnosis more difficult. Individuals with type IIB FH do not have the xanthomas seen in FH. Broad beta disease (type III) is caused by a defect in the metabolism of VLDL remnants, due to abnormal Apo E or hypothyroidism. Affected people may have palmar xanthomas and develop premature CAD. Both total cholesterol and triglycerides are elevated. This is noted in 1 of 10,000 individuals.

Familial hypertriglyceridemia (type IV) is characterized by elevated triglycerides and VLDL, and is associated with obesity but not CAD. Triglyceride levels are greater than 1,000 with normal LDL levels. Type IV FH can sometimes be mistaken for type I disease, although since that is very rare, isolated elevations of triglycerides are usually felt to be type IV. Type IV FH occurs in 16% of adults. Primary mixed hyperlipidemia (type V) is characterized by marked increases in triglycerides, chylomicrons, and VLDL. Pancreatitis, xanthomas, and hepatosplenomegaly can occur. Onset is in midlife and does not appear to affect children or adolescents. They do, however, have a higher risk of atherosclerosis. Both type IV and type V FH may exist secondary to uncontrolled diabetes mellitus, excessive ethanol intake, and use of glucocorticoids as well as estrogens. This is noted 1 in 1,000.

Secondary hyperlipidemia

Most secondary causes of hyperlipidemia are phenotypically similar to type IIA or IIB FH. In hypothyroidism, hepatic LDL receptors are decreased, causing an elevation in LDL cholesterol. Hypothyroidism can increase triglycerides by lowering LPL activity.

In diabetes, glycosylation of apoprotein B causes increased VLDL synthesis with a concomitant rise in LDL levels. Insulin regulates LPL such that a deficiency (type 1 diabetes) or relative deficiency due to increased resistance (non-insulin dependent diabetes mellitus, renal disease, liver disease, Cushing disease, etc.) can cause hypertriglyceridemia. Treatment of secondary hyperlipidemia should be primarily directed at treating the underlying condition, although lipid-lowering medication can be used in the interim.

The National Cholesterol Education Program (NCEP) and the American Academy of Pediatrics (AAP) have published guidelines for cholesterol screening (7,8). Both groups recommend a targeted approach to individuals at higher risk, rather than broad population screening. Children and adolescents whose parents have cholesterol measurements of >250 mg/dL or unknown family history should be screened with non-fasting total cholesterol testing. Children with family history of dyslipidemia, or who are at risk for secondary dyslipidemia, should have a fasting lipid profile performed.

If hyperlipidemia is noted, then repeat testing is warranted and the two cholesterol values should be averaged. In addition, with the second lipid profile, thyroid studies, liver and renal function tests and glucose or fasting insulin levels should be tested to evaluate for secondary causes of elevated cholesterol.

Management

Treatment of hyperlipidemias should start with dietary modifications for 6 to 12 months, especially for obese individuals. In adolescents with FH, nonpharmacologic measures usually are not sufficient and most specialists will prescribe statins along with dietary management. The American Heart Association (AHA) has abandoned the Step 1 and Step 2 diet in favor of a more uniform recommendation (9). Dietary reductions in cholesterol to <200 mg/day, <30%

total fat, and <7% saturated fat are recommended by the NCEP (7). Calories should be 55% from carbohydrates, 20% from protein and 25% from fat in a developing child. Consultation with a nutritionist is helpful, especially if caloric restriction is also indicated.

The goal of treatment is to reduce total cholesterol to <200 mg/dL, LDL to <130 mg/dL, and triglycerides to <125 mg/dL. Patients with dyslipidemias, such as FH, have stricter guidelines. The NCEP and AAP still recommend cholesterol-binding agents as the initial medication; however, problems with palatability and side effects usually limit compliance in most adolescents (7,8).

Statins have rapidly become the mainstay of pharmacologic treatment of dyslipidemia in both adults and children (see table 3).

Table 3. Statins

Statin	Adult Dose	Pediatric Dose
Lovastatin (Mevacor)	Initial: 20 mg/d orally every bedtime Followed by: 10-80 mg/d orally every bedtime or divided twice daily	10-17 years: 10-20 mg/d orally every bedtime initially; maintenance dosage ranges from 10-40 mg/d
Simvastatin (Zocor)	Initial: 5-10 mg/d orally every bedtime Followed by: 5-40 mg/d orally every bedtime or divided twice daily Simvastatin dosages of 80 mg have been associated with higher risk of rhabdomyolysis	10-17 years: 10 mg/d orally every bedtime initially; maintenance dosage ranges from 10-40 mg/d
Pravastatin (Pravachol)	Initial: 10-20 mg/d orally every bedtime Followed by: 5-40 mg/d orally every bedtime	8-13 years: 20 mg orally every day 14-18 years: 40 mg orally every day
Fluvastatin (Lescol)	Initial: 20-30 mg/d orally every bedtime Followed by: 20-80 mg/d orally every bedtime; for 80 mg/d, divide twice daily	10-16 years: 20 mg orally every day initially; maintenance dosage ranges from 20-80 mg/d
Atorvastatin (Lipitor)	Initial: 10 mg/d orally every bedtime Followed by: 10-80 mg/d orally every bedtime	10-17 years: 10 mg orally every day initially; maintenance dosages not to exceed 20 mg/d
Rosuvastatin (Crestor)	10-20 mg orally every day initially; maintenance dosage range is 5-40 mg/d	Not established

Numerous studies have shown statins to be both safe and efficacious in children older than 10 years (10). According to the 2007 AHA and 2008 AAP guidelines, treatment with statins could be recommended in boys older than 10 years and girls who have started their menses and have regular periods. Female patients should be counseled regarding the potential teratogenic effects of statin therapy and the need for appropriate contraception, if warranted. Statins can be started in patients as young as 8 years old who have severe dyslipidemia (e.g.,

FH or type 1 diabetes mellitus) who have failed nonpharmacologic therapy (8). Recent studies suggest that statins may also up-regulate endothelial nitric oxide (NO) synthase, thereby increasing the availability of endothelial nitrous oxide, which may have beneficial effects on endothelial vasomotor function (11).

In the adolescent, statins are indicated if the LDL is >190 mg/dL without other risk factors, or if he LDL is >160 mg/dL but <190 mg/dL and one of the following conditions applies: 1) a family history of premature cardiovascular disease (CVD), 2) two or more other CVD risk factors after vigorous attempts to control CVD risk factors (i.e., overweight, hypertension, insulin resistance, or smoke exposure), or 3) a primary disease associated with a moderate or mild increased risk of CVD. Statins can also be used if the LDL is >130 mg/dL and the patient has moderate risk underlying disease, such as heterozygous FH, or type II diabetes mellitus, or if the LDL is >100 mg/dL and the patient has high-risk underlying disease, such as homozygous FH or diabetes mellitus type I.

Currently only lovastatin (Altocor, Altoprev, Mevacor), simvastatin (Zocor), pravastatin (Pravachol) and atorvastatin (Lipitor) are approved by the United States Food and Drug Administration (FDA) for use in children. Pravastatin, simvastatin and lovastatin are available in generic forms.

Statins should be started at the lowest dose and given at bedtime to take advantage of the fact that most LDL synthesis occurs at night. The patient should be reassessed within a month to monitor the effectiveness of the medication and its side effects. Major side effects of statins include rhabdomyolysis (breakdown of muscle tissue resulting in renal impairment) and hepatic dysfunction. Creatine phosphokinase (CPK) levels and liver function should be monitored during initiation of therapy and if symptoms develop. Although all statins affect the same pathway, there are subtle differences in how individuals respond.

Typically, a parent or sibling of the young patient is also on a statin, so the clinician starts with the same one if it is working for the relative. The efficacy of the different statins in summarized in Table 4. The ability to lower LDL level does not necessarily equate to reduced risk for CAD. However, statins have other beneficial effects, such as improved arterial compliance, reduction in inflammatory response, decrease in thrombus formation, and improved plaque stability. Lovastatin and simvastatin are generic and less expensive. Atorvastatin and fluvastatin are not eliminated by the kidneys and can, therefore, be used in patients with renal impairment.

All statins have similar safety profiles. The risk of rhabdomyolysis occurs in less than 1 in 10,000 patients. Higher doses (particularly of simvastatin) and renal impairment can increase the levels of statins and place the individual at greater risk. Fluvastatin and pravastatin are recommended in individuals who are taking other medications, because they have the fewest drug interactions.

Ezetimibe (Zetia) acts on the brush border of the small intestine, inhibiting the absorption of cholesterol. It is available alone or in combination with simvastatin (as Vytorin). Typical adult dose is 10 mg once a day; no pediatric dose is available. Bile acid sequestrants (Table 5) have the advantage of no systemic absorption, but palatability decreases patient compliance. These should be offered but, realistically, are not used as much as other medications.

Niacin is usually used in cases of hypertriglyceridemia or mixed hyperlipidemia and usually in conjunction with a statin.

Table 4. Percentage Lowering of LDL-Cholesterol by Statins

Statin	Name Of Drug	Daily Dose of Drug				
		5 mg	10 mg	20 mg	40 mg	80 mg
Atorvastatin	Lipitor Torvast	31%	37%	43%	49%	55%
Fluvastatin	Lescol	10%	15%	21%	27%	33%
Lovastatin	Mevacor Altocor	-	21%	29%	37%	45%
Pravastatin	Pravachol Lipostat Selektine	15%	20%	24%	29%	33%
Rosuvastatin	Crestor	38%	43%	48%	53%	58%
Simvastatin	Zocor Lipex	23%	27%	32%	37%	42%

(Law MR, 2003).

Table 5. Bile Acid Sequestrants

Bile Acid Sequestrant	Adult Dose	Pediatric Dose
Cholestyramine	Begin with 1 scoop (4 g) or pouch mixed with water or juice; advance slowly to 8-16 g/d (usually divided twice daily immediately before major meals)	240 mg/kg/d divided in 2-3 doses, not to exceed 8 g/d
Colestipol	2 g once or twice daily, with increases of 2 g once or twice daily over periods of 1-2 months	1 g once or twice daily, with increases of 1 g once or twice daily over periods of 1-2 months

Side effects of flushing, headaches, and liver toxicity tend to limit its use. Aspirin (325 mg) given 30 minutes before the niacin does help diminish the flushing. Niacin is indicated in type IV and type V hyperlipidemias with an adult dose of 100 to 250 mg 3 times per day, then increased 100 mg/day each week as tolerated based on liver function testing. The dosage for extended release is 500 mg at bedtime.

Anticoagulants

Advances in pediatric cardiac surgery and interventional cardiology have dramatically increased the use of anticoagulants (12). Coumadin has been the standard oral anticoagulant, while aspirin is commonly used for its antiplatelet effect (see chapter 24). Enoxaparin (Lovenox) achieves more stable levels than Coumadin; though patients may be reluctant to give injections, most youth and parents quickly adapt.

Newer oral anticoagulants that act via direct thrombin inhibition (ximelegatran, Exanta) or direct Factor Xa inhibition (rivaroxaban, Xarelto) offer stable pharmokinetics similar to enoxaparin but as oral agents. These are not used as frequently, so experience and safety data are not as extensive as for the other medications.

Warfarin

Warfarin (Coumadin, Jantoven, Marfarin) is the oldest and most commonly used Vitamin K antagonist (VKA) (see chapter 24). Warfarin interferes with the cyclic interconversion of vitamin K and its 2, 3 epoxide. Vitamin K is a cofactor for the carboxylation of glutamate residues of coagulation proteins (factors II, VII, IX and X). Warfarin can inhibit carboxylation of the regulatory anticoagulant proteins C and S and, therefore, has the potential to exert a procoagulant effect.

Dosages for warfarin range from 0.3 mg/kg in infants to 0.09 mg/kg in older children. Improved hepatic metabolism as a child develops is responsible for the difference between doses for infants and older children, which may also explain the lower doses needed in patients with Fontan circulation (13). Bleeding is the most serious side effect with a relative risk of 0.5% per patient year. Warfarin is titrated to achieve an international normalized ratio (INR) in the range of 2 to 3 in most instances (Table 6). Patients with mechanical prosthetic mitral valves usually have an INR range of 2.5 to 3.5. Warfarin dosages usually need to be decreased by 10% to 15% when antibiotics are taken. Many electronic medical record systems have the ability to track INR levels and warfarin dosages, making following a patient's anticoagulant therapy easier.

Aspirin

Aspirin is used to decrease platelet adhesion in Kawasaki disease and after hemi-Fontan and Fontan palliation. Aspirin is also frequently used in patients with arterio-pulmonary shunts and as an adjunct to other anticoagulants. Dosage ranges from 3 to 10 mg/kg/day, with dose rounded up to the most convenient dose.

Table 6. INR dosing and schedules

International Normalized Ratio (INR)	Dose
Loading dose if INR 1-1.3	0.2 mg/kg (maximum10 mg)
Day 2-4 dependent on INR	
1.1-1.3	Repeat loading dose
1.4-3	Repeat 50% loading dose
3.1-3.5	Repeat 25% loading dose
>3.5	Hold dose till INR <3.5
Maintenance dose after day 5	
1.1-1.4	Increase dose 20%
1.5-1.9	Increase dose 10%
2-3	No change
3.1-3.5	Decrease dose 10%
>3.5	Hold dose till <3.5 then restart dose decreased by 20%

Typical doses range from 40.5 mg, 81 mg, 162 mg, up to maximum dose of 325 mg. Since the effects of aspirin are irreversible for the life of the platelet, therapy can be easily suspended for up to a week with no significant increased risk of coagulation. This is beneficial as many physicians will halt aspirin therapy when the patient has influenza to decrease the risk of Reye's syndrome.

Table 7. Reasons for cardiology referral in syncope

Recurrent	If there is a history of recurrent syncope
Exercise related	If dizziness or syncope occurs during exercise. Frequently there may be dizziness or syncope after running if the adolescent does not keep moving.
Family history	Many of the cardiac causes of syncope are due to autosomal dominant conditions, so a family history of syncope, sudden death, arrhythmia, cardiomyopathy, etc., is important. Family history is second only to the history of the event in importance when working up syncope.
ECG or exam abnormal	If there are abnormalities on the ECG or examination, the risk of cardiac disease as a cause of syncope increases.
Rapid onset	Vagally mediated syncope usually has identifiable prodrome of nausea, pallor, dizziness, and visual changes. Any syncope that occurs without a prodrome should be suspected to be cardiac in origin.

Other anticoagulants

Dipyridimole also decreases platelet adhesion but through a different mechanism than aspirin. It can be used as adjunctive therapy to other oral anticoagulants and aspirin. Dosage is 3 to 6 mg/kg/day divided in three doses. Newer oral anticoagulants ximelegatran acts by direct thrombin inhibition. It is dosed twice daily and has the advantage of a predictable, stable anticoagulant effect. Ximelegatran has not been studied in pediatric patients. Rivaroxaban is another oral anticoagulant that acts by direct inhibition of activated Factor X.

Syncope

Syncope is defined as a temporary loss of consciousness secondary to a decrease in cerebral blood flow. It is one of the more common complaints of adolescents seen in the office and the incidence ranges from 0.03% to 0.5%.

According to one survey, 20% of males and 50% of females have had at least one syncopal episode by the age of 20 (14). In 90% of cases, syncope is mediated by the vagal response and though benign, it can cause considerable anxiety in both the adolescent and parents, thereby generating more testing and expense for reassurance. History is the key factor in evaluating syncope, with the physical examination and testing usually being normal. Orthostatic blood pressure measurement and a 12-lead ECG are considered standard in the work-up of syncope. Reasons for referral of an adolescent with syncope to a pediatric cardiologist are noted in table 7.

Management

Treatment of dizziness and syncope is largely supportive by increasing fluid and salt intake, as well as recognizing and avoiding precipitating factors. Clinicians should also encourage the youth to avoid skipping meals and eliminate caffeine intake. If patients become dizzy, maneuvers to increase venous return (such as squatting, sitting, or lying down) will help alleviate the symptoms and avoid syncope. When supportive measures are insufficient, especially when a history of injury is associated with syncope, then pharmacologic intervention may be indicated.

Fludrocortisone (Florinef) is the most commonly used medication in treating autonomic syncope. As a mineralocorticoid, it increases sodium reabsorption in the distal loops of the kidney, thereby decreasing water loss and increasing the circulating blood volume. Fludrocortisone at the appropriate dosages does not have significant glucocorticoid effect, but at higher dosages, may cause problems. The recommended dosage is 0.1 to 0.2 mg twice daily. Patients should continue to increase the salt and water intake and other supportive measures while on fludrocortisone. Since adolescents with dizziness and syncope tends to improve with age, a 6-month to 1-year trial on medication can be followed by a trial without medication. Drug discontinuation is best accomplished during the summer when school is not in session.

Midodrine (Amatine, Gutron) can be used either instead of or in addition to fludrocortisone. As an alpha agonist, midodrine increases vasomotor tone and does not stimulate cardiac beta-adrenergic receptors; thus it does not cause tachycardia. Also, midodrine does not cross the blood brain barrier to exert effects on the central nervous system. Midodrine is very effective in treating orthostatic hypotension, but can also be useful as therapy for vasovagal syncope. Oral dosage is 0.1 to 0.2 mg four times daily. In addition, the selective serotonin uptake inhibitors (SSRIs), such as paroxetine (Paxil), fluoxetine (Prozac), and sertraline (Zoloft), have been used to treat vasovagal syncope, possibly by reregulating the autonomic nervous system.

Postural orthostatic tachycardia syndrome (POTS) is one of the dysautonomias and can be similar to vasovagal syncope. We view it as an exaggerated response to orthostatic changes. Individuals with POTS have an increased heart rate of over 30 bpm when going from supine to standing, and frequently have standing heart rates over 120 bpm. Similar to vasovagal syncope, 80% of patients with POTS are female and are 13 to 40 years of age. Individuals can be very symptomatic and anxiety can increase those symptoms.

A combination of counseling, lifestyle changes, and medications can effectively treat many of these individuals with POTS. In addition to fludrocortisone and midodrine, beta blockers can be used to treat the tachycardia. Care should be taken as beta blockers may worsen hypotension, especially if the patient is hypovolemic and has significant orthostatic hypotension. For that reason, clinicians usually use beta blockers in conjunction with other medications. Propranolol (Inderal) can be helpful, especially if migraines are part of the constellation. Start with at a dose of 10 mg twice daily and titrate upward, based on symptoms. Once the adolescent is stable, longer acting propranolol (Inderal LA) 60 to 80 mg daily usually is sufficient. Atenolol can also be used at a dose of 25 to 50 mg daily.

Cardiac evaluation for ADHD medication

Attention deficit hyperactivity disorder (ADHD) is the most common neurobehavioral disorder of childhood and adolescents, with a prevalence of 4% to 12% in community samples of American school children (see chapter 10). More than 2.5 million children take medications for ADHD yearly. The disorder is more prevalent in children with cardiac disease than in the general pediatric population without heart disease. Mahle et al. reported abnormal attention scores in 45% of children with heart disease (15) while Kishbom reported that 50% of children with total anomalous pulmonary venous return displayed evidence of hyperactivity or attention deficit (16). Also, ADHD reportedly affects 35% to 55% of children with 22q11 microdeletion (17).

Between 1999 and 2004, 19 children prescribed ADHD medications died suddenly, according to the FDA voluntary reporting system, and 26 children reportedly experienced cardiovascular events, including heart palpitations, strokes, and cardiac arrests (see chapter 10). The amount of accurate information about the cause of death, dose of medication, and duration of therapy varied considerably among cases. Some patients had underlying cardiac abnormalities, a family history of ventricular tachycardia, or other medical conditions.

Based upon the data, the estimated rate of sudden death among the 2.5 million children taking stimulant medication in the United States would be 1.9 per 1 million children <18 years of age, which is substantially lower than the estimated rate in the general pediatric population of 10 to 20 per 1 million children <18 years of age (18). In a large cohort study 241,417 patients ages 3 to 17 years using amphetamine, atomoxetine (Strattera), or methylphenidate were matched by gender, database, state and age to 965,668 nonusers.

No statistically significant difference was noted in sudden death, ventricular arrhythmia, stroke, myocardial infarction, and all causes of death, even though the ADHD medication users had a higher incidence of cardiac conditions and/or cardiac risk factors (19).

The American Academy of Pediatrics (AAP) and the American Heart Association (AHA) differ in their opinions regarding screening electrocardiograms (ECGs) for children and adolescents before ADHD medication is prescribed. The AHA published a statement in 2008 saying that screening ECGs may increase the sensitivity for detecting underlying heart disease, and calling for routine ECGs as an indication for starting ADHD medications (class IIA, level of evidence C). The organization subsequently corrected that statement, recommending ECGs but not requiring them before starting ADHD medications (20).

The AAP statement that same year reported the incidence of cardiac events as extremely low and no higher than that seen in the general population, It classified routine ECGs as supported by class IIB, level of evidence D (21). Both groups agree that a careful history and physical examination directed to the cardiac system is needed. The author of this discussion agrees that with the extremely low incidence of sudden death due to stimulant medication, the low positive predictive value of ECGs make them a poor screening tool. The practitioner is encouraged to follow the AAP guidelines, obtaining a careful history and physical exam, and using an ECG when there is suspicion of heart disease (see chapter 10).

Even in children or adolescents with known palliated congenital heart disease, ADHD medications can frequently be used without undue concern. There are no studies that have demonstrated an increased risk of sudden cardiac death (SCD) in pediatric patients with congenital heart disease on stimulant medication.

The AHA felt stimulant medication was reasonable in patients with known risk factors for SCD (long QT syndrome, hypertrophic cardiomyopathy) even with history of arrhythmia requiring cardiopulmonary resuscitation [CPR]) after other methods have been considered or attempted.(20). Nevertheless, one should try to avoid stimulant medication in patients with long QT intervals, known tachyarrhythmia, or cardiac conditions that place them at a high risk for arrhythmia. Consultation with the cardiologist taking care of the adolescent is warranted before starting, or if planned dosages are in the high therapeutic range.

Conclusion

Many advances have occurred in the field of pediatric cardiology that has remarkable benefit for adolescents with cardiac disease. An important part of this progress is the development of pharmacologic approaches to disorders that have profound impact on the adolescents themselves and the adults they will become in later life. Though often off-label, these drugs are beneficial. This paper reviews pharmacologic approaches to dyslipidemias, anticoagulation, and syncope. Also considered is the controversial role of stimulant medication in youth with both cardiac disorders and attention-deficit/hyperactivity disorder.

Acknowledgments

This paper is an adapted version of a chapter in the book “Adolescent medicine: Pharmacotherapeutics in medical disorders” edited by Donald E Greydanus, Dilip R Patel, Cynthia Feucht, Hatim A Omar, Joav Merrick and published with permission by Walter de Gruyter, Berlin and New York.

References

[1] Pasquali SK, Hall M, Slonim AD, Jenkins KJ, Marino BS, Cohen MS, et al. Off-label use of cardiovascular medications in children hospitalized with congenital and acquired heart disease. Circ Cardiovasc Qual Outcomes 2008;1:74-83.

[2] Alexander DC, Bundy DG, Shore AD, Morlock L, Hicks RW, Miller MR. Cardiovascular medication errors in children. Pediatrics 2009;124:324-32.

[3] Newman WP III, Freedman DS, Voors AW, Gard PD, Srinivasan SR, Cresanta JL, et al. Relation of serum lipoprotein levels and systolic blood pressure to early atherosclerosis: the Bogalusa Heart Study. N Engl J Med 1986;314(3):138-44.

[4] Berenson GS, Srinivasan SR, Bao W, Newman WP III, Tracy RE, Wattigney WA. Association between multiple cardiovascular risk factors and atherosclerosis in children and young adults. The Bogalusa Heart Study. N Engl J Med 1998;338(23):1650-6.

[5] McMahan CA, Gidding SS, Malcom GT, Tracy RE, Strong JP, McGill HC, Jr. Pathobiological determinants of atherosclerosis in youth risk scores are associated with early and advanced atherosclerosis. Pediatrics 2006;118(4):1447-55.

[6] Kanani PM, Sperling MA. Hyperlipidemia in adolescents. Adolesc Med 2002;13:37-52.

[7] Third Report of the National Cholesterol Education Program (NCEP) Expert Panel on Detection, Evaluation, and Treatment of High Blood Cholesterol in Adults (Adult Treatment Panel III) final report. Circulation 2002;106(25):3143-421.

[8] Daniels SR, Greer FR and the Committee on Nutrition. Lipid screening and cardiovascular health in childhood. Pediatrics 2008;122:198-208.

[9] American Heart Association. Heart Disease and Stroke Statistics: 2006 Update. Dallas, TX: American Heart Association; 2006.

[10] de Jongh S, Lilien MR, op't Roodt J, Stroes ES, Bakker HD, Kastelein JJ. Early statin therapy restores endothelial function in children with familial hypercholesterolemia. J Am Coll Cardiol 2002;40(12):2117-21.

[11] Laufs U, LaFata V, Plutzky J, Liao K. Upregulation of endothelial nitric oxide synthase by HMG CoA reductase inhibitors. Circulation 1998;97:1129-35.

[12] Jain S, Vaidyanathan B. Oral anticoagulants in pediatric cardiac practice: A systemic review of the literature. Ann Pediatr Cardiol 2010;3:31-4.

[13] Streif W, Andrew M, Marzinotto V, Massicotte P, Chan AKC, Julian JA, et al. Analysis of warfarin therapy in pediatric patients: A prospective cohort study of 319 patients. Blood 1999;94(9):3007-14.

[14] Ganzeboom KS, Colman N, Reitsman JB. Prevalence and triggers for syncope in medical students. Am J Cardiol 2003;91:1006-8.

[15] Mahle WT, Clancy RR, Moss EM, Gerdes M, Jobes DR, Wernovsky G. Neurodevelopmental outcome and lifestyle assessment in school-aged and adolescent children with hypoplastic left heart syndrome. Pediatrics 2000;105:1082-9.

[16] Kirshborm PM, Flynn TB, Clancy RR, Ittenbach RF, Hartman DM, Paridon SM, et al. Late neurodevelopmental outcome after repair of total anomalous pulmonary venous connections. J Thorac Cardiovasc Surg 2005;129:1091-7.

[17] Gothelf D, Gruber R, Presburger G, Dotan I, Brand-Gothelf A, Burg M, et al. Methylphenidate treatment for attention-deficit/hyperactivity disorder in children and adolescents with the velocardiofacial syndrome: An open-label study. J Clin Pschiatry 2003;64:1163-9.

[18] Nissen SE. ADHD drugs and cardiovascular risk. N Engl J Med 2006;354:1445-8.

[19] Schelleman H, Bilken WB, Strom BL, Kimmel SE, Newcomb C, Guevara JP, et al. Cardiovascular events and death in children exposed and unexposed to ADHD agents. Pediatrics 2011;127:1102-10.

[20] Vetter VL, Elia J, Erickson C. Cardiovascular monitoring of children and adolescents with heart disease receiving medications for attention deficit disorder. Circulation 2008;117(18):2407-23.

[21] Perrin JM, Friedman RA, Knilans TK, The Black Box Working Group. The Section on Cardiology and Cardiac Surgery. Cardiovascular monitoring and stimulant drugs for Attention-Deficit/Hyperactivity Disorder. Pediatrics 2008;122:451-3.

Submitted: November 01, 2011. *Revised:* December 05, 2011. *Accepted:* December 20, 2011.

In: Child and Adolescent Health Yearbook 2013
Editor: Joav Merrick
ISBN: 978-1-63117-658-6

Chapter 2

PULMONARY DISORDERS IN ADOLESCENCE

John H Marks, MD*
Pediatrics and Human Development,
Michigan State University College of Human Medicine,
Division of Pediatric Pulmonology, Pediatrics Program,
Michigan State University/Kalamazoo Center for Medical Studies,
Kalamazoo, Michigan, United States of America

ABSTRACTS

Pulmonary disorders in adolescents represent an important cause of morbidity and mortality and thus appropriate care of these conditions is critical to the overall health of these individuals. The most common pulmonary condition in youth is asthma, a problem that continues to increase in prevalence and severity around the world. other disorders that are considered include community-acquired pneumonia and cystic fibrosis. The management is generally based on national or international guidelines developed by expert panels and published in professional journals.

Keywords: Adolescence, pulmonary disease

INTRODUCTION

This chapter reviews the pharmacologic management of paramount respiratory conditions in the adolescent patient: community-acquired pneumonia, asthma, and cystic fibrosis. A brief discussion of the definition, epidemiology, and differential diagnosis precedes consideration of pharmacologic management of each disorder. The management is generally based on national or international guidelines developed by expert panels of professional groups that

* Correspondence: John H Marks MD, Associate Professor, Pediatrics and Human Development, Michigan State University College of Human Medicine, Division of Pediatric Pulmonology, Pediatrics Program, Michigan State University/Kalamazoo Center for Medical Studies, 1000 Oakland Drive Kalamazoo, MI 49008-1284 United States. E-mail: Jhmarks@kcms.msu.edu or Marks@kcms.msu.edu

include the American Thoracic Society, the U.S. Infectious Disease Society and the British Thoracic Society for community-acquired pneumonia, the U.S. National Asthma Education and Prevention Program (NAEP) of the National Institutes of Health, and the U.S. Cystic Fibrosis Foundation.

COMMUNITY ACQUIRED PNEUMONIA

Community-acquired pneumonia (CAP) is defined as pneumonia acquired outside of the hospital setting as opposed to nosocomial pneumonia acquired in the hospital (1). Streptococcus pneumoniae, Mycoplasma pneumoniae and Chlamydophila (formerly Chlamydia) pneumoniae appear to be the most frequently encountered pathogens in CAP. These organisms also cause CAP in adults. Other bacterial pathogens that can cause CAP include Staphylococcus aureus and Haemophilus influenzae. Legionella pneumophila is a less common pathogen.

"Atypical pneumonia" refers to pneumonia that does not present with the usual clinical picture of “typical” pneumonia due to S pneumoniae infection that includes high fever, productive cough, and chills. The term atypical pneumonia is frequently used to describe adolescents with CAP. The clinical presentation of CAP can be highly variable, depending on the causative agent. However, the clinical picture does not always predict the infecting organism. It is probably inaccurate to use the term atypical pneumonia and preferable instead to refer to more atypical pathogens as common causes of CAP.

CAP may also be caused by several viruses, which cause 20% of CAP cases. The most common viruses are influenza, parainfluenza, respiratory syncytial virus, metapneumovirus, and adenovirus. Less common viruses causing significant illness include chicken pox, severe acute respiratory syndrome (SARS) virus, avian flu, and hantavirus.

Epidemiology

The incidence of pneumonia caused by specific pathogens is not well known for the adolescent population with CAP. Adolescents are often grouped together with young children or adults in epidemiologic studies, which may obscure the results (2). Wide variability in diagnostic testing methods may also affect the incidence reported in studies (3).

An estimated annual incidence of CAP in older children and adolescents is 6 to 12 cases per 1000. In patients between 10 and 16 years of age, S pneumoniae cause approximately 30% of cases of CAP. Mycoplasma pneumoniae is the cause in 15% to 40% of cases and C. pneumoniae comprise 14% to 35% of cases. Non-typable H influenzae, influenza A or B, adenovirus, metapneumovirus and other respiratory viruses are found less frequently.

Diagnosis

The diagnosis of CAP is based on clinical history, physical examination, radiographic studies, and laboratory evaluation (1,4). For teaching purposes, clinical features have been classified to differentiate between bacterial pneumonia, atypical bacterial pneumonia, or viral pneumonia. However, the clinical features of pneumonias caused by different microorganisms frequently overlap and cannot be used reliably to establish etiology. In addition, as many as 50% of infections may be mixed bacterial/viral infections.

"Typical" bacterial pneumonia, usually resulting from S. pneumoniae infection, is abrupt in onset, with fever, and an ill-appearing, sometimes toxic patient. Respiratory distress may be moderate or severe; auscultation may reveal crackles and egophony, limited to the involved anatomic segment. Pleural involvement with pleuritic pain and pleural friction rub on auscultation are suggestive of bacterial etiology, as these findings are rarely present in nonbacterial pneumonia. These symptoms may follow days of upper respiratory tract infection symptoms.

"Atypical" bacterial pneumonia, resulting from M. pneumoniae or C. pneumoniae infection, often presents with abrupt onset of fever, malaise and myalgia, headache, photophobia, sore throat, and gradually worsening nonproductive cough, despite improvement of other symptoms. Although hoarseness may be seen in disease caused by both agents, it is more frequently seen with C. pneumoniae infection. Wheezing is a frequent finding in atypical bacterial and viral pneumonias.

Differential diagnosis

The differential diagnosis of CAP includes conditions that may present with fever, cough, dyspnea, chest pain, hypoxemia, crackles on auscultation, and radiographic infiltrates. Possible diagnoses include noninfectious lower respiratory syndromes such as asthma, hypersensitivity pneumonitis, pulmonary involvement in collagen vascular disease (see chapter 31), aspiration, and cardiac causes of tachypnea and crackles.

Pharmacologic management

When considering pharmacologic management of CAP the first decision is whether the patient can be managed as an outpatient or is ill enough to require hospitalization. This determination is based on clinical presentation, severity of symptoms, and, in some cases, laboratory and radiologic evaluation. Administration of an oral macrolide antibiotic (eryth¬romycin, clarithromycin, or azithromycin) is acceptable for treatment of the outpatient who is not seriously ill. Doxycycline is also acceptable for these patients (see table 1). These drugs will treat most of the common causes of CAP in adolescents, including the atypical pathogens (4-7).

It should be noted that up to 50% of S pneumoniae strains are resistant to macrolides. Patients should be monitored for response to therapy and if they are not improving or are worsening, a change should be made in antibiotic coverage. For outpatients a beta-lactam (amoxicillin or cephalosporin) should be instituted (see table 2). Oral fluoroquinolones (levofloxacin or moxifloxacin) are alternatives in stable outpatients, even with penicillin-resistant S pneumoniae (see table 3). Adolescents with CAP who are ill enough to be hospitalized should be treated with an intravenous penicillin or cephalosporin (Table 4).

Table 1. Antibiotic treatment of suspected atypical organisms (*Mycoplasma pneumoniae, Chlamydophila pneumoniae)* in outpatients not seriously ill. All are given for 7-10 days

Medication	Dose
Erythromycin	50 mg/kg per day divided every six hours; maximum dose 2 g/day as base, 3.2 g/day as ethyl succinate
Clarithromycin	15 mg/kg per day divided every 12 hours; maximum dose 1 g/day
Azithromycin	10 mg/kg administered once on day one [maximum dose 500 mg] followed by 5 mg/kg once daily on days two to five [maximum dose 250 mg/day]
Doxycycline	4 mg/kg per day in two divided doses; maximum 200 mg/day

Table 2. Antibiotic treatment of suspected drug resistant *Streptococcus pneumoniae.* All are given for 7-10 days

Medication	Dose
Amoxicillin	80 to 100 mg/kg per day by mouth in three divided doses; maximum dose 2 to 3 g/day; this regimen is preferred because of superior in vitro activity against S. pneumoniae
Cefdinir	14 mg/kg per day by mouth in one or two divided doses; maximum dose 600 mg/day
Cefpodoxime	10 mg/kg per day by mouth in one or two divided doses; maximum dose 800 mg/day

Table 3. Antibiotic treatment of suspected atypical organisms or possible drug resistant *Streptococcus pneumoniae.* All are given for 7-10 days

Medication	Dose
Levofloxacin	500 mg, once per day
Moxifloxacin	400 mg, once per day

Table 4. Antibiotics for treatment of hospitalized adolescents with CAP. All are given for 7-10 days

Medication	Dose
Cefuroxime	150 mg/kg/day given every 8 hours
Ceftriaxone	50-75 mg/kg/day once daily
Ampicillin	50 mg/kg/day given every 6 hours
Vancomycin	40-60 mg/kg/day given every 6 hours
Linezolid	600 mg (IV/PO) every 12 hours

For treatment of penicillin-resistant S. pneumoniae, vancomycin or linezolid can be used.

These antibiotics also cover methicillin-resistant S. aureus (MRSA). Oral or intravenous azithromycin should be added to cover the possibility of an atypical pathogen. Whether the adolescent with CAP is treated as an outpatient or is hospitalized, the importance of monitoring clinical response cannot be stressed too much.

The role of immunomodulatory agents (i.e., macrolides, statins, aspirin, corticosteroids) requires further research to elucidate (8)

CYSTIC FIBROSIS

Cystic fibrosis (CF) is an autosomal recessive disorder in which the gene that codes for a protein called the cystic fibrosis transmembrane conductance regulator (CFTR) is defective (9). The CFTR facilitates the transport of chloride ions across the apical membrane of epithelial-lined cells.

The altered chloride transport results in altered sodium and water distribution, causing thickened, dehydrated epithelial secretions and mucus.

As a result, CF has pulmonary, gastrointestinal, pancreatic and hepatic manifestations. Obstructive pulmonary disease is the leading cause of morbidity and mortality in CF patients.

The pulmonary aspect of cystic fibrosis has four major components: airway obstruction, infection, inflammation, and, ultimately, lung tissue damage. Because of the extremely thick mucous secretions, airway clearance is impaired.

The thick, stagnant mucus facilitates the growth of bacteria and other pathogens that colonize the airways. The presence of bacteria such as S. aureus, Pseudomonas aeruginosa, H. influenzae, and Burkholderia cepacia, contribute to the destruction of lung tissue and compound the inflammatory process.

Cellular debris becomes trapped and accumulates in the sputum, resulting in more inflammation. As neutrophils die, they release large amounts of DNA, which contributes to the viscosity of the already thick sputum.

Manifestations of CF include bronchiectasis, frequent exacerbations, air trapping with an increase in the anterior-posterior chest diameter (barrel chest), a flattened diaphragm, pulmonary hypertension, and, ultimately, right-sided heart failure (6). Common signs are decreased hemoglobin oxygen saturation, leukocytosis, tachypnea, and fever. Serious complications include hemoptysis and pneumothorax. Digital clubbing and nasal polyps are common in CF patients.

Epidemiology

The incidence of CF varies according to ethnic group. This disease is the most common lethal autosomal recessive disorder in Caucasians, who make up an estimated 90% of the patients diagnosed with CF. Hispanics represent 5% of the diagnosed cases, while African-Americans account for approximately 4%. Cystic fibrosis occurs in 1 of every 2500 Caucasian infants and 1 of every 17,000 African-American infants.

The disease has been reported in Asians as well as Native Americans, but is rare in these groups. Life expectancy for patients with CF is now longer than 35 years and death is often due to such causes as infection (Pseudomonas) and pulmonary hypertension (10).

Differential diagnosis

Cystic fibrosis is now diagnosed routinely by newborn screening; however, in older children and adolescents born before implementation of newborn screening, diagnosis was based on clinical suspicion, sweat chloride and/or gene mutation analysis.

Differential diagnosis includes conditions causing chronic cough and progressive obstructive lung disease, such as immune deficiency, primary ciliary dyskinesia, and recurrent aspiration. CF-related diabetes mellitus (CFRD) is a common co-morbid condition (see chapter 21) (11). Also, chronic (polypoid) sinusitis is a near universal aspect of CF due to chronic bacterial infection, but also allergic mechanisms to some extent (12).

Pharmacologic management

Acute pulmonary exacerbations

Acute exacerbations occur because of a flare-up of infection within the airways. Frequent signs and symptoms of an acute exacerbation include cough with sputum production, weight loss, a decrease in pulmonary function, and reduced energy levels. Treatment of pulmonary exacerbations consists of airway clearance techniques, nutritional support, and antibiotic therapy. The specific antibiotics used in treatment are determined by the known or suspected organisms in the most recent sputum culture (13-17). S aureus and P aeruginosa are the most common pathogens in adolescents and adults. Often, sputum samples reveal different strains of P aeruginosa with varying degrees of susceptibility.

Another highly resistant organism that eventually emerges as CF progresses is B. cepacia. Patients colonized with this pathogen generally have a faster rate of pulmonary decline and a shorter lifespan. Evolving data suggest that the pathogenicity of this organism depends on the specific genomovar (subspecies of microbe) present. Preliminary epidemiological data indicate that B cepacia (genomovar III) carries the greatest risk for increased morbidity and mortality.

Initial treatment generally consists of 2 to 3 weeks of antibiotic therapy (9,18,19). The patient is hospitalized if symptoms are moderate to severe, while mild exacerbations often are managed in the home setting. Table 5 lists frequently prescribed intravenous antibiotics and their dosing regimens. Ampicillin/sulbactam or cefuroxime are reasonable empiric choices when S. aureus and H. influenza are suspected pathogens. Treatment of exacerbations involving S aureus typically includes a first-generation cephalosporin (cefazolin, cephalothin) or a penicillinase-resistant penicillin such as nafcillin (20). When MRSA is the causative agent, vancomycin or linezolid may be used.

Treatment of exacerbations involving P. aeruginosa requires a combination of an antipseudomonal beta-lactam (piperacillin, ceftazidime, cefepime, imipenem or meropenem) and an aminoglycoside (gentamicin or tobramycin) or fluoroquinolone (ciprofloxacin or levofloxacin). Combination therapy is used to provide synergistic activity and reduce the potential for development of resistance. Oral ciprofloxacin or levofloxacin are widely used in the management of mild exacerbations involving P. aeruginosa; however, due to increased resistance over the past decade, they may no longer be effective as monotherapy.

The antibiotic doses for CF patients tend to be higher than those for non-CF patients for a number of reasons. Patients with CF possess an increased clearance and volume of distribution for the aminoglycosides and many beta-lactam compounds. In addition, due to chronic colonization and frequent antibiotic courses, antibiotic resistance is inevitable. Also, the microenvironment within the airways contains mucin, DNA, cations and other factors that interfere with antibiotic activity. These factors explain the rationale for more aggressive therapy when exacerbations occur.

The larger volume of distribution, expressed as L/kg of body weight, may be a result of the patient's nutritional status. Beta-lactams and aminoglycosides are distributed into lean body mass. Patients with CF tend to have an increased lean body mass and relatively low amounts of adipose tissue because of weight loss and malnutrition. The increased clearance of certain drugs exhibited by CF patients may be the result of other mechanisms, including increased renal clearance, increased nonrenal clearance, and decreased protein binding.

Management of chronic cystic fibrosis

Anti-inflammatory agents

The presence of bacterial organisms within the airway creates a chronic inflammatory state that leads to the eventual destruction of the airways themselves (21). Early studies showed low-dose oral corticosteroids given on alternate days slow the pulmonary decline in CF patients. Because doses of 1 mg/kg every other day were used, adverse events were dramatically decreased but not totally eliminated. In a 4-year, multicenter trial, 285 patients were randomly assigned to receive prednisone 1 mg/kg, 2 mg/kg, or placebo every other day (7,17). The study demonstrated evidence of a significant increase in glucose intolerance among patients receiving 2 mg/kg compared to those receiving 1 mg/kg.

A significant increase in growth retardation was also observed in both treatment groups vs. the placebo group. The beneficial effects of alternate-day prednisone, as measured by a decrease in serum IgG and pulmonary function (FEV1 and FVC) and a decline in hospitalization, reached a plateau after 6 months of therapy. The authors recommended that therapy be limited to less than 1 year to decrease the risk of adverse effects (growth retardation and glucose intolerance) (7,17,88,21). Prednisone 2 mg/kg could not be recommended because of adverse effects (17,18,21).

In general, chronic therapy with prednisone is not a common event, simply because the risks appear to outweigh the benefits. Studies examining the use of inhaled corticosteroids (ICSs) have shown conflicting results. At this point the role of inhaled steroids for maintenance therapy in CF patients is not clearly defined. As a result, there is general consensus that ICSs should not be used unless the patient is concurrently diagnosed with asthma.

Nonsteroidal anti-inflammatory drugs (NSAIDs) are used in the treatment of CF to inhibit neutrophil activation and migration (21). The effects of high-dose ibuprofen were examined in a 4-year clinical trial of 85 patients with mild lung disease (17). The study resulted in a slower rate of decline in pulmonary function in patients treated with ibuprofen. However, the most benefit was noted in patients ages 5 to 13, who only showed a 2% decline in FEV1 over the 4-year period, vs. a 15% decline during the same period in the placebo group.

Patients treated with ibuprofen also maintained their body weight while patients in the placebo group lost weight. Despite the significant efficacy demonstrated in this study, ibuprofen is not routinely prescribed in all centers due to concerns for serious bleeding or renal insufficiency, especially when given with an aminoglycoside. In patients who are started on ibuprofen, blood testing is recommended to ensure optimal therapy.

Table 5. IV Antibiotic dosage recommendations for treatment of pulmonary exacerbations in CF

Antibiotic	Dosage (mg/kg/day)	Doses per day	Maximum daily dose (g) or Desired serum concentration
Amikacin	30	2-3	Peak 25-30 Trough <5
Ampicillin-sulbactam	100-150	4	9g
Aztreonam	150-200 100	3-4 c.i.	8g 8g
Cefepime	150-200	3-4	8g
Ceftazidime	150-200 100	3-4 c.i.	8g 8g
Cefuroxime	100-150	3	4.5g
Ciprofloxacin	20-30	2-3	1.2
Colistin	5-8	3	0.45
Gentamicin	10	2-3	Peak 8-12 Trough <2
Imipenem-cilastatin	50-100	4	4g
Nafcillin	100-200	4	12g
Piperacillin, ± tazobactam	400**	4	18g
Ticarcillin, ± clavulanate	400**	4	18g
Tobramycin	10-15	2-3 1	Peak 8-12 Trough <2
Trimethoprim/ Sulfamethoxazole	10-15	2	0.64 (TMP)

c.i. = continuous infusion regimen ** Refers to dosing of piperacillin and ticarcillin components.

Azithromycin, an antibiotic with both antimicrobial and anti-inflammatory activity, has been shown to be beneficial in treating CF. Although the mechanism of action of azithromycin in CF is not understood, 4 randomized, placebo-controlled trials have been conducted in adults and children with CF, most of whom had chronic infection with P aeruginosa (17,18). These studies demonstrated that azithromycin was associated with reduced pulmonary exacerbations, increased weight gain, and improved lung function. Azithromycin is currently recommended for people with CF, 6 years of age or older, who have P aeruginosa in their sputum for at least 1 year. The dose is 250 mg or 500 mg, based on body weight, taken 3 days per week.

Aerosolized antibiotics

The purpose of aerosolized antibiotics is to deliver large quantities of medication to the lungs while decreasing the risk of side effects from systemic absorption. Aerosolized antibiotics have been used as adjunctive treatment with intravenous antibiotics for acute pulmonary exacerbations, as chronic suppressive therapy in patients colonized with P aeruginosa, and, more recently, as early treatment to eradicate P aeruginosa after initial positive sputum culture.

Tobramycin solution for inhalation (TOBI) was introduced in 1998. The efficacy and safety of chronic maintenance therapy were established based on a large, multicenter, randomized controlled trial in CF patients persistently colonized with P aeruginosa (17,18,22). Patients were treated with aerosolized tobramycin 300 mg twice a day, in 3 cycles of 28 days on therapy, followed by a period of 28 days off therapy. This study showed a significant increase in pulmonary function over baseline measurements. The greatest effect was seen in patients aged 13 to 17 years. The secondary endpoints of the study were to evaluate the need for hospitalization and antipseudomonal antibiotics. Patients who received aerosolized tobramycin had fewer hospitalizations and required less use of antipseudomonal antibiotics (17,22). The use of TOBI did not result in significant increases in ototoxicity or nephrotoxicity.

Aztreonam for inhalation solution (Cayston--75 mg) is an inhaled antibiotic for patients with CF who have P aeruginosa infection. Aztreonam has potent in vitro activity against gram-negative aerobic pathogens, including P. aeruginosa. Cayston contains aztreonam formulated with lysine, a proprietary formulation developed specifically for inhalation. The medication was approved by the U.S. FDA in 2010 after reviewing results of safety and efficacy studies. Cayston had positive effects on maintenance of pulmonary function and delayed onset of acute pulmonary exacerbations. It is administered 3 times a day using a proprietary nebulizer system that delivers the dose in 2 to 3 minutes. Therapy is given daily for a 28-day course, followed by 28 days off. Other antibiotics delivered by inhalation aerosol are being studied for the treatment of pulmonary infection in patients with CF. These include levofloxacin, ciprofloxacin, amikacin, and fosfomycin/tobramycin.

Mucolytic agents

Mucolytic agents loosen sputum by cleaving DNA remnants left behind by degenerating neutrophils (23). Currently dornase alpha (Pulmozyme) is the only FDA-approved mucolytic agent in the United States (24). A mucolytic is a well-accepted adjunct to standard airway clearance and antibiotic therapy. By using this agent, clinicians hope to prevent or delay the bronchiectasis that results from obstruction of the airways. The typical dose is 2.5 mg nebulized daily over a period of 15 to 20 minutes. Side effects include rash, pharyngitis, laryngitis, chest pain, and conjunctivitis. Dornase alpha received approval from the U.S. FDA when safety and efficacy were established in a Phase III clinical trial involving 968 patients with mild-to-moderate lung disease (17). Compared to the control group, patients receiving 2.5 mg of dornase alpha daily showed a 5.8% increase in pulmonary function, as measured by mean FEV1, and a 31% decrease in the risk of pulmonary exacerbations (17).

Hypertonic saline (7%) inhalation has been found in controlled clinical trials to improve lung function and decrease the number of pulmonary exacerbations compared to normal saline (0.9%) (25). It is thought to increase airway surface liquid by osmosis, thus aiding airway clearance. Side effects are cough and bronchospasm; thus, a nebulized bronchodilator should be used prior to saline inhalation. Mannitol, a non-ionic osmotic agent, has been shown to be as effective as hypertonic saline when given as a dry-powder inhalation. As of this writing it has not been approved by the FDA.

Potential newer treatments

Several agents that modulate CFTR function or stimulate chloride secretion via non-CFTR pathways are being investigated. These agents are meant to return the airway surface liquid to normal or near-normal, thereby limiting the degree of airway obstruction, infection and inflammation in the lungs of patients with CF (13-17). Although caring for adolescents with CF is challenging, the prospect of newer therapies that will improve the quality of life and survival of these patients is exciting. Dealing with co-morbid depression and anxiety is important as well as ensuring proper transitioning to adult care (26-29).

Asthma

Asthma is the most common chronic disease of children and adolescents (30). It is characterized by recurrent episodes of reversible airway obstruction, hyperreactivity, and inflammation (31-33). Increased airway responsiveness to a variety of immunologic challenges (e.g., pollen, dust mites) and nonimmunologic stimuli (e.g., exercise, smoke, cold air, viral respiratory infection) is characteristic of asthma. Exposure results in release of inflammatory mediators, such as leukotrienes, from eosinophils, causing bronchial smooth muscle constriction, airway mucosal edema, and mucus secretion. This leads to symptoms of wheezing, coughing, chest tightness, and dyspnea. Recurrent episodes lead to bronchial smooth muscle hypertrophy, subepithelial fibrosis, and often airway remodeling, with collagen deposition in the basement membrane.

Epidemiology

Nine million children under the age of 18 years in the United States have been diagnosed with asthma (30). In 2005, 8.9% of children in the United States currently had asthma. Children and adolescents with asthma miss about 10 school days per year, and account for 3 million sick visits to health care providers and 200,000 hospitalizations annually. Asthma prevalence and morbidity are higher in poor, disadvantaged minority children and adolescents living in urban areas. Research is identifying a link between asthma and obesity, two conditions that are both increasing in prevalence (34).

Differential diagnosis

The differential diagnosis of asthma in adolescents includes conditions that cause acute or chronic respiratory symptoms, such as wheezing, coughing, dyspnea, and chest pain. These include CF, pneumonia, aspiration, pulmonary edema, airway compression from tumors or lymph nodes, vocal cord dysfunction, and anxiety-hyperventilation.

Pharmacological management

Treatment of asthma is based on a classification of severity based on symptom frequency and pulmonary function (31-33). Asthma management guidelines were initially published by the

National Institutes of Health, National Heart, Lung, and Blood Institute Expert Panel Report 1 in 1991 as the National Asthma Education and Prevention Program (NAEPP). The latest revision of the Report was published in 2007 (33). Asthma severity is classified as intermittent, mild persistent, moderate persistent, or severe persistent as illustrated in Table 6. Severity is usually classified initially, before long-term controller medications are started. After asthma classification, the NAEPP recommends a stepwise approach to therapy (Figure 1), with aggressive attempts to control symptoms quickly and subsequent adjustment of therapy in a stepwise fashion as symptoms require. The principal goals of treatment of asthma are to minimize symptoms, normalize pulmonary function, prevent exacerbations, and improve health-related quality of life.

Table 6. Classifying asthma severity and initiating treatment in youths greater than or equal to 12 years of age and adults

Components of severity		Classification of asthma severity (≥12 years of age)			
		Intermittent	Persistent		
			Mild	**Moderate**	**Severe**
Impairment Normal FEV_1/FVC: 8-19 yr 85 percent 20-39 yr 80 percent 40-59 yr 75 percent 60-80 yr 70 percent	Symptoms	≤2 days/week	>2 days/week but not daily	Daily	Throughout the day
	Nighttime awakenings	≤2x/month	3-4x/month	>1x/week but not nightly	Often 7x/week
	Short-acting $beta_2$-agonist use for symptom control (not prevention of EIB)	≤2 days/week	>2 days/week but not daily, and not more than 1x on any day	Daily	Several times per day
	Interference with normal activity	None	Minor limitation	Some limitation	Extremely limited
	Lung function	• Normal FEV_1 between exacerbations • FEV_1 >80 percent predicted • FEV_1/FVC normal	• FEV_1 ≥80 percent predicted • FEV_1/FVC normal	• FEV_1 >60 but <80 percent predicted • FEV_1/FVC reduced 5 percent	• FEV_1 <60 percent predicted • FEV_1/FVC reduced >5 percent
Risk	**Exacerbations requiring oral systemic corticosteroids**	**0-1/year (see footnote)**	**≥2/year (see footnote)**		
		Consider severity and interval since last exacerbation			
		Frequency and severity may fluctuate over time for patients in any severity category			
		Relative annual risk of exacerbations may be related to FEV_1			
Recommended step for initiating treatment		Step 1	Step 2	Step 3	Step 4 or 5
				And consider short course of oral systemic corticosteroids	
		In 2-6 weeks, evaluate level of asthma control that is achieved and adjust therapy accordingly.			

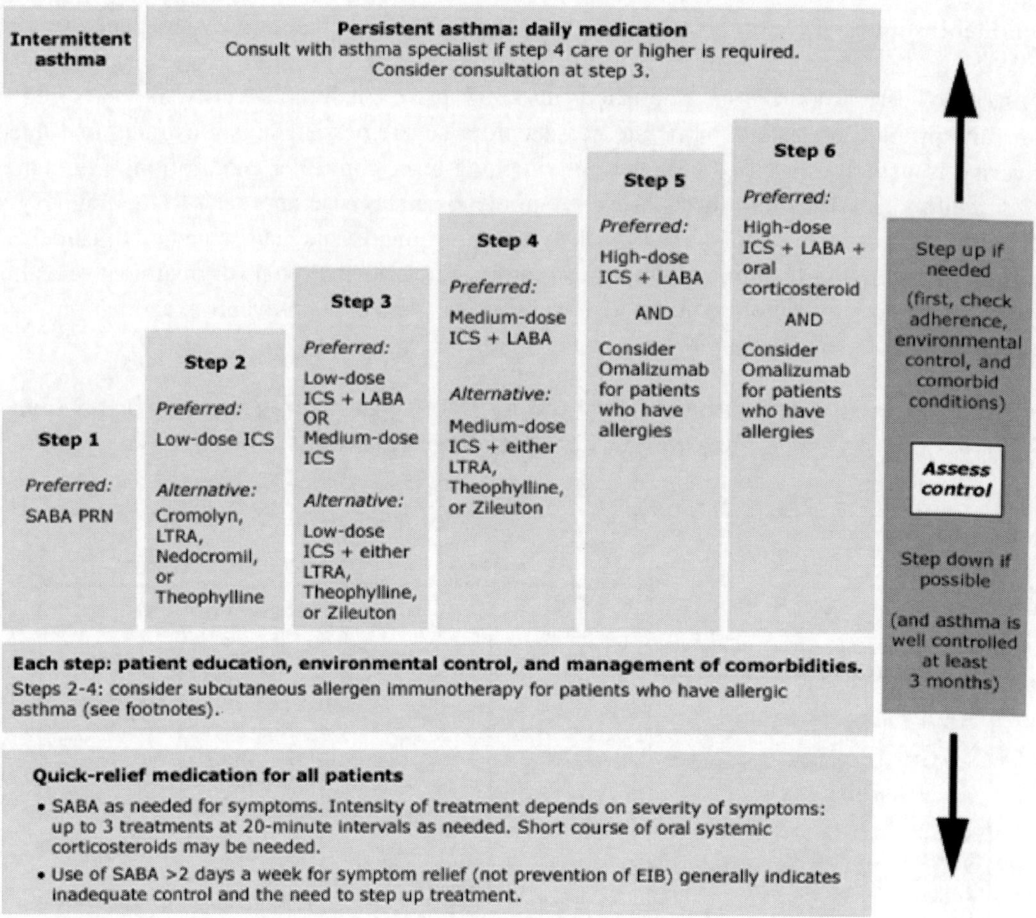

Figure 1. Stepwise approach for managing asthma in youths greater than or equal to 12 years of age and adults.

A theoretical goal is to prevent long-term consequences of airway inflammation, particularly airway remodeling and chronic persistent airway obstruction. Dealing with asthma, co-morbidities (i.e., depression, anxiety, post-traumatic stress disorder) is important to improve compliance with recommended treatment guidelines (35,36).

Intermittent asthma does not require daily controller medications, and is usually managed with as-needed use of a short acting beta-agonist (SABA), such as albuterol, given by metered-dose inhaler (37). Available SABAs are shown in table 7. A patient with intermittent asthma may have exacerbations requiring anti-inflammatory medications such as oral corticosteroids.

When the adolescent with asthma presents with decreased lung function and poorly controlled symptoms, a short course or "burst" of an oral corticosteroid such as prednisone or prednisolone is started at a dose of 1 to 2 mg per kg given for 5 to 7 days. This is done while starting an aggressive program of anti-inflammatory controller medications in addition to SABA rescue medication. Inhaled corticosteroids are the daily controller medications of choice. Several randomized, prospective studies demonstrate that inhaled ICSs improve lung function, diminish symptoms, decrease need for SABAs, and improve airway responsiveness to methacholine in patients with all levels of persistent asthma (17).

Table 7. Short acting inhaled beta agonists

Drug	Approved age range	Formulation	Adult dosage
Short-acting, inhaled beta-2 agonists			
Albuterol			
Proventil®,Ventolin®, or generic solution	≥2 years old	Nebulizer solutions: 0.021 percent (0.63 mg/3 mL), 0.042 percent (1.25 mg/3 mL), 0.083 percent (2.5 mg/3 mL), 0.5 percent (0.5 mg/20 mL)	2.5 mg every 4-6h, PRN
Proventil-HFA®, Ventolin-HFA®, or ProAir®	≥4 years old	MDI: 90 mcg/puff	2 puffs every 4-6h, PRN
Levalbuterol			
Xopenex® solution	≥6 years old	Nebulizer solution: 0.31, 0.63 or 1.25 mg/3 mL	0.63 to 1.25 mg, 2 to 4 times daily, PRN
Xopenex-HFA®	≥6 years old	45 mcg/puff	2 puffs every 4-6 h, PRN
Pirbuterol			
Maxair Autohaler®	≥12 years old	Breath-actuated MDI: 200 mcg/puff	2 puffs every 4-6h, PRN
Long-acting, beta-2 agonists			
Salmeterol			
Serevent® Diskus	>4 years old	DPI: 50 mcg/inhalation	1 inhalation every 12h
Formoterol			
Foradil® Aerolizer	≥5 years old	DPI: 12 mcg/inhalation	1 inhalation every 12h

MDI: metered-dose inhaler; DPI: Dry-powder inhaler; HFA: hydrofluoroalkane; h: hour.

In patients with stable but not well controlled asthma, a medium-dose ICS is prescribed initially. Several ICSs are available in metered-dose inhalers or dry-powder inhalers (table 8). If daily ICS is not achieving adequate control of symptoms, an additional controller should be added, such as a long-acting beta-agonist (LABA, formoterol or salmeterol) or a leukotriene modifier (montelukast or zafirlukast) (17). Short-acting beta-agonist "rescue" inhalers are prescribed to all patients with persistent asthma.

Inhaled LABAs help maintain bronchodilation for 8 to 12 hours and are taken twice daily (table 9) (38,39). Salmeterol has a slow onset of action, while formoterol has a rapid onset of action, 5 to 15 minutes, similar to albuterol. The LABAs should not be prescribed as rescue medications, and should not be used without concurrently using an ICS. These medications have an FDA "black box" warning due to results of a placebo-controlled study of salmeterol that showed a significantly increased risk of asthma-related deaths in the salmeterol group (17). This risk was greater in African-Americans; however, only 38% of African-Americans in the study were using an inhaled ICS (17).

Table 8. Estimated comparative daily doses for inhaled glucocorticoids in adolescents and adults

Drug	Low dose	Medium dose	High dose
Beclomethasone HFA	80-240 mcg	240-480 mcg	>480 mcg
40 mcg/dose	(2-6 puffs)		
80 mcg/dose	(1-3 puffs)	(3-6 puffs)	(>6 puffs)
Budesonide DPI (Flexhaler®)	180-600 mcg	600-1200 mcg	>1200 mcg
90 mcg/dose	(2-6 inhalations)		
180 mcg/dose	(1-3 inhalations)	(4-6 inhalations)	(>6 inhalations)
	200-600 mcg	600-1200 mcg	>1200 mcg
100 mcg/dose	(2-6 inhalations)		
200 mcg/dose	(1-3 inhalations)	(3-6 inhalations)	(>6 inhalations)
400 mcg/dose	(1 inhalation)	(2-3 inhalations)	(>3 inhalations)
Ciclesonide HFA	80-320 mcg	320-640 mcg	>640 mcg
80 mcg/puff	(1-4 puffs)	(4-8 puffs)	(>8 puffs)
160 mcg/puff	(1-2 puffs)	(2-4 puffs)	(>4 puffs)
Flunisolide HFA*	320 mcg	320-640 mcg	>640 mcg
80 mcg/puff	(4 puffs)	(4-8 puffs)	(>8 puffs)
Flunisolide CFC*	500-1000 mcg	1000-2000 mcg	>2000 mcg
250 mcg/puff	(2-4 puffs)	(4-8 puffs)	(>8 puffs)
Fluticasone HFA	88-264 mcg	264-440 mcg	>440 mcg
44 mcg/puff	(2-6 puffs)		
110 mcg/puff	(2 puffs)	(3-4 puffs)	(>4 puffs)
220 mcg/puff			(>2 puffs)
Fluticasone DPI	100-300 mcg	300-500 mcg	>500 mcg
50 mcg/dose	(2-6 inhalations)		
100 mcg/dose		(3-5 inhalations)	(>5 inhalations)
250 mcg/dose			(>2 inhalations)
Mometasone DPI	220 mcg	440 mcg	>440 mcg
110 mcg/dose	(2 inhalations)		
220 mcg/dose	(1 inhalation)	(2 inhalations)	(>2 inhalations)

Table 9. Long acting inhaled beta agonists

Long-acting, beta-2 agonists			
Salmeterol			
Serevent® Diskus	>4 years old	DPI: 50 mcg/ inhalation	1 inhalation every 12h
Formoterol			
Foradil® Aerolizer	≥5 years old	DPI: 12 mcg/ inhalation	1 inhalation every 12h

DPI: Dry-powder inhaler; h: hour.

Combination inhalers containing both an ICS and a LABA can be prescribed for patients not controlled on medium- or high-dose ICSs alone. The combination of a LABA plus an inhaled ICS is more effective than higher doses of inhaled ICSs in most patients. The combinations include fluticasone and salmeterol, budesonide and formoterol, and mometasone and formoterol as shown in Table 10. Combination inhalers are preferred to separate ICS and LABA inhalers, because they ensure that patients will not omit the ICS leaving them on LABA monotherapy.

Leukotriene modifiers may be added to obtain better asthma control with lower doses of ICSs. Montelukast and zafirlukast are leukotriene D4 receptor antagonists, and zileutin is a 5-lipoxygenase inhibitor (Table 11). Leukotriene modifiers may be slightly less effective than a LABA when added to an ICS.

Table 10. Usual doses of combination inhaled glucocorticoids and long-acting beta-agonists for the treatment of asthma in adolescents age 12 and older and adults

Medication	Low dose	Medium dose	High dose
Budesonide/formoterol HFA			
80 mcg-4.5 mcg	2 puffs twice a day		
160 mcg-4.5 mcg		2 puffs twice a day	
Fluticasone/salmeterol DPI			
100 mcg-50 mcg	1 inhalation twice a day		
250 mcg-50 mcg		1 inhalation twice a day	
500 mcg-50 mcg			1 inhalation twice a day
Fluticasone/salmeterol HFA			
45 mcg-21 mcg	2 puffs twice a day		
115 mcg-21 mcg		2 puffs twice a day	
230 mcg-21 mcg			2 puffs twice a day
Mometasone/formoterol HFA			
100 mcg-5 mcg		2 puffs twice a day	
200 mcg-5 mcg			2 puffs twice a day

By convention, doses from metered dose inhalers are expressed as puffs, and doses from dry powder inhalers are expressed as inhalations. HFA: metered dose inhaler with hydrofluoroalkane propellant; DPI: dry powder inhaler.

Table 11. Usual doses of agents affecting 5-lipoxygenase pathway

Medication	Dose form	Age 12 through adult
Montelukast (Singulair®)	Granules: 4 mg/packet Tablet: 10 mg Chewable tablets: 4 mg, 5 mg	10 mg tablet once daily in evening
Zafirlukast (Accolate®)	Tablets: 10 mg, 20 mg	20 mg twice daily
Zileuton (Zyflo CR®)	Extended-release tablet: 600 mg	1200 mg twice daily

Theophylline in an oral sustained-release form may be added as a long-term controller in some patients. Once a commonly used first-line treatment, theophylline is now used only in selected patients, such as those who cannot tolerate a LABA. Blood levels of the drug need to be monitored to avoid side effects.

Table 12. Assessing asthma control and adjusting therapy in youths greater than or equal to 12 years of age and adults

Components of control		Classification of asthma control (≥12 years of age)		
		Well-controlled	**Not-well controlled**	**Very poorly controlled**
Impairment	Symptoms	≤2 days/week	>2 days/week	Throughout the day
	Nighttime awakenings	≤2x/month	1-3x/week	≥4x/week
	Interference with normal activity	None	Some limitation	Extremely limited
	Short-acting beta$_2$-agonist use for symptom control (not prevention of EIB)	≤2 days/week	>2 days/week	Several times per day
	FEV_1 or peak flow	>80 percent predicted/personal best	60-80 percent predicted/personal best	<60 percent predicted/personal best
Risk	**Exacerbations requiring oral systemic corticosteroids**	**0-1/year**	**≥2/year (see footnote)**	
		Consider severity and interval since last exacerbation		
	Progressive loss of lung function	Evaluation requires long-term follow-up care		
	Treatment-related adverse effects	Medication side effects can vary in intensity from none to very troublesome and worrisome. The level of intensity does not correlate to specific levels of control but should be considered in the overall assessment of risk.		
Recommended action for treatment		• Maintain current step. • Regular follow-ups every 1-6 months to maintain control. • Consider step down if well controlled for at least 3 months.	• Step up 1 step and • Reevaluate in 2-6 weeks. • For side effects, consider alternative treatment options.	• Consider short course of oral systemic corticosteroids, • Step up 1-2 steps, and • Reevaluate in 2 weeks. • For side effects, consider alternative treatment options.

Assessing control

Assessment of "control," rather than severity, is used to adjust therapy. Control is based on impairment over the past 2 to 4 weeks (based on history or a validated questionnaire), current FEV1 or peak flow, and estimates of risk, as shown in table 12. If asthma is not well-controlled, therapy should be "stepped-up." If the asthma is well-controlled, therapy can be continued or possibly "stepped-down" to minimize medication side effects. Most patients who are compliant with therapy achieve control of their asthma within a few weeks or months. Achieving control is emphasized because patients with poor control of asthma symptoms are more likely to require urgent care for asthma than those whose asthma is well-controlled. The use of complementary and alternative medical strategies, though commonly used by patients with asthma, requires further research to identify any potential efficacy (40).

CONCLUSION

Pulmonary disorders are important yet challenging conditions to treat in adolescents. Three key pulmonary disorders are considered: community-acquired pneumonia, cystic fibrosis, and asthma (17). Improvement in morbidity and mortality includes attention to behavioral issues as well as ever-changing pharmacologic management. Antibiotic resistance presents an on-going dilemma in managing pulmonary infections. Attention to co-morbid conditions is also important.

Improving compliance with recommended treatments remains a challenge for clinicians caring for youth with acute and chronic pulmonary disorders. Successful transitioning to accepting adult care providers is also a critical component in caring for youth with chronic disorders.

ACKNOWLEDGMENTS

This paper is an adapted version of a chapter in the book "Adolescent medicine: Pharmacotherapeutics in medical disorders" edited by Donald E Greydanus, Dilip R Patel, Cynthia Feucht, Hatim A Omar, Joav Merrick and published with permission by Walter de Gruyter, Berlin and New York.

REFERENCES

[1] American Thoracic Society. Guidelines for the initial management of adults with community-acquired pneumonia: diagnosis, assessment of severity, and initial antimicrobial therapy. Am J Resp Crit Care Med 2001;163:1730-54.

[2] Kronman MP, Hersh Al, Feng R, Huang YS. Lee GE, Shah SS. Ambulatory visit rates and antibiotic prescribing for children with pneumonia, 1994-2007. Pediatrics 2011;127:411-8.

[3] Bartlett JG. Diagnostic tests for agents of community-acquired pneumonia. Clin Infect Dis 2011;52(Suppl 4):S296-304.

[4] British Thoracic Society Standards of Care Committee. British Thoracic Society guidelines for the management of community acquired pneumonia in childhood. Thorax 2002;57(suppl 1):i1.

[5] Community acquired pneumonia guideline team, Cincinnati Children's Hospital Medical Center. Evidence-based care guidelines for medical management of community acquired pneumonia in children 60 days to 17 years of age. Accessed 2011 Jun 08. URL: www.cincinnatichildrens.org /svc/alpha/h/health-policy/ev-based/pneumonia.htm.

[6] File TM, Niederman MS. Antimicrobial therapy of community-acquired pneumonia. Infect Dis Clin North Am 2004;18:993-1016.

[7] Mandell LA, Wunderink RG, Anzueto A, Bartlett JG, Campbell GD, Dean NC, et al. Infectious Diseases Society of America/American Thoracic Society consensus guidelines on the management of community-acquired pneumonia in adults. Clin Infect Dis 2007;44(suppl 2):S27-S72.

[8] Corrales-Medina VF, Musher DM. Immunomodulatory agents in the treatment of community-acquired pneumonia: A systemic review. J Infect 2011 Jul 5. [Epub ahead of print]

[9] Nasr SZ. Cystic fibrosis in adolescents and young adults. Adolesc Med 2000;11:589-603.

[10] Baghale N, Kalilzedeh S, Hasssanzad M, Parsanejad N, Velayati A. Determination of mortality from cystic fibrosis. Pneumologia 2010; 59(3):170-3.

[11] Laguna TA, Nathan BM, Moran A. Managing diabetes in cystic fibrosis. Diabetes Obes Metabol 2010;12:858-64.

[12] Schraven SP, Wehrmannn M, Wagner W, Blumenstock G, Koitschev A. Prevalence and histopathology of chronic polypoid sinusitis in pediatric patients with cystic fibrosis. J Cyst Fibros 2011; 10:181-6.

[13] Davis SD, Ferkol TW. Hitting the target: new treatments for cystic fibrosis. Am J Respir Crit Care Med 2010;182:1460-1.

[14] Bais R, Hubert D, Tümmler B. Antibiotic treatment of CF lung disease: from bench to bedside. J Cyst Fibros 2011;10(Suppl 2): S146-51.

[15] Van Westreenen M, Tiddens HA. New antimicrobial strategies in cystic fibrosis. Paediatr Drugs 2010;12:343-52.

[16] Rogers GB, Hoffman LR, Döring G. Novel concepts in evaluating antimicrobial therapy for bacterial lung infections in patients with cystic fibrosis. J Cyst Fibros 2011 Jul 11. [Epub ahead of print]

[17] Light MJ, Blaisdell Cj, Homnick DN, Schechter MS, Wienberger MM, eds. Pediatric pulmonology. Elk Grove Village, IL: American Academy of Pediatrics, 2011.

[18] Flume PA, O'Sullivan BP, Robinson KA, Goss CH, Mogayzel PJ, Willey-Courand DB, et al. Cystic Fibrosis Foundation, Pulmonary Therapies Committee. Cystic fibrosis pulmonary guidelines: chronic medications for maintenance of lung health. Am J Respir Crit Care Med 2007;176(10):957-69.

[19] Breen L, Aswani N. Elective versus symptomatic intravenous antibiotic therapy for cystic fibrosis. Cochrane Database Syst Rev 2001;1:CD001747.

[20] Goss CH, Muhlebach MS. Review: Staphylococcus aureus and MRSA in cystic fibrosis. J Cyst Fibros 2011 Jun 28. [Epub ahead of print]

[21] Chmiel JF, Konstan MW. Inflammation and anti-inflammatory therapies for cystic fibrosis. Clin Chest Med 2007;28(2):331-46.

[22] Konstan MW, Flume PA, Kappler M, Chiron R, Higgins M, Brockhaus F, et al. Safety, efficacy and convenience of tobramycin inhalation powder in cystic fibrosis patients: The EAGER trial. J Cyst Fibros 2011;10:54-61.

[23] Jones AP, Wallis CE. Recombinant human deoxyribonuclease for cystic fibrosis. Cochrane Database Syst Rev 2003;3:CD001127.

[24] Dentice R, Elkins M. Timing of dornase alfa inhalation for cystic fibrosis. Cochrane Database Syst Rev 2011;5:CD007923.

[25] Donaldson SH, Bennett WD, Zeman KL, Knowles MR, Tarran R, Boucher RC. Mucus clearance and lung function in cystic fibrosis with hypertonic saline. N Engl J Med 2006;354(3):241-50.

[26] Modi AC, Driscoll KA, Montaq-Leifling K, Acton JD. Screening for symptoms of depression and anxiety in adolescents and young adults with cystic fibrosis. Pediatr Pulmonol 2011;46:153-9.

[27] Casier A, Goubert L, Theunis M, Huse D, De Baets F, Matthys D, et al. Acceptance and well-being in adolescents and young adults with cystic fibrosis: a prospective study. J Pediatr Psychol 2011;36:476-87.

[28] Barker DH, Driscoll KA, Modi AC, Light MJ, Quittner AL. Supporting cystic fibrosis disease management during adolescence: the role of family and friends. Child Care Health Dev 2011 Jul 19. [Epub ahead of print]

[29] Towns SJ, Bell SC. Transition of adolescents with cystic fibrosis from paediatric to adult care. Clin Respir J 2011;5:64-75.

[30] Centers for Disease Control and Prevention. Vital signs: asthma prevalence, disease characteristics, and self-management education: United States, 2001-2009. MMWR 2011;60:547-52.

[31] Bateman ED, Boushey HA, Bousquet J, Busse WW, Clark TJ, Pauwels RA, Pedersen SE. Can guideline-defined asthma control be achieved? The Gaining Optimal Asthma ControL study. GOAL Investigators Group Am J Respir Crit Care Med 2004;170(8):836-44.

[32] Global Initiative for Asthma (GINA). Global strategy for asthma management and prevention: NHLBI/WHO Workshop Report: Bethesda, MD: National Heart Lung Blood Institute, 02-3659, 2002.

[33] National Asthma Education and Prevention Program: Expert panel report III: Guidelines for the diagnosis and management of asthma. Bethesda, MD: 08-4051, 2007.

[34] Jensen ME, Collins CE, Gibson PG, Wood LG. The obesity phenotype in children with asthma. Paediatr Respir Rev 2011; 12:152-9.

[35] Sadof M, Kaslovsky R. Adolescent asthma: A developmental approach. Curr Opin Pediatr 2011;23:373-8.

[36] Arellano FM, Arana A, Wentworth CE, Vidaurre CF, Chipps BE. Prescription patterns for asthma medications in children and adolescents with health care insurance in the United States. Pediatr Allergy Immunol 2011;22;469-76.

[37] Panontin E, Longo G. Treatment of mild persistent asthma in children. Lancet 2011;377:1743-4.

[38] Ducharme FM, Lasserson TJ, Cates CJ. Addition to inhaled corticosteroids of long-acting beta2-agonists versus anti-leukotrienes for chronic asthma. Cochrane Database Syst Rev 2011;5:CD003137.

[39] Robinson PD, Van Asperen P. Update in paediatric asthma management: Where is evidence challenging current practice? J Paediatr Child Health 2011 Apr 6. [Epub ahead of print]

[40] Cotton S, Luberto CM, Yi MS, Tsevat J. Complementary and alternative medicine behaviors and beliefs in urban adolescents with asthma. J Asthma 2011;48:531-8.

Submitted: November 02, 2011. *Revised:* December 07, 2011. *Accepted:* December 20, 2011.

In: Child and Adolescent Health Yearbook 2013
Editor: Joav Merrick

ISBN: 978-1-63117-658-6

Chapter 3

ADOLESCENCE, MUSCULOSKELETAL DISORDERS AND SPORTS INJURIES

Cynthia L Feucht**, PharmD, BCPS
and Dilip R Patel, MD, FAAP, FACSM, FAACPDM, FSAM
Department of Pharmacy Practice, Ferris State University, Kalamazoo,
Borgess Ambulatory Care, Kalamazoo, Pediatrics and Human Development,
Michigan State University College of Human Medicine,
Michigan State University/Kalamazoo Center for Medical Studies,
Kalamazoo, Michigan, United States of America

ABSTRACT

Musculoskeletal injuries account for most sports-related injuries. Overuse musculoskeletal injuries account for more than half of all sport-related injuries in adolescents and young adults. Overuse injuries can result in chronic or intermittent symptoms depending on the athlete's level of activity. Acute muscle injuries (strains, contusions, and lacerations) can lead to significant structural or functional damage to the muscle. Non-pharmacological approaches are often considered as first-line treatment for musculoskeletal injuries and may include relative rest, ice, compression, and elevation. Treatment options include analgesics such as nonsteroidal anti-inflammatory drugs (NSAIDs), acetaminophen, and topical over-the-counter (OTC) preparations. These classes of drugs are reviewed in this paper, including their mechanisms of action, side effects, and efficacy in treating pain and inflammation associated with acute and overuse musculoskeletal injuries.

Keywords: Adolescence, muscoloskeletal disorder, injury, sports

---

* Correspondence: Cynthia L Feucht, PharmD, BCPS, Department of Pharmacy Practice, Ferris State University, Kalamazoo, MI, United States, Borgess Ambulatory Care, 1701 Gull Road, Kalamazoo, MI, 49048, United States. E-mail: cynthia.feucht@gmail.com

INTRODUCTION

Musculoskeletal injuries account for most sports-related injuries (1). Overuse musculoskeletal injuries account for more than half of all sport-related injuries in adolescents and young adults. Overuse injuries can result in chronic or intermittent symptoms depending on the athlete's level of activity. Acute muscle injuries (i.e., strains, contusions, and lacerations) can lead to significant structural or functional damage to the muscle (1-11). Delayed-onset muscle soreness (DOMS) (exercise-induced muscle damage [EIMD]), typically associated with new or unaccustomed exercise, often results from intense eccentric muscle activity and manifests with pain, discomfort, and decreased performance 24 to 48 hours after exercise (1,4).

Nonpharmacological approaches are often considered as first-line treatment for musculoskeletal injuries and may include relative rest, ice, compression, and elevation (3). Moderate to severe injuries to the athlete may result in several weeks of an inability to train or compete. Even after resuming the physical activity or sport, the athlete may continue to experience difficulties with muscle weakness and decreased flexibility (1). As a result, treatment is often sought to alleviate pain, restore function, and allow the athlete to resume activities more quickly. Treatment options include analgesics such as nonsteroidal anti-inflammatory drugs (NSAIDs), acetaminophen, and topical over-the-counter (OTC) preparations. These classes of drugs are reviewed in this chapter, including their mechanisms of action, side effects, and efficacy in treating pain and inflammation associated with acute and overuse musculoskeletal injuries.

MECHANISM OF ACTION

Arachidonic acid is released from cellular membranes as a result of tissue injury. Arachidonic acid is broken down by cyclooxygenase (COX) to produce prostaglandins and thromboxane A2, and by lipoxygenase (LOX) enzymes to produce leukotrienes. Prostaglandins are localized hormones that, once released within the intracellular space, can produce fever, inflammation, and pain (12). Thromboxanes are released in response to tissue injury and are responsible for producing platelet aggregation as well as clot formation, and for regulation of vascular tone (12). Pain relief and decreased inflammation occur from the blockade of COX enzymes, thereby inhibiting prostaglandin E2 and prostacyclin (PGI2) formation (12,13).

Two forms of COX enzymes are cyclooxygenase-1 (COX-1) and cyclooxygenase-2 (COX-2). COX-1 is expressed in most normal tissues and cells, and is the predominant form within gastric epithelial cells (12,14). Prostaglandin production within the gastrointestinal tract protects the gastrointestinal mucosa from gastric acidity. COX-2 is expressed when tissue damage occurs, and its release is induced by cytokines and inflammatory mediators during inflammation (12,14). NSAIDs are a heterogeneous class of medications that are chemically unrelated but known to have similar therapeutic effects, including antipyretic, analgesic, and anti-inflammatory activity. Their primary therapeutic effect is due to inhibition of prostaglandin synthesis by inhibiting COX-2 activity, and a correlation exists between COX-2 inhibition and anti-inflammatory activity (15). Bradykinin and cytokines (i.e., tumor necrosis factor-a [TNF-a] and interleukin-1 [IL-1]) are thought to be responsible for inducing pain with inflammation and releasing prostaglandins that enhance pain sensitivity (16). Other mediators, such as neuropeptides (i.e., substance P) are also involved in inducing pain. The gastrointestinal adverse effects of NSAIDs are predominantly, but not exclusively, due to inhibition of COX-1 enzyme. NSAIDs are considered competitive, reversible inhibitors of COX enzymes (unlike aspirin, which is considered an irreversible inhibitor of COX enzymes) and do not affect the LOX pathway (17).

Salicylated NSAIDs

Derivatives of salicylic acid include aspirin (acetylsalicylic acid), diflunisal (difluorophenyl derivative), salsalate, magnesium salicylate, and choline magnesium salicylate (tables 1 and 2). Aspirin continues to be the most widely used drug and is the standard to which other NSAIDs are compared (18). Due to its widespread availability, aspirin's potential for toxicity often goes under-recognized, and it continues to be a cause of fatal poisonings in children (14).

Salicylates are rapidly absorbed from the gastrointestinal tract, are widely distributed throughout the body, and are highly protein bound (especially albumin) (16).

Due to their high protein binding, salicylates may compete for binding with other compounds, including thyroxine, penicillin, phenytoin, bilirubin, uric acid, and other NSAIDs such as naproxen (14). Salicylates are metabolized in the liver and excreted by the kidneys, with free salicylate excretion dependent on urinary pH and salicylate dose (16).

Gastrointestinal adverse effects are common with salicylates and may include dyspepsia, nausea, vomiting and, more seriously, gastric ulceration, gastrointestinal hemorrhage, and erosive gastritis (14,16).

Table 1. Salicylated NSAIDS

Drug	Onset of Action and Duration of Effect (hours)	Comments
Diflunisal	Onset: ~1 Duration: Analgesic: 8-12 Anti-inflammatory: ≤12	~4-5 times more potent analgesic and anti-inflammatory effects than aspirin; fewer platelet/GI side effects compared with aspirin; not metabolized to salicylic acid
Salsalate	Onset: N/A Duration: N/A	Fewer platelet and GI side effects than aspirin
Choline magnesium trisalicylate	Onset: ~2 Duration: N/A	Less effect on platelet aggregation and fewer GI side effects than aspirin; avoid or use with caution in renal insufficiency due to magnesium content
Magnesium salicylate	Onset: N/A Duration: 4-6	Available OTC; less effect on platelet aggregation and fewer GI side effects than aspirin; avoid or use with caution in renal insufficiency due to magnesium content

Abbreviations: GI, gastrointestinal; N/A, no data available OTC, over-the-counter.
Data from Refs. (13,14,40).

Table 2. Common doses of salicylated NSAIDs

Generic Name	Trade Name	Adult Dose	Comments
Diflunisal		1000 mg, then 500 mg every 12 h Age ≥ 12 y: same as adult	Do not crush or chew tablet; maximum 1.5 g daily
Salsalate	Amigesic	1 g 3 times daily	Do not crush tablets; urinary acidification can decrease clearance and increase risk for toxicity
Choline magnesium trisalicylate	Trilisate	500 mg-1.5 g 2-3 times daily	Maintenance dose: 1-4.5 g daily; available as liquid formulation; urinary acidification can decrease clearance and increase risk for toxicity
Magnesium salicylate	Doan's Extra Strength Keygesic	Doan's (467 mg): 2 caplets every 6 h as needed Keygesic (650 mg): 1 tablet every 4 h as needed Age ≥ 12 y: same as adult	Available OTC; Doan's maximum 8 caplets in 24 h Keygesic: maximum 4 tablets in 24 h

Data from Refs. (19,40).

Aspirin irreversibly inhibits platelet aggregation and leads to a prolongation in the bleeding time. Gastrointestinal and platelet effects are less likely to occur with nonacetylated salicylates (i.e., salsalate, magnesium salicylate, and so forth) because they cannot acetylate COX (16). Owing to aspirin's effect on platelet aggregation, it should be avoided in patients with hepatic impairment, hypoprothrombinemia, vitamin K deficiency, hemophilia, and within 1 week of a surgical procedure (14).

Salicylates have been shown to have a dose-dependent effect on uric acid excretion, and in elevated doses can result in pulmonary edema, hepatotoxicity, and hyperglycemia (14). Hypersensitivity to salicylates can result in hives, flushing, bronchoconstriction, angioedema, low blood pressure, and shock (14). Hypersensitivity is thought to be due to COX inhibition, and cross-sensitivity occurs with other agents in the class as well as with nonsalicylated NSAIDs (14). Patients with asthma, nasal polyps, and sensitivity to tartrazine dyes are at an increased risk for salicylate sensitivity (19). In general, salicylates are avoided during pregnancy, especially the third trimester, due to an increased risk for perinatal death, anemia, antepartum and postpartum hemorrhage, prolonged gestation, and premature closure of the ductus arteriosus (14).

Drug interactions can occur from salicylates displacing other agents from plasma-binding proteins. Dosages of NSAIDs, sulfonylureas, and methotrexate may need to be adjusted to prevent toxicity due to displacement.

NSAIDs given concurrently with corticosteroids and warfarin may increase the risk for bleeding. NSAIDs should not be given concomitantly with the following herbals due to their anticoagulant or antiplatelet activity and increased risk for bleeding: danshen, dong quai, evening primrose, feverfew, garlic, ginger, ginkgo, red clover, horse chestnut, green tea, policosanol, and willowbark (19,20). In addition, NSAIDs decrease the effectiveness of angiotensin-converting enzyme (ACE) inhibitors because of the blockade of renal prostaglandin production.

Salicylates have fallen out of favor for use in adolescents and young adults because of their association with Reye syndrome. Reye syndrome is characterized by toxic hepatitis and has been associated with encephalopathy, prolonged prothrombin time, fatty infiltration of the liver, and intracranial hypertension in advanced stages (21). Aspirin and other salicylates are contraindicated in children and young adults younger than 20 years who have a fever associated with a viral illness (14).

Nonsalicylated NSAIDs

Various classes of nonsalicylated NSAIDs (Tables 3 and 4) are among the most widely used drugs, with yearly sales in the United States for OTC drugs estimated at $30 billion (13,22). Nonsalicylated NSAIDs are considered effective for mild to moderate pain, and have been used for a variety of musculoskeletal disorders including osteoarthritis, rheumatoid arthritis, and sports-related injuries. The choice of a particular nonsalicylated NSAID depends on its onset of action, tolerability, cost, and insurance coverage. An agent with a short onset of action, minimal adverse effects, low cost, and wide acceptability would make for an ideal nonsalicylated NSAID.

As a class, nonsalicylated NSAIDs are usually well absorbed and highly bound to plasma proteins, and are excreted via either glomerular filtration or tubular secretion (14).

These agents accumulate at sites of inflammation, and most exhibit nonselectivity for COX-1 and COX-2 enzymes. The last decade has seen the emergence of COX-2 selective inhibitors designed to minimize gastrointestinal effects that occur due to COX-1 inhibition.

Other older nonsalicylated NSAIDs have also been found to have COX-2 selectivity similar to the currently available celecoxib, based on whole blood assays (14). Most studies on nonsalicylated NSAIDs are done in adults; however, some findings are of relevance to the adolescent age group.

Side effects of nonsalicylated NSAIDs

Gastrointestinal

Gastrointestinal adverse effects are common with nonsalicylated NSAIDs and are often the leading reason for their discontinuation. The gastrointestinal toxicity is often dose dependent and associated with chronic use (14).

Dyspeptic symptoms are frequently experienced by patients and may include anorexia, epigastric pain, nausea, bloating, and heartburn. These symptoms have been associated with both selective and nonselective nonsalicylated NSAIDs (13,23).

Gastrointestinal toxicity may be related to prostaglandin inhibition, which is important for enhancing mucosal blood flow, mucus and bicarbonate production, and inhibition of acid production. Nonsalicylated NSAIDs also may contribute to gastrointestinal toxicity from local irritation to the gastric mucosa.

Table 3. Nonsalicylated NSAIDs

Drug	Onset of Action and Duration of Effect	Comments
Propionic acids		
Fenoprofen	Onset: ~72 h Duration: 4-6 h	~15% of patients will have side effects but few stop therapy
Flurbiprofen	Onset: ~1-2 h Duration: variable	Strong inhibitor of CYP 450 2C9 isoenzyme; substrate CYP 2C9 (minor)
Ibuprofen	Onset: Analgesic: 0.5-1 h Anti-inflammatory: ≤7 d Duration: 4-6 h	Strong inhibitor of CYP 450 2C9 isoenzyme; substrate CYP 2C9 and 2C19 (minor); equal efficacy to aspirin; ~10%-15% of patients stop therapy due to side effects
Ketoprofen	Onset: 0.5 h Duration: 6 h	~30% of patients develop side effects with GI as the most common
Naproxen	Onset: Analgesic: 1h Anti-inflammatory: 2 weeks Duration: Analgesic: ≤7 h Anti-inflammatory: ≤12 h	Available as OTC product; more potent than aspirin in vitro, likely better tolerated than aspirin; may provide cardioprotection for some individuals with heart disease
Oxaprozin	Onset: ~0.5-4 h Duration: variable	Slower onset of effects compared with others; longer half-life allows for once a day dosing
Acetic acids		
Diclofenac	Onset: 1-4.5 h Duration: 12-24 h	More potent than aspirin; side effects experienced by ~20% and 2% stop therapy; ~15% of patients will experience an increase in liver function test; available as topical patch and gel as well as in combination with misoprostol
Etodolac	Onset: Analgesic: 2-4 h Anti-inflammatory: several days Duration: N/A	In vitro COX-2 selectivity; 100 mg of etodolac provides similar efficacy to aspirin 650 mg but may have fewer side effects
Sulindac	Onset: N/A Duration: N/A	Similar efficacy to aspirin; active metabolite; side effects experienced ~ 20% GI and ~10% CNS
Tolmetin	Onset: Analgesic: 1-2 h Anti-inflammatory: days to weeks Duration: variable	Similar efficacy to aspirin; side effects experienced by ~25%-40% and 5%-10% stop therapy
Indomethacin	Onset: ~0.5 h Duration: 4-6 h	Compared with aspirin 10-40 times more potent; incidence of side effects 3%-50%; ~20% of patients stop therapy due to side effects
Ketorolac	Onset: Analgesic: ~10 min (IM) Duration: Analgesic: 6-8 h	Maximum duration of 5 d (oral and parenteral); strong analgesic activity but weak anti-inflammatory activity; may be given parenterally for acute pain
Oxicams		
Meloxicam	Onset: N/A Duration: N/A	CYP 450 inhibitor of isoenzyme 2C9 (weak); substrate CYP 2C9 and 3A4 (minor); some COX-2 selective action at lower end of dosing range

Drug	Onset of Action and Duration of Effect	Comments
Piroxicam	Onset: ~ 1 h Duration: variable	Equal efficacy to aspirin; may be better tolerated than aspirin; ~20% of patients will experience side effects and 5% will stop therapy
Naphthylalkanone		
Nabumetone	Onset: ~72 h Duration: variable	Prodrug; some COX-2 selectivity; has less GI toxicity than most NSAIDs
Fenemate		
Meclofenamate	Onset: <1 h Duration: ≤6 h	Equal efficacy to aspirin; ~25% of patients will experience gastrointestinal adverse events
Mefenamic acid	Onset: N/A Duration: ≤6 h	CYP 450 inhibitor of isoenzyme 2C9 (strong); substrate CYP 2C9 (minor)
COX-2 inhibitor		
Celecoxib	Onset: Analgesic: ~0.75 h to several months Duration: ~4-8 h	CYP 450 inhibitor of isoenzymes 2C8 (moderate) and 2D6 (weak); substate CYP 2C9 (major) and 3A4 (minor); does not inhibit platelet aggregation

Data from Refs.(13,14,40).

Table 4. Common doses of nonsalicylated NSAIDs

Generic Name	Trade Name	Adult Dose	Comments
Propionic acids			
Fenoprofen	Naflon	200 mg every 4-6 h as needed	Maximum: 3.2 g/d; do not crush tablets
Flurbiprofen	Ocufen	50-100 mg 2-3 times daily	Maximum: 300 mg/d; maximum single dose 100 mg; do not crush tablets
Ibuprofen	Motrin Advil	200-400 mg every 4-6 h Maximum: 3.2 g/d	Available OTC; available in tablets (regular and chewable), capsule, suspension and infant drops; chewable tablets may contain phenylalanine
Ketoprofen	Oruvail	25-50 mg every 6-8 h as needed	Extended-release formulation is not recommended for acute pain; maximum (immediate release) 300 mg/d; maximum (extended release): 200 mg/d
Naproxen sodium	Aleve Anaprox Anaprox DS	500 mg initially, then 250 mg every 6-8 h as needed OTC label: 200 mg every 8-12 h as needed	Available OTC; dosage recommendations expressed as naproxen base; maximum (adult): 1250 mg/d (naproxen base); OTC formulation not indicated for age <12 y
Naproxen	Naprosyn Naprelan	500 mg initially, then 250 mg every 6-8 h as needed	Available as immediate-release, extended-release and suspension; extended release not recommended for acute pain; do not break, crush, or chew extended-release formulation; maximum (adult): 1250 mg/d
Oxaprozin	Daypro	600-1200 mg daily	Patients with low body weight should start with 600 mg daily; do not crush tablets

Table 4. (Continued)

Generic Name	Trade Name	Adult Dose	Comments
Acetic acids			
Diclofenac	Voltaren	50 mg 3 times daily	Available as immediate, extended-release formulation and powder for solution; do not crush or chew tablets; mix powder in 30-60 mL of water and drink immediately; maximum: 200 mg daily
Diclofenac patch	Flector patch	Apply 1 patch twice daily	Apply patch to most painful area of intact skin; wash hands after applying and after removal; may tape edges of patch if peeling occurs; do not wear while sunbathing; fold used patches before disposal
Etodolac	Lodine	200-400 mg every 6-8 h	Maximum: 1000 mg daily (immediate-release) and 1200 mg daily (extended-release formulation); do not crush tablets or break capsules
Sulindac	Clinoril	150-200 mg twice daily	Maximum: 400 mg daily
Tolmetin	Tolectin	400 mg 3 times daily	Maximum: 1800 mg daily; taking with food decreases bioavailability; do not crush tablets or break capsules
Indomethacin	Indocin	25-50 mg 2-3 times daily Age ≥15 y; same as adult	Available as immediate- and extended-release capsules and suspension; maximum (adult): 200 mg/d (immediate-release) and 150 mg/d (extended-release); do not crush, break or chew capsules
Ketorolac	Toradol	20 mg, then 10 mg every 4-6 h as needed <50 kg: 10 mg, then 10 mg every 4-6 h as needed	Not to exceed 5 d in duration (injection and oral combined); maximum: 40 mg daily; oral dosing intended to be a continuation of IM/IV therapy; not indicated for minor or chronic pain conditions
Oxicams			
Meloxicam	Mobic	7.5-15 mg once daily	Available as oral suspension
Piroxicam	Feldene	10-20 mg once daily	Maximum: 20 mg/d; do not break capsules
Naphthylalkanone			
Nabumetone	Relafen	1000 mg daily in 1-2 divided doses	Maximum: 2 g/d; do not crush tablets
Fenamate			
Meclofenamate		50-100 mg every 4-6 h as needed Age > 14 y: same as adult	Maximum: 400 mg/d
Mefenamic acid	Ponstel	500 mg, then 250 mg every 4 h as needed Age > 14 y: same as adult	Maximum duration: usually 1 week
COX-2 inhibitor			
Celecoxib	Celebrex	200 mg twice daily as needed	Contents of capsule may be sprinkled onto applesauce for administration; poor metabolizers of CYP 2C9 start at half the recommended dose

Data from Refs. (19,40).

More serious complications include gastric and duodenal ulcers, which may occur in up to 15% to 30% of regular nonsalicylated NSAID users (24,25). Complications from ulcers include bleeding, perforation, and obstruction. Patients may present with a serious gastrointestinal event but have had no symptoms before presentation (13).

Factors that may increase the risk for gastrointestinal complications include the presence of Helicobacter pylori, advanced age, concomitant use of aspirin, anticoagulants, or corticosteroids, and duration of NSAID use (greatest within the first month) (13,26). Lifestyle factors such as smoking and alcohol use also contribute to an increased risk for side effects, but are not independent risk factors (13,26). For those patients at risk, a proton pump inhibitor (PPI) has been shown to be effective at reducing the frequency and severity of upper gastro¬intestinal symptoms (13,27).

COX-2 inhibitors were developed with the aim of reducing gastrointestinal complications associated with nonselective nonsalicylated NSAIDs. COX-2 inhibitors do not inhibit the COX-1 enzyme, which is responsible for prostaglandin production in the gastrointestinal mucosa, and therefore should have less risk for gastrointestinal toxicity.

The benefit of COX-2 inhibitors with regard to less gastrointestinal toxicity remains controversial. In patients with gastrointestinal disease or risk factors for gastrointestinal complications, risk versus benefit should be assessed, and if nonsalicylated NSAIDs are used, the lowest dose for the shortest time period should be considered (24-28).

Hepatotoxicity

Hepatotoxicity from NSAID use appears to be rare, with estimates between 3 and 23 cases per 10,000 patient years (29,30). Two older agents (benoxaprofen and bromfenac) have been withdrawn in the United States due to reports of serious hepatotoxicity (13). Rostom and colleagues (31) in a systematic review, found the rate of hospitalization due to nonsalicylated NSAID-related hepatotoxicity to be 2.7 per 100,000 patients and the rate of death to be 1.9 per 100,000 patients.

A recent case report by Bennett and colleagues details a 16-year-old who was previously healthy and found to be taking ibuprofen for 6 weeks before presentation (29). The first 2 weeks of ibuprofen use was scheduled dosing and the subsequent 4 weeks was sporadic use. The adolescent presented with dark-colored urine, jaundice, and pruritus. Laboratory results were significant for an elevated bilirubin and minimal elevation in liver enzymes (29). The results of a liver biopsy revealed intrahepatic and canalicular cholestasis and histology was suggestive of drug-induced hepatotoxicity (29). Over the following 4 months, the patient's symptoms resolved and laboratory values returned to normal.

Liver dysfunction related to nonsalicylated NSAIDs is rare in otherwise healthy adolescents, but should be considered in a patient with recent nonsalicylated NSAID use and presenting with cholestasis (29). Thorough medication histories are important in determining the cause and effect in such situations. Despite the potential for hepatotoxicity, current data do not support routine monitoring of liver enzymes in individuals receiving nonsalicylated NSAIDs.

Renal toxicity

Renal insufficiency is well known with nonsalicylated NSAID use and is likely the result of inhibition of renal prostaglandins. Renal insufficiency is estimated to occur in approximately 1% to 5% of patients, and is usually reversible on discontinuation of the NSAID (13,32).

Renal prostaglandins serve an important role in maintaining renal circulation, including vasodilation, renin secretion, and sodium as well as water excretion (13). The disruption in balance between vasoconstriction and vasodilation within the kidneys may predispose a patient to renal failure. Those at the greatest risk for renal toxicity associated with nonsalicylated NSAIDs include patients with heart failure, cirrhosis, chronic kidney disease, and hypovolemic states (13,14). Renal toxicity is characterized by elevated serum creatinine, sodium and water retention, hyperkalemia, proteinuria, interstitial nephritis, papillary necrosis, acute renal failure, acute glomerulitis, vasculitis, acute tubular necrosis, and papillary necrosis (13,33,34). In patients at risk for renal toxicity, the risk versus benefit in using a nonsalicylated NSAID should be carefully considered and, if at all possible, NSAIDs, including COX-2 inhibitors, should be avoided.

There have been several case reports of renal toxicity in adolescents with nonsalicylated NSAID use. Nakahura and colleagues (35) discuss 5 adolescents (13-19 years old) who developed renal toxicity with the use of nonsalicylated NSAIDs. The first case was a 16-year-old girl who took ibuprofen intermittently over 9 months. Kidney biopsy results were consistent with interstitial nephritis and the patient was treated with corticosteroids. At 1 year she was asymptomatic with a decrease in serum creatinine; however, 2 years later her serum creatinine had risen and results of a repeat kidney biopsy revealed chronic interstitial fibrosis (35). Case 3 in this report describes a 15-year-old girl who used ibuprofen every other day for 6 months. The patient was found to have proteinuria, and results of renal ultrasonography were reported normal. The patient discontinued the nonsalicylated NSAID and was asymptomatic after 1 month (35). The other 3 cases describe adolescents who used naprosyn (1 week before hospitalization), ibuprofen (daily use for several weeks), and ketorolac (intermittently for 4 months), who all developed an increase in serum creatinine and were found to have urine eosinophilia indicative of nonsalicylated NSAID-associated nephrotoxicity (35). In 2 of the cases nephrotoxicity resolved, and the other case reported resolution of symptoms at 1 month but continued elevation in serum creatinine.

These case reports illustrate that nonsalicylated NSAID nephrotoxicity can occur in healthy adolescents. Given the fact that several nonsalicylated NSAIDs are available as OTC preparations, adolescents should be aware of their potential adverse effects. It is important to use the lowest dose of the nonsalicylated NSAID for the shortest time period necessary, and to maintain adequate hydration while on nonsalicylated NSAIDs.

Cardiovascular toxicity

Cardiovascular toxicity related to nonsalicylated NSAID use is generally not of concern in otherwise healthy adolescents. Cardiovascular toxicity came to light with the emergence of the selective COX-2 inhibitors. It has been theorized that the disruption in the balance between prostacyclin and thromboxane formation by selective COX-2 inhibitors may increase this risk. The selective COX-2 inhibitors, via their inhibition of prostacyclin formation, favor increased thromboxane formation and subsequent platelet aggregation.

Current data suggest that selective nonsalicylated NSAIDs may increase cardiovascular risk, but data are conflicting (24,36-38). Heterogeneity of the studies including patient selection, duration of study, agents used, study design, and cardiovascular risk at baseline makes it challenging to summarize the cardiovascular risks associated with nonsalicylated NSAIDs. Rofecoxib was voluntarily withdrawn from the United States market in September 2004, and the U.S. Food and Drug Administration (FDA) requested Pfizer to voluntarily remove valdecoxib from the market in April 2005 because of cardiovascular risks (39). In addition, in 2005 the FDA requested the makers of prescription and OTC nonsalicylated NSAIDs to include a boxed warning highlighting the increased risk for cardiovascular events as well as gastrointestinal toxicity, including the risk for life-threatening gastrointestinal bleeding (39).

Drug interactions

Drug interactions are similar to those already described for salicylated NSAIDs as well as the following additional drug interactions. Nonselective nonsalicylated NSAIDs may decrease the effectiveness of aspirin if given concomitantly due to blockade of the platelet COX-1 site (14). It is recommended that the nonsalicylated NSAIDs be given at least 2 hours after the dose of aspirin to achieve irreversible platelet inhibition by aspirin (13). Nonsalicylated NSAIDs may also decrease the effectiveness of thiazide and loop diuretics through blockade of renal prostaglandins (40).

In addition, nonsalicylated NSAIDs can reduce renal clearance of lithium, resulting in elevated lithium plasma levels, and the efficacy of nonsalicylated NSAIDs can be reduced with cholestyramine and colestipol due to blockade of absorption (40). Drug interactions can occur with mefenamic acid, celecoxib, meloxicam, ibuprofen, and flurbiprofen due to their metabolism via cytochrome P450 isoenzymes. With a wide variety of drug interactions, each patient's medication profile should be reviewed, including prescription, OTC, and herbal products, to evaluate for drug-drug interactions before initiating an nonsalicylated NSAID.

Efficacy of NSAIDs in musculoskeletal injuries

NSAIDs have been purported to help in decreasing pain and inflammation, restore musculoskeletal function, decrease time to healing, and allow faster return to previous activity level. The benefit of using NSAIDs in the prevention of myositis ossificans traumatica following deep muscle contusions remains controversial. Concern has been raised that by inhibiting the inflammatory response, NSAIDs may slow phagocytic function and time for muscle regeneration and healing. Animal studies have been conflicting as to the effects of NSAIDs in the musculoskeletal model. Human studies have not always shown a consistent benefit of NSAIDs in treating musculoskeletal injuries. Studies have been limited at times by small sample sizes, lack of placebo group, subjective assessment, differing patient populations, and lack of control for confounding factors.

A recent review by Mehallo and colleagues summarized data regarding use of NSAIDs for acute ligament and muscle injuries (3). Rat models for ligament sprains have shown that piroxicam strengthens the medial collateral ligament of the knee at 14 days versus celecoxib, which was found to weaken the medial collateral ligament at 14 days compared with placebo. Other animal studies have not found any benefit with selective and nonselective NSAIDs versus placebo (3). Human studies have provided evidence for a more consistent benefit of NSAIDs in ligament sprains. A variety of NSAIDs have been shown to decrease pain and inflammation associated with acute ankle sprains (3). Several studies have documented the efficacy of NSAIDs in decreasing pain, increasing functional ability, and allowing for a more rapid return to training (3).

Although NSAIDs have been shown to be effective for treating the pain associated with injured ligaments, their efficacy in improving joint stability remains unknown (3). In 2 animal model studies, piroxicam was shown to improve contractile force and greater maximal failure force early post injury, but also slowed deposition of collagen and regeneration of muscle tissue (3). Studies examining NSAIDs in human muscle strains are limited. One trial evaluated meclofenamate and diclofenac versus placebo along with physiotherapy in treating acute hamstring injuries, and found no differences among the groups with respect to pain, swelling, and isokinetic muscle performance (3).

Howatson and van Someren reviewed the use of NSAIDs in the treatment and prevention of DOMS (5). In one study, ketoprofen used prophylactically was found to decrease muscle soreness and enhance muscle function, while another study evaluated ibuprofen before and after exercise and demonstrated a decrease in muscle damage. In contrast, a study evaluated ibuprofen 45 minutes before downhill running and scheduled dosing for 3 days after the activity, and found no effect on muscle soreness or strength (5). Additional studies with oxaprozin and ibuprofen with acetaminophen post exercise failed to provide benefit (5). NSAIDs were found to attenuate loss of muscle strength and muscle soreness in 2 studies post exercise and in one study failed to provide evidence of benefit compared with placebo after elbow flexor eccentric muscle injury (3). Conflicting evidence to support the use of NSAIDs in DOMS may be the result of differences in study methodology, patient selection, and study limitations. NSAIDs may provide benefit in decreasing muscle soreness and improving short-term muscle recovery (3,41). Given the potential ability of NSAIDs to impair muscle healing, risk versus benefit should be considered and, if used, a short course of 3 to 7 days should be considered (3).

Topical NSAIDs

In addition to oral NSAIDs, topical formulations of NSAIDs have been used for treating musculoskeletal injuries. A systematic review conducted by Moore and colleagues (42) evaluated 37 placebo-controlled trials of topical NSAIDs in the treatment of acute soft tissue injury, sprains, strains, or trauma. Twenty-seven of the trials demonstrated a significant benefit of the topical NSAID over placebo (42). The pooled relative benefit for all trials was 1.7 (95% confidence interval [CI]: 1.5–1.9) (42). For topical NSAIDs evaluated in 3 or more studies, pooling of data for the individual agents showed ketoprofen, felbinac, ibuprofen, and piroxicam to be superior to placebo (42). Local skin reactions were reported in 3% or fewer, systemic adverse effects in less than 1%, and discontinuation due to adverse effects in 0.6% or less, with no significant difference noted between active treatment and placebo groups (42). The authors note that due to the small sample size of most of the trials, publication bias may have influenced the results of the systematic review.

Diclofenac gel and topical patch were the first topical NSAIDs approved in 2007 in the United States by the FDA. Diclofenac gel (Voltaren gel) is currently approved for treatment of osteoarthritis and diclofenac topical patch (Flector patch) for the treatment of acute minor sprains, strains, and contusions (19). When applied to the skin, diclofenac accumulates under the application site, leading to a tissue reservoir for localized effects (43). With its topical application, systemic plasma concentrations are in the range of 1 to 3 ng/mL and relative systemic bioavailability compared with oral administration is approximately 1% (13). The diclofenac patch is relatively safe, with skin reactions as the most common adverse event (43). Thus, the risk for systemic adverse effects is minimal due to low plasma concentrations.

A randomized, double-blind, placebo-controlled trial using topical diclofenac in ankle sprains found it to provide a greater reduction in pain on rest and movement from day 2 and faster joint swelling reduction from day 3 (44). Five percent of the patients in the placebo group discontinued treatment due to lack of efficacy compared with none in the topical diclofenac group (44). Another randomized, double-blind, placebo-controlled study compared topical diclofenac to placebo in patients with traumatic blunt soft tissue injury (44). Tenderness at the center of the injured area was produced by pressure applied from calibrated calipers. The primary end point was the area under the curve (AUC) for tenderness over the first 3 days of treatment (44). The patch was found to be significantly more effective than placebo for the primary end point ($P<0.0001$) (44). Topical diclofenac also produced a greater pain intensity reduction at rest and with activity (44). There were no significant differences between the groups with respect to adverse events, and topical diclofenac was well tolerated (44). Additional single-blinded or nonrandomized trials have assessed the topical diclofenac patch in acute injuries and have found it to be superior to placebo in relieving pain (44).

Studies support the use of topical diclofenac in alleviating pain related to acute injuries, but its ability to improve muscle recovery and allow participants to return to activity more quickly remains to be appropriately evaluated. Topical diclofenac, because of its low systemic bioavailability, may be beneficial in those patients who are at risk for gastrointestinal or cardiovascular toxicity from oral NSAIDs.

Acetaminophen

Acetaminophen (Tylenol) was initially used in 1893 but did not gain wide acceptance until 1949 (14). Acetaminophen is the active metabolite of phenacetin, which was widely used until the 1980s when it was withdrawn from the market due to its association with analgesic-abuse nephropathy and hemolytic anemia (14). Acetaminophen, along with NSAIDs, has largely replaced aspirin as the analgesic of choice in children, adolescents, and young adults, because of aspirin's association with Reye syndrome. Acetaminophen is known to have analgesic and antipyretic activity similar to aspirin; however, acetaminophen has poor anti-inflammatory effects. At typical doses of 1,000 mg, acetaminophen has been shown in whole blood assays of healthy volunteers to inhibit only approximately 50% of COX-1 and COX-2 enzymes (14).

Acetaminophen has good bioavailability and is evenly distributed throughout most body fluids (14). Protein binding of acetaminophen is variable, and it undergoes extensive hepatic metabolism with glucuronidation and sulfation to form inactive metabolites that are excreted by the kidneys (14). A small percentage (about 5%-15%) of acetaminophen is metabolized to N-acetyl-p-benzoquinoneimine (NAPQI), which normally reacts with glutathione sulfhydryl groups, is further metabolized, and then excreted (45). When excessive amounts of acetaminophen are consumed, conjugation pathways become saturated and larger amounts of acetaminophen are converted to NAPQI (14,45). With the shift to NAPQI, glutathione stores become depleted and the excessive NAPQI can lead to hepatotoxicity (14,45).

Acetaminophen has mild to moderate analgesic properties as well as antipyretic activity. Acetaminophen has been used for a wide variety of indications, including fever and pain associated with many different conditions (45). Contributing to acetaminophen's widespread use is its easy tolerability. Unlike NSAIDs, acetaminophen does not affect platelet function or uric acid levels, nor is it associated with significant gastrointestinal toxicity (45). Acetaminophen is felt to be safe in patients with peptic ulcer disease and aspirin hypersensitivity, but is not a reasonable alternative to NSAIDs in patients with inflammatory conditions such as rheumatoid arthritis (14). Side effects that have been reported, albeit infrequently, include rash, hypersensitivity reactions, blood dyscrasias, and renal toxicity (45).

The most serious adverse event that may occur with acetaminophen is the risk for hepatotoxicity that occurs with overdose. The maximum adult dose of acetaminophen is 4,000 mg per day and for those with chronic alcohol use, 2,000 mg daily (Table 5) (14). Because of the vast number of preparations that contain acetaminophen, including prescription and OTC, accidental overdose can occur due to consumption of multiple products (i.e., prescription analgesic agents as well as OTC cough and cold preparations). Whether accidental or intentional, acetaminophen overdose is a medical emergency (14). Overdose can occur with single doses of 10 to 15 g, and doses of 20 to 25 g can be lethal (14). Acetaminophen toxicity is divided into 4 stages.

The first stage can occur within several hours of acute ingestion, is typically associated with nausea, vomiting, and stomach pain, and may resolve within 24 hours (14,45). The second stage can start approximately 12 to 36 hours after acute ingestion, and is significant for right upper quadrant pain and elevated liver enzymes (45).

Table 5. Acetaminophen formulations and dosing

Formulation	Regular: 80 mg, 160 mg, 325 mg, 500mg Extra strength: 500 mg Extended release: 650 mg Liquid: 80 mg/0.8 mg, 160 mg/5 mL, 500 mg/15 mL Rectal suppository: 80 mg, 120 mg, 325 mg, 650 mg
Dosage (adult and adolescent)	325-650 mg every 4-6 h as needed 1000 mg 3-4 times daily Not to exceed 4 g/d
Comments	80 mg and 160 mg available in chewable, oral disintegrating, and meltaways Shake suspension well before dispensing Avoid chronic use in hepatic impairment Chewable tablets may contain phenylalanine Avoid or limit alcohol to <3 drinks per day Avoid other products with acetaminophen

Data from Ref. (19).

Stage 3 occurs 72 to 96 hours after ingestion of toxic doses, and hepatomegaly, jaundice, and coagulopathy may be present (14,45). Liver enzyme levels peak during this time period and renal failure can be present. The onset of encephalopathy or worsening coagulopathy after this time period indicates a poor prognosis (14). Stage 4 is the recovery period for those who make it past stage 3 (45). Acetaminophen overdose is best managed when early diagnosis and treatment can occur. It has been estimated that about 10% of those who do not receive proper treatment will develop severe hepatic impairment, and 10% to 20% of those may eventually die from liver failure (14,45).

Several studies have evaluated acetaminophen and compared it with an NSAID for treating pain. A study by Dalton and Schweinle (46) compared acetaminophen extended-release to ibuprofen in 260 patients who presented with grade I or II lateral ankle sprains. At the end of the study, acetaminophen was found to be not inferior to ibuprofen; 78% to 80% of patients had resumed normal activities, and mean time to resumption was approximately 4 days in both groups (46).

A study by Woo and colleagues (47) recruited 300 patients who presented to an emergency room with an isolated painful limb injury. Patients were randomized to a 3-day course of acetaminophen, indomethacin, diclofenac, or acetaminophen and diclofenac. Pain reduction was seen in all treatment arms, with score reductions not found to be clinically or statistically significant among the 4 groups over the course of the 3 days (47). The combination therapy group had the greatest reduction in pain scores at each time point but also produced more side effects, including abdominal pain (47). Although the literature is not as extensive as for NSAIDs regarding the use of acetaminophen for treating musculoskeletal injuries, there is evidence to support its use.

Topical nonprescription analgesics

Nonprescription, or OTC, analgesic agents and external counterirritants are widely used in the United States, with more than $2 billion spent on them each year (48). Due to their easy access without a prescription, OTC topical analgesics are often first used in treating acute injuries before scheduling a visit to the physician. Topical analgesics can have one of several different properties; those with counterirritant effects are indicated for the acute treatment of minor aches and pains. Counterirritants exert their effect by producing a less intense pain than the pain the individual is experiencing (48).

The perception of another sensation distracts the person from the original pain produced by the injury. Counterirritants can fall into 1 of 4 categories based on their mechanism: (1) act as rubefacients, (2) production of a cooling sensation, (3) producing vasodilation, and (4) causing irritation without rubefaction (48). A classification of topical analgesics with counterirritant properties is outlined in Table 6.

Table 6. Classification of topical analgesics with counterirritant properties (48)

Group Classification	Mechanism	Counterirritant
I	Rubefacients	Methyl salicylate Turpentine oil Ammonia water
II	Cooling sensation	Camphor Menthol
III	Vasodilation	Histamine dihydrochloride Methyl nicotinate
IV	Irritation without rubefaction	Capsaicin Capsicum oleoresin[a]

[a]Capsaicin is the major ingredient in capsicum oleoresin. (*Data from* Wright E. Musculoskeletal injuries and disorders. In: Berardi R, Ferreri S, Hume A, et al., editors. Handbook of nonprescription drugs, an interactive approach to self-care. 16th edition. Washington, DC: American Pharmacists Association; 2009. p. 95-113).

The FDA has approved these agents for use in treating minor aches and pain for both adults and children 2 years or older (48). Counterirritants from different categories are often combined in various preparations to enhance the efficacy of the product.

Methyl salicylate

Methyl salicylate is a commonly used rubefacient that is available naturally in wintergreen oil, or it can be produced by esterification of salicylic acid with methyl alcohol (48). Methyl salicylate is thought to exert its effect by producing a local vasodilation, and the counterirritant effect results from the local increase in skin temperature (48). Most of the effects of methyl salicylate are locally mediated; however, systemic absorption can increase with the use of multiple applications, and use with local application of heat and occlusive dressings (48). The most common adverse effects are skin irritation and rash, but more severe skin reactions along with systemic toxicity can occur (48).

The use of heating pads should be avoided while using topical methyl salicylate because tissue and muscle necrosis along with interstitial nephritis have been reported when topical methyl salicylate and menthol were used (49). Methyl salicylate should be avoided in children and in individuals with aspirin sensitivity and asthma, due to the risk for systemic absorption (48). Drug interactions with warfarin have been reported with typical and high-dose topical methyl salicylate, resulting in an elevation of the prothrombin time/international normalized ratio (50,51).

Camphor

Most camphor is synthetically produced and exerts a counterirritant effect via a cooling sensation. Camphor stimulates skin nerve endings producing mild pain, which allows for a masking of the deeper-seated pain (48). The major toxicity associated with camphor is tonic-clonic seizures. The risk for toxicity correlates with the amount and extent of the camphor ingested (48). In addition to seizures, high doses have also been associated with nausea, vomiting, dizziness, delirium, coma, and death (48).

Concentrations of camphor oil at 20% and as little as 5 mL can be lethal when ingested by children (48). As a result, in 1982 the FDA ruled that camphorated oil products could no longer be produced and products containing camphor must have concentrations less than 11% to be considered safe for nonprescription use (52). Unfortunately, pediatric cases of toxicity from acute ingestions have continued to be reported with OTC preparations containing camphor (48,52,53).

Menthol

Menthol, prepared synthetically or derived from peppermint oil, is another counterirritant when used at concentrations greater than 1.25% (48). Menthol exerts its cooling effect by activating the transient receptor potential, TRPM8, in sensory neurons (54). Menthol has also been associated with an increase in local blood flow at the application site, resulting in a warm sensation (54). Menthol has been associated with a low incidence of hypersensitivity reactions including itching, erythema, and skin lesions, and postmarketing data indicate minimal toxicity (54).

Capsaicin

Capsaicin, which is derived from hot chili peppers, produces an analgesic effect due to its direct irritant properties. Topical application of capsaicin produces a warm sensation locally due to activation of the TRP vanilloid (TRPV1); this effect decreases with repeated administration due to tachyphylaxis (55,56). Capsaicin depletes substance P (neurotransmitter for pain communication) from unmyelinated type C sensory neurons, which can produce an initial burning or itching sensation (57). Blockade of further synthesis of substance P with repeated application leads to persistent desensitization (57). The burning sensation diminishes with repeated use, but can lead to an increase in nonadherence and discontinuation of its use.

Topical capsaicin has been recommended for use in osteoarthritis, and pain relief is usually seen within several weeks. Capsaicin is applied routinely 3 to 4 times daily to sustain its effect. Gloves should be used to minimize contact with mucous membranes (48). As with other topical analgesics, capsaicin should not be applied to open wounds and should be discontinued if skin breakdown occurs (48). Capsaicin has not been studied in acute sports-related injuries, and given that its analgesic effects may not be seen for several weeks, may make it less ideal for treatment.

Others

Other counterirritants not widely used include turpentine oil, histamine dihydrochloride, and ammonia water (48). The efficacy of these agents is difficult to evaluate, because they are often used in combination with other counterirritant agents. Little data exist to support the use of eucalyptus oil and trolamine salicylate; however, trolamine salicylate continues to be available in a variety of topical analgesics. Trolamine salicylate is not a counterirritant and has been shown to be systemically absorbed (48). In general, for trolamine salicylate 10% to 15%, is applied to the skin 3 to 4 times daily (48). Contraindications, precautions, and drug interactions are similar to those of salicylates. Trolamine may be beneficial for those who are unable to tolerate other counterirritants or find them unacceptable.

Counterirritants are available in a wide variety of single and combination products as nonprescription analgesic agents (table 7). Counterirritants are indicated for the treatment of mild aches and pains related to acute injury, and provide a useful option for self-treatment. General guidelines for use of topical counterirritant agents are outlined in Box 1.

Box 1. General guidelines for the use of topical analgesics

Apply to affected areas of intact skin 3 to 4 times daily
Massage or rub gently into the affected area
Wash hands thoroughly with soap and water after application
For patch application, clean and dry the affected areas and remove film before application
Consider using gloves, especially for capsaicin application
Capsaicin is contraindicated for those younger than 18 years
Follow directions for each product carefully

Use and abuse of analgesics

OTC (over-the-counter) medications are widely available and used in the United States. It is not uncommon for individuals to self treat for a wide variety of ailments, including acute musculoskeletal injuries. It has been estimated that 30% of adults have used one or more OTC medications within the past 2 days (59). Children and adolescents are also consumers of OTC medications for cough and cold, headache, fever, menstrual, and joint and muscle pain. Chambers and colleagues (59), administered a questionnaire to 651 junior high school students in Nova Scotia to evaluate the use of OTC medications, indications, and self-administration. Of those who used an OTC medication, 88% reported using it for muscle, joint, and back pain; acetaminophen was the most common medication used for each type of pain assessed (59). Self-administration was common, with 58% to 76% reporting taking medication within the past 3 months without consulting any knowledgeable professional (59).

With increasing self-administration and easy accessibility, factors that influence consumption of OTC medications have been evaluated. Van den Bulck and colleagues (60) evaluated the association between watching television and analgesic use in 2,545 Belgian students (aged 13-16 years). Using a questionnaire, the investigators found that the use of analgesics differed among school years and between gender. A significant correlation was found between regular OTC analgesic use (at least monthly) and viewing of television (odds ratio [OR] 1.16, 95% CI: 1.08-1.24) (60). Playing video games and internet use was not significantly associated with analgesic use. The authors note that this study did not evaluate the extent to which adolescents were exposed to advertisements during television viewing (60).

Self-administration of medications by children and adolescents can be influenced by multiple factors and is potentially dangerous. Huott and Storrow (61) surveyed 203 adolescents aged 13 to 18 years who presented to an emergency room or acute care clinic. The adolescents completed a 1-page survey assessing their knowledge of OTC medication toxicity.

An informal survey of the investigators' colleagues and standard texts served as the reference point regarding medication toxicity (61). Survey results of the adolescents indicated that 63% considered aspirin, 57% acetaminophen, 24% iron, 22% camphor, and 17% to 21% methyl salicylate to be nonlethal, which was contradictory to the faculty's viewpoint (61). The results of this study emphasize that education regarding the toxicity of OTC medications needs further emphasis.

While analgesic use is common among adolescents in general, the pattern of their use among student athletes in particular has not been clearly elucidated. Many student athletes experience muscle aches and pains as well as sports-related injuries; thus, they may self-medicate with OTC analgesic agents including NSAIDs. Evidence indicates that many adolescents are unaware of the potential toxicity or risk for side effects associated with nonprescription analgesic medications. Warner and colleagues distributed a self-administered questionnaire to 604 high school football athletes to compare users with nonusers of NSAIDs and discern differences in attitudes regarding daily use of NSAIDs (62). The study found that 75% had used NSAIDs in the past 3 months while 15% considered themselves daily users of NSAIDs (62). After controlling for confounding variables, those who perceived that NSAIDs enhanced performance (adjusted odds ratio [AOR] 2.4; 95% CI 1.4-4.1), those who used prophylactic NSAIDs (AOR 2.5; 95% CI 1.5-4.3), and those who self-administered NSAIDs (AOR 2.2; 95% CI 1.01-4.9), were more likely to take NSAIDs on a daily basis (62).

Often in athletes, student as well as elite, studies focus on medications of abuse rather than common prescription and nonprescription medications. Alaranta and colleagues (63) used a questionnaire to determine the frequency of prescribed medications in a group of elite athletes.

Table 7. Topical analgesic agents

Preparation	Product	Ingredients
Menthol preparations	ActivOn Topical Analgesic Ultra Strength Joint and Muscle	Menthol 4.127%
	Icy Hot Extra Strength Medicated Patch	Menthol 5%
	Ben Gay Ultra Strength Pain Relieving Patch	Menthol 5%
	Absorbine Jr. Pain Relieving Liquid	Menthol 1.27%
	Aspercreme Heat Pain Relieving Gel	Menthol 10%
	Flexall Maximum Strength Relieving Gel	Menthol 16%
Camphor preparations	JointFlex Arthritis Pain Relieving Cream	Camphor 3.1%
Capsaicin preparations	Capzasin Arthritis Pain Relief No Mess Applicator	Capsaicin 0.15%
	Zostrix Arthritis Pain Relief Cream	Capsaicin 0.025%
	Zostrix HP Arthritis Pain Relief Cream	Capsaicin 0.075%
	WellPatch Natural Capsaicin Pain Relief Patch	Capsaicin 0.025%
Trolamine preparations	Aspercreme Analgesic Creme Rub	Trolamine 10%
	Mobisyl Maximal Strength Arthritis Pain Relief Cream	Trolamine 10%
	Sportscreme Deep Penetrating Pain Relieving Rub	Trolamine 10%
Combination preparations	Tiger Muscle Rub ActiveOn Topical Analgesic Ultra Strength Arthritis Salonpas Pain Relieving Patch Icy Hot Extra Strength Pain Relieving Chill Stick Icy Hot Extra Strength Relieving Balm Flexall Plus Maximum Strength Pain Relieving Gell Freeze It Advanced Therapy Roll On	Methyl salicylate 15% Menthol 5% Camphor 3% Histamine dihydrochloride 0.025% Menthol 4.127% Camphor 1.12% Menthol 5.7% Methyl salicylate 6.3% Methyl salicylate 30% Menthol 10% Methyl salicylate 29% Menthol 7.6% Camphor 3.1% Methyl salicylate 10% Menthol 16% Camphor 0.2% Menthol 3.5%

Data from Ref. (58).

In 2002, 446 athletes, supported by the U.S. National Olympic Committee, completed the survey and were matched to 1503 controls obtained from a population-based study done by the National Public Health Institute (63). Among athletes, within the previous 7 days 34.5% were using a prescription medication compared with approximately 25% of the controls (63).

NSAIDs were among the most frequently prescribed medications (8.1%) in athletes, with an AOR of 3.63 (95% CI: 2.25–5.84) for use within the past 7 days (63). Adverse events were reported in 20% of NSAID users (63).

Conclusion

The idea of ''no pain, no gain'' is a common misperception that should be dispelled. Muscle soreness can be expected with strenuous activity or due to an unaccustomed activity, but significant pain is the body's response that rest should occur to allow for healing (6). Too often, athletes do not take the time off from training or competition to allow for adequate healing (64). By using analgesics, in particular NSAIDs, pain may subside but further damage can result from continued exercise. Also, NSAIDs, via their inhibition of prostaglandins, may impede the healing process and muscle regeneration after an acute injury. While these agents are relatively safe they are not without side effects, and caution is warranted. There is only limited evidence (albeit conflicting) in DOMS that NSAIDs can provide a benefit as prophylactic therapy.

Overall, analgesic agents (including NSAIDs, acetaminophen, and topical OTC agents) can effectively relieve pain associated with acute or chronic musculoskeletal injury. Data regarding the ability of NSAIDs to improve muscle recovery and allow a faster return to activity remains controversial.

This area of focus has not been adequately studied with acetaminophen and topical OTC analgesics. When considering an analgesic for alleviating pain, the lowest dose for the shortest time interval should be used. Risk for side effects should be considered and compared with the benefits of the medication. Long-term use for symptoms of sport-related injuries should be avoided, especially with NSAIDs, due to their side effect profile and concern for their impeding the healing process. Data do not adequately support the use of prophylactic NSAIDs prior to sporting events, and should be avoided.

ACKNOWLEDGMENTS

Adapted with permission from: Feucht CL, Patel DR. Analgesics and anti-inflammatory medications in sports: use and abuse. Pediatr Clin North Am 2010;57;(3):751-774. The authors thank Kim Douglas and Amy Esman, Kalamazoo Center for Medical Studies, for assistance in the preparation of this article.

This paper is an adapted version of a chapter in the book "Adolescent medicine: Pharmacotherapeutics in medical disorders" edited by Donald E Greydanus, Dilip R Patel, Cynthia Feucht, Hatim A Omar, Joav Merrick and published with permission by Walter de Gruyter, Berlin and New York.

REFERENCES

[1] Almekinders L. Anti-inflammatory treatment of muscular injuries in sport, an update of recent studies. Sports Med 1999;28(6):383-8.

[2] Garrett WE. Muscle strain injuries: clinical and basic aspects. Med Sci Sports Exerc 1990;22:436-43.

[3] Mehallo C, Drezner J, Bytomski J. Practical management: nonsteroidal anti-inflammatory drug (NSAID) use in athletic injuries. Clin J Sport Med 2006;16:170-4.

[4] Micheli L. Common painful sports injuries: assessment and treatment. Clin J Pain 1989;5(Suppl 2):S51-60.

[5] Howatson G, van Someren K. The prevention and treatment of exercise-induced muscle damage. Sports Med 2008;38(6):483-503.

[6] Smith B, Collina S. Pain medications in the locker room: to dispense or not. Curr Sports Med Rep 2007;6:367-70.

[7] Almekinders LC, Gilbert JA. Healing of experimental muscle strains and the effects of non-steroidal anti-inflammatory medication. Am J Sports Med 1986;14:303-8.

[8] Crisco JJ, Jokl P, Heinen GT, et al. A muscle contusion injury model: biomechanics, physiology and histology. Am J Sports Med 1994;22:702-10.
[9] Tidball JG. Inflammatory cell response to acute muscle injury. Med Sci Sports Exerc 1995;27:1022-32.
[10] Kuipers H. Exercise-induced muscle damage. Int J Sports Med 1994;15:132-5.
[11] Jarvinen TA, Jarvinen TL, Kaariainen M, et al. Muscle injuries biology and treatment. Am J Sports Med 2005;33:745-64.
[12] Maroon J, Bost J, Borden M, et al. Natural anti-inflammatory agents for pain relief in athletes. Neurosurg Focus 2006;21(4):E11.
[13] Herndon C, Hutchinson R, Berdine H, et al. Management of chronic nonmalignant pain with nonsteroidal anti-inflammatory drugs. Pharmacotherapy 2008;28(6):788-805.
[14] Burke A, Smyth E, FitzGerald G. Analgesic-antipyretic and anti-inflammatory agents; pharmacotherapy of gout. In: Brunton L, Lazo J, Parker K, editors. Goodman and Gilman's, the pharmacological basis of therapeutics. 11th edition. New York: McGraw-Hill; 2006. p. 671-715.
[15] Vane J, Botting R. Mechanism of action of nonsteroidal anti-inflammatory drugs. Am J Med 1998;104(3A):2S-8S.
[16] Furst DE, Ulrich RW, Varkey-Altamirano C. Nonsteroidal anti-inflammatory drugs, disease-modifying antirheumatic drugs, nonopioid analgesics, drugs used in gout. In: Bertram GK, Susan BM, Anthony JT, eds. Katzung's basic and clinical pharmacology, 11th ed. New York: McGraw-Hill, 2009:621-42.
[17] Smyth EM, FitzGerald GA. The eicosanoids: prostaglandins, thromboxanes, leukotrienes, related compounds. In: Bertram GK, Susan BM, Anthony JT, eds. Katzung's basic and clinical pharmacology, 11th ed. New York: McGraw-Hill, 2009:313-30.
[18] Vane J, Botting R. The mechanism of action of aspirin. Thromb Res 2003;110:255-8.
[19] Lexi-Comp, Inc (Lexi-Drugs®). Lexi-Comp. Accessed 2011 Jun 21.
[20] Natural medicines comprehensive database [database on the Internet]. Stockton (CA): Therapeutic Research Faculty; c1995–2009. Antiplatelet. Accessed 2011 Jun 21. URL: http://www.naturaldatabase.com/(S(wqklte55rbhkbvzskfpaim45))/nd/Search.aspx?cs5MHSLA%7ECP ands5NDandpt59andProduct5antiplatelet
[21] Kirchain W, Allen R. Drug-induced liver disease. In: DiPiro JT, Talbert RL, Yee GC, Matzke GR, Wells BG, Posey LM, eds. Pharmacotherapy: A pathophysiologic approach, 7th ed. New York: McGraw-Hill, 2008:652.
[22] Scheiman JM, Fendrick AM. Practical approaches to minimizing gastrointestinal and cardiovascular safety concerns with COX-2 inhibitors and NSAIDs. Arthritis Res Ther 2005;7(Suppl 4):S23-9.
[23] Golstein JL, Eisen GM, Burke TA, et al. Dyspepsia tolerability from the patients' perspective: a comparison of celecoxib with diclofenac. Aliment Pharmacol Ther 2002;16(4):819-27.
[24] Goldstein JL, Eisen GM, Burke TA, Peña BM, Lefkowith J, Geis GS. Comparison of upper gastrointestinal toxicity of rofecoxib and naproxen in patients with rheumatoid arthritis. N Engl J Med 2000;343:1520-8.
[25] Laine L. Nonsteroidal anti-inflammatory drug gastropathy. Gastrointest Endosc Clin North Am 1996;6:489-504.
[26] Gabriel SE, Jaakkimainen L, Bombardier C. Risk for serious gastrointestinal complications related to use of nonsteroidal anti-inflammatory drugs: a meta-analysis. Ann Intern Med 1991;115:787-96.
[27] Ekström P, Carling L, Wetterhus S, Wingren PE, Anker-Hansen O, Lundegårdh G, et al. Prevention of peptic ulcer and dyspeptic symptoms with omeprazole in patients receiving continuous nonsteroidal anti-inflammatory drug therapy: a Nordic multicentre study. Scand J Gastroenterol 1996;31(8):753-8.
[28] Hippisley-Cox J, Coupland C, Logan R. Risk of adverse gastrointestinal outcomes in patients taking cyclo-oxygenase-2 inhibitors or conventional non-steroidal anti-inflammatory drugs: population based nested case-control analysis. BMJ 2005;331:1310-6.
[29] Bennett W, Turmelle Y, Shepherd R. Ibuprofen-induced liver injury in an adolescent athlete. Clin Pediatr 2009;48(1):84-6.
[30] Rubenstein JH, Laine L. Systematic review: the hepatotoxicity of non-steroidal anti-inflammatory drugs. Aliment Pharmacol Ther 2004;20:373-80.

[31] Rostom A, Goldkind L, Laine L. Nonsteroidal anti-inflammatory drugs and hepatic toxicity: a systematic review of randomized controlled trials in arthritis patients. Clin Gastroenterol Hepatol 2005;3:489-98.

[32] Whelton A. Nephrotoxicity of nonsteroidal anti-inflammatory drugs: physiologic foundations and clinical implications. Am J Med 1999;106(Suppl 5B):S13-24.

[33] Clive DM, Stoff JS. Renal syndromes associated with nonsteroidal anti-inflammatory drugs. N Engl J Med 1984;310:563-72.

[34] Henrich WL. Nephrotoxicity of nonsteroidal anti-inflammatory agents. Am J Kidney Dis 1983;2:478-84.

[35] Nakahura T, Griswold W, Lemire J, Mendoza S, Reznik V. Nonsteroidal anti-inflammatory drug use in adolescents. J Adolesc Health 1998;23(5):307-10.

[36] Solomon SD, McMurray JJ, Pfeffer MA, Wittes J, Fowler R, Finn P, et al. Cardiovascular risk associated with celecoxib in a clinical trial for colorectal adenoma prevention. N Engl J Med 2005;352(11):1071-80.

[37] Bresalier RS, Sandler RS, Quan H, Bolognese JA, Oxenius B, Horgan K, et al. Cardiovascular events associated with rofecoxib in a colorectal adenoma chemoprevention trial. N Engl J Med 2005;352(11):1092-102.

[38] McGettigan P, Henry D. Cardiovascular risk and inhibition of cyclooxygenase, a systematic review of the observational studies of selective and nonselective inhibitors of cyclooxygenase 2. JAMA 2006;296:1633-44.

[39] COX-2 selective (includes Bextra, Celebrex, and Vioxx) and non-selective non-steroidal anti-inflammatory drugs (NSAIDs). U.S. Food and Drug Administration, Drug Safety and Availability. Accessed 2011 Jun 21. URL: http://www.fda.gov/Drugs/DrugSafety/PostmarketDrugSafety InformationforPatientsandProviders/ucm103420.htm

[40] Drug Facts and Comparisons [database on the Internet]. Facts and comparisons. Indianapolis (IN). 4.0; 2009. Nonsteroidal anti-inflammatory agents; [about 21 pages]. Accessed 2011 Jun 21. URL: http://0-online.factsandcomparisons.com.libcat.ferris.edu/ MonoDispaspx?id5570727andbook5DFC.

[41] Lanier A. Use of nonsteroidal anti-inflammatory drugs following exercise-induced muscle injury. Sports Med 2003;3:177-86.

[42] Moore RA, Tramèr MR, Carroll D, Wiffen PJ, McQuay HJ. Quantitative systematic review of topically applied non-steroidal anti-inflammatory drugs. BMJ 1998;316(7128):333-8.

[43] Peterson B, Rovati S. Diclofenac epolamine (Flector®) patch, evidence for topical activity. Clin Drug Investig 2009;29(1):1-9.

[44] Zacher J, Altman R, Bellamy N, Brühlmann P, Da Silva J, Huskisson E, et al. Topical diclofenac and its role in pain and inflammation: an evidence-based review. Curr Med Res Opin 2008;24(4):925-50.

[45] Drug Facts and Comparisons [database on the Internet]. Facts and comparisons. Indianapolis (IN). 4.0; 2009. Acetaminophen; [about 5 pages]. Accessed 2011 Jun 11. URL:: http:// 0-online.factsandcomparisons.com.libcat.ferris.edu/MonoDisp.aspx?monoID5fandc-hcp10022andquick 5acetaminophenandsearch5acetaminophenanddisease5

[46] Dalton J, Schweinle J. Randomized controlled noninferiority trial to compare extended release acetaminophen and ibuprofen for the treatment of ankle sprains. Ann Emerg Med 2006;48:615-23.

[47] Woo WW, Man SY, Lam PK, Rainer TH. Randomized double-blind trial comparing oral paracetamol and oral nonsteroidal anti-inflammatory drugs for treating pain after musculoskeletal injury. Ann Emerg Med 2005;46(4):352-61.

[48] Wright E. Musculoskeletal injuries and disorders. In: Berardi R, Ferreri S, Hume A, Kroon LA, Newton GD, Popovich NG, et al., eds. Handbook of nonprescription drugs, an interactive approach to self-care, 16th ed. Washington, DC: American Pharmacists Association, 2009:95-113.

[49] Heng MC. Local necrosis and interstitial nephritis due to topical methyl salicylate and menthol. Cutis 1987;39(5):442-4.

[50] Yip A, Chow W, Tai Y, Cheung KL. Adverse effect of local methylsalicylate ointment on warfarin anticoagulation: an unrecognized potential hazard. Postgrad Med J 1990;66(775):367-9.

[51] Joss J, LeBlond R. Potentiation of warfarin anticoagulation associated with topical methyl salicylate. Ann Pharmacother 2000;34(6):729-33.

[52] Love J, Sammon M, Smereck J. Are one or two dangerous? Camphor exposure in toddlers. J Emerg Med 2004;27(1):49-54.

[53] Gouin S, Patel H. Unusual cause of seizure. Pediatr Emerg Care 1996;12(4):298-300.

[54] Patel T, Ishiuji Y, Yosipovitch G. Menthol: A refreshing look at this ancient compound. J Am Acad Dermatol 2007;57:873-8.

[55] Vyklický L, Nováková-Tousová K, Benedikt J, Samad A, Touska F, Vlachová V. Calcium-dependent desensitization of vanilloid receptor TRPV1: a mechanism possibly involved in analgesia induced by topical application of capsaicin. Physiol Res 2008;57(Suppl 3):S59-68.

[56] Knotkova H, Pappagallo M, Szallasi A. Capsaicin (TRPV1 agonist) therapy for pain relief farewell or revival? Clin J Pain 2008;24:142-54.

[57] Mason L, Moore A, Derry S, Edwards JE, McQuay HJ. Systematic review of topical capsaicin for the treatment of chronic pain. BMJ 2004;328(7446):991.

[58] Drugstore. Topical analgesics. Accessed 2013 Jan 23.. URL:http://www.drugstore.com/medicine-and-health/sore-muscle-relief/qxg183118-7bf3f43

[59] Chambers C, Reid G, McGrath P, Finley GA. Self-administration of over-the-counter medication for pain among adolescents. Arch Pediatr Adolesc Med 1997;151(5):449-55.

[60] Van den Bulck J, Leemans L, Laekeman G. Television and adolescent use of over-the-counter analgesic agents. Ann Pharmacother 2005;39:58-62.

[61] Huott M, Storrow A. A survey of adolescents' knowledge regarding toxicity of over-the-counter medications. Acad Emerg Med 1997;4:214-8.

[62] Warner D, Schnepf G, Barrett M, Dian D, Swigonski NL. Prevalence, attitudes, and behaviors related to the use of nonsteroidal anti-inflammatory drugs (NSAIDs) in student athletes. J Adolesc Health 2002;30(3):150-3.

[63] Alaranta A, Alaranta H, Heliövaara M, Airaksinen M, Helenius I. Ample use of physician-prescribed medications in Finnish elite athletes. Int J Sports Med 2006;27(11):919-25.

[64] Alaranta A, Alaranta H, Helenius I. Use of prescription drugs in athletes. Sports Med 2008;38(6):449-63.

In: Child and Adolescent Health Yearbook 2013
Editor: Joav Merrick

ISBN: 978-1-63117-658-6

Chapter 4

ADOLESCENCE AND RHEUMATOID DISORDERS

Donald E Greydanus*, MD, Dr HC (ATHENS), Mary D Moore, MD and Cynthia L Feucht, D Pharm, BCPS

Department of Pediatric & Adolescent Medicine,
Western Michigan University School of Medicine, Kalamazoo, Michigan,
Department of Pharmacy Practice, Ferris State University,
Kalamazoo and Borgess Ambulatory Care, Kalamazoo, United States of America

ABSTRACT

Rheumatoid diseases (RDs) are both common and rare conditions of adolescents that present with a wide variety of features due to inflammation in joints, muscles, and other tissues. The hallmark of the rheumatic disorders is the presence of a chronic inflammatory process that if left uncontrolled, often leads to significant morbidity and even mortality. The most common of these autoimmune diseases are juvenile idiopathic arthritis (JIA) and systemic lupus erythematosus (SLE). JIA, SLE, and other related rheumatoid conditions are considered in this review. Medications for RDs can have significant adverse effects. Management of these conditions is complex, must be individualized, and coordinated with appropriate subspecialists.

Keywords: Adolescence, rheumatoid disorders

INTRODUCTION

Rheumatic diseases (RDs) are conditions with inflammation and pain in connective tissues and supporting body structures: joints, ligaments, tendons, and muscles (1-7). The primary presentations involve joint pain, swelling, and stiffness (especially morning type) with resultant and variable disability complicated by underlying autoimmune dysfunction. RDs are

* Correspondence: Professor Donald E Greydanus, MD, Chair, Department of Pediatric & Adolescent Medicine, Western Michigan University School of Medicine, 1000 Oakland Drive, Kalamazoo, MI 49008-1284 United States. E-mail: donald.greydanus@med.wmich.edu

also complicated by the involvement of other organs in the body. More than 100 RDs have been identified that involved nearly 50 million people in the United States (see table 1). RDs are a more common cause of limitation of activity than diabetes mellitus, cancer, and heart disease. Most RDs are more common in females, though some (such as gout) are seen more commonly in males. The most common rheumatic disorders are juvenile idiopathic arthritis and the spondyloarthropathies that are seen in 0.5 to 2.0 per 1,000 children and adolescents.

Table 1. Rheumatic and related disorders

Juvenile Idiopathic Arthritis (JIA); Juvenile Rheumatoid Arthritis (JRA)
Rheumatic Fever
Spondyloarthropathies
Enthesitis-related arthritis
Ankylosing spondylitis
Reiter syndrome (Reactive arthritis)
Psoriatic arthritis
Arthritides of inflammatory bowel disease
Unclassified (undifferentiated) types
Systemic Lupus Erythematosus
Scleroderma (systemic or localized forms)
Dermatomyositis
Heredity syndromes with musculoskeletal manifestations
Benign joint hypermobility syndrome (BJHS)
Ehlers-Danlos Syndrome
Marfan Syndrome
Marfanoid hypermobility syndrome
Multiple epiphyseal dysplasias
Osteogenesis imperfecta
Williams syndrome
Inborn errors of metabolism (homocystinuria, hyperlysinemia)
Vasculitis
Churg-Strauss disease
Henoch-Schönlein purpura (HSP)
Hypersensitivity (Leukocytoclastic) Vasculitis
Kawasaki disease
Polyarteritis Nodosa
Sjögren’s syndrome
Takayasu's Arteritis
Wegener's Granulomatosis
Infectious Joint Disease
Bacterial arthritis/osteomyelitis
Viral arthropathy
STD arthritis
Lyme Disease
Pain amplification syndromes
Complex regional pain syndrome
Joint Hypermobility syndrome
Reflex sympathetic dystrophy (RSD)
Fibromyalgia

Sarcoidosis
Miscellaneous Arthropathies
Traumatic arthritis
Congential hip dislocation
Legg-Calvé-Perthes disease
Osgood Schlatter Disease
Patellofemoral syndromes
Slipped femoral epiphyhsis
Any poorly healed fracture or inadequately treated infection
Systemic disorders often complicated by arthritis
Hemophilia
Secondary Gout and pseudogout
Serum sickness
Sickle cell disease
Neoplastic disease
Hypertrophic osteoarthropathy
Miscellaneous/Rare
Mixed Connective Tissue Disease
Weber-Christian Disease
Jaccoud's Arthritis
Behçet's syndrome
Relapsing polychronritis
OTHERS

*Modified with permission from: Greydanus DE: Rheumatoid disorders and other. Miscellaneous disorders. In: Hofmann AD, Greydanus DE: (eds): Adolescent Medicine, 3rd Ed. Stamford, CT: Appleton & Lange, Ch 20:433, 1997.

SYMPTOMATOLOGY

Rheumatoid diseases can present with a myriad of signs and symptoms in addition to those involving the joints and muscles. Any body system can be involved and there can be dermatological conditions (rashes, skin or mucosal ulcers, alopecia), pain (joints, muscles, chest, abdomen, headaches, generalized), eye involvement (conjunctivitis, iritis), gastrointestinal (anorexia, dysphagia, weight loss), pulmonary (shortness of breath, hemoptysis), vasomotor instability, fatigue, fever, and others.

A careful medical history seeks to identify the cause of the pain, such as bony pain or neuropathic pain. Stiffness after rest (night sleep, long naps, long car rides, others) is a classic feature of RD inflammation and may be due to reduced hyaluronic acid in inflamed synovial fluid. RDs can change over time and thus meticulous, regular re-evaluations over time is important.

A variety of conditions must be considered if the youth presents with musculoskeletal complaints, including RDs, vasculitides, connective tissue infections, bone cancer (Ewings sarcoma, osteogenic sarcoma—see chapter 25), psychosomatic and/or chronic pain syndromes, peripheral neuropathies, primary muscle disorders, overuse injuries, and others. Table 2 lists conditions to consider in youth who present with monoarthritis (acute versus chronic) and polyarthritis.

Table 2. Conditions presenting as Arthritis*

Acute Monoarthritis
Enthesitis-related arthritis
Hemophilia
Leukemia
Neuroblastoma
Oligoarthritis
Psoriatic arthritis
Reactive arthritis
Septic arthritis
Trauma
Chronic Monoarthritis
Enthesitis-related arthritis
Episodic fever syndromes
Hemophilia
Hemangioma
Juvenile Idiopathic Arthritis (JIA)
Juvenile psoriatic arthritis
Lyme arthritis
Oligoarthritis
Sarcoidosis
Synovial chondromatosis
Tuberculosis
Villonodular synovitis
Polyarthritis
Spondyloarthropathies
Enthesitis-related arthritis
Arthritis with Inflammatory bowel disease
Juvenile idiopathic polyarthritis
Lyme disease (usually monoarticular)
Malignancies
Periodic Fever Syndromes
Polyarthritis related to infection
Psoriatic juvenile idiopathic arthritis
Reactive arthritis
Rheumatic fever (migratory joint involvement)
Sarcoidosis
Serum Sickness, Systemic juvenile idiopathic arthritis, SLE, Vasculitis, Viral arthritis

* Modified with permission from: Patel DR, Moore MD: Concepts of Rheumatology In: Handbook of Clinical Pediatrics: An Update for the Ambulatory Pediatrician. Eds: DE Greydanus, DR Patel, VN Reddy, AN Feinberg, HA Omar. New Jersey; World Scientific, Ch 25: page 702, 2010.

RD studies

A variety of laboratory and imaging studies are important depending on the specific conditions being evaluated (8). There are signs of inflammation, such as an elevated erythrocyte sedimentation rate (ESR) or C-reactive protein (CRP). The finding of autoantibodies in rheumatoid diseases can be very helpful in specific conditions and must be interpreted carefully. These include rheumatoid factor (RF), various antinuclear antibodies (ANA), cyclic citrullinated peptide (CCP), and antineutrophil cytoplasmic antibody (ANCA).

For example, RF is commonly found in rheumatoid arthritis (RF-positive polyarticular juvenile idiopathic arthritis), Sjögren syndrome, and hepatitis C-induced cryoglobulinemia. RF may occasionally be found in other conditions such as dermatomyositis, SLE, scleroderma, mixed connective tissue disease, and chronic bacterial infections. CCP is found in RF positive polyarticular JIA.

Other tests include joint fluid examination, HLA (Human Leukocyte Antigen) typing, complement analysis, and measurement of cryoglobulins. Imaging involves judicious use of CT and MRI which have higher diagnostic yield than plain radiography and ultrasound. Consultation with rheumatology specialists is needed to successfully navigate the complex world of RDs and RD laboratory interpretation.

Juvenile idiopathic arthritis (JIA)

Different terms have been used over the past decades to refer to a heterogenous group of chronic inflammatory arthritides in childhood. These terms include including JRA (juvenile rheumatoid arthritis), JCA (juvenile chronic arthritis), JA (juvenile arthritis), and in this text, JIA--based on the ILAR system of classification (7). JIA involves the development of arthritis in which there is persistent (over 6 weeks) joint swelling and/or painful joint movement restriction versus arthralgia in which there is joint pain with or without inflammation. The tem, juvenile, refers to the onset of the condition before 16 years of age.

Three historic subtypes of JIA are recognized: Pauciarticular, Polyarticular (RF positive and RF negative), and systemic-onset (Stills Disease). The ILAR classification for JIA also includes psoriatic arthritis, enthesitis related arthritis, and undifferentiated arthritis. The work-up must exclude other causes of arthritis (table 2) including septic arthritis, reactive arthritis, post infectious arthritis, Lyme arthritis, and other rheumatoid disorders.

JIA typically presents with stiffness after a prolonged rest (i.e., morning stiffness) with mild aching and variable joint swelling (9,10). Fortunately, severe pain is not the norm. Those with pauciarticular JIA are at increased risk for the development of uveitis (iritis) that is usually insidious and typically found only on eye screening; some may present with more overt eye symptoms, such as eye pain, redness, photophobia, and/or vision changes. Patients with polyarthritis are at less risk for chronic uveitis.

In pauciarticular JIA (oligoarthritis) there is a limp with non-painful swelling of four or less joints within 6 months of disease onset and the onset is typically under 8 years of age. In polyarticular JIA the joint swelling involves five or more joints within 6 months of disease onset; the age of onset is bimodal—age 1 to 6 years of age and 11 to 16 years of age. In the polyarthritis JIA, there are two types: RF negative and RF positive (i.e., 2 or more positive RF tests during the first 6 months of disease onset at least 3 months apart) (11).

In the systemic-onset JIA there is arthritis in one or more joints with variable age onset that occurs with or is preceded by fever with high spikes of 2 weeks or more duration that is daily (quotidian) for 3 days or more. In addition there is one or more of these features: recurrent rash (evanescent, erythematous), hepatosplenomegaly (one or both), generalized lymphadenopathy, and serositis (pericarditis and/or pleuritis and/or peritonitis).

Laboratory tests in JIA are either normal or only mildly elevated, the RF is negative in over 90% of JIA patients, and there is a low ANA titer in 70 to 90%. There is no test or combination of laboratory tests to conclusively pinpoint JIA from other disorders. Laboratory testing is used to exclude other conditions such as septic arthritis or malignancy. Joint aspiration (Table 3) is useful in this differential process and includes a gram stain, culture, cell count, fluid glucose, and other tests in selective situations (i.e., fungal or acid-fast bacillus evaluation, cytology, crystal examination).

Table 3. Synovial fluid analysis

Normal	White Blood Count (WBC) 200 -500	Synovial Glucose 2/3 of serum	Sterile fluid
Inflammatory	WBC: 10,000 to 50,000	Synovial Glucose is variable; can be very low	Sterile fluid
Septic	>50,000	Synovial Glucose is very low	Positive culture from synovial fluid, blood, other
Hemorrhagic	WBC: 200-500	Synovial glucose is normal	Sterile fluid

Differential diagnosis

A wide variety of disorders must be considered in the differential of common rheumatic conditions that can manifest as musculoskeletal pain. For example, benign hypermobility syndrome presents as intermittent pains at night more commonly in females with an age of onset of 3 to 10 years and often with a positive family history. There may be hyperextended metacarpophalangeal joints, elbows or knees. The clinician should rule out Ehlers-Danlos syndrome and Marfan syndrome. Benign nocturnal limb pains of childhood (growing pains of childhood) presents as cramping, lower-leg pain in evenings or at night with an age of onset between 3 and 10 years; the examination and laboratory tests are normal. Systemic lupus erythematosus (SLE) is discussed in the next section.

Acute rheumatic fever (ARF) or streptococcal infection-related arthritis presents as migratory arthritis 2 to 3 weeks after streptococcal pharyngitis usually during the school age years with a distribution related to streptococcal infection risk. A persistent arthritis may indicate streptococcal infection-related arthritis or post-streptococcal reactive arthritis (PSRA). Also, the streptococcus can directly invade the joint causing a bacterial arthritis distinct from the type of arthritis seen in ARF and PSRA. The characteristic rash is called erythema marginatum and carditis is a serious complication; additional features of the revised Jones criteria for ARF include subcutaneous nodules and chorea. There is evidence for an antecedent streptococal infection. Treatment of streptococcal pharyngitis is reviewed in table 2 of chapter 17.

Malignancy includes osteosarcoma, leukemia, lymphoma, Ewing's tumor, rhabdomyosarcoma, and others (see chapter 25). The presentation includes painful joints, bone pain, and variable constitutional symptoms. The youth may be ill appearing with joint swelling, malignant effusions, abnormal CBCs, elevated ESR, and abnormalities noted by radiographs and imaging studies. Henoch-Schönlein purpura (HSP) is the second most common vasculitis in children and adolescents that presents with a purpuric rash and abdominal pain often triggered by an upper respiratory tract infection in school age children with a median age of 4 years (2-11 years of age).

There is non-specific swelling of joints and hematuria as well as proteinuria develop; in addition, hypertension may occur. Management is supportive (i.e., hydration, nutrition, pain relief). Corticosteroids are used if necessary and severe disease may require the use of various other rheumatic disease medications as reviewed later. Long-term outcome is dependent on the underlying renal involvement and approximately 8% develop end-stage renal disease (ESRD).

Spondyloarthropathies include arthritis with enthesitis, ankylosing spondylitis, reactive arthritis (Reiter syndrome), psoriatic arthritis, and arthritides of inflammatory bowel disease. Arthritis with enthesitis presents with ankle pain, heel pain, Achilles apophysitis, and back (lumbosacral) or hip stiffness. The pain is usually worse at the day's end and there is often a positive family history for spondyloarthropathy. There is inflammation and tenderness at sites of tendon insertion and it is often diagnosed as overuse syndrome for many years before this diagnosis is made. Acute, symptomatic uveitis may develop and the HLA-B27 antigen is often positive.

Ankylosing spondylitis (AS) presents with insidious, chronic low (lumbar) back pain and stiffness in males usually 13 years of age and older. Painful iritis is common. There can be enthesitis and peripheral arthritis. Classic radiographic AS spinal changes may not be evident for years. One should observe for vertebral compression fractures. Laboratory data shows a positive HLA-B27 antigen, negative ANA, and the platelet count as well as ESR are elevated.

Reiter syndrome (reactive arthritis) presents with painful joints with swelling following a genitourinary or gastrointestinal infection in a teenager 13 and older. The classic triad is arthritis, urethritis, and uveitis (conjunctivitis); most present only with arthritis that is usually acute, asymmetric, and lower-limb. Evidence of ankylosing spondylitis occurs in 10% and there can be mouth ulcers as well. The HLA-B27 is typically positive while the ANA is usually negative.

Psoriatic arthritis presents with a psoriatic rash that may occur after the arthritis (mono- or polyarthitis) develops. The arthropathy can take a variety of forms and it is more common in males.. There may also be dactylitis, nail pitting or onycholysis, and a positive family history for psoriasis in a first-degree relative. The HLA-B27 is often positive. See chapter 20 for a discussion of psoriasis and its management.

Arthritides of inflammatory bowel disease (IBD) involve large-joint polyarthritis with chronic or recurrent abdominal pain, weight loss or lack of normal weight gain, malaise, positive HLA-B27, and negative ANA. It occurs in about one-third with IBD and tends to resolve with control of the IBD (see chapter 23). There can be spinal disease, ankylosing spondylitis, mouth ulcers, skin lesions (pyoderma gangrenosa, erythema nodosum), and uveitis.

JIA complications

The natural history of children and adolescents with JIA is quite varied and fortunately, most do well with early diagnosis and appropriate management by experts in rheumatoid diseases. Some, however, have chronic and recalcitrant disease. There can be joint destruction, growth

inhibition with resultant short stature, contractures, bony overgrowth, and cervical spine involvement with spinal cord compression that includes the cervical spine.
Eye involvement is noted in up to half with oligoarticular JIA, 10% in polyarticular disease, and is rare in systemic-onset JIA. The most common eye condition is uveitis (also referred to as iritis or iridocyclitis) that is often painless and progressive. It can lead to many eye complications including secondary glaucoma, cataracts, band keratopathy, posterior synechiae with papillary complications, vision loss, and blindness. The severity of the arthropathy does not correlate with the risk of uveitis. Regular screening visits for eye disease is important for RD patients since the eye damage can be insidious and progressive, especially if undertreated.

Death from JIA arises as a result of complications from pharmacologic management, infections, traumatic C-spine injury, or the rare MAS—macrophage activation syndrome. MAS is a form of hemophagocytic lymphohistiocytosis syndrome that may be precipitated by viral infections or drugs. Those with MAS develop rapid severe illness with fever, adenopathy, organomegaly, petchiae, pancytopenia, bleeding, rapidly lowering ESR, and very high ferritin levels. Supportive care is necessary and there may be improvement with high dose corticosteroids, cyclosporine, and tumor necrosis factor inhibitors (See below). Mortality in MAS can exceed 30%.

JIA management

Each youth with arthritis needs an individual plan managed by a clinician skilled in arthropathy management (4). Conservative measures can be helpful for pain such as use of moist heat, joint support (i.e., casting, splinting, canes, crutches), rest, and appropriate physical activity.

Non-narcotics are also helpful for pain and narcotics used very judiciously for severe pain keeping in mind the problematic potential for addiction (see chapter 9). Attention to co-morbid sleep problems, mood disturbances, and anxiety conditions is very important. Many adolescents with rheumatoid disorders find help on-line via chat rooms (see chapter 2) and other types of support from local RD chapters.

Non-pharmacologic treatments include relaxation therapy, physical therapy, occupational therapy, heat and cold applications, hydrotherapy, transcutaneous electrical nerve stimulation (TENS), and others. Also, corticosteroid intra-articular infections can be very useful in JIA management, especially in children and adolescents with involvement of only a few joints. Surgery may be helpful as well that includes arthroscopic surgery, bone fusion, osteotomy, and arthroplasty.

The use of nutritional supplements remains controversial and unproven. This includes proposed use of glucosamine and chondroitin sulfate, or SAM-e (S-adenosylmethionine) for osteoarthritis, SAM-e for fibromalgia, or DHEA (dehydroepiandrosterone) for SLE. Hyaluronic acid substitutes mimic a natural body substance that lubricates joints and some adults with osteoarthritis receive intra-articular injections in attempts to relieve pain and provide better joint motion. However, hyaluronic acid substitutes are not useful in inflammatory arthritis and are not U.S. FDA-approved in the pediatric population.

RD medication: general considerations

The specific medication used for arthropathy depends on the specific condition and the specific patient (12,13). Drugs used for rheumatoid disorders are generally used to control the pain, reduce inflammation and joint damage and limit RD symptoms as well as functional decline. Medications may slow the disease course and limit or prevent more damage to joints or other body parts. Cure is not possible except in select situations, such as correct use of antibiotics in infectious arthritis or early use of antibiotics in Lyme disease.

Analgesics

Non-steroidal anti-inflammatory drugs (NSAIDs) are the most commonly used medications for management of inflammatory arthropathy, non-inflammatory musculoskeletal disorders, and many other conditions. They have become very popular analgesics since their introduction in the 1960s (See the Preface). These medications with dosages are listed in Table 4 and potential side effects are noted in Table 5. These drugs do not affect the long-term outcome but can control pain, stiffness, swelling, and fever. Table 6 lists components of common topical analgesics (chapter 30).

Table 4. Systemic analgesics and anti-inflammatory drugs (see chapter 30, Tables 1-4)

Generic Name	Adult Dosage	Pediatric Dosage
Diclofenac sodium	100-200mg daily (2-4 divided doses) *ER given 1-2x daily*	2-3 mg/kg/day (2-4 divided doses)
Diclofenac potassium	100-200mg daily (2-4 divided doses)	2-3 mg/kg/day (2-4 divided doses)
Diclofenac epolamine	180mg patch every 12 hr	N/A
Etodolac	600-1000mg daily (2-3 divided doses)	20-30kg: 400mg daily 31-45kg: 600mg daily 46-60kg: 800mg daily >60kg: 1000mg daily *Age 6-16 yrs* *Based on ER product*
Fenoprofen calcium	200-600mg 3-4 x/day Max 3200mg/day	N/A
Flurbiprofen	200-300mg daily (2-4 divided doses)	N/A
Ibuprofen	1200-3200mg daily (3-4 divided doses)	4-10 mg/kg/dose 3-4x/day Max 40mg/kg/day
Indomethacin	50-200mg daily (2-3 divided doses)	1-2 mg/kg/day (2-4 divided doses) Max 4mg/kg/day, NTE: 150-200mg/day *Age >2 yrs*
Ketoprofen	IR: 150-300mg daily (3-4 divided doses) ER: 100-200mg daily	N/A

Table 4. (Continued)

Generic Name	Adult Dosage	Pediatric Dosage
Ketorolac tromethamine	20mg initially, 10mg 4x/day Max 5 day duration	N/A
Meclofenamate sodium	200-400mg daily (3-4 divided doses)	N/A
Mefenamic acid	500mg initially, 250mg every 6hr as needed (NTE: 1 week)	N/A
Meloxicam	7.5-15mg daily	0.125 mg/kg/day Max 7.5mg daily *Age ≥2 yrs*
Nabumetone	500-2000mg daily (1-2 divided doses)	N/A
Naproxen	Naproxen: 250-500mg 2x/day Naproxen sodium: 200-500mg 2x/day Naproxen DR: 375-500mg 2x/day	*Analgesia: 5-7 mg/kg/dose every 8-12 hrs *Inflammatory disease: 10-15mg/kg/day (2 divided doses) Max 1000mg/day *Age >2 yrs*
Oxaprozin	600-1200mg daily Max 1800mg daily (in divided doses)	22-31kg: 600mg daily 32-54kg: 900mg daily ≥55kg: 1200mg daily *Age 6-16 yrs*
Piroxicam	10-20mg daily	0.2-0.3 mg/kg/day Max 15mg daily
Sulindac	150-200mg 2x/day	2-4 mg/kg/day (2 divided doses) Max 6mg/kg/day, NTE: 400mg/day
Tolmetin sodium	600-1800mg daily (3 divided doses) Max 2000mg daily	*Analagesia: 5-7 mg/kg/dose every 6-8 hrs *Inflammatory disease: 15-30mg/kg/day (3-4 divided doses) NTE: 1800mg/day *Age ≥2 yrs*
Celecoxib	100-400mg daily (1-2 divided doses)	10-25kg: 50mg 2x/day > 25kg: 100mg 2x/day *Age ≥2 yrs*
Diflunisal	500-1000mg daily (2-3 divided doses) Max 1500mg daily	N/A
Magnesium salicylate	Novosal®: 600mg 3-4x day, Max 4800mg daily Doan's®: 934mg every 6hr as needed	N/A
Salsalate	3000mg daily (2-4 divided doses)	N/A
Choline magnesium trisalicylate	500-1500mg 2-3x/day	30-60mg/kg/day (3-4 divided doses)

IR: immediate-release; ER: extended-release; DR: delayed-release, NTE: not to exceed.

Table 5. (See Text; see chapter 30)

Adverse effects of non-steroidal anti-inflammatory drugs
Acute renal insufficiency
Anaphylaxis
Bone marrow suppression
Bronchospasm
Bruising
Dizziness
Fluid retention or peripheral edema
Gastritis
Gastrointestinal ulceration and bleeding (see text)
Headache
Hepatotoxicity (see text)
Hyperkalemia
Hypersensitivity reactions
Increased risk of cardiovascular thrombotic events, myocardial infarction & stroke
Indigestion, heartburn
Interstitial nephritis
Nausea, vomiting
Peptic ulcer
Photosensitivity
Rash (see text)
Tinnitus

Table 6. Over the counter topical counterirritant analgesic agents (see chapter 30, Table 7)

Active Ingredients Used Alone	Active Ingredients Often Used in Combination	Combination Product Examples
Camphor	Turpentine oil	Camphor 3%, menthol 5% & methyl salicylate 15%
Menthol	Histamine dihydrochloride	Camphor 3.6%, oleoresin capsicum 0.25%, methyl salicylate 18%
Capsaicin	Ammonia water	Camphor 1.2%, menthol 5.7%, methyl salicylate 6.7%
Trolamine salicylate	Allyl isothiocyanate	Menthol 4.127%, histamine dihydrochloride 0.025%
	Methyl salicylate	Menthol 7.6%, methyl salicylate 29%
	Methyl nicotinate	Menthol 10%, methyl salicylate 30%

Despite the convenience of topical agents and minimal systemic absorption, some youth do not like or tolerate the burning sensation or the texture of some topical medications.

Traditional NSAIDs include ibuprofen, naproxen, acetylsalicylic acid, indomethacin, sulinac, tolmetin sodium and others (see chapter 30). They non-selectively inhibit cyclooxygenase 1 and 2 (COX-1 and COX-2) and this contributes to their adverse effects. For example, the COX-1 enzyme is expressed in various organ systems such as renal, gastrointestinal (GI), and hematologic (i.e., platelets) (Table 5). NSAIDs can lead to drowsiness, headache, and dizziness; these effects tend to stop with discontinuing the NSAID.

More recent selective COX-2 inhibitors (i.e., celecoxib, valdecoxib, rofecoxib) produce less GI adverse effects but increase the risk for cardiovascular toxicity. However, valdecoxib and rofecoxib were removed from the market due to the increased risk of cardiovascular adverse effects in adults taking these agents. Celecoxib has been approved by the FDA for use in JIA.

Table 7. Corticosteroid side effects

Acute effects (usually reversible)
Swelling (sodium and fluid retention)
Increased appetite
Weight gain ("moon facies"; Cushinoid appearance)
Emotional lability
Acne (steroid acne)
Sleep disturbances
Severe muscle weakness (rare)
Psychosis (rare)
Effects from chronic use
Striae
Dyslipidemias
Accelerated atherogenesis
Osteoporosis
Osteonecrosis of hips (2% for most; up to 25% in SLE)
Excessive hair growth
Growth failure
Hypertension
Damage to arteries
Hyperglycemia
Cataracts
Pseudotumor cerebri
Infections

Acetylsalicyclic acid (Aspirin) has a historical background as an analgesic but has been replaced by the traditional NSAIDs in JIA management. Concern is raised with the small but well-known risk of Reye syndrome and other aspirin (ASA)-adverse effects (see chapter 30). Salicylates should be avoided in youth who also have active infection with varicella or influenza. Salicylates (particularly ASA) are the only NSAIDs which results in less platelet aggregation with clinical relevance; this effect can last for 4-6 days in as small a dose as 80 mg. Selective COX-2 inhibitors do not reversibly inhibit platelet aggregation. Salicylates have increased frequency of side effects and more toxic result from an overdose compared to other NSAIDs.

The adverse effects of NSAIDs result from a complex mix of various factors including the specific drug, duration of use, dose, degree of COX-1 inhibition, co-morbid disorders, and use of other medications. NSAIDs should be avoided in youth with asthma if they are aspirin sensitive. Use of misoprostol or proton pump inhibitors can decrease the GI toxicity of NSAIDs including those at high risk of GI toxicity (i.e., history of GI disorders, additional use of cortocosteroids).

Dermatologic side effects range from urticaria to Stevens-Johnson syndrome. Chronic use of naproxen can lead to pseudoporphyria, a photosensitive rash especially seen in fair complexion persons; chronic scarring may result. Hepatotoxicity is possible with NSAIDs including increased liver transaminases (3% with chronic use including 5% with salicylates) and rare liver toxicity that can be fatal. Renal toxicity may occur in some that includes hyperkalemia, proteinuria, and even interstitial nephritis. Leukopenia may arise that is typically mild and resolves when the NSAID is discontinued; however, it may be severe and permanent in rare situations. Aseptic meningitis can occur in patients on NSAIDs particularly in those with SLE; reports have included the following NSAIDS: ibuprofen, naproxen, diclofenac, ketoprofen, tolmetin, sulindac and rofecoxib.

NSAIDs approved by the US FDA for use in children include aspirin, ibuprofen, naproxen, oxaprozin, etodolac SR, meloxicam, indomethacin, and celecoxib. Some persons note more benefit from one versus another NSAID and sometimes a trial and error method is needed to find the best one for each person. An NSAID that can be given once or twice a day is best for youth to minimize difficulties in school and improve compliance. Some are available in liquid form (i.e., ibuprofen, naproxen, meloxicam, indomethacin, and various salicylate preparations); also, some are available for parenteral administration (ketorolac and indomethacin)and diclofenac is available in a topical gel and patch formulation. Those on chronic NSAID treatment should receive periodic (i.e., every 3 months) screening for renal, GI, and hematopoietic toxicity. Screen for GI toxicity by evaluating for melena and abdominal pain; add a proton pump inhibitor as previously noted. Serum levels of NSAIDs are not clinically usefully except for monitoring of salicylate levels in those on chronic salicylate management.

Corticosteroids

Corticosteroids are strong anti-inflammatory agents that have been around for many decades (see the Preface). These drugs (i.e., prednisone, cortisone, hydrocortisone, methylprednisolone, others) are commonly used for rheumatoid disorders because they reduce inflammation and powerfully suppress the immune system. They can be given orally, topically, intraarticularly, intramuscularly, or intravenously (4).

They are potent drugs with great benefit but also have the potential for significant adverse effects (Table 7). Because of potentially severe adverse effects, oral or parenteral corticosteroids are often only used for refractory RDs and used for severe JIA complications (such as anemia, pericarditis, others). The lowest effective dose should be used as well as alternate day dosing to reduce adverse effects. Doses vary and oral doses can range from 1-3 mg per kilogram per day.

Side effects include infections that range from typical bacterial microbes to increased risk of Mycobacterium tuberculosis and various opportunistic infections. Youth on chronic corticosteroids should receive appropriate calcium and Vitamin D intake (supplementation) and counseled about the importance of weight bearing exercise. Annual bone density studies should be done and clinicians should consider use of a bisphosphonate to prevent osteoporosis for those receiving chronic steroid therapy.

Intra-articular injections of corticosteroids are beneficial especially in those with minimal joint involvement and may ameliorate the need for regular systemic corticosteroid or chronic NSAID use. The amount of the steroid varies with the joint size and synovitis may be controlled for several months after an injection. Large joints (i.e., sacroiliac or hip) require that the injection be performed under fluoroscopy or with ultrasound guidance. A short-acting sedative may be necessary for youth with severe anxiety about the procedure and general anesthesia is needed if several joints are injected. Sometimes joint injection is difficult due to infection, bony changes, or fibrosis; if severe synovial hypertrophy is present, dispersal of the injection throughout the joint may be compromised. There may also be minor atrophy along the needle tract area due to steroid leakage into adjacent tissue.

Disease-modifying anti-rheumatic drugs (DMARDS)

DMARDs are used to treat rheumatoid arthritis, ankylosing spondylitis, and other inflammatory arthropathies with the attempt to control the inflammatory process. The result may be less swelling, joint destruction and pain for these individuals. DMARDs do not reverse damage that has already occurred. They include methotrexate, hydroxychloroquine, intramuscular gold salts, sulfasalazine, D-penicillamine, and leflunomide (Table 8) (4,6,13-17). Methotrexate is the DMARD most often used by rheumatologists treating these disorders. For example, methotrexate is often begun in youth with polyarthritis, oligoarticular conditions refractory to other measures, and chronic uveitis that is severe and refractory to corticosteroids. Due to excess toxicity, gold salts are rarely used, if at all. Similarly, leflunomide is used infrequently in adolescent females due to its long half life and risk of teratogenesis.

Methotrexate in moderate doses may be combined with hydroxychloroquine, sulfasalazine or biologic response modifiers (see below) to control inflammation and joint destruction more that noted with use of a single agent. Exact combinations of medications and dosages should be determined in each patient by an experienced clinician. As noted with many chronic conditions, there is no "cook book" approach that covers all situations. Leflunomide has similar benefit and toxicity to methotrexate; however, as noted, it has a long half-life and detoxification is required if a patient wishes to become pregnant.

Cytotoxic agents

Cytotoxic drugs are used infrequently for RD individuals with very severe disease that have failed other treatments. They include cyclophosphamide, chlorambucil, and azathioprine. They may part of protocols involving autologous bone marrow transplantation. Other drugs that may be used for such refractive situations include immune modulating agents such as cyclosporine and mycophenolate mofetil. These are less utilized due to the high incidence of adverse effects and availability of alternative agents. Live vaccine administration should be avoided while on these drugs. Cytotoxic agents are briefly reviewed in Table 9 but should only be used by experts experienced in the use of these medications (18).

Biologic response modifiers

Biologics or biologic response modifiers are a group of drugs that are genetically engineered to block identified pathways in the immune system that are involved in the inflammatory process (4,6,19).

Table 8. DMARDs for Rheumatoid Disorders

Generic Name	Adult Dosage	Adverse Effects	Monitoring
Methotrexate	10 to 15 per week; usually given IM or orally Add folic acid 1mg daily	Anorexia, nausea, emesis, abdominal cramps, hepatotoxicity, hepatic fibrosis, bone marrow suppression, allergic pneumonitis, opportunistic infections. Teratogenic; abortifacient; avoid with renal insufficiency (CrCl < 30ml/min); increased toxicity if given with NDSAIDs, trimethoprim, sulfamethoxazole/trimethoprim	LFTs, hepatitis B & C serologies for those with risk factors for infection, CBC with platelets, Scr
Leflunomide	Initial: 100 mg/day for 3 days. Maintenance: 10 to 20 mg per day. Add folic acid 1mg daily.	Diarrhea, nausea, reversible hair loss, rash, bone marrow suppression, hepatoxocity, interstitial lung disease, peripheral neuropathy, anaphylaxis, severe dermatological reactions, weight loss. Teratogenic	LFTs, CBC with platelets Drug elimination procedure: stop leflunomide and administer cholestyramine 8gm 3x/day for 11 days. Verify plasma level is < 0.02 mg/L.
Hydroxy-chloroquine	400 to 600 mg per day; maintenance is 200-400 mg per day; also used as anti-malaria drug	Dermatological reactions including skin & mucosal pigmentation (blue/black), nausea, epigastric pain, retinal damage, blurred vision, keratopathy, central nervous system toxicity, hemolysis with G6PD deficiency	Ophthalmic exams, CBC with platelets, G6PD
Gold Salts Gold sodium thiomalate (Solganol; Myochrysine)	IM: 10 mg as an initial dose, followed by 25 mg on week 2, then 25-50mg weekly until 1 gm total dose achieved. Maintenance: 25-50mg every 2-4 weeks.	Nausea, diarrhea, stomatitis, decreased appetite, exfoliative dermatitis, proteinuria, hepatitis, interstitial pneumonitis, enterocolitis, blood dyscrasias with bone marrow suppression. "Nitroid" reaction: flushing, fainting, sweating and dizziness within 30 minutes of injection	CBC with platelets, urinalysis
Sulfasalazine	500 mg daily increasing to a maximum daily dose of 3,000 mg (in 2 divided doses). Consider adding folic acid 1mg daily. Also used for inflammatory bowel disease	Nausea, anorexia (use enteric coated form to reduce), rash, headache, hepatitis, bone marrow suppression, hemolytic anemia with G6PD deficiency, oligospermia (reversible), aplastic anemia, hypersensitivity reactions, renal toxicity	CBC with platelets, LFTs, urinalysis, G6PD
D-penicillamine	Initial: 125-250mg/day, increase by 125-250mg/day at 1-3 month intervals. Maintenance: 500-750mg/day. Consider addition of pyridoxine 25mg/day. Also used to treat Wilson's disease, cystinuria, arsenic poisoning	Aplastic anemia, lupus-like syndrome, pruritis/rash, proteinuria, membranous glomerunephritis, elastosis performans serpiginosa, myasthenic syndrome, bone marrow suppression, drug fever, mouth ulcers, GI distress, altered taste, neuropathy, intrahepatic cholestasis Contraindicated during pregnancy. Avoid in renal insufficiency. Avoid concomitant use with gold therapy, antimalarial & cytotoxic agents Do not coadminister with antacids, iron or food	CBC with platelets, urinalysis, LFTs

Table 9. Cytotoxic and immune modulating agents for Rheumatoid Disorders

Generic Name	Adult Dosage	Adverse Effects	Monitoring
Cyclo-phosphamide	1-3.5 mg/kg/day Nitrogen mustard alkylating agent. Indications: SLE, JIA, nephrotic syndrome, neoplasms, others Cytotoxic agent	Nausea, emesis, anorexia, lethargy, diarrhea, rash, hair loss, weakness, bone marrow suppression, hemorrhagic cystitis, hematuria, proteinuria, amenorrhea, nail & skin pigmentation, fertility impairment, anaphylaxis. Teratogenic. Dosage adjustment required for hepatic and renal dysfunction. Metabolized by CYP 450 system: potential for drug interactions.	CBC with platelets, urinalysis, Scr, LFTs, bilirubin
Chlorambucil	to 0.2 mg/kg/day (4-10 mg per day on average) Nitrogen mustard alkylating agent. Indication: treatment of various cancers. Cytotoxic agent	Agitation, confusion, peripheral neuropathy, bone marrow suppression, tremor, hypersensitivity reactions, interstitial pnemonitis, hepatotoxicity, fertility impairment, sterility. Low emetogenic potential. Teratogenic. Adjust dosage in renal insufficiency.	CBC with platelets, Scr
Azathioprine	Variable. 1 mg/kg/day orally for 6-8 weeks. May increase by 0.5 mg/kg/day every 4 weeks up to a maximum of 2.5 mg/kg/day. Antagonizes purine metabolism. Indications: RA and organ transplant rejection.	Nausea, emesis, fatigue, hair loss, fever, bone marrow suppression (especially with TPMT deficiency), acute pancreatitis, hepatotoxicity, increased neoplasm risk, increased risk of serious infections, fertility impairment. Teratogenic.	CBC with platelets, LFTs, thiopurine S-methyltransferase (TPMT)
Cyclosporine	Variable; initial: 2.5 mg/kg/day orally divided into 2 doses up to a maximum of 4 mg/kg/day (Neoral & Gengraf only). Inhibits production & release of interleukin 2; immuno-suppressive agent. Indications: psoriasis, prevent organ transplant rejection, RA Not all cyclosporine products are interchangeable.	Acne, nausea, abdominal pain, headache, tremor, dizziness, increased hair growth, nephrotoxicity, hepatotoxicity, hypertension, malignancy, increased risk of serious infections, encephalopathy. Avoid use in patients with renal impairment, uncontrolled hypertension & malignancy. Avoid concomitant use of other nephrotoxic agents. Metabolized by and inhibitor of CYP 450 enzyme system.	Scr, electrolytes, LFTs, CBC with platelets, blood pressure
Mycophenolate	Variable. 1 gram orally twice a day. Inhibits guanosine nucleotide synthesis pathway. Indications: prevent organ transplant rejection.	Anorexia, nausea, emesis, weakness, cough, headache back pain, rash, increased infection risk, reactivation of latent viral infections, possible increased risk for lymphoma & other cancers, leucopenia, pure red cell aplasia, others. Teratogenic. Multiple drug interactions including decreased efficacy of oral contraceptives	CBC with platelets

Table 10. Biologic response modifiers for RDs

Generic Name	Adult Dosage	Adverse Effects	Monitoring
Etanercept	25 mg SQ twice a week or 50 mg SQ once a week Indications: RA, JIA, psoriatic arthritis, ankylosing spondylitis (AS), others.	Inhibits tumor necrosis factor (TNF). Side effects: increase risk of serious infection, reactivation of latent TB & hepatitis B, neoplasm (rare lymphoma), injection site reactions, allergic reactions, pancytopenia, new or worsening heart failure, hepatotoxicity	Tuberculin skin test, CBC, LFTs, Scr, hepatitis B & C serology for those with risk factors for infection
Infliximab	IV infusion: 3 mg/kg at 0, 2, & 6 weeks, then every 8 weeks thereafter Indications: RA, JIA, inflammatory bowel disease, psoriasis, AS. May premedication with H2 blocker, acetaminophen &/or corticosteroids	Anti-TNF monoclonal antibody. Inhibits tumor necrosis factor (TNF). Often used in combination with methotrexate. Side effects similar to etanercept including increased risk for autoantibody formation & increased risk for demyelinating disease.	Tuberculin skin test, CBC, LFTs, Scr, hepatitis B & C serology for those with risk factors for infection
Abatacept	IV infusion: 500 to 1,000 mg at 0, 2, & 4 weeks, then monthly (dosage based on body wt) Indications: RA, JIA.	Fusion protein that inhibits costimulation of T cells. Side effects include nausea, headache, cough, dizziness, infusion-related reactions, serious infections, reactivation of latent TB & hepatitis B, antibody formation, malignancy	Tuberculin skin test, hepatitis B C serology for those with risk factors for infection.
Rituximab	IV infusion: 1000 mg on days 1 & 15 in combination with methotrexate. Premedication with corticosteroid recommended Indications: RA & non-Hodgkin's lymphoma	Monoclonal antibody that selectively binds to CD20. Side effects: severe infusion-related reactions (occasionally fatal), anaphylactic reaction, rash, weakness, nausea, cough, hematological toxicity, hyper or hypotension, arrhythmias, tumor lysis syndrome, serious viral infections, reactivation of hepatitis B, fatal mucocutaneous reactions	CBC with platelets, hepatitis B & C serology for those with risk factors for infection.
Adalimumab	40 mg subcutaneously every other week Indications: RA, JIA, Crohn disease, AS, psoriasis.	Anti-TNF monoclonal antibody. Inhibits tumor necrosis factor (TNF). Side effects similar to other TNF inhibitors (see above)	Tuberculin skin test, CBC, LFTs, Scr, hepatitis B & C serology for those with risk factors for infection
Anakinra	100 mg subcutaneously per day Indications: RA	Antagonizes the interleukin-1 receptor. Side effects: nausea, diarrhea, headache, serious infections (predominantly bacterial), injection site reactions, neutropenia, antibody formation, hypersensitivity reactions. Adjust dose when CrCl < 30 ml/min.	CBC with platelets, Scr

Table 10. (Continued)

Generic Name	Adult Dosage	Adverse Effects	Monitoring
Certolizumab pegol	400mg (2 SQ injections of 200mg) at weeks 0, 2 & 4 and then 200mg every other week. Indications: Crohn disease, RA	Selective inhibitor of TNFα. Side effects: Headache, fatigue, hypertension, back pain, rash, upper respiratory tract infections. Same class warnings as noted with other TNFα inhibitors (see above). Risk of malignancy similar to placebo in clinical trials.	Tuberculin skin test, CBC, LFTs, Scr, hepatitis B & C serology for those with risk factors for infection
		Conjugated with polyethylene glycol to extend duration.	
Golimumab	50mg SQ once monthly. Indications: RA, psoriatic arthritis, AS	Monoclonal antibody that binds to TNFα. Side effects: dizziness, hypertension, upper respiratory tract infections, injection site reactions. Same class warnings as noted with other TNFα inhibitors (see above).	Tuberculin skin test, CBC, LFTs, Scr, hepatitis B & C serology for those with risk factors for infection
Tocilizumab	4mg/kg IV infusion every 4 weeks. May increase to 8mg/kg. Maximum single dose of 800mg. Indications: RA, JIA Indicated after inadequate response to one or more TNFα inhibitors.	Interleukin-6 receptor monoclonal antibody. Side effects: increased risk of serious infections, latent viral reactivation, bone marrow suppression, anaphylaxis, bowel perforation, increased LFTs, increased risk of malignancy, hypertension, increased LFTs, hyperlipidemia, antibody formation, infusion reactions. Do not initiate if ANC < 2000/mm^3, platelets < 100,000/mm^3 or AST/ALT > 1.5 X upper limit of normal. Dosage modifications required for increased LFTs, neutropenia & thrombocytopenia (see manufacturer recommendations). May increase metabolism of drugs that are CYP 450 substrates.	Tuberculin skin test, Hepatitis B & C serology for those with risk factors for infection, CBC with platelets, LFTs, fasting lipid profile, blood pressure

RDs represent complex dysfunction of the immune system and thus, biologics are beneficial to some with RDs including inflammatory joint disease and bowel disease. However, their immune blocking mechanism can lead to an increase in infections (including reactivation of latent tuberculosis and hepatitis B) as well as certain types of cancer (including lymphoma). These drugs may be given via home injection or infusion in clinics. Biologics include such drugs as etanercept, infliximab, abatacept, rituximab, adalimumab, certolizumab pegol, golimumab and tocilizumab. (Table 10).

These biologic agents are extremely expensive in the U.S. health care system and long term safety is still a concern, with the possible increased risk of malignancies like lymphoma and demyelinating disorders.

Biologic response modifiers may be used alone or in combination with other DMARDs (most commonly methotrexate) and are often utilized for those with moderate to severe disease or have failed previous trials of other DMARDs. Combination therapy using more than one biologic is not recommended due to the high risk for adverse effects and lack of additive benefit. Antibody production against the biologic may occur which may result in a lower response rate to therapy.

Patients receiving biologic agents may receive vaccines but should avoid live vaccines. Guidelines for rheumatoid arthritis and juvenile idiopathic arthritis have been published by the American College of Rheumatology (2008 and 2011, respectively—3,5). Guideline recommendations focus on duration of disease, disease activity and presence or absence of features indicative of poor prognosis in determining drug therapy. These medications should only be used by experts in RDs and their management.

Management of spondyloarthropathies

Management of these conditions with enthesitis-inflammation is similar to that used for JIA. Treatment is based on pain control with NSAIDs as well as rest and exercise. Depending on the specific condition, exercise is recommended to protect back flexibility and inserts to protect heels and plantar fascia.

The addition of doxycycline for an acute exacerbation of reactive arthritis may be helpful by reducing the number of days of the acute episode.

The judicious use of additional drugs for chronic or recalcitrant spondyloarthropathy include methotrexate, sulfasalazine, chronic NSAIDs use, low dose prednisone, and even the newer biologic agents. Corticosteroid injection into involved joints can be very helpful. The treatment of associated or underlying conditions, such as psoriasis or inflammatory bowel disorder, is important.

Management miscellaneous RD and related disorders

Table 11 provides a list of various RDs, related conditions, and comments on overall pharmacologic management (4, 20, 21). SLE is discussed below.

Table 11. Miscellaneous RDs and related conditions

Name	Comments	Pharmacologic Treatment
Dermatomyositis	Rare autoimmune disorder involving the skin and striated muscles. Myopathic and neuropathic muscle weakness. Complement-mediated microangiopathy with muscle fiber destruction. Red or violaceous dermatitis in butterfly pattern; neck and shoulder pattern seen also. May see heliotrophe rash over eyelids with periorbital edema. Positive Gottron sign/papules. Variable lab work.	RD medications including corticosteroids and good skin care. Avoid sun exposure and use daily high SPF sunscreen Physical therapy and occupational therapy for optimal muscle function. Use of steroids can include high dose pulse methylprednisolone (maximum dose of 1 gram per day for 3 days). Other meds can include methotrexate, hydroxy-chloroquine, IV immunoglobulin, mycophenolate mofetil, or cyclosporine.. If on long-term steroids: calcium and vitamin D supplementation.
Fibromyalgia	Seen in 3-5% of older teen females. Present with chronic, diffuse pain of various body sites with sleep disturbance, emotional lability, long history of chronic complaints, fatigue. Often see positive family history for fibromalgia and/or irritable bowel syndrome. Exam notes tender points over the back and anterior chest wall. Lab tests are usually normal. Can use official criteria with major and minor criteria.	Variable treatments based on presenting concerns. Management focuses on pain control (avoid narcotics), improve sleep dysfunction, reduced stress (psychotherapy as needed), judicious use of psycho-pharmacologic agents (low dose amitryptyline, nortriptyline fluoxetine, sertraline, anxiolytics, anticonvulsants). Pregabalin is an anticonvulsant that is US FDA approved for adults with neuropathic pain. Also, use physical therapy and active exercise program.
Hypersensitivity vasculitis	Diverse group of vasculitides with deposits of immune complexes in capillaries,venules, and sometimes arterioles. Antigen stimulation can be many factors—infections, drugs, others. Can include serum sickness, Henoch-Schönlein syndrome, mixed cryoglobulinemia.	Treat specific syndrome. Remove the offending antigen if possible. Antihistamine treatment for urticaria and immunosuppressive medications as needed, such immunosuppressive drugs for progressive renal disease.
Granulomatosis of (Allergic angiitis and granulomatosis of) Churg and Strauss	Rare systemic vasculitis (fibrinoid necrosis of small to medium sized vesssels) mostly in the skin, lungs, and peripheral nerves. Any organ can be involved. Eosinophilia and asthma often noted. See increased IGE and various allergies.	Supportive and corticosteroids are key treatment principles. Cyclophosphamide may reduce relapse incidence. Others include methotrexate, azathioprine, infliximab, or interferon-α (21).

Name	Comments	Pharmacologic Treatment
Joint Hypermobility syndrome (JHS)	12% have hyperextensible joints; most prevalent in dancers, gymnasts, instrumental musicians; JHS diagnosis based on showing joint hyperextension in testing of 5 joint maneuvers. Rule out Marfan's or Ehler's Danlos syndrome; joint laxity can lead to arthralgias, dislocations, transient joint effusions, pain syndromes as fibromyalgia. See higher incidence of mitral valve prolapse	Limit activities that cause pain, physical therapy (strengthening, bracing, pain control), analgesics (NSAIDs), avoid narcotics. Hypermobility tends to improve over time.
Kawasaki Disease	Acute systemic vasculitis developing mostly in children under age 5 (most under age 2) with highest rates noted in Japan. Etiology is unknown. Can develop fever with polymorphous rash (classic: groin/buttocks), bilateral conjunctivitis (non-purulent), oral changes (dry lips with cracking, bleeding, peeling, strawberry tongue), cervical lymphadenopathy, extremity changes (palmar redness, swollen hands/feet, dequamation. A variety of other features including coronary aneurysms detected on echocardiograms.	IV immune globulin (IVIG): 2 gram/kig over 12 hours; can be repeated. Aspirin (80-100 mg/kg/day and reduced to 3-5 mg/kg'day in children when the fever subsides. Aspirin is a good anti-inflammatory and anti-platelet agent. Follow-up with echocardiograms. Anticoagulation is prescribed in the presence of abnormal coronary arteries. Other medications used in resistant situations include IV methyl-prednisolone, plasmapheresis, cyclophosphamide, and infliximab.
Mixed Connective Tissue Disease	Overlap syndrome with features of SLE, systemic slcerosis, arthritis, and mysoitis. Teens usually present with Raynauds, puffy hands, and arthritis. See less renal disease than children with SLE. Pulmonary hypertension (with anticardio-lipin antibodies) and infections are the most common cause of death. See antibodies to extractable nuclear antigen ribonucleoprotein (anti-RNP) and against U1-70 kd smRNP. May evolve into more classic RD or systemic sclerosis.	Supportive, corticosteroids; other RD drugs as necessary.
Osteoporosis	Decreased bone mass can develop due to many conditions including use of steroids for RDs. It can be seen with chronic amenorrhea, eating disorders, renal disorders, GI disorders, metabolic disorders, chronic use of other drugs (as anticonvulsants), and others. Osteomalacia can arise in renal disease, vitamin D deficiency states, and inborn errors of vitamin D metabolism.	Careful use of drugs that can induce osteomalacia or osteoporosis. Follow with bone marrow measurements (DEXA). Dietary counseling for adequate and if supplemental calcium and vitamin D. Judicious use of bisphosphonates (i.e., alendronate or risedronate).
Panarteritis nodosa (PAN)	Uncommon in adolescents; necrotizing fasculitis of medium size vessels involving many tissues: kidneys, lungs, skin, joints, intestinal tract, peripheral nerves. Cutaneous PAN is mainly skin involvement. Lab results depending on what organs are involved but show signs of inflammation. Screen for streptococcal infection.	Supportive; use of corticosteroids (oral and IV pulse) and other RD drugs depend on specific involvement. These include cyclophosphamide (IV or oral), methotrexate, azathioprine, dapsone, cyclosporine, and anti-TNF agents. Antibiotic prophylaxis is provided if there is an infectious trigger for the PAN.

Table 11. (Continued)

Name	Comments	Pharmacologic Treatment
Raynaud's Phenomenon	Episodes of vasospasm stimulated by cold or stress. Fingers can turn white, then a dusky blue, and with rewarming—bright red. Primary form has no underlying disorders. Nail fold changes include telangietasias. Some develop evidence of RDs over time. 10% of those with dermatomyositis , SLE and adult RD develop Raynaud's Phenomenon..	Avoid cold exposure and use warm clothes. Avoid or manage emotional stress. Avoid tobacco since this can stimulate episodes. Severe situations require use of calcium channel blockers (nifedipine SR [30-60 mg per day] or amlodipine [2.5-10 mg per day]). Others drugs include losartan, bosentan, sildenafil, prazosin. ACE inhibitors are used for hypertension with renal disease: captopril or enalapril. Treat disorders associated with Raynauds. Methotrexate or mycophenolate mofetil used for skin involvement. Cyclophosphate for pulmonary alveolitis.
Reflex Sympathetic Dystrophy (RSD) (Complex Regional Pain Syndrome Type I) Old names include causalgia, Sudeck's atrophy, reflex neurovascular dystrophy.	Trauma (even mild)-induced extremity that is very painful ("pins & needles"), mottled, swollen, cool. Overlying skin has increased sweating; sometimes-dry. Often confused with inflammatory arthritis. Lab work is usually normal. Bone scan or thermography can be helpful. May be secondary to underlying diabetes or degenerative cervical spine disease in adults.	Pain control , prompt mobilization of affected extremity in acute episode, analgesics (as NSAIDs), Physical therapy, biofeedback, counseling (cognitive behavior therapy-chapter 8). Most resolve over time. Severe disorder can lead to contractures and disability. Low dose amitriptyline (10-50 mg orally ½ hour before bedtime). Trial of anti-convulsant (as gabapentin). Give analgesic prior to a nerve block (sympathetic or epidural)
Secondary gout	Abnormal purine metabolism with hyperuricemia, urate crystal deposition in cartilage or joints that leads to arthritis. Mainly seen in adults. Seen in youth with neoplasms, blood dyscrasias, adverse effects of some drugs. Initial attack is one joint and later attacks can occur with many joints: first metatarsophalangeal joint, ankle, mid-foot, or knee.	Management of acute attack: NSAIDs (indomethacin), colchicine, steroids. Chronic Hyperuricemia: Remove offending drugs; use anti-hyperuricemia drugs: allopurinol, probenecid.
Systemic Vasculitis	Group of idiopathic disorders with different clinical manifestations and involvement of different sizes of vessels. Common vasculitides of adolescents include Kawasaki disease and Henoch-Schönlein purpura.	Supportive, steroids, other RD medications depending on specific issues

Name	Comments	Pharmacologic Treatment
Takayasu's arteritis	Inflammation of the aorta and major brances. Called "pulseless" disease. Most are postpubertal females, especially of Asian (Japanese) descent. There is anorexia, fatigue, poor weight gain, growth inhibition, hypertension. There can be acute hypertensive encephalopathy with seizures, cerebral ischemia, congestive heart failure due to renal and systemic arterial occlusion. See increased ESR and gamma globulin. Blood vessel studies reveal the abnormality.	High dose corticosteroids, methotrexate, azathioprine; cyclophosphamide, mycophenolate mofetil, anti-TNF-α therapy. Treat hypertension. Vascular surgery if possible. Poor prognosis
Weber-Christian Disease (Relapsing nodular non-suppurative Panniculitis)	Rare idiopathic disorder or collection of disorders with systemic vasculitis and successive crops of tender, red nodules in subcutaneous fat of breasts, trunk, or thighs. Nodules appear over months to years and undergo fat liquefaction with release of oily material.	Supportive; corticosteroids
Wegener's Granulomatosis	Necrotizing, granulomatous angiitis involving upper & lower respiratory tract (90%), kidneys (>75%), joints (60%), and other organs. See fever & polyarthritis followed by lung or upper airway involvement. Extensive symptomatology. Varied neurologic features up to 50%. Lab data reflect inflammation; increased serum antineutrophil cytoplasma antibody. Biopsy is diagnostic. Limited Wegener's refers to lesions in the orbi and respiratory tract but not the kidneys or vascular system.	High, rapid mortality rate in untreated individuals. Steroids, cyclophosphamide, other cytotoxic agents (i.e., azathioprine) and other RD drugs (i.e., methotrexate). Antibiotics may be helpful. Subglottic stenosis usually does not improve with use of systemic drugs; use frequent intratracheal dilation and injection of long-acting glucocorticoids that may prevent the need for tracheostomy (21).
Systemic sclerosis (diffuse scleroderma)	Localized form involves linear scleroderma or morphea in the skin. Systemic form: rare in teens with multisystem inflammatory changes. Most also develop Raynaud's Phenomenon. Variant is the CREST syndrome.	Physical therapy to maintain joint function and keep the skin soft. Methotrexate may be helpful. Other RD medications (i.e., methotrexate plus steroids) are helpful depending on specific issues. Use steroids cautiously in systemic sclerosis to avoid triggering a renal crisis. Superficial morphea: topical steroids or ultraviolet (UV) therapy.

Systemic Lupus Erythematosus (SLE)

Systemic lupus erythematosus (SLE) is the second most common rheumatoid disease in adolescence, second to JIA (1-6, 22-27). It is found in 15 to 50 in 100,000 and has a female to male ratio of 8:1. SLE is more common in Hispanic, Asian, and African-Americans.

Clinical features

Common features include arthritis, arthralgia, fever, fatigue, headache, and weight loss. It can have many other clinical features and specific diagnosis is based on the presence of 4 of 11 specific classification criteria (Table 12) that includes rash, arthritis, nephritis, serositis, neurological or hematologic abnormalities, and specific serologic markers (table 13).

Table 12. Diagnostic criteria for Systemic Lupus Erythematosus (SLE)[A]

Criteria	Comment
1. Facial butterfly rash	Flat or raised malar erythema with or without edema. May develop vesicles, crusting, or ulcerations. Present in half of all cases. Non specific for SLE.
2. Discoid lupus	Scaly erythematous plaques predominating on face and scalp with or without scarring, atrophy, pigment changes, and telangiectasia. May be an isolated cutaneous disorder or part of a systemic disease. Other skin lesions that may be seen with SLE include urticaria, tender nodules on palms, fingertips, and soles, digit gangrene, and periungual erythema. See Text.
3. Photosensitivity	Includes sun-exposure induced urticarial plaques on the skin.
4. Oral or nasopharyngeal ulceration	May result in epistaxis or perforation of the septum.
5. Nephritis or nephrotic syndrome	Renal involvement occurs in half of cases, involving persistent proteinuria, hematuria, or cellular casts (glomerular or tubular) - See Table 6A.
6. Joint swelling	Polyarthritis (two or more peripheral joints) similar to juvenile rheumatoid arthritis but without joint destruction. Present in nine of ten cases. See Text.
7. Pleuritis or pericarditis	Also may develop peritonitis, myocarditis, endocarditis (Libman-Sacks), or parenchymal lung disease. Cardiac tamponade is rare.
8. Psychosis or convulsions	Other CNS manifestations that may be seen include mononeuritis, cranial nerve neuropathy, chorea, myelopathy, aseptic meningitis, and cerebrovascular accidents.
9. Hemolytic anemia, leukopenia, lymphopenia, and/or thrombocytopenia	Coombs' test will be positive if hemolytic anemia is present. Splenomegaly is also seen.

Classic features include the SLE butterfly malar rash, alopecia, cutaneous vasculitis (livedo reticularis, palpable purpura), generalized photosensitivity, and others. SLE renal disease is noted in 50 to 70% and ranges from minimal mesangial proliferation to diffuse proliferative glomerulonephritis based on kidney biopsy. SLE inflammatory lesions can develop in the CNS with resultant seizures, stroke, psychosis, and even coma.

SLE arthritis can resemble JIA or more commonly be seen as small joint swelling and stiffness in hands or feet; it is usually non-disfiguring and usually overshadowed by other SLE features. The term Jaccoud's arthritis refers to distinctive and reversible hand involvement see in SLE.

The etiology of this autoimmune disease is unknown, though there are a number of drugs that can induce a SLE reaction (Table 14). The presence of anti-dsDNA and various antibodies to cytoplasmic antigens are more specific and sensitive than a positive ANA test. The combination of depressed complement with elevated anti-dsDNA is 100% specific for SLE; these titers are also useful to monitor disease activity as well as prediction for an acute episode. One-third have anti-phospholipid antibodies or other lupus anticoagulants (Table 13).

Table 13. Laboratory features of SLE

Positive ANA (good as screening test; lacks specificity)
Antibodies to double-stranded DNA (anti-dsDNA) and cytoplasmic antigens
Low C3 and C4 levels
Leukopenia
Low platelet count
Coombs-positive hemolytic anemia
Anti-phospholipid antibodies
Other lupus anticoagulants

Table 14. Drugs association with SLE

Hydralazine	Captopril
Propylthiouracil	Isoniazide
Chlorpramazine	Quinidine
Alphamethyldopa	Beta-blockers
Lithium	Penicillamine
Sulfasalazine	Procainamide
Antibiotics	Oral contraceptives
Anticonvulsants	
a. Diphenylhydantoin	
b. Ethosuximide	
c. Trimethadone	

Management

Specific management is based on organ involvement and response to medication. All patients are advised to use sunscreen with high sun protective factor (SPF). Arthritis and mucocutaneous involvement is treated with NDAIDs and hydroxychloroquine. Systemic steroids are used for visceral disease including severe hematologic complications. Steroids can be started at 2 mg/kg/day of prednisone up to 60 to 80 mg per day. Alternative-day dosing is used when possible to reduce steroid side effects (Table 7). Twenty-five percent on steroids develop avascular necrosis of hips.

Severe disease (i.e., progressive renal or pulmonary insufficiency, systemic vasculitis, or CNS disease) require larger steroid doses: intravenous pulse methylprednisolone at 30 mg/kg up to 1,000 mg. Immunosuppressive medications are used for refractory SLE disease. Other medications used to treat SLE include methotrexate, azathioprine, cyclophosphamide, cyclosporin A, intravenous gammablobulin and others (26). Anti-CD20 Mab is used to threat SLE hemolytic anemia and thrombocytopenia.

Diffuse proliferative glomerulonephritis is treated with monthly intravenous cyclophosphamide since steroids are often not enough to prevent significant renal progression. Methotrexate, azathioprine, and cyclosporine A are also used and can be used to lower steroid doses (26). Autologous bone marrow transplantation is used for refractory SLE disease.

Those with antiphospholipid antibodies or lupus anticoagulant are at increased risk for arterial and venous thromboses with resultant strokes, thrombophlebitis, and miscarriages. If contraception is requested, estrogen-based contraceptives are contraindicated. These youth may be placed on low dose aspirin. Life-long anticoagulation is needed for those with a significant thrombotic event. Death in SLE patients occurs due to infection, renal failure, pulmonary hemorrhage, severe CNS disease, and early myocardial infarction. The degree of renal involvement directly affects morbidity and mortality.

Conclusion

Rheumatoid (rheumatic) disorders (RDs) are a wide variety of complex autoimmune disorders (4, 28-33). The hallmark of the rheumatic disorders is the presence of a chronic inflammatory process that if left uncontrolled, often leads to significant morbidity and even mortality. The most common RD is juvenile idiopathic arthritis while SLE is the second most common RD.

Management includes non-pharmacologic measures (as physical therapy, occupational therapy, splints, braces, assistive devices) and pharmacologic measures as reviewed in this chapter. A wide range of pharmacologic agents are available to the specialist in rheumatology including analgesics (as NSAIDs), corticosteroids, DMARDs (disease-modifying antirheumatic drugs), and biologic response modifiers. Concepts of other RDs as well as SLE are also presented.

ACKNOWLEDGMENTS

This paper is an adapted version of a chapter in the book "Adolescent medicine: Pharmacotherapeutics in medical disorders" edited by Donald E Greydanus, Dilip R Patel, Cynthia Feucht, Hatim A Omar, Joav Merrick and published with permission by Walter de Gruyter, Berlin and New York.

REFERENCES

[1] Cassidy JT, Petty RE, eds. Textbook of pediatric rheumatology, 5th ed. Philadelphia, PA: Saunders Elsevier, 2005.
[2] Junnila JL, Cartwright VW. Chronic musculoskeletal pain in children: Part II. Rheumatic causes. Am Fam Physician 2006;74:293-300.
[3] Klippel JH, Crofford LJ, Stone JH, Weyand CM, eds. Primer on the rheumatic diseases, 12th ed. Atlanta, GA: Arthritis Foundation, 2001.
[4] Moore MD. Rheumatic diseases, In: Greydanus DE, Patel DR, Pratt HD, eds. Essential adolescent medicine. New York: McGraw Hill, 2006:201-34.
[5] National Institute of Arthritis and Musculoskeletal and Skin Diseases. Arthritis and rheumatic diseases. Bethesda, MD: National Institutes Health Publication, 08-4999, 2008.
[6] Patel DR, Moore MD. Concepts of rheumatology. In: Greydanus, Patel DR, Reddy VN, Feinberg An, Omar HA, eds. Handbook of clinical pediatrics: An update for the ambulatory pediatrician. Singapore: World Scientific, 2010:697-713.
[7] Petty RE, Southwood TR, Manners P, Baum J, Glass DN, Goldenberg J, et al. International League of Associations for Rheumatology classification of juvenile idiopathic arthritis, second revision, Edmonton, 2001. J Rheumatol 2004;31(2):390-2.
[8] Agarwal M, Sawhney S. Laboratory tests in pediatric rheumatology. Indian J Pediatr 2010;77(9): 1011-6.
[9] Hilderson D, Corstijens F, Moons P, Wouters C, Westhovens R. Adolescents with juvenile idiopathic arthritis: who cares after the age of 16? Clin Exp Rheumatol 2010;28(5):790-7.
[10] Martini A, Lovell DJ. Juvenile idiopathic arthritis: state of the art and future perspectives. Ann Rheum Dis 2010;69(7):1260-3.
[11] Singh S, Mehra S. Approach to polyarthritis. Indian J Pediatr 2010; 77(9):1005-10.
[12] Hashkes PJ, Laxer RM.: Medical treatment of juvenile idiopathic arthritis. JAMA 2005;294(13):1671-84.
[13] Hayward K, Wallace CA. Recent developments in anti-rheumatic drugs in pediatrics: Treatment of juvenile idiopathic arthritis. Arthritis Res Ther 2009;11(1):216-20.
[14] Beresford MW, Baildam EM. New advances in the management of juvenile idiopathic arthritis-1: non-biological therapy. Arch Dis Child Educ Pract Ed 2009;94(5):144-50.
[15] Holzinger D, Frosch M, Föll D. Methotrexate in the therapy of juvenile idiopathic arthritis. Z Rheumatol 2010;69(6):496-504.
[16] Ruperto N, Martini A. Pediatric rheumatology: JIA, treatment and possible risk of malignancies. Nat Rev Rheumatology 2011;7(1):6-7.
[17] Neovius M, Simard JF, Askling J. ARTIS study group. Ann Rheum Dis 2011;70(4):624-9.
[18] Quartier P. Current treatments for juvenile idiopathic arthritis. Joint Bone Spine 2010;77(6):511-6.
[19] Lamot L, Bukovac LT, Vidovic M, Frieta M, Harjacek M. The head to head comparison of etanercept and infliximab in treating children with juvenile idiopathic arthritis. Clin Exp Rheumatol 2011;29(1): 131-9.
[20] Kimura Y, Walco GA. Treatment of chronic pain in pediatric rheumatic disease. Nature Clin Pract Rheumatol 2007;3:210-8.

[21] Light MJ, Blaisdell CJ, Homnick DN, Schechter MS, Weinberger MM, eds. Pediatric pulmonology. Elk Grove Village, IL: American Academy of Pediatrics, 2011.

[22] Pineles D, Valente A, Warren B, Peterson MG, Lehman TJ, Moorthy LN. Worldwide incidence and prevalence of pediatric onset systemic lupus erythematosus. Lupus 2011 Jul 18. [Epub ahead of print]

[23] Mikita N, Ikeda T, Ishiquro M, Furukawa F. Recent advances in cytokines in cutaneous and systemic lupus erythematosus. J Dermatol 2011 July 18. [Epub ahead of print]

[24] Manson JJ, Rahman A. Systemic lupus erythematosus. Orphanet J Rare Dis 2006;1(6):22-6.

[25] Kalunian K, Joan TM. New directions in the treatment of systemic lupus erythematosus. Curr Med Res Opin 2009;25(6):1501-14.

[26] Szer IS, Kimura Y, Malleson PN, Southwood TR, eds. Arthritis in children and aolescents: Juvenile idiopathic arthritis. Oxford: Oxford University Press, 2006.

[27] Aringer M, Hiepe F. Systemic lupus erythematosus. Z Rheumatol 2011;70(4):313-23.

[28] Wright E. Musculoskeletal injuries and disorders. In: Berardi R, ed. Handbook of nonprescription drugs, an interactive approach to self-care. Washington DC: American Pharmacists Association, 2009:95-113.

[29] Drugstore. Topical analgesics. Accessed 2011 Jun 02. URL: http://www.drugstore.com/search/search_results.asp?N50andNtx5mode%2BmatchallpartialandNtk5Allandsrchtree5 5andNtt5topical1analgesics. Accessed July 5, 2011.

[30] Facts and comparisons. Drug information full monographs. Wolters Kluwer Health, Incorporated. Accessed 2011 Jun 02. URL:: http://0-online.factsandcomparisons.com.libcat.ferris.edu/index.aspx.

[31] Pediatric Lexi-drugs. Lexi-Comp, Inc. 2011. Accessed 2011 Jun 02. URL: http://www.lexi.com/

[32] Drugs for rheumatoid arthritis. Treatment guidelines. Med Letter 2009;7(81):37-46.

[33] Beukelman T, Patkar NM, Saag KG, Tolleson-Rinehart S, Cron RQ, DeWitt EM, et al. 2011 American college of rheumatology recommendations for the treatment of juvenile idiopathic arthritis: initiation and safety monitoring of therapeutic agents for the treatment of arthritis and systemic features. Arthritis Care Res 2011;63(4):465-82.

Submitted: November 05, 2011. *Revised:* December 07, 2011. *Accepted:* December 20, 2011.

In: Child and Adolescent Health Yearbook 2013
Editor: Joav Merrick
ISBN: 978-1-63117-658-6

Chapter 5

ADOLESCENCE AND METABOLIC DISORDERS

Donald E. Greydanus*, MD, Dr. HC (ATHENS), Cynthia L Feucht, PharmD, BCPS, and Mary D Moore, MD

Department of Pediatric & Adolescent Medicine,
Western Michigan University School of Medicine, Kalamazoo, Michigan,
Department of Pharmacy Practice, Ferris State University,
Kalamazoo and Borgess Ambulatory Care, Kalamazoo, United States of America

ABSTRACT

Inborn errors of metabolism (IEMs) or metabolic disorders are complex conditions involving abnormalities in biochemical and metabolic pathways necessary for healthy human existence. They are often caused by partial or total deficiency of key enzymes and these conditions usually present in infancy or early childhood. Some may not be identified until adolescence or even during the adult years. This discussion reviews some of the IEMs that can become evident in the adolescent years, such as adrenoleukodystrophy, glycogen storage diseases, lysosomal storage diseases, urea cycle disorders, and others. Management focuses on symptomatic treatment and when available as well as affordable, enzyme replacement therapies. Gene therapy and stem cell transplantation are options under current research in addition to finding more replacement enzymes.

Keywords: Adolescence, metabolism

INTRODUCTION

Inborn errors of metabolism (IEMs) or metabolic disorders are unusual, complex conditions involving abnormalities in biochemical and metabolic pathways necessary for human life.

* Correspondence: Professor Donald E Greydanus, MD, Dr. HC (ATHENS), Chair, Department of Pediatric & Adolescent Medicine, Western University School of Medicine 1000 Oakland Drive, D48G, Kalamazoo, MI 49008-1284 United States. E-mail: donald.greydanus@med.wmich.edu

Though often identified in infancy or childhood, some may not be diagnosed until adolescence or adulthood. The initial term, inborn errors of metabolism, was introduced by Sir Archibald Garrod in 1902 and referred to cystinuria, albinism, alkaptonuria, and benign pentosuria (1). Phenylketonuria (PKU) was identified in 1934 by Ivar Asbjørn Følling (1888-1973) and in the second half of the 20st century, over 500 IEMs have been identified (2). Table 1 presents a partial list of IEMs (2).

IEMs are complex conditions that are usually genetic, typically inherited in an autosomal recessive manner, though a few are X-linked recessive conditions (i.e., Fabry disease, ornithine carbamylase deficiency, or pyruvate dehydrogenase deficiency). Autosomal dominance is noted in Marfan syndrome, familial hypercholesterolemia, and acute intermittent porphyria. Some IEMs are caused by mitochondrial genome mutations and there can be enzyme deficiencies or problems with cellular transporters.

Table 1. Inborn Errors of Metabolism (IEMs) (2)

Aminoacidurias (disorders of amino acid metabolism)

- Homocystinuria
- Maple syrup urine disease
- Nonketotic hyperglycemia
- PKU (phenylketonuria)
- Tyrosinemia

Carbohydrate metabolism disorders

- Galactosemia
- Glycogen storage diseases

Fatty acid oxidation disorders

- Short-chain acyl coenzyme A (CoA) dehyrogenase (SCAD)
- Medium-chain acyl CoA dehyrogenase (MCAD)
- Long-chain acyl CoA dehyrogenase (LCAD)
- Very long-chain acyl CoA dehyrogenase (VLCAD)

Lipid Storage disorders

- Gaucher' disease
- Metachromatic leukodystrophy
- Tay-Sachs disease

Lysosomal disorders

- Combined defects
- Glycoproteinosis
- I-cell disease
- Sphingolipidosis
- Mucopolysaccharidoses (MPS)
    - ◊ MPS I (Hurler and Scheie disease)
    - ◊ MPS II (Hunter disease)
    - ◊ MPS III (Sanfilippo disease)
    - ◊ MPS IV (Morquio disease)
    - ◊ MPS VI
    - ◊ MPS VII

Mitochondrial metabolisms disorders

- Glutaric aciduria

- MELAS (**m**itochondrial **m**yopathy, **e**ncephalopathy, **l**actic **a**cidosis, and **s**troke-like episodes)
- Pyruvate dehydrogenase deficiency

Metal metabolism disorders
- Hemochromatosis
- Menkes disease
- Wilson disease

Organic acidemias (organic acid metabolism disorders)
- Methylmalonic acidemia
- Propionic acidemia

Peroxisomal disorders
- Adrenoleukodystrophy
- Adult Refsum disease
- Chondrodysplasia punctata
- Zellweger syndrome

Purine transport metabolism disorder
- Lesch-Nyhan syndrome

Steroid pathway disorders
- Congenital adrenal hyperplasia
- Smith-Lemli-Opitz syndrome

Transport disorders
- Cystinosis
- Hypercholesterolemia

Urea cycle disorders
- Arginosuccinate deficiency
- Carbamoyl phosphate synthetase deficiency
- Ornithine transcarbamylase deficiency

Miscellaneous
- Hemoglobinopathies
- Hypothyroidism

INCIDENCE

The incidence of IEMs varies to a considerable extent depending on the specific condition. For example, congenital hypothyroidism is noted in 1:4,500, congenital adrenal hyperplasia in 1:10,000, medium chain acyl CoA dehydrogenase (MCAD), phenylketonuria in 1:15,000, and galactosemia in 1:30,000.

A number of IEMs are much rarer and noted in 1:100,000—such as fatty acid oxidation disorders, organic acidemias, homocystinuria, maple syrup urine disease (MSUD), and others (2). Some IEMs are seen in increased incidence among certain populations such as Tay Sachs in the Ashkenazi Jewish population or maple syrup urine disease (MSUD) in United States Pennsylvania Mennonites. Consanguinity is a factor in some of these conditions.

PRESENTATION

IEMs may present with *metabolic* syndromes (acute acidotic or hypoglycemia crises), *hepatic* syndromes (liver disease with abnormal liver function tests), *cardiac* syndromes (acute cardiac myopathy or cardiovascular collapse), or *neurological* syndromes (altered mental status or neurological functioning). The neurological syndromes can have acute or chronic presentations and involve seizures, sensory dysfunctions, coma, changes of tone, intellectual deterioration, behavioral dysfunction, psychosis, and others. In the metabolic presentations, there can be acidosis, hypoglycemia, or hyperammonemia (i.e., urea cycle defects). There can also be progressive, chronic cellular storage disorders with variable presentations.

Some can present later on in childhood, such as metachromatic leukodystrophy, Tay-Sachs disease, Gaucher's disease, lysosomal storage disorders, and others (2). There can be progressive neurological deterioration and some conditions result in mental subnormality that have an onset in adolescence or adulthood (Table 2) (3). A wide variety of features can be seen including dysmorphic phenotypes as well as abnormalities in different organ systems, such as gastrointestinal, dermatological, hematological, and others.

Table 2. Adult (Adolescent-onset) Metabolic Disorders with MR

A. Amino acid disorder: Homocystinuria
B. Lipid Storage Disorders
1. Juvenile Metachromatic Leukodystrophy
2. Adult Metachromatic Leukodystrophy
3. Mannosidosis
4. Niemann-Pick C
5. GM1 Gangliosidosis
6. GM2 Gangliosidosis
C. Mucopolysaccharidoses: Sanfillipo Disease, types B and D
D. Peroxisomal disorder: X-linked adrenoleukodystrophy
E. Urea cycle disorders: Ornithine transcarbamylase deficiency

Unique odors can be present such as burnt sugar or maple syrup –like in MSUD, fruity odor in acidemias (propionic or methylmalonic), mousy (musty) in PKU, cheese-like (sweaty socks) in isovaleric academia, malt-like in methionine malabsorption, fish-like in trimethylaminuria or carnitine excess, cat urine-like (3-methylcrotonic academia or 3-hydroxy-3-methyl glutaric aciduria) or cabbage-like in tyrosinemia (2). Thus, a careful evaluation along with a high index of clinical suspicion is necessary to make the correct diagnosis, often in consultations with experts in genetics, metabolic disorders, and other specialists. The diagnosis may be delayed for many years if the presentation of the condition is non-specific or mild often due to a partial enzyme deficiency.

MENTAL SUBNORMALITY

As noted, IEMs can result in variable levels of intellectual and developmental disability (IDD) and severe to profound IDD is usually diagnosed in early childhood. Routine metabolic screening is usually not helpful in a youth with IDD unless clues are found in the evaluation, such as new onset psychiatric or neurological features (4,5). Selective metabolic disorder testing may be helpful including laboratory work such as blood studies (i.e., lactate, quantitative amino acids, aldolase, creatine kinase, acylcarnitine, lipid profile), urine studies (i.e., quantitative amino acids, organic acids, myoglobin), imaging (MRI of the brain, echocardiogram), muscle and/or skin biopsies, and genetic studies.

Chromosome abnormalities are the most common identifiable causes in evaluations for IDD in adolescents; aneuploidy is the most common defect found in evaluations followed by abnormal X-linked genes such as in fragile X syndrome or X-linked adrenoleukodystrophy (3). Over 200 genes causing X-linked mental retardation conditions have been identified (3).

Finding a specific cause for an adolescent's mental retardation can be beneficial to both the family and youth with closure being brought to the many years if searching to find a reason for the IDD. The youth and his normal–IQ siblings may have worries regarding their reproductive futures and may request a full genetic evaluation.

Phenylketonuria (PKU)

This discussion now presents comments about a number of IEMs that can present in the adolescent or even adult years. Sometimes the paucity of symptoms hides the diagnosis for many years often due to a partial and not absolute deficiency of the responsible enzyme (s). For example, PKU is usually identified in infancy and is caused by a defect of phenylalanine hydroxylase that converts phenylalanine to tyrosine. A plasma amino acid screen reveals very high levels of phenylalanine levels and the urine contains phenylpyruvic acid. Though normal at birth, the toxic levels of phenylalanine result in an infant with emesis, irritability, and eventual neurologic injury with mental retardation; the urine has a *musty* or *mousy* odor. PKU can also lead to generalized hypopigmentation leading to the classic blond and fair skinned PKU child due to the block of phenylalanine to tyrosine.

A newborn screen identifies the PKU and allows treatment that traditionally has consisted of restricting dietary intake of phenylalanine for the life of the individual so that plasma phenylalanine is at a safe level (i.e., not too high or not too low). Medication is now also available--sapropterin dihydrochloride (Kuvan), that is a synthesized normal cofactor for phenylalanine hydroxylase (tetrahydrobiopterin [BH4]) and boosts phenylalanine levels residual enzyme activity in those with mild PKU mutations.

Thus, the clinician will usually encounter an adolescent with PKU who has been diagnosed in infancy and is on the proper diet management and perhaps Kuvan, if a mild PKU condition is present (Table 3). If this youth goes off the diet plan, neurologic injury may develop and include concentration problems, cognitive impairment, psychosocial problems, and even psychosis.

Maple Syrup Urine Disease (MSUD)

MSUD is a disorder of branch-chain amino acid metabolism caused by deficiency of four different enzymes leading to oxidative decarboxylation of ketoacids. It is usually diagnosed in infancy and the plasma amino acid screen reveals an increase in allo-isoleucine (pathognomonic for MSUD), isoleucine, leucine, and valine. The infant develops an acute metabolic crisis with metabolic acidosis and massive urine ketonuria. A variety of symptoms develop including feeding difficulties, lethargy, emesis, abnormal breathing, seizures, opisthotonos, rigidity, cerebral edema, mental retardation, and death. The maple syrup smell of the urine led to the name of this disease first identified in 1934 (2).

Treatment is early diagnosis with lifetime dietary restriction of branch chain amino acids that is low in isoleucine, leucine, and valine; the levels of these amino acids should be in the "Goldilocks level"—not to low and not to high for normal growth and development. As with PKU, the clinician normally encounters an adolescent with MSUD who has been diagnosed in infancy and is on the proper diet management. Rare situations do arise in which a mild mutation of one of the four MSUD responsible enzymes allows a later presentation and perhaps more elusive symptoms. A minority of PKU patients are also thiamine responsive.

Adrenoleukodystrophy (ALD)

ALD (Schilder disease) is an X-linked recessive disorder due to dysfunction of β-oxidation of VLCFA (very long-chain fatty acids). It is the most common peroxisomal disorder; peroxisomes are organelles present in all cells except red blood cells with many roles in key enzymes including oxidation of very long chain fatty acids (VLCFAs). ALD is the result of mutations in the gene that encodes ALDP and affects 1 in 21,000 males; if female heterozygotes are included, the overall frequency is 1 in 16,800. Females who carry the gene can develop features of ALD that usually are milder than noted with males. The ALDP protein is involved in the breakdown of VLCFAs (12-18 carbons in length) found in normal diet. Lack of this protein leads to high levels of VLCFAs with damage to the peripheral nervous system, the brain, and the adrenal gland.

Evaluation reveals increased levels of VLCFAs (especially C26:0) and MRI can identifies evidence of demyelination; cultured skin fibroblasts note the dysfunction of β-oxidation of VLCFAs. Technology for the prenatal diagnosis of ALD is available and useful for prevention of disease transmission in affected persons.

The onset is usually between 3 and 10 years of age and it may begin with ADHD-like or behavioral symptoms. Youth with this neurodegenerative, demyelinating disorder develop a myriad of symptoms including dementia, epilepsy, sensory loss (vision [optic atrophy] and hearing), spastic quadriplegia with ataxia, joint pains, dysphagia, and others. Adrenal insufficiency may develop with hypoglycemia and salt wasting episodes as well as hyperpigmentation similar to Addison's disease (6). Death will occur if this is not treated.

Management of ALD is based on restriction of dietary very long-chain fatty acids and ingestion of shorter chain fatty acids. However, restriction of VLCFAs does not stop cerebral deterioration once it develops. Correction of the adrenal insufficiency is important. Adding Lorenzo's oil (4:1 combination of glycerol trioleate and glycerol trierucate) can lower VLCFA levels in half of patients; however, it does not lead to significant improvement or prevention of the overall disease (Table 3).

Research is focusing on bone marrow transplantation in boys with childhood onset and also stem cell gene therapy (7,8). Hematopoietic stem cell transplantation can stabilize or even reverse cerebral demyelination if performed early but after differentiation of mild from severe disease can be made.

Table 3. Medications for Inborn Errors of Metabolism (Part II)

Medication	Indication	Adult Dosage	Side Effects	Comments
Penicillamine	Cystinuria	Initial: 250mg/day Usual dose: 2gm/day (1-4gm/day) Also administer: pyridoxine 25mg/day	Same as in Part I. Avoid during pregnancy and lactation. Avoid interruption in therapy due to risk of sensitivity reactions with reinstitution. Avoid in renal insufficiency.	*The greater the fluid intake the lower the dose required *Administer 1hr before or 2 hrs after meals *Administer at least 1hr apart from other drugs, food or milk
Pyridoxine (Vitamin B6)	Homocystinuria	Usual: 300-600 mg/day Range: 25-600 mg/day	Sensory neuropathic syndromes, ataxia, paraesthesia, unstable gait, photoallergic reactions	*May be given in conjunction with vitamin B12 and folate *Drug interactions with levodopa and phenytoin
Betaine	Homocystinuria	3gm orally twice daily	GI distress, nausea	*Dissolve in 4-6 ounces of water and immediately administer *Monitor plasma homocysteine levels
Glycine	Isovaleric acidemia	150 mg/kg/day (orally)	Nausea, vomiting	*Avoid in anuric patients
Biotin	Multiple carboxylase deficiency	Usual dose: 10-40mg daily	GI upset	*Anticonvulsants may impair biotin absorption *Dietary supplement: no standard regulation in the U.S.
Lorenzo's oil	Adrenoleukodystrophy	Pediatric: 2-3 ml/kg/day (based on one study)	Thrombocytopenia, purpura, petechiae, bleeding, GI upset, gingivitis, increased LFTs	*Triglyceride mixture of glycerol trierucate and glycerol trioleate in 1:4 ratio *May reduce risk of developing cerebral disease
Pyrimethamine	GM2 gangliosidosis	25-100 mg/day (based on one open-label Phase I/II clinical trial in adults)	Folic acid deficiency, hemolytic anemia (with G6PD deficiency), severe hypersensitivity reactions, anorexia,	*Increased incidence of adverse events with escalating dose in trial *Administer with food to minimize vomiting

Table 3. (Continued)

Medication	Indication	Adult Dosage	Side Effects	Comments
		Consider addition of daily folinic acid supplement	vomiting, atrophic glossitis, bone marrow suppression,, hyperphenylalaninemia. May be carcinogenic. Use with caution in renal and hepatic impairment.	*Drug interactions with myelosuppressive agents and antifolate drugs
Genistein	Sanfilippo syndrome	5 mg/kg/day in divided doses Dosage based on two open-label trials	Constipation, nausea, bloating, diarrhea, insomnia, rash	*Studies utilized a genistein rich soy isoflavone extract *No adverse effects reported in the two trials *Supplements are not regulated by the FDA *Isoflavone content can vary among the different forms of soy
Sapropterin	Phenylketonuria (mild)	Initial: 10 mg/kg/day Maintenance: 5-20 mg/kg/day	Abdominal pain, headache, diarrhea, nausea, vomiting, cough, pharyngolaryngeal pain, rhinorrhea, bruising, neutropenia Use with caution in hepatic and renal impairment (not evaluated)	*Used in conjunction with a phenylalanine restricted diet *Monitor phenylalanine blood levels to determine response to therapy *Administer with food to increase absorption *Dissolve tablets in 4-8 oz. water/apple juice and take within 15 min of dissolution *Drug interactions with levodopa , antifolate drugs and PDE-5 inhibitors

References:

Facts and Comparisons. Drug information full monographs. Wolters Kluwer Health, Incorporated. Available at: http://0-online.factsandcomparisons.com.libcat.ferris.edu/index.aspx. Accessed August 15, 2011.

AltMedDex System (electronic version). Thomson Reuters, Greenwood Village, Colorado, USA. Available at http://www.thomsonhc.com. Accessed August 17, 2011.

DRUGDEX System (electronic version). Thomson Reuters, Greenwood, Village, Colorado, USA. Available at http://www.thomsonhc.com. Accessed August 17, 2011.

Delgadillo V, O'Callaghan M, Artuch R, Montero R, Pineda M. Genistein supplementation in patients affected by sanfilippo disease. J Inherit Metab Dis. 2011; May 10 [Epub ahead of print].

Piotrowska E, Jakobkiewicz-Banecka J, Tylki-Symanska A, Libereck A, Mary naik A, et al. Genistein-rich soy isoflavone extract in substrate reduction therapy for sanfilippo syndrome: an open-label, pilot study in 10 pediatric patients. Curr Ther Res 2008;69(2):166-179.

Natural Medicines Comprehensive Database. Evidence-based monographs. Therapeutics Research Faculty, Stockton, CA, USA. Available at http://0-naturaldatabase.therapeuticresearch.com.libcat.ferris.edu/home.aspx?cs=MHSLA~CPands=ND. Accessed August 19, 2011.

Testai F, Gorelick F. Inherited metabolic disorders and stroke part 2, homocystinuria, organic acidurias and urea cycle disorders. Arch Neurol 2010;67(2):148-153.

Clarke J, Mahuran D, Sathe S, Kolodny E, Rigat B, Raiman J, et al. An open-label phase I/II clinical trial of pyrimethamine for the treatment of patients affected with chronic GM2 gangliosidosis (Tay-Sachs or Sandhoff variants). Mol Genet Metab 2011;102(1):6-12.

The development of modern gene therapy viral vectors is underway that seeks to allow the targeting of the leukodystrophy disease gene into oligodendrocytes or astrocytes to treat various forms of leukodystrophies (8).

Another variant, adrenomyeloneuropathy (AMN), may develop in adolescents or adults with urinary dysfunction and spastic paraparesis due to distal axonopathy, mostly of the spinal cord. AMN may also be seen in female who are heterozygotes for ALD.

AMN patients can also develop adrenal insufficiency and may be the cause of adrenal insufficiency in one out of three with Addison's disease. Features also noted include psychosis, mania, and depression.

Metachromatic Leukodystrophy (MLD)

Adolescents may develop the juvenile or adult form of MLD that is an autosomal recessive lysosomal storage disease due to deficiency of the enzyme arylsulfatase A which can be identified in white blood cells or cultured skin fibroblasts; there is also increased sulfatide in the urine (9). There is intra-lysosomal storage of sulfatides (sphingolipid cerebroside 3-sulfates) which are found in high amounts in myelin and neurons (10).

Symptoms are due to demyelination and neurodegeneration; these include ataxia, painful joints, pain with swallowing, peripheral neuropathy, spasticity, personality changes (social withdrawal, obsessive features), deterioration in school work, and others. There is also a heterozygote state. Research is focusing on hematopoietic stem cell gene therapy and intracerebral gene transfer (brain gene therapy) (10).

Refsum disease

Classic or adult Refsum disease is a rare disorder due to impaired alpha-oxidation of branched chain fatty acids that leads to increase of phytanic acids and its derivatives in plasma and various tissues.

It is also called *heredopathia atactica polyneuritiformis*. It should not be confused with infantile Refsum disease which is a peroxisomal disorder seen in infants. Adult Refsum disease can present in the school age child or adolescent with retinopathy, night blindness, cataracts, peripheral neuropathy, ataxia, anosmia, and sensorineural hearing loss.

Skin changes may arise that resemble eczema or ichthyosis. Treatment includes placing the individuals on phytanic acid restricted diet that includes avoidance of fats from ruminant animals and some fish. Plasmapheresis has also been tried in some situations.

Glycogen storage disease Type I

Glycogen storage disease type I (GSD I or von Gierke's disease) is the most common of the several types of glycogen storage diseases and is due to deficiency of the enzyme glucose-6-phosphatase leading to hypoglycemia, lactic acidosis, hyperlipidemia, and hyperuricemia. It is an autosomal recessive condition with three subtypes: GSD Ia (mutations of G6PC), GSD Ib (mutations of G6PT1), and GSD Ic (other mutations).

Growth failure and developmental delay (including mental retardation) occurs in children in poor, chronic metabolic control (11). Other problems include recurrent episodes of metabolic acidosis, neutropenia, impaired platelet aggregation (with epistaxis), and hepatomegaly.

Additional problems may arise in adolescents and adults, such as depression, pancreatitis, hyperuricemic gout, hepatic adenomas, chronic renal failure, and premature atherosclerosis (12). The hepatic adenomas present in most adults and can bleed or undergo malignant transformation. Proteinuria develops with renal hypertension, renal stones, and eventual development of focal segmental glomerulonephritis. Treatment involves prevention of hypoglycemia, metabolic acidosis, hyperlipidemia, and increased uric acid levels.

Diet control is important in this respect and an inexpensive manner to help is with cornstarch that provides gradually digested glucose. Allopurinol may be needed to manage hyperuricemia (Table 4) and statin medications for hyperlipidemia. Liver transplantation has been used in selected cases.

Glycogen storage disease Type II

Glycogen storage disease Type II (GSD II, Pompe disease, or acid maltase deficiency) is due to deficiency of acid alpha-glucosidase (GAA) enzyme in an autosomal recessive manner. Laboratory data include increased serum creatine kinase and urinary oligosaccharides along with complete or partial deficiency of GAA. The *infantile* type presents *in utero* or infancy with failure to thrive.

Late-onset (childhood, juvenile or adult) presents with respiratory dysfunction with proximal muscle weakness without cardiac disease. Death typically occurs in the adolescent to young adult years in the juvenile form. The adult form typically presents after age 20 (up to the 60s). GSD II is also a lysosomal storage disease (not GSD I) and most with late-onset disease show characteristic muscle biopsy changes.

Management includes attention to specific dysfunctions such as respiratory insufficiency, cardiomyopathy (in the infantile type), physical therapy for muscle weakness, surgery for contractures, wheelchair if necessary, and ventilator support as needed. Enzyme replacement therapy is available with alglucosidase alfa which is given intravenously and tends to work best with the adult or milder form of disease.

Gaucher disease

This is a rare autosomal recessive disorder due to a deficiency of the enzyme glucocerebrosidease (acid β-glucosidase) that results in lipid accumulation in cells (especially white blood cells) and various organs (i.e., brain, bone marrow, kidneys, lungs, liver, and spleen) (13).

It is the most common of the lysosomal storage diseases and is due to a gene located on chromosome 1. Gaucher disease is increased in incidence in the Ashkenazi Jewish population and low enzyme activity is noted in leukocytes or cultured skin fibroblasts. Bone marrow aspiration reveals “Gaucher storage cells” (onion-skin morphology in histiocytes).

Table 4. Medications for Inborn Errors of Metabolism

Medication	Indication	Adult Dosage	Side Effects	Comments
Penicillamine	Wilson's disease	0.75-1.5 gm/day Maximum: 2 gm/day Also administer: pyridoxine 25mg/day	Aplastic anemia, pruritis/rash, hypersensitivity reactions, proteinuria, membraneous glomerulopathy, increased skin friability, myasthenic syndrome, neurological toxicity, bone marrow suppression, drug fever, mouth ulcers, GI distress, anorexia, altered taste, neuropathy, intrahepatic cholestasis Avoid interruption in therapy due to risk of sensitivity reactions with reinstitution. Avoid in renal insufficiency.	*Optimal dosage determined by measurement of urinary copper excretion & free copper in serum *Administer 1hr before or 2 hrs after meals *Administer at least 1hr apart from other drugs, food or milk *Therapy protects against relapse during pregnancy: reduce dose to 750mg/day.
Trientine	Wilson's disease	Initial: 750-1250mg daily in 2-4 divided doses Maximum dose: 2gm daily	Hypersensitivity reactions, iron deficiency anemia, anorexia, dyspepsia, epigastric pain, muscle spasm, systemic lupus erythematosus, dystonia, myasthenia gravis	*Take on an empty stomach at least 1 hr before or 2 hrs after a meal *Administer at least 1 hr apart from all medicines *Do not give mineral supplements *If contact with capsule contents, wash with water due to risk for contact dermatitis
Sodium phenylbutyrate	Urea cycle disorder Orinthine transcarbamylase deficiency	Powder (>20kg): 9.9-13 $gm/m^2/day$ in 4-6 equally divided doses Tablets (>20kg): 9.9-13 $gm/m^2/day$ in 3 equally divided doses	Menstrual dysfunction, altered taste, body odor, decreased appetite, GI upset, fatigue, sedation, depression, headache, increased LFTs, metabolic abnormalities (acidosis, hyperchloremia, hypophosphatemia, hyperuricemia), hypoalbuminemia, bone marrow suppression	*Mix powder with solid or liquid foods; avoid acidic beverages *Level teaspoon provides 3.2gm of powder & 3gm of sodium phenylbutyrate *Level tablespoon provides 9.1gm of powder & 8.6gm of sodium phenylbutyrate
Arginine	Urea cycle disorder	Initial: 200 mg/kg IV over 90-120 min Maintenance: 200 mg/kg/day IV continuous infusion Maximum dose: 30gm	Extravasation, skin necrosis, hypersensitivity reactions, anaphylaxis Excessive rate can lead to local irritation, flushing, nausea, vomiting, headache	*Hyaluronidase may be used empirically for extravasation
Phenylacetate and sodium benzoate	Hyperammonemia associated with urea cycle disorder	Initial: 5.5 gm/m^2 IV over 90-120 min	Extravastation, skin necrosis, injection site reactions, pyrexia, nausea, vomiting, hyperglycemia, hypokalemia, convulsions,	*Use in conjunction with caloric supplementation and dietary protein restriction *Dilute prior to infusion

Medication	Indication	Adult Dosage	Side Effects	Comments
		Maintenance: 5.5 gm/m^2 IV over 24 hrs	mental impairment, brain edema, agitation, hypotension Use caution in hepatic and renal impairment	*Administer through a central line *Do not administer repeat loading doses *Drug interactions with penicillin, probenecid & valproic acid
Carnitine	Organic acidemia	Oral solution initial: 1 gm/day Oral solution maintenance: 1-3 gm/day Tablets: 990mg 2-3 times per day	Nausea, vomiting, abdominal cramps, diarrhea, body odor, seizures Decreasing dose can reduce drug-related body odor or GI symptoms	*Solution may be given alone or placed in drink/liquid food *Space doses evenly apart *Administer during or after meals *Consume slowly to maximize tolerance
Allopurinol	Hyperuricemia	100-800 mg/day >300mg/day: administer in divided doses	Acute gouty attacks, sedation, headache, rash, severe hypersensitivity reactions, increased liver function tests, nausea, diarrhea, peripheral neuropathy, bone marrow suppression	*Adjust dose according to serum uric acid levels *Dosage adjustment required with renal insufficiency *Administer after meals *Prophylactic colchicine may be needed when initiating treatment to prevent acute gouty attacks *Multiple drug interactions

Reference: Facts and Comparisons. Drug information full monographs. Wolters Kluwer Health, Incorporated. Available at: http://0-online.factsandcomparisons.com.libcat.ferris.edu/index.aspx. Accessed August 15, 2011.

Four types are identified with type 2 usually dying during the first few years of age from failure to thrive and neurologic features as ataxia, spasticity, dementia, seizures, myoclonus, and supranuclear ophthalmoplegia. Those with type 4 usually die within a few weeks of birth. Type 3 is a variant that is common in Scandinavian countries with type 3a resulting in death in the adolescent or young adult years.

Type 1 (non-neuropathic) is the most common form of Gaucher disese, is relatively mild, and may not be diagnosed due to subclinical features. It is the most common lysosomal storage disease and has increased incidence in the Ashkenazi Jewish population. Most diagnosed type 1 patients present in the adolescent or early adult years. Painless hepatosplenomegaly develops leading to abdominal distention and thrombocytopenia with excessive bleeding as well as anemia. The bone marrow expands due to the abnormal cells with bone remodeling and chronic bone pain that may severe, occur at night, and may be misdiagnosed as growing pains. Pathological fractures and avascular necrosis of the hips may arise. Pulmonary infiltration may develop leading to restrictive lung disease in adulthood.

Enzyme replacement therapy (intravenous recombinant glucocerebrosidase [imiglucerase; Veraglucerase alfa]) is used for type 1 and most of type 3 Gaucher patients. Bone marrow transplantation can cure non-neurological features of Gaucher's but carries high risk of complications. Other potential treatment options include splenectomy, blood transfusions, joint replacement, antibiotics, anti-epileptics, bisphosphonates, and liver transplantation. Splenectomy is a less frequent procedure now for these patients because it can lead to bone disease deterioration. Research is also evaluating such therapies as substrate reduction therapy (for type 2), gene therapy, and pharmacological chaperoning with drugs that work at a molecular level—such as miglustat and isofagomine tartrate.

Nieman-Pick Disease (NPD)

This is a rare, fatal, autosomal recessive lysosomal storage disease with a deficiency of acid sphingomyelinase. NPD is classified as a lipid storage disease (sphingolipidosis) with high levels of lipids accumulating in tissues such as brain, bone marrow, lungs, spleen, and liver. Types A (infantile) and B NPD are due to mutations in the SMPD1 gene while type C is due to mutations in NPC1 and NPC2 (14). NPD A and B are increased in the Ashkenazi Jewish population.

Type A is a severe degenerative disease in infants while Type B disease can present in mid to late childhood or later with a progressively enlarged spleen. Cirrhosis and pulmonary insufficiency can also develop. Bone marrow examination reveals characteristic "foamy storage" cells and enzyme deficiency can be seen in white blood cells ("sea blue" histiocytes) or cultured skin fibroblasts.

Treatment remains limited at this time and those with type B and C disease may live to their teenage or adult years (15). Organ transplant has been attempted for type B NPD with limited efficacy. Research is focusing on such drugs as zavesca (miglustat) for type C disease with progressive neurological disease. Research is also evaluating enzyme replacement and gene therapy.

Late-onset GM1 gangliosidosis

This is an autosomal recessive lysosomal storage disease due to the deficiency of lysosomal hydralase, acid β-galactosidase (beta-galactosidase enzyme), leading accumulation of GM1 ganglioside, oligosaccharides, and the mucopolysaccharide keratin sulfate (and deriviates) (16). Over 100 mutations have been reported in the beta-galactosidase gene (GLB1) (17). The enzyme deficiency leads to GM1 gangliosidosis and mucopolysaccharidosis type IVB (Morquio disease type B).

Three types of GM1 gangliosidosis are noted: *infantile (type 1), juvenile (type 2),* and *adult (type 3)*. It is lethal in types 1 and 2 disease. In the adult type there is an onset between 3 and 30 years of age. Features include early neurologic development with the gradual development of dementia, muscle atrophy, angiokeratomas, corneal clouding, extrapyramidal features, dystonia, and Parkinsonian features. Intellectual disability may be seen in an adolescent with this GM1 gangliosidosis. There is no specific treatment for this disorder at this time. Research is focusing on bone marrow transplantation, stem-cell transplantation, gene therapy, and enzyme replacement.

Late-onset GM2 gangliosidosis

This is due to deficiency of β-hexosaminidase A or A *and* B with a typical presentation in childhood between ages 2 and 10 years of age in an autosomal recessive pattern. Symptoms include ataxia, seizures, spasticity, dystonia, choreoathetosis, muscle wasting, blindness with retinal pigmentary features, pes cavus, psychomotor dysfunction, and others.

GM2 gangliosidosis may also develop in the adolescent years with severe mental health disorders---psychotic depression, paranoria, or acute schizophrenia. Enzyme deficiency is noted in serum, white blood cells, or cultured skin fibroblasts. The GM2 gangliosidoses include Tay-Sachs disease, AB variant, and Sandhoff disease; these are generally fatal by early childhood. Treatment options are limited and research is looking at such options as pyrimethamine (Table 3), leukovorin, enzyme replacement therapy, or gene therapy (18).

Fabry disease

Fabry disease (*angiokeratoma corporis diffusum*) is a rare x-linked recessive lysosomal storage disease. It is a sphingolipidosis due to deficiency of α-galactosidase that usually presents in later childhood or around puberty in a male with episodes of severe burning pain of feet and hands that may be misdiagnosed as "growing pains." The pain is out of proportion to the examination and there may be a history of hypohydrosis and periodic fevers. Joint pain develops that is similar to pauciarticular arthritis and abdominal pain may resemble inflammatory bowel disease (19). Laboratory tests reveal α-galactosidase deficiency (blood, white blood cells, cultured skin fibroblasts) and increased urinary excretion of ceramide trihexoside; urine examination reveals birefringent lipid globules ("Maltese Crosses"). It is often difficult to diagnose in females though heterozygous females may have similar pain episodes to males.

By ages 15 to 20 years, males develop angiokeratomata over buccal mucosa, umbilicus, and genital areas (bathing suit area). These angiokeratomas are small red/purple papules with a vascular appearance and may bleed but without additional symptoms. There can be periodic gastrointestinal distress with post-prandial discomfort, constipation, or diarrhea. Adolescent males also develop cardiac arrhythmias while slit-lamp examination reveals corneal verticillata. Transition to later adolescence and adulthood can lead to peripheral neuropathy (with pain episodes as well as loss of vibration sense and somatosensation), hypertrophic cardiomyopathy, proteinuria, renal disease, transient ischemic attacks, and cerebrovascular accidents. Males can have renal failure in their 20s to 40s.

Treatment includes use of various supportive medications such as antiepileptic drugs (i.e., gabapentin or carbamazepine), ace-inhibitors (for renal protection), aspirin or clopidogrel bisulfate (for stroke prophylaxis), NSAIDs, and other analgesics. Infusion of enzyme replacement therapy (agalsidase alpha, agalsidase beta) is a very expensive treatment modality that allows the patient to develop normal metabolism, prevent worsening of the disease, and perhaps symptom reversal (20).

Alpha-mannosidosis

This is a rare, autosomal recessive lysosomal storage disease caused by deficiency of the enzyme alpha-D-mannosidase that can range from mild to severe clinical subtypes (21). Deficient enzyme is noted in peripheral white blood cells or fibroblasts. MAN2B1 is a gene associated with this disorder. A severe type leads to prenatal or early infancy death while a moderate type leads to a variety of features before age 10, such as progressively skeletal abnormalities and myopathy.

The mild form may be identified in adolescence or adulthood without skeletal or muscle features. However, the mild subtype can have CNS disease (cerebellar dysfunction with ataxia), immunodeficiency, intellectual disability (mild to moderate), hearing impairment, psychiatric symptoms, skeletal abnormalities, and others. Disease progression can lead to hepatosplenomegaly, destructive arthritis, corneal opacities, and metabolic myopathy.

Management of alpha-mannosidosis involves carefully addressing specific issues as they arise including treating infections, hydrocephalus, hearing loss, and others. Genetic counseling for this autosomal recessive disorder is needed. Research is focusing on gene therapy, bone marrow or peripheral blood stem cell transplantation, and enzyme replacement therapy.

Late-onset urea cycle disorders

A urea cycle disorder or urea cycle defect results from a deficiency of one or more enzymes in the human urea cycle that takes ammonia out of the blood. Nitrogen is a waste product of protein, converted to urea, and removed from the body via the urine.

A number of urea cycle disorders are noted including deficiencies of these enzymes: N-acetylglutamate synthetase (with increased ammonia), carbamoyl phosphate synthetase I (with increased ammonia), argininosuccinic acid synthetase (increased citrulline--*citrullinemia*), arginase (increased arginine-*argininemia*), argininosuccinase acid lyase (increased argininosuccinic acid and citrulline—*argininosuccinic aciduria*), and ornithine transcarbamylase (with increased ornithine, uracil, and orotic acid—see below). They are autosomal recessive disorders except for the X-linked recessive ornithine transcarbamylase deficiency (see below).

Urea cycle disorders are generally identified in infancy or early childhood. However, some are diagnosed in adolescents or adults probably due to less severe degrees of enzyme deficiencies. In late onset urea cycle disorders there can be episodes of hyperammonemia caused by viral illnesses, lethargy, high-protein diets, childbirth, and even consumption of valproic acid (22). There is also increased glutamine in urea cycle defects along with alanine or asparagine as well as other amino acids depending on the specific defect. It can lead to lethargy, emesis, psychiatric illness symptoms, cerebrovascular accident-like symptoms, coma, and death (23). Some female carriers are asymptomatic until later in adulthood and exposed to metabolic challenge (such as pregnancy).

Management involves providing required protein in the diet without inducing hyperammonemia. Supplementation is provided with amino acid formulas as well as intravenous arginine hydrochloride (except in argininemia) (Table 4) along with vitamins, minerals, trace elements, and calcium depending on the specific deficiency (24). Some medications can lower ammonia levels and increase long-term survival via an alternative pathway. Drugs that reduce ureagenesis include sodium phenylacetate and sodium benzoate (Table 4) and they conjugate with nitrogen-containing amino acids to allow increased excretion of nitrogen in urine (25). Hemodialysis is needed for refractory situations and liver transplantation has been used in select cases. Improved newborn screening for urea cycle defects and other inborn errors of metabolism will allow early treatment and improved outcomes in these disorders.

Ornithine transcarbamylase deficiency

This rare X-linked recessive disorder is the most common of the urea cycle conditions and is due to deficiency of the enzyme ornithine transcarbamylase leading to an increase in serum ammonia, uracil, and orotic acid (26). Some males die shortly after birth while half or more die by age 5 years. Some are not diagnosed until adolescence or at variable times in adulthood (27,28). A variety of symptoms can arise including developmental delay, mental retardation, brittle hair, liver dysfunction, poor school performance, mood swings, encephalitis, and others. Some female carriers may not develop symptoms until subject to metabolic stress induced by starvation, malnutrition, pregnancy, surgery, or others.

Since the individual cannot process a high nitrogen load, treatment involves a low-protein diet to reduce nitrogen intake and reduce excessive body protein breakdown during acute illnesses with hydration and appropriate nutrition. Medications such as sodium phenylbutyrate (Table 4) or sodium benzoate may (Table 4) be helpful in this regard (29). For example, sodium benzoate combines with glycine to produce hippurate and remove an ammonium group (Table 3). Supplemental amino acids are helpful such as leucine, isoleucine, valine, citrulline, and arginine (Table 4). Biotin may benefical since it can stimulate ornithine transcarbamylase and may reduce ammonia levels (Table 3). Liver transplantation has been used in some patients.

Alkaptonuria

This is a rare autosomal recessive disorder of phenylalanine and tyrosine metabolism due to a defect in the enzyme homogentisate 1,2-dioxygenase, a liver enzyme that catalyzes oxidation of homogentisic acid which is the third step of tyrosine metabolism. Increased levels of homogentisic acid are noted in blood as well as urine and non-freshly voided urine will oxidize to a brown/black-blue color. It was the first IEM identified by professor Sir Archibald E Garrod (1857-1936) in 1902 and this condition is increased in frequency in Slovakia (1).

Though usually without symptoms in childhood or adolescence, extensive pigmentation may develop in adolescence or young adulthood or later with the deposition of pigment (bluish or brownish) in ears, sclera, heart valves, and others (ochronosis). Valvular heart disease (aortic and mitral calcification and regurgitation), hip or spinal damage, and ochronotic arthritis may develop that is similar to symptoms of rheumatoid arthritis or osteoarthritis in adults. Renal stones may also develop.

Treatment includes joint or heart valve replacement and treatment of coronary artery disease that may occur prematurely. There is no specific treatment for the defect of this disorder. Dietary restrictions of phenylalanine and tyrosine are recommended as well as increased doses of vitamin C. Research is evaluating the effectivenss of nitisinone that inhibits an enzyme that generates homogentisic acid (30).

Sanfillipo disease

Mucopolysaccharidoses (MPS) are a group of metabolic disorders due to the lack of or defects in various lysosomal enzymes used to metabolize glycosaminoglycans. A variety of MPS are noted (Table 2). Sanfillipo disease is a rare autosomal recessive lysosomal storage disease that is also called mucopolysaccharidosis III (MPS-III) and is due to deficiency in one of the enzymes required for metabolism of glycosaminoglycan heparin sulfate that is found in extracellular tissue and on cell surface glycoproteins.

Four types are identified: *MPS-III A* (deficiency of heparan N-sulfatase located on 17q25.3), *MPS-III B* (deficiency of N-acetyl-alpha-D-glucosaminidase located on 17q21), *MPS-III C* (deficiency of acetyl-CoA:alpha-glucosaminide acetyltransferase located on 8p11-q13), and *MPS-III D* (deficiency of N-acetylglucosamine-G-sulfate sulfatase located on 12q14). These four types are difficult to separate out on clinical grounds and the specific diagnosis is made with assay of the specific deficient enzyme in tissues via gene sequencing; prenatal diagnosis can be also accomplished.

Sanfillipo disease usually presents in young childhood but may not be seen until later in childhood or adolescence. A variety of behavioral and developmental problems can develop with intellectual decline (31). There can be hyperactivity, sleep disorders, aggressive behaviors, and others. Some MPS features (i.e., coarse hair, stiff joints, hirsuitism) may present later.

Mental retardation may be seen in adolescents with types B and D disease and some conditions present in adolescence with psychosis. Eventually other features also develop including hepatosplenomegaly, diarrhea, carious teeth, osteonecrosis of the hips, progressive scoliosis, immobility (with need for a wheelchair), swallowing problems, and epilepsy (32). Most do not live beyond the early twenties.

Treatment is mainly dealing with the specific complications that arise and bone marrow transplantation may be beneficial in early disease. Pharmacologic treatment of behavioral or psychiatric problems is usually not helpful. Replacement of the deficient enzymes does not penetrate the blood brain barrier and neurological features of MPS are not improved.

Research is focusing on gene therapy, development of replacement enzymes to penetrate the blood brain barrier, improvement of defective enzymes, and use of stem cell therapy. Improved neonatal screening would allow very early diagnosis which would improve outcome of management plans. Research is also evaluating the potential benefit of the flavonoid genistein (Table 3).

Homocystinuria

This is an autosomal recessive aminoaciduria due to methionine metabolism dysfunction because of cystathionine beta synthase deficiency (33,34). It is a defect of sulfur-containing amino acids (i.e., cysteine, methionine) with increased levels of homocysteine that are found in serum and urine while also eventually leading to a multisystem condition affecting the cardiovascular system, central nervous system, connective tissue, and muscles. At least 150 different mutations have been seen in the cystathionine β-synthase gene (33).

A classic feature is the development of Marfanoid appearance, ocular lens dislocation, and developmental delay (mental retardation). The Marfanoid habitus can include increased height, thin physique, dolichostenomelia, pes cavus, genu valgum, pectus excavatum (or carinatum), ectopia lentis, lens subluxation, myopia, glaucoma, and/or optic atrophy. The lens dislocation is usually downward versus an upward dislocation in Marfan syndrome. Homocystinuria is part of a differential diagnosis for tall stature in adolescents that includes Marfan syndrome, hyperthyroidism, obesity, Kleinfelter's syndrome, cerebral gigantism, pituitary gigantism, XYY syndrome, constitutional tall stature, and others. Patients with homocystinuria have tight joints and not the loose joints or aortic root dilatation as well as dissection noted with the Marfan syndrome.

There can be the development of atheroma of many arteries and intravascular thromboses due to increased homocystine in the blood which can lead to death in young adulthood or even earlier. Variable mental illness can develop as well. The adolescent with homocystinuria may have scoliosis, epilepsy, and mental subnormality (60%); the cognitive dysfunction may be due to S-adenosylhomocysteine accumulation in the CNS and/or repeated strokes. There can also be osteoporosis, vertebral collapse, and scoliosis.

Approximately half of those with homocystinuria improve with high doses of pyridoxine (vitamin B_6) (Table 3) and are called vitamin B_6 responders; others can be placed on a low methionine diet. Treatment options also include a high cystine diet, use of trimethylglycine, folic acid supplement, and even cystine. Betaine (N,N,N-trimethylglycine) can be used to lower homocystine levels because it stimulates conversion of homocysteine to methonine (Table 3); it is used with a low protein diet (low in methionine). Folate is added if the serum homocysteine level is increased with identified MTHFR gene mutation.

Cystinuria

This is caused by a defective kidney amino acid transporter protein in which the kidney is not able to reabsorb basic, positively charged amino acids in filtration. It is autosomal recessive and affects one in 10,000 persons. It may be subclinical and may not present until adolescence or adulthood. The urine shows marked increase in amino acids that are not absorbed such as cysteine, ornithine, lysine, arginine, and to some extent--histidine. A urinalysis shows hexagonal cystine crystals precipitating in the urine. Cystine stones develop in the kidney leading to symptomatic nephrolithiasis. Management is with hydration, urine alkalinization (with citrate supplementation), and dietary changes to lower salt and protein intake. Chelation therapy may be needed with such agents as penicillamine (Table 3). Surgery may be needed to remove renal stones.

Wilson's Disease

Wilson's disease (hepatolenticular degeneration) is an autosomal recessive condition due to copper metabolism dysfunction that leads to impaired biliary excretion of copper with copper accumulation in various tissues (i.e., liver, brain, cornea) and neurodegeneration (35).

Copper is toxic to these tissues. The genetic defect is on chromosome arm 13q and it affects copper-transporting adenosine triphosphatase (ATPase) gene (ATP7B) in the liver (36).

First noted in 1912, half of patients develop symptoms by mid-adolescence though the copper accumulation in tissues starts in infancy. It is unusual for symptoms to appear before 6 years of age. The urinary copper level is increased (>100 μg/24 hour) and a liver biopsy shows increased copper deposits. Ceruloplasmin is the protein that binds copper and serum ceruloplasmin is typically low in WD; the serum copper is also low. The serum ceruloplasmin can be normal in up to 20% of homozygotes for Wilson's disease and low in 10% of homozygotes who do not have the overt disease symptomatology.

The classic disease triad is due to copper deposits and includes hepatic disease, neuropsychiatric symptoms (Parkinson-like symptoms, schizophrenia, bipolar disorders), and Kayser-Fleisher rings (corneal copper deposits with golden discoloration in the membrane of Descemet at the limbic regions). However, manifestations of WD can be protean and the diagnosis difficult (37). There can be dystonia, dystonic posturing, incoordination, arm "wing-beating," dysphagia, dysarthria (nearly all), and even anarthria. The clinical and histologic picture of Wilson's disease can be identical to that of chronic active hepatitis.

Adolescents with unexplained recurrent liver disease and neurologic symptoms should be evaluated for Wilson's disease (36). The differential diagnosis includes cystic fibrosis, α_1-antitrypsin deficiency, sclerosing cholangitis (usually due to inflammatory bowel disease), chronic active hepatitis, and childhood cirrhosis. *Menkes disease* is an X-linked copper excretion disorder in boys due to a different copper transporter than WD in the Golgi apparatus; it starts in early infancy and leads to seizures, hypothermia, hypotonia, "wire-like" hair (*pili torti*), spasticity, failure to thrive, skin looseness, bladder diverticula, and death usually before age 3 years. There are no Keyser-Fleischer rings in Menkes disease and copper chelation does not benefit these patients.

Wilson's disease is fatal without effective therapy. The adolescent with Wilson disease should be on a low copper diet and avoid such foods as dried fruits, nuts, shellfish, liver, mushrooms, chocolate, and cocoa. Treatment involves early diagnosis and copper chelation with D-penicillamine or trientine (Table 4). Penicillamine is the most frequently used chelation agent for WD.

Usually the clinician begins with a low dose of 250 mg per day since rapid loss of copper from tissues may lead to neurological dysfunction or an acute hemolytic crisis. One can raise the dose 250 mg per week up to 1,000-1,200 mg per day. Adverse effects include gastric irritation that reduces compliance with the D-penicillamine. Pyridoxine is added to avoid the development of phosphate deficiency. Other potential side effects include proteinuria, nephrotic syndrome, bone marrow suppression, fever, pemphigus, lymphadenopathy, and collagen disease-like symptoms. The addition of corticosteroids may improve many of these side effects.

After ½ to 1 year after treatment, the daily urine copper excretion should be one third or less of values seen before staring chelation. If this is not seen, non-compliance with the D-penicillamine may be the reason. If the treatment is successful, the Kayser-Fleischer corneal rings disappear in one to two years. The progress is greatly improved if an early diagnosis is made and effective chelation occurs; some may even become asymptomatic. Chelation is also given to asymptomatic patients since treatment can prevent the onset of symptoms. Zinc acetate can be used after successful chelation or in the individual with asymptomatic WD disease. Mutational analysis is used to screen family members of one with known WD causative mutation; haplotype analysis is also used in genetic screening (35).

CONCLUSION

Inborn errors of metabolism (IEMs) are rare, complex, and often poorly understood disorders that typically involve deficiencies of enzymes needed for healthy maintenance of normal biochemical and metabolic pathways of human existence. There are hundreds of IEMs and their volume, complexity, and rarity result in limited understanding by clinicians and the high expense of their treatment.

Though many are identified *in utero* or early infancy, some present in later childhood, adolescence, or even various times in the adult years. A confusing myriad of features can be noted also adding to the complexities of accurate as well as timely diagnosis and successful management. IEMs present society with considerable challenges including how much care and research will be allotted for such often rare, complicated, and costly disorders of human physiology.

This discussion focuses on some of the known IEMs presenting in the adolescent years, such as adrenoleukodystrophy, glycogen storage diseases, lysosomal storage diseases, urea cycle disorders, and others. Management is often symptomatic or non-specific dealing with the numerous problems that can arise over the lifetime of these individuals. Enzyme replacement therapy (ERT) is provided if available and affordable since ERT is very expensive. Research is also looking at gene therapies, stem cell transplantation, and bone marrow transplantation.

Acknowledgments

This paper is an adapted version of a chapter in the book "Adolescent medicine: Pharmacotherapeutics in medical disorders" edited by Donald E Greydanus, Dilip R Patel, Cynthia Feucht, Hatim A Omar, Joav Merrick and published with permission by Walter de Gruyter, Berlin and New York.

References

[1] Garrod AE. The incidence of alkaptonuria: a study in chemical individuality. Lancet 1902;2:1616-20.

[2] Kamboj MK. Inborn errors of metabolism. In: Patel DR, Greydanus DE, Omar HA, Merrick J, eds. Neurodevelopmental disabilities: Clinical care for children and young adults. Dordrecht: Springer, 2011:53-67.

[3] Greydanus DE, Pratt HD. Syndromes and disorders associated with mental retardation. Indian J Pediatr 2005;72(10):859-64.

[4] Curry CJ, Stevenson RE, Aughton D. American College of Medical Genetics: Evaluation of mental retardation: Recommendations of a consensus conference. Am J Med Genet 1997;72:468-77.

[5] Shevell M. Practice parameter: Evaluation of the child with global developmental delay: Report of the Quality Standards Subcommittee of the American Academy of Neurology and the Practice Committee of the Child Neurology Society. Neurology 2003;60:367-80.

[6] Hsieh S, White PC. Presentation of primary adrenal insufficiency in childhood. J Clin Endocrinol Metab 2011;96(6):E925-8.

[7] Salzman A. Adrenoleukodystrophy patient perspective: turning despair into a gene therapy. Hum Gene Ther 2011;22(6):647-8.

[8] Biffi A, Aubourg P, Carter N. Gene therapy for leukodystrophies. Hum Mol Genet 2011; 20:R42-53.

[9] Hayashi T, Nakamura M, Ichiba M, Matsuda M, Kato M, Shiokawa N, et al. Adult-type metachromatic leukodystrophy with compound heterozygous ARSA mutations: A case report and phenotypic comparison with a previously reported case. Psychiatr Clin Neurosci 2011;65(1):105-8.

[10] Sevin C, Cartier-Lacave N, Aubourg P. Gene therapy in metachromatic leukodystrophy. Int J Clin Pharmacol 2009;47(Suppl 1):S128-31.

[11] Storch E, Keeley M, Merlo L, Jacob M, Correia C, Weinstein D. Psychosocial functioning in youth with glycogen storage disease type I. J Pediatr Psychol 2008; 33(7):728-38.

[12] Talente GM, Coleman RA, Alter C, Baker L, Brown BI, Cannon RA, et al. Glycogen storage disease in adults. Ann Int Med 1994;120(3):218-26.

[13] Grabowski GA. Phenotype, diagnosis, and treatment of Gaucher's disease. Lancet 2008; 372:1263-71.

[14] Xiong H, Bao XH, Zhang YH, Xu YN, Qin J, Shi HP, et al. Nieman-Pick disease type C: analysis of 7 patients. World J Pediatr 2011;8(7):10-5.

[15] Sévin M, Lesca G, Bauman N, Millat G, Lyon-Caen O, Vanier MT, et al. The adult form of Niemann-Pick disease type C. Brain 2007;130(Pt 1):120-33.

[16] Brunetti-Pierri N, Scaglia F. GM1 gangliosidosis: review of clinical, molecular, and therapeutic aspects. Mol Genet Metab 2008;94(4):391-6.

[17] Caciotti A, Garman SC, Rivera-Colón Y, Procopio E, Catarzi S, Ferri L, et al. GM1 gangliosidosis and Morquio B disease: An update on genetic alterations and clinical findings. Biochim Biophys Acta 2011;12(7):782-90.

[18] Tsuji D, Akeboshi H, Matsuoka K, Yasuoka H, Miyasaki E, Kasahara Y, et al. Highly phosphomannosylated enzyme replacement therapy for GM2 gangliosidosis. Ann Neurol 2011;69(4):691-701.

[19] Marchesoni CL, Roa N, Pardal AM, Neumann P, Caceres G, Martinez P, et al. Misdiagnosis in Fabry disease. J Pediatr 2010;156(5):828–31.

[20] Hoffmann B, Beck M, Sunder-Plassmann G, Borsini W, Ricci R, Mehta A. Nature and prevalence of pain in Fabry Disease and Its response to enzyme replacement therapy. A retrospective analysis from the Fabry Outcome Survey. Clin J Pain 2007;23(6):535-42.
[21] Malm D, Nilssen O. Alpha-mannosidosis. Orphanet J Rare Dis 2008;3(1):21-4.
[22] Summar ML, Barr F, Dawling S, Smith W, Lee B, Singh RH, et al. Unmasked adult-onset urea cycle disorders in the critical care setting. Crit Care Clin 2005;21(Suppl 4):S1-8.
[23] Gropman A, Batshaw M. Cognitive outcome in urea cycle disorders. Mol Genet Metab 2004;81(Suppl 1): 58-62.
[24] Scaglia F. New insights in nutritional management and amino acid supplementation in urea cycle disorders. Mol Genet Metab 2010;100(Suppl 1):572-6.
[25] Enns GM, Berry SA, Berry GT, Rhead WJ, Brusilow SW, Hamosh A. Survival after treatment with phenylacetate and benzoate for urea-cycle disorders. N Engl J Med 2007;356(22):2282-92.
[26] Tuchman M, Jaleel N, Morizono H, Sheehy L, Lynch MG. Mutations and polymorphisms in the human ornithine transcarbamylase gene. Hum. Mutat 2002;19(2): 93–107.
[27] Rohininath T, Costello DJ, Lynch T, Monavari A, Tuchman M, Treacy EP. Fatal presentation of ornithine transcarbamylase deficiency n a 62-year old man and family studies. J Inherit Metab Dis 2004;27(2):285-8.
[28] Brajon D, Carassou P, Pruna L, Feillet F, Kaminsky P. Ornithine transcarbamylase deficiency in an adult. Rev Med Interne 2010;31(10):709-11.
[29] Marini JC, Lanpher BC, Scaglia F, O'Brien WE, Sun Q, Garlick PJ, et al. Phenylbutyrate improves nitrogen disposal via alternative pathway without eliciting an increase in protein breakdown and catabolism in control and ornithine transcarbamylase deficient patients. Am J Clin Nutr 2011;93(6):1248-54.
[30] Suwannarat P, O'Brien K, Perry MB, Sebring N, Bernardini I, Kaiser-Kupfer MI, et al. Use of nitisinone in patients with alkaptonuria. Metab Clin Exp 2005;54(6):719–28.
[31] Valstar MJ, Marchal JP, Grootenhuis M, Colland V, Wijburg FA. Cognitive development in patients with Mucopolysaccharidosis type III (Sanfilippo syndrome). Orphanet J Rare Dis 2011;6:43-46.
[32] White KK, Karol LA, White DR, Hale S. Musculoskeletal manifestations of Sanfilippo syndrome (mucopolysaccharidosis type III). J Pediatr Orthop 2011;31(5):594-8.
[33] Mudd SH. Hypermethioninemias of genetic and non-genetic origin: A review. Am J Med Genet C Semin Med Genet 2011;157(1):3-32.
[34] Maillot F, Kraus JP, Lee PJ. Environmental influences on familial discordance of phenotype in people with homocystinuria: a case report. J Med Case Reports 2008;2(1): 113-6.
[35] Ferenci P. Wilson's disease. Clin Gastroenterol Hepatol 2005;3(8):726-33.
[36] Hancu A, Mihai MC, Axelerad AD. Wilson's disease: A challenging diagnosis. Clinical manifestations and diagnostic procedures in 12 patients. Rev Med Chir Soc Med Nat Iasi 2011;115(1):58-63.
[37] Pfeiffer RF. Wilson's disease. Handb Clin Neurol 2011;100:681-709.

Submitted: November 10, 2011. *Revised:* December 10, 2011. *Accepted:* December 21, 2011.

In: Child and Adolescent Health Yearbook 2013
Editor: Joav Merrick

ISBN: 978-1-63117-658-6

Chapter 6

KIDNEY DISEASES IN ADOLESCENCE

Alfonso D Torres, MD and
Donald E Greydanus, MD, Dr HC (ATHENS)*
Department of Pediatric & Adolescent Medicine,
Western Michigan University School of Medicine, Kalamazoo,
Michigan, United States of America

ABSTRACT

The renal system is a critically important and complex organ system needed for normal growth and health in the adolescent. This paper reviews paramount issues in this regard including urinary tract infections, proteinuria, hematuria, and glomerulonephritis. This discussion considers the nephrotic syndrome, minimal changes disease (MCD), collapsing focal segmental glomerulosclerosis, IgA nephropathy, post-streptococcal glomerulonephritis, Henoch-Schönlein Purpura (HSP) Nephritis, hemolytic-uremic syndrome, lupus nephritis, and other renal disorders in adolescents. Concepts of diagnosis and management are presented. Consultation with colleagues in nephrology is recommended for adolescents with complex and refractory renal conditions.

Keywords: Adolescence, kidney diseases

INTRODUCTION

Urinary tract infections are common conditions in adolescent females. Glomerular diseases represent the most characteristic abnormalities affecting the kidney in adolescents. The clinical manifestations range from asymptomatic, incidental findings during a routine medical assessment such as proteinuria or microscopic hematuria to life-threatening condition with rapid deterioration of multiple organ function including acute kidney injury. The clinical

* Correspondence: Professor Donald E Greydanus, MD, Dr. HC (ATHENS), Chair, Department of Pediatric & Adolescent Medicine, Western Michigan University School of Medicine, 1000 Oakland Drive, D48G Kalamazoo, MI 49008-1284 United States. E-mail: donald.greydanus@med.wmich.edu

evaluation rests in a comprehensive history, physical examination and other investigations aimed to assess renal function and to the presence of extrarenal disease. Asymptomatic urine abnormalities are the most frequent conditions reported. The incidence is related to the community or country practices for routine urinalysis. In the United States a urinalysis is requested for adolescents who enroll in organized sports at high school or at college level and for individuals that join the Armed Forces. In Japan and other Asian Countries urinalysis is routinely performed at school.

Some definitions

The definition of microscopic hematuria in children is 3 or more red blood cells (RBC) /high power fields in the centrifuged sediment from 10 ml of freshly voided midstream urine collection, with the RBC usually dysmorphic. In the adult the upper normal limit of RBC in the urine is 2 per high power field in the spun urinary sediment.

Proteinuria can detected by the ubiquitous use of the dipstick or the use of sulfosalicylic acid test and be semi-quantitatively assessed methods such as the ratio of urine protein concentration in mg/dl to urine creatinine concentration in mg/dl, with the accepted normal value of < 0.2 for older children, adolescents and adults; this is also by 24 hours urine collection for the determination of urine protein, with values of $150/1.73m^2$ mg in 24 hours accepted as upper normal values in boys and in girls. The presence of proteinuria and hematuria particularly with dysmorphic reb blood cells (RBCs) and cast is an indication of glomerular involvement. Macroscopic hematuria or gross hematuria (usually brown or red in color) with proteinuria and no clots, that is sometimes recurrent, is seen in adolescents with IgA nephropathy.

The nephrotic syndrome is defined as heavy proteinuria, that causes hypoalbuminemia; in the adult the proteinuria is > 3.5 g a day and in the child 50 mg/kg of protein excretion a day, in association with edema, hypercholesterolemia, and lipiduria. The Nephritic Syndrome is usually characterized by sudden onset of oliguria, hematuria, red cell casts moderated proteinuria, oliguria hypertension and edema, usually preceded by an infection; in general, it is self limited.

Rapid progressive glomerulonephritis is characterized by rapid deterioration of renal function in a matter of days or weeks, associated with moderated, non severe proteinuria, usually of < 3g/day; the blood pressure may be normal or moderately elevated. Often, extrarenal manifestations of vasculitis are also observed. The renal biopsy usually demonstrated crescentic glomerulonephritis in high percentage of the glomeruli. Rapid therapeutic intervention is needed in order to preserve renal function. Chronic glomerulonephritis is characterized by decreased renal function, hypertension, proteinuria of variable severity, and usually small kidneys.

Clinical symptoms of an underlying acute or chronic renal parenchymal disorder, when present, usually relates to the dominant physiologic disturbance. For instance, adolescents with chronic reflux nephropathy and moderately severe hypertension may complain of blood pressure-related headaches or visual disturbances. By contrast, patients with acute nephritis may experience flank pain while those with the severe anemia characteristic of nephronophthisis/ medullary cystic disease, may be most concerned about their fatigue and diminished mental performance. In many youth, the clinical course of the kidney disease is silent until the process is sufficiently advanced as to produce findings such as diminished growth, edema, uremia, oliguria, hypertension, or colic from urolithiasis. Therefore, many of those cases with initially silent clinical courses may only be discovered at the time of routine health screening examinations.

Many serious renal disorders which present in childhood may, for the adolescent, progress to become the problems of chronic or even end-stage renal disease, dialysis, and transplantation. Other disorders do not appear until the teenage years, with diagnostic and early treatment issues as the principal clinical concerns. The importance of chronic renal insufficiency in adolescents is reflected in the finding that between 25%–27% of chronic renal failure in pediatric patients is reported in adolescents between 13 and 17 years. This section will primarily focus upon those renal disorders that may arise and require evaluation during the teenage years. However, we will start with a discussion of urinary tract infections.

URINARY TRACT INFECTION

Epidemiology

Urinary tract infections (UTIs) are common infections identified throughout the life span, particularly for females. Infection of the bladder (cystitis) is 3 to 5 times more common in the female versus the male and typically develops as a primary infection in a healthy individual (1-3). The first episode incidence decreases during the first 10 years of life and gradually increases over time, especially in the female.

Table 1 lists factors noted as risk factors for UTI occurrence and include vesicoureteral reflux (VCR), voiding dysfunction, constipation (i.e., causes voiding dysfunction), and others. Five percent or more of females who are 5 to 18 years of age develop a UTI with an incidence of 2% in adolescent females, and over 20% of females experience at least one UTI during their reproductive years. Approximately 30% of females have recurrent UTIs. The incidence of UTI in males is highest in the first year of life and after 55 years of age (due to prostatic hypertrophy) and it is at its lowest during the young adult years.

Etiology

The main uropathogens of cystitis in adolescents are enterobacteriaceae (particularly *Escherichia coli*) and coagulase negative staphylococci, though others may be causative as well (see table 2) (4). A number of factors place the individual at risk for UTIs as noted in table 1. This includes coital behavior in females that may result in incomplete bladder emptying. Approximately 20% of females with bacteriuria have vesicoureteral reflux (VUR). The virulence of the E coli strain can be enhanced by pili or fimbriae (type I and type II) on the outer surface of the bacteria that increase its adherence to epithelial cells leading to more invasive infections. Virulence factor genes are associated with persistence or recurrence of infections. Urogenital abnormalities increase the incidence of infection leading to an upper urinary tract infection (pyelonephritis) due to E coli, drug-resistant enteric pathogens, and others-- especially in those with chronic or recurrent diseases. Recurrent infection may occur as a relapse (with the same organism as before) versus a reinfection with a different organism. Multiple antibiotic usage may lead to infection with two or more pathogenic strains. A relapse may be due to incomplete treatment of an initial infection and/or complication of underlying urolithiasis or a structural urogenital abnormality.

Table 1. Factors Contributing to the Risk of UTI*

Females
Anatomic short urethra
Poor perineal hygiene
Coital irritation, change of coital patterns, new sexual partner ("honeymoon cystitis")
Vulvovaginitis
Vaginal or rectal colonization with pathogenic bacterial serogroups (viz. *E. coli*)
Pregnancy (abnormal ureteral peristalsis)
Bladder contamination secondary to douching
Vaginal foreign body
Diaphragm and/or spermicide use (controversial for disease)
Males
Urethral strictures (extremely rare in girls who have not had prior surgery, trauma, or radiation)
Posterior urethral valves
Phimosis
Meatal stenosis
Sexual practices exposing the urethra to fecal flora
UTI is increased in uncircumcised versus circumcised males
Males or Females
Urologic abnormality with stasis and/or obstruction (dysfunctional bladder [neurogenic or other], ectopic ureter, nephrolithiasis, etc.)
Vesicoureteral reflux
Urethral instrumentation (catheters, foreign bodies, masturbatory)
Urethral trauma
Other foci of infection (direct extension from kidney, prostate, vagina or hematogenous spread from distant site)
Lowered host resistance to infection (including due to HIV infection)
Multiple antibiotic usage and development of resistant organisms
Infrequent or incomplete voiding
Voluntary urinary retention
Chronic illnesses such as diabetes

*Reprinted with permission from: Greydanus DE, Torres, AD, Wan JH: "Genitourinary and renal disorders" in: Essential Adolescent Medicine. Editors: DE Greydanus, DR Patel, DH Pratt, NY: McGraw Hill Medical Publishing Division, Ch 16: 330, 2006.

Table 2. Etiologic agents in UTIs

Escherichia coli (E. coli: 80%-90%)
Staphylococcus saprophyticus (15%)
Enterobacter aerogenes
Enterococcus species
Klebsiella pneumoniae
Proteus mirabilis
Pseudomonas aeruginosa
Serratia marcescens
Gastrointestinal pathogens (i.e., Salmonella, Shigella, Campylobacter)
Adenovirus (types 11 and 21)
Rare: Staphylococcus aureus (consider other source of infection), Group B Streptococcus, Mycobacterium tuberculosis, Haemophilus influenzae B
Nosocomial Infection (Yeasts [Candida albicans], Staphylococcus aureus, Gram-negative rods)
Human papovavirus BK

Diagnosis

Clinical manifestations of UTIs can range from being asymptomatic to fulminant systemic infections. Typical symptoms of a simple cystitis or lower urinary tract infection are listed in Table 3. Pain on urination (dysuria) along with other UTI symptoms suggests a lower URI; suprapubic pain may be present These features may also be present in the acute urethral syndrome and urethritis. Dysuria may also occur in those with vaginitis though there is usually less urinary frequency and urgency along with the presence of vulvovaginal inflammation. Examination may reveal phimosis in males, labial adhesions in girls, or evidence of sexual abuse or trauma in both. There may be a dimple over the back or other defects noted with neurogenic bladder and spinal cord involvement.

Frequency and urgency can result from viral cystitis and also from irritation induced by consumption of chocolate, caffeine, or carbonated beverages. Chemical irritation can occur from female hygiene products. Bedwetting in a previous toilet trained child and/or foul smelling urine in a developmentally disabled child or adolescent may suggest a UTI as well.

Table 3. Urinary Tract Symptoms

Dysuria
Urinary frequency
Hesitancy
Urgency
Nocturia
Urination produces small amount of urine (can be turbid or bloody)
Low abdominal pain including suprapubic pain
Low grade temperature elevation
Hematuria (gross or microscopic)

Acute hemorrhagic cystitis may occur due to E coli, adenovirus (types 11 and 21), or human papovavirus BK. Adenovirus-induced hemorrhagic cystitis is more commonly seen in boys, is self-limiting, and usually resolves in four days or so. Interstitial cystitis is noted in adolescent females with UTI-like symptoms including bladder/pelvic pain improved with voiding but with negative urine cultures. Cystoscopy reveals bladder distention with mucosal ulcers. It is an idiopathic condition with no specific beneficial treatment.

Sometimes distinguishing a lower UTI from an upper urinary tract infection (acute pyelonephritis [involvement of renal parenchyma]) can be difficult because the symptoms may be similar. In pyelonephritis there may be fever, chills, and variable costovertebral tenderness. Confusion may occur with other causes of abdominal pain, such as appendicitis, cholecystitis, hepatitis, and others. The risk of developing pyelonephritis increases in those with functional or structural urinary tract abnormalities. It is usually an ascending infection from the urethra to the bladder and upper urinary tract; rarely, it may be blood-borne. Potential complications of pyelonephritis include renal scarring (pyelonephritic scarring), renal abscess, septic shock, hypertension, proteinuria with or without FSGS (focal segmental glomerulosclerosis), pregnancy-related complications, renal impairment, and end-stage renal failure.

Laboratory

Classic supportive laboratory data include pyuria of over 10 white blood cells per high power microscopic field of spun urine sediment, a positive Gram stain with one or more bacteria per high power field of uncentrifuged urine, and/or a positive urine culture with antibiotic sensitivities to identify the etiologic microbe and the most effective antibiotic treatment based on results of sensitivity testing. A urine dipstick typically includes tests of leukocyte esterase and nitrite for white blood cells and gram-negative bacteria respectively. Sensitivity of the leukocyte esterase (LE) test is 76 to 85% and sensitivity of the nitrite reaction is variable, from 29 to 70%.

It should be noted that negative results from symptomatic patients require cautious interpretation since false negative results can be common while gram-positive and non-bacterial infections can be missed. A positive nitrite test performed on freshly voided urine specimen is highly suggestive of a UTI while negative microscopy for bacteria with a negative LE test has high negative predictive value for a UTI. A negative Gram stain of urine for bacteria with the presence of fewer than 10 WBCs/mm3 essentially rules out a UTI.

Traditionally a bacterial colony count $>10^5$ CFU/mL of a specific bacteria from a clean voided specimen defines the etiologic agent that allows effective treatment for cystitis or pyelonephritis. This correlates with actual infection in 80% with a false positive rate of 20%; two positive cultures of the same microbe correlate with true infection in 95%. Youth with symptoms of cystitis or even pyelonephritis can have colony counts as low as 10^4/mL while counts as low as 10^2/mL may be noteworthy in situations of urethritis or when the urine was gathered via suprapubic aspiration or catheterization. Symptomatic urethritis may have counts between 10^2 and 10^5especially in males.

A negative urine culture in sexually active adolescents with symptoms suggestive of a UTI should prompt evaluation for urethral infection with such STD agents as Chlamydia trachomatis, Neisseria gonorrhoeae, Trichomonas vaginalis or herpes simplex virus. The growth of mixed cultures, even with high counts, usually suggests contamination of the specimen.

Approximately 70% with a significant culture have infections localized to the bladder while 30% will have dual infection in the lower and upper urinary tracts. An elevated white blood count (leukocytosis, neutrophilia), elevated erythrocyte sedimentation rate, and elevated C-reactive protein may be seen in pyelonephritis.

Recurrent or complex UTIs

A single episode of a UTI in a male or repeated UTIs in female adolescents (i.e., 2-3 episodes of cystitis over 1-2 years) would warrant further investigation for underlying factors. Renal ultrasonography may reveal a urogenital abnormality such as hydronephrosis, renal cysts, or renal calculi. A CT (computed tomography) scan and intravenous urography can reveal renal calculi with a negative sonography.

Voiding cystourethrography (isotope or contrast) can detect vesicoureteral reflux (VCU) as well as bladder and/or urethral abnormalities. Renal magnetic resonance imaging (MRI) is an effective tool for the diagnosis and follow-up of acute pyelonephritis.

In subclinical or overt pyelonephritis a technetium ^{99}m-dimercaptosuccinic acid (DMSA) renal scan can detect infectious foci in the renal parenchyma and/or renal scarring from previous renal infection. A CT scan or ultrasound can identify a renal abscess.

Management

Successful treatment of a UTI involves knowledge of the *specific* causative agent based on culture and sensitivity results (1-3,5,6). Prompt treatment reduces risks for recurrence and complications. Adolescent females with an acute, uncomplicated cystitis can usually be adequately treated with a three day course of an oral trimethoprim-sulfamethoxazole, trimethoprim, or a fluoroquinolone (see table 4). Treatment of urinary tract infections can also include use of oral analgesics (as NSAIDs) and urinary analgesics as phenazopyridine hydrochloride. This urinary analgesic is given at 200 mg three times a day for two days and may partially relieve urinary burning, frequency, or urgency. Adverse effects include headaches, gastric irritation and rash; the urine may turn orange or red and there can be staining of clothes or contact lens.

Table 4. Antibiotic treatment of simple UTIs

Ciprofloxacin: 250 mg twice daily for three days *
(used off label for patients who are prepubescent)
Levofloxacin: 250 mg once a day for three days
Nitrofurantoin: 50 mg-100 mg four times daily for seven days
Trimethoprim-sulfamethoxazole Double Strength
(160 mg/800 mg): Twice daily for three days
Trimethroprim: 100 mg twice daily for three days
Others: See text

Research suggests that fluoroquinolones (i.e., ciprofloxacin) may induce cartilage damage in children but it has been effective against pseudomonas infection. Oral cefixime and parenteral ceftriaxone can be effective against Gram-negative microbes except for pseudomonas. Aminoglycosides can have nephrotoxic and ototoxic effects but can be effective against pseudomonas.

Ampicillin and cephalosporins alter periurethral and fecal flora with the resultant encouragement of multidrug resistance. Recent studies note the emergence of extended-spectrum β–lactamase-producing E coli leading to increased resistance to β-lactam antibiotics (i.e., amoxicillin-clavulanic acid, trimethoprim-sulfamethoxazole, quinolones) in addition to the ineffectiveness of cephalosporins and vancomycin against enterococci. Additional antibiotics include nitrofurantoin, fosfomycin (single dose in cystitis), daptomycin, linezolid, and others. Nitrofurantoin does not achieve effective renal tissue levels.

A longer course of antibiotics may be necessary with complicating factors, such as diabetes mellitus, pregnancy, use of a diaphragm, or history of frequent UTIs (6-10). Cystitis in the male is treated for 7 to 10 days and mild cases of pyelonephritis may be managed on an ambulatory basis with 7 to 10 days of oral antibiotics. Those with severe disease and/or situations complicated by urosepsis, severe illness, or others may need hospitalization with intravenous antibiotic coverage that can include third generation cephalosporins; an alternative treatment is ampicillin plus gentamicin or an antipseudomonal penicillin After the patient is improved, antibiotic switch therapy can be used in switching from intravenous to oral antibiotics in selective situations.

Recurrent UTI management

The female with recurrent cystitis despite absence of any genitourinary abnormality may see less infections if on antibiotic prophylaxis for 4 to 6 months (11-13). Examples include taking these antibiotics and doses at night: nitrofurantoin 50 mg to 100 mg, trimethoprim 100 mg, or trimethoprim-sulfamethoxazole (80 mg/400 mg)—half a tablet. If coital activity seems to be a factor, she can take an antibiotic immediately after coitus; examples include 100 mg of nitrofurantoin, ½ tablet (or 1 tablet) of trimethoprim-sulfamethoxazole (double-strength), or 250 mg of ciprofloxacin.

Avoidance of coitus may also be helpful. Other measures that may be beneficial include proper perineal hygiene (particularly post-defecation) and postcoital voiding. If use of a diaphragm and spermicide are underlying factors, a different form of birth control may be helpful. Recent research is looking at the efficacy of intravesical instillation of hyaluronic acid and chondroitin sulfate in adult females with recurrent UTIs (14). Cranberry juice has not been shown to prevent recurrent UTIs (15). Circumcision may help if phimosis is a precipitating factor.

Bacteriuria

Epidemiologic studies note that 3% to 5% of adolescent females without UTI symptoms have $>10^5$ CFU/mL of a specific bacterial microbe on repeat urine cultures. Evaluation reveals a normal upper urinary tract, bladder function, and normal VUR studies. The impact of this is unclear, though some do eventually clear themselves of the bacteria. Antibiotic coverage can transiently clear the bacteria, but the bacteriuria recurs when antibiotics are stopped. Distinguishing between asymptomatic bacteriuria and a UTI can be difficult in some situations. Progressive renal injury is usually not seen in adolescents or young adults with histories of childhood bacteriuria.

There is increased risk of bacteriuria recurrence (asymptomatic or symptomatic) during pregnancy and those not treated in childhood with antibiotics may develop reduced renal adaption to later pregnancy (16). Though controversial, treatment of adolescent females with asymptomatic bacteriuria and normal studies is not recommended if she is not pregnant and may be problematic because of possible alteration of the urinary flora from low-virulence microbes to higher-virulence. The work-up should rule out incontinence (day or night) and perineal discomfort. If she has post-coital cystitis, treatment may be warranted. Also, if she becomes pregnant, antibiotic treatment is recommended because of the increased risk for pyelonephritis, miscarriage, and fetal infection.

Proteinuria

Clinically asymptomatic proteinuria is a frequent finding in adolescents and young adults. The vast majority of patients with asymptomatic proteinuria will be found to have orthostatic (postural) or intermittent proteinuria. Orthostatic proteinuria has a good prognosis and intermittent proteinuria is carefully followed up to ensure it does not become persistent. Also, proteinuria is a common hallmark of many renal diseases; unless it is sufficiently severe as to cause nephrotic syndrome, clinical findings may be scant. The situation may become more clouded since fever, strenuous exercise, dehydration, extreme cold, and, possibly, emotional stress, often increase the rate of protein excretion both in normal individuals and patients with kidney disease-associated proteinuria.

False-positive dipstick results for urine protein should be considered in all asymptomatic patients with unexplained proteinuria; these include highly buffered urine from alkaline medications or storage, urine contamination by quaternary ammonium cleaning agents. urine pH>7.0, leaving dipstick in the urine too long (i.e., washing out the buffer), and use of phenazopyridine (for some dipstick brands). Also note that urine proteins other than albumin are not readily detected by standard dipstick testing. Thus, gamma globulins, Bence Jones proteins, hemoglobin, lysozyme, and others may produce negative results. Detection of non-albumin urinary proteins can be routinely accomplished using sulfosalicylic acid and most specifically by protein electrophoresis in urine. A positive dipstick for proteinuria is an indication for quantification of proteinuria.

Quantification of proteinuria

The traditional method for quantification of proteinuria has been the 24-hour urine collection, expressed as g/L or g/24 hour. Normal values range between 30–150 mg/24/hours.in adults and around 100 $mg/m^2/day$ in children.

A more practical alternative is the measurement of the protein to creatinine ratio expressed as gram of protein per gram of creatinine in a randomly collected urine sample. It has an excellent correlation with the 24-hour urine collection. Normal values are <0.2 after 5 years of age.

Orthostatic proteinuria

Orthostatic proteinuria is a condition most generally described as the presence of abnormally high rates of protein excretion occurring in the upright position only. When unassociated with any other urinary abnormality (i.e., hematuria), long term follow-up studies have demonstrated that the risk of underlying significant renal disease is not increased for the normal population. Since the majority of adolescents evaluated for protein in the urine will be found to have intermittent or orthostatic proteinuria, the clinician's first task is to screen out those patients with a benign diagnosis.

Normal males excrete 20–26 mg/kg/day of creatinine while normal females excrete 14–22 mg/kg/day. The upper limit of normal protein excretion is approximately 100 $mg/m^2/24$ hours (150–200 mg/24 hours). The diagnosis of orthostatic proteinuria is based upon first-morning recumbent urine protein testing by dipstick that is negative or trace, increased values during daytime activity, and less than 1,000 mg of protein/24 hours (some authors suggest an upper limit of 2,000 mg/24 hours). A number of different algorithms for the diagnosis of orthostatic proteinuria have been proposed. A useful approach is described below which can be applied to the adolescent found to have proteinuria and no historical or physical finding suggestive of underlying renal or urologic disease; this method allows one to demonstrate the orthostatic component of the proteinuria.

In this method a 24-hour "split" urine collection is recommended. The test requires two clean containers, usually provided by the laboratory performing the test. On the day of the test, the first voided urine specimen is discarded and the time is noted. All the urines voided the rest of the day are collected in one container and labeled "daytime urine collection". Before retiring to bed, the adolescent should rest, reclining for 1–2 hours. Just before going to bed the teen should urinate, place the urine in the daytime urine collection container, note the time, and the teen retires to bed for the night. The following morning, the teen should urinate, if possible by the bed side. The urine is collected in the second container and labeled "night time urine collection". Both containers are taken to the laboratory for determination of volume, protein and creatinine content; also, the ratio of grams of protein to grams of creatinine excretion in each container is established. The normal urine protein to urine creatinine excretion ratio is <0.2; an elevated protein excretion during the day time in the presence of normal protein excretion during the night establishes the presence of orthostatic or postural proteinuria (17).

The general consensus among nephrologists is that orthostatic proteinuria has a good prognosis and that renal biopsy is not necessary; it seems prudent to follow these patients at yearly or every 2-year intervals. Indications for renal biopsy vary according to the considerations of the ethnicity, age and geographic characteristics of the population studied. Most common indications for renal biopsy are listed in table 5 (18).

Rapid deterioration of renal function requires an emergency renal biopsy to exclude or confirm crescentic glomerulonephritis. Isolated microscopic hematuria in which all other studies are normal require follow-up, but the need for prompt renal biopsy is less clear.

Few contraindications for renal biopsy exist and include uncontrolled bleeding diathesis, uncontrolled hypertension, uncooperative patient, renal neoplasm, and renal infection multiple cyst; a solitary kidney is a relative contraindication. Contraindications for renal biopsy are noted in table 6.

Table 5. Indications for renal biopsy (18)

Nephrotic Syndrome: in prepubertal children only if the clinical presentation is atypical for MCD; renal biopsy is indicated in adolescents and adult patients, because the other than MCD causes of nephrotic syndrome are common
In acute kidney injury after obstruction, reduced renal perfusion, acute tubular necrosis, acute post streptococcal glomerulonephritis have been rule out
Systemic disease with renal dysfunction: small vessels vasculitis, anti-glomerular basement membrane disease, systemic lupus erythematosus. Those with diabetes only if atypical features are present.
Isolated microscopic hematuria only in unusual circumstances
Non- nephrotic range proteinuria, > 1g/day
Unexplained chronic kidney disease, may be diagnostic: IgA nephropathy, Nephronophthisis
Familial renal disease: Biopsy of one affected member may be diagnostic and minimize clinical investigation of other affected members
Renal transplant dysfunction: indicated if ureteral obstruction, infection, vascular thrombosis calcineurin toxicity are **not** present.

Laboratory studies

Adolescents with persistent proteinuria particularly associated with one or more of renal factors listed above, should be considered for referral to a subspecialist for further evaluation and possible renal biopsy. Although many tests for underlying renal disease may be performed by the primary care physician, tests beyond quantitative protein excretion measurements and basic renal function studies are oftentimes best done in the context of a formal nephrology evaluation. Once the proteinuria has been characterized as a non-orthostatic, persistent proteinuria (see above) and appropriate measures taken, serial quantitative changes of protein excretion may be approximated without the need of repeated 24-hour urine collections.

The technique for this estimate uses a random daytime specimen of urine in which protein and creatinine concentrations are measured. The protein concentration divided by the creatinine concentration (in the same units, e.g., mg/dL, g/L) multiplied by the factor 0.63, gives the result in grams of protein excreted/m^2/24 hours. This method of long-term reevaluation is an attractive alternative to task of 24-hour urine collections, one the often-dreaded by adolescents attending school or working.

Urinalysis is an important aspect in the evaluation of any patient with proteinuria; unfortunately, the microscopic evaluation of the urinary sediment is becoming an infrequent exercise for many physicians. A simple estimation of renal function can be obtained by measuring BUN, creatinine, electrolytes, and CO_2 in serum. Adolescents with non-orthostatic proteinuria require renal ultrasound evaluation to detect structural abnormalities, such as number of renal units, cystic diseases, renal asymmetry, or hydronephrosis. These basic studies can be performed by the primary care physician; however, adolescents with non-orthostatic proteinuria, need to be referred to a nephrologist for further evaluation and management.

NEPHROTIC SYNDROME

Etiology

Advances that occurred in the last decade in the knowledge of the structure and function of the filtering mechanism of the glomerulus has facilitated the understanding of familial and secondary forms of severe proteinuria manifested as the nephrotic syndrome, a generic term describing the concomitant presence of proteinuria, > 50 mg/kg in children a day, or an urine albumin to urine creatinine ratio > 2mg of protein /mg of creatinine, hypoalbuminemia of 25 gm of albumin /L, edema and hypercholesterolemia that is secondary to hypoalbuminemia.

In brief, the glomerular filtering barrier is made up of a fenestrated endothelium, the endothelial surface layer, glomerular basement membrane, a slit diaphragm between interdigitating foot processes, and the sub-podocyte space. The disruptions of the filtration barrier will results in loss of the permiselectivity, loss of protein in the urine that can be severe, leading to development of the nephrotic syndrome (19). There is evidence that support the relative importance of each component of the filtering barrier in maintaining its integrity. Identification of mutations in a number of these genes causing familial forms of FSGS has resulted in significant advances (20).

There are multiple causes of nephrotic syndrome including genetic causes, secondary causes that are immunologically mediated or secondary to infections, metabolic disease and idiopathic. The traditional classification of the nephrotic syndrome has been based in the histopathologic alterations of the glomerulus as describe in the International Study of Kidney Disease in Children (ISKDC). Glomerulopathies are now considered (see table 7).

Minimal Change Disease (MCD)

In children less than 10 years of age the nephrotic syndrome has a sudden onset with edema of the face and lower extremities, nephrotic range proteinuria, and hypoalbuminemia. On renal biopsy, the findings are that of normal histology by light microscopic examination and by immunofluorescence (IF). The abnormal findings are only detected by electron microscopic (EM) examination, demonstrating generalized foot processes effacement. From here the designation of *minimal change disease* (MCD).

In those < of 10 years of age, MCD is observed in 80%-90% of idiopathic nephrotic syndrome. MCD is seen in up to 50% of those older than 10 years and between 10%-15% of non diabetic adults who present with sudden onset of idiopathic nephrotic syndrome. Based on this knowledge, a renal biopsy is not indicated in young children < 10 years of age with the nephrotic syndrome. These children usually respond well to treatment with corticosteroids (21). On the other hand, in non diabetic adults with sudden onset of nephrotic syndrome, unless contraindicated, a renal biopsy in necessary to determine the underlying pathologic lesion.

In the majority of cases of MCD, there is not an identifiable etiology. Recently the expression of CD80 on the podocytes and urinary excretion of CD80 in the urine in MCD has been reported (22). The initial treatment of MCD is with corticosteroids, in pediatric, adolescent, and as well adults ((23). The initial dose of prednisone for the adolescent patient likely to have MCD is 60 mg m^2/day until the proteinuria disappears, usually by two weeks. Prednisone is continued at the same daily dose for 6 weeks of daily prednisone, at which time the patient is switched to alternated day, same dose of prednisone for another six weeks. Prednisone is then tapered by 15 mg/ m^2 every 2 weeks.

Relapse occurs in up to 60% within the year of initiation of treatment and 30% to 40% will have frequent relapses (i.e., four or more relapses in one year).

The treatment of a relapse consist of administration of prednisone at 60 mg/m^2/ day divided in 3 doses until the proteinuria disappears for 3 to 5 days; thereafter, the prednisone is decreased to 40 mg/m^2/a day divided in 3 doses every other day for 1 month and then discontinued. There are some other regimes for the treatment of frequent relapses and steroid dependent treatment. Experience indicates that longer duration of initial prednisone treatment decreases the number of relapses, and in the long term results in less exposure to prednisone (24,25). When a patient continues to have frequent relapses or is steroid dependent, this youth is at an increased risk of steroids side effects and may require the use of different medications before the steroid toxicity manifests. The conventional treatment of MCD in the adult is the same as the treatment in children or adolescents. The initial dose of prednisone is 1 mg/Kg/ day with maximal dose of 80 mg a day.

The response to prednisone may be delayed up to 3-4 months of treatment and 25% will fail to respond. The dose of prednisone is decrease in half after remission as observed by the disappearance of protein in the urine as shown by dipstick, and continued for 4 to 6 more weeks. Relapses are less frequent in the adult than in the pediatric or adolescent patient. Relapses are less frequent in the adult than in the pediatric or adolescent patient.

Table 8 lists important definitions for evaluation and treatment of nephrotic syndrome. When the use of steroids is ineffective or the side effects become intolerable, alternative pharmacologic therapy becomes necessary. Table 9 lists the most frequently used nonsteroidal immunosuppressive agents available for the treatment of glomerular diseases. Only physicians familiar with the use of immunosuppressive medication should prescribe them. During the second decade of life the prevalence of minimal changes disease decreases and nephrotic syndrome is increasingly associated with other forms of glomerular diseases. Most frequently in the United States are focal segmental glomerulosclerosis (FSGS) and other forms of glomerular diastases as listed in table 10.

The concurrent findings of hypertension and hematuria in adolescents with new-onset nephrotic syndrome are unusual in minimal change disease.

Table 6. Contraindications for renal biopsy (18)

Kidney status	Patient status
Multiple cysts	Uncontrolled bleeding diathesis
Solitary kidney (relative contraindication)	Uncontrolled blood pressure
Acute pyelonephritis/perinephric abscess	Uremia
Renal neoplasm	Obesity; uncooperative patient.

Table 7 Frequent glomerulopathies in adolescents

Minimal Changes disease (MCD)	Mesangioproliferative glomerulonephritis
Focal segmental glomerulosclerosis (FSGS)	Post streptococcal glomerulonephritis
Membranous Nephropathy (MN)	Goodpasture's disease
Membranoproliferative glomerulonephritis (MPGN)	ANCA associated Vasculitis
Dense deposits disease (DDD)	Lupus nephritis

Table 8. Useful definitions for management of the nephrotic syndrome

Term	Adult	Adolescent/Child
Relapse	Proteinuria ≥ 1g day1	Albustix 3+ or proteinuria >40 mg $^{m2-h-1}$ occurring on 3 days within 1 week
Frequently relapsing 2	2+ relapses within 6 months	2 + relapses within 6 months
Complete remission	Reduction of proteinuria ≤0.20 g day and serum albumin > 35 g/l	< 4 mg $m^{2h\ -1}$ on at least 3 occasions within 7 days. Serum albumin > 35 g/l-1
Partial remission	Reduction of proteinuria to 0 .21g /day and serum albumin > 35 g/l ± decrease in proteinuria of 50% from base line	Disappearance of edema. Increase in serum albumin > 35 g/l and persisting proteinuria > 4mg m $^{2h-1}$ or > 100 mg m^2/day
Steroid- resistant	Persistence of proteinuria despite prednisone therapy 1mgkg-day-1 X4 months	Persistence of proteinuria despite prednisone therapy of 60 mg m^2X 4 weeks and 3 methylprednisolone pulses
Steroid- dependent-nephrotic syndrome	Two consecutive relapses that occurring during therapy or within 14 days of completing steroid therapy	Two relapses of proteinuria 14 days after stopping or during alternated steroid therapy

Focal segmental glomerulosclerosis

Focal segmental glomerulosclerosis (FSGS) is defined as a clinicopathologic syndrome characterized by proteinuria and focal and segmental glomerulosclerosis pattern of injury by microscopic examination that is common to many different conditions (see table 10). A rigorous analysis of the characteristics and localization of the glomerular lesions and knowledge of clinical circumstances provides more specificity and clinical relevant information for the evaluation and treatment of patients. With the advancement in the knowledge of the structure and function of the filtering mechanism in the glomerular basement membrane, many forms of genetically determined causes of FSGS have been identified. In addition, increasing recognition of secondary causes of FSGS are also becoming more commonly encounter including low birth weight, prematurely born individuals, obesity, and the use of anabolic steroids in adolescents and young adults (26).

Primary focal segmental glomerulosclerosis (FSGS) is of particular concern to the physician caring for adolescents. It is the most common cause of glomerular disease resulting in end stage renal disease (ESRD) in this age group, particularly in African American adolescent males. It is now recognized that the prevalence of primary FSGS in nephrotic black patients is two to four times that of the Caucasian population. The incidence of FSGS in children and in adults is increasing in all ethnic groups.

Table 9. Non steroid immunosuppressive agents use in glomerular diseases

Drug	Pediatric Dose	Adult Dose	Problem	Comment
Levamisol	2.5 mg/k; limited experience in USA	Limited experience in adult patients in the USA	No readily available in USA	Causes neutropenia
Cyclo-phosphamide	2-3 mg/Kg/day for 12 weeks	In refractory nephrotic syndrome Oral 2.5-3 mg /k/ day every day for 60 to 90 days. In proliferative lupus nephritis: 500mg to1g I.V. m^2 every month for 6 months then quarterly for 2 years	Need to monitor for bruising, bleeding, red urine, dysuria, rash.	Hemorrhagic cystitis, risk of sterility particularly in adolescents boys > than in adolescent girls; premature ovarian failure in women Repeated cycles not recommended
MMF (mycophenolate mofetil)	600 mg m^2 day ÷ 2 doses 12.5 to18 mg/kg/dose twice a day	0.5 to 3 g a day ÷ 2 doses (lupus nephritis). Usual adult dose for other conditions 2 g) a day.	Gastrointestinal distress	Risk of immunosuppression reactivation of latent viral infections, progressive multifocal leukoencephalopathy, lymphoproliferative disease.
Cyclosporin-A (Neoral)	6 /mg/kg day ÷ every 12h monitor through levels to lower therapeutic range	3-5 mg k/day ÷ 2 doses keep through level low therapeutic range (150 to 225 µg /L	Therapeutic levels are needed	May cause interstitial renal fibrosis, hypertension (calcineurin nephrotoxicity) and decrease GFR
Tacrolimus	0.075 to 0.2 mg/Kg/day ÷ 2 doses		Therapeutic levels to be monitored	May cause calcineurin nephrotoxicity increased risk of diabetes mellitus in overweight patients
Rituximab	375 mg/m^2 I.V. weekly 2-4 doses	375 mg/m2 weekly 4 doses	US Boxed waning	A CD20 depleting agent is primarily used for treatment of hematologic malignancies. Its use has been extended to immune mediated diseases including renal diseases.
Eculizumab	It is use for treatment of Paroxysmal nocturnal hemoglobinuria. Is an investigational drug for kidney diseases	Has been use "off label" in some forms of atypical hemolytic uremic syndrome and in kidney transplantation.	US Box Warning Increases susceptibility to meningococcal disease.	Monoclonal humanized IgG antibody that binds to complement protein C5,preventing cleavage intoC5a and C5b, preventing formation of membrane attack complex (MAC)

Treatment of primary focal segmental glomerulosclerosis

The response to treatment of primary FSGS is difficult to predict; however, based on the experience of the use of immunosuppression protocols, some patients do respond to medical management. Current treatment recommendations for primary FSGS include treatment of hypertension, use of antiproteinuric medication such as ACEs/ARBs, treatment of hyperlipidemia, administration of immunosuppressive medications including steroids, calcineurin inhibitors: Cyclosporin- A, Tacrolimus, and other medication as listed in tables 9 and 11. The recurrence of primary FSGS in the graft after transplantation is 23 percent to 40 percent and is treated with plasmapheresis and intensification of immunosuppression. Response to Plasmapheresis is well documented.

Table 10. Etiologic classification of focal segmental glomerulosclerosis

Primary FSGS or idiopathic associated with vascular permeability factor
Secondary forms of FSGS Familial/Genetic mutations in nephrin, podocin, α- actin-4, mutation in transient receptor potential cation 6 channel (TRPC6), mutations in WT1,
Viral infection associated HIV, Parvovirus 18
Drug induced Heroin, interferon, lithium, Pamidronate, sirolimus
Post adaptive response Reduced renal mass very low birth weight. Unilateral renal agenesis, renal dysplasia, reflux nephropathy, sequel to cortical necrosis, surgical renal ablation, any advance renal disease with reduction of functioning nephrons Initial normal renal mass hypertension, obesity, increased lean body mass, anabolic steroids, cyanotic congenital heart disease

Table 11. Drugs commonly used to treat glomerular diseases

Immunomudulatory agents	Proposed mechanism of action
Glucocorticoids	Steroids suppress B cell and T cell function inactivate NF-ƘBa, thereby decreasing cytokines generation
Cyclophosphamide	An alkylating agent that covalently links DNA, RNA and proteins leading to either cell death or protein function. Cyclophosphamide causes neutropenia and Lymphopenia.
Mycophenolic acid	Inhibits T and B cell proliphrtation by blocking purine synthesis by inhibition of inosine monophosphate dehydrogenase.
Cyclosporin A/Tacrolimus	Inhibits the phosphatase calcineurin, preventing the translocation of nuclear factor of activated T cells (NFAT) leading to reduced transcriptional activation of early cytokines genes. Cyclosporin may also stabilize the actin cytoskeleton of podocytes maintaining podocytes function.
Rituximab	Murine/human chimeric anti-CD20 monoclonal antibody that depletes B cells
Azathioprine	Inhibits T and B cells proliferation by blocking purine synthesis
Chlorambucil	An alkylating agent that cross links DNA it reduces the number of both T and B cells
Eculizumab	Monoclonal antibody to the complement protein C5. It blocks cleavage of C5, thereby preventing the formation of C5 and the membrane attack complex.
Plasma exchange	Removes large molecular weight substances such as antigen antibody complexes, cryoglobulins myeloma light chains–from the plasma.
Nonimmunomodulatory Agents: ACE/ARBs	Decrease intraglomerular pressure. May also have antifibrotic properties

An important form of familial FSGS nephrotic syndrome presenting in adolescents follows an autosomal dominant pattern of inheritance and these patients are resistant to immunosuppression. Though no immune suppression medication is indicated, they need to have their hypertension and dyslipidemia treated. Many affected family members' progress to end stage renal disease (ESRD). Families with inherited forms of FSGS will benefit from genetic counseling. After renal transplantation, the disease does not reoccur in the renal graft. Patients with obesity and metabolic syndrome induced-FSGS will respond to weight reduction, diet and exercise, and antihypertensive medication (27). There are reports of beneficial effects of bariatric surgery for morbid obese patients with nephrotic range proteinuria (28).

Collapsing focal segmental glomerulosclerosis

The term *collapsing focal segmental glomerulosclerosis* was initially used in 1986 by Weiss et al. (17) to describe six African- Americans who presented with febrile illness, severe nephrotic syndrome, rapidly progressive renal failure leading to end stage renal disease. Histopathologic findings include FSGS with glomerular capillaries membranes that are wrinkled, collapsed, with hyperplasic podocytes obliterating the urinary space.

Although the clinical and pathological findings suggested HIV infection, only one patient in this group went on to develop acquired immunodeficiency syndrome. There is a striking racial disparity in the predisposition of African-American and European-American populations for the development of FSGS and HIV infection.

Research notes a genetic predisposition linking variants in the nonmuscle myosin heavy chain 9 gene (MYH9) that seems to play a major role in both FSGS and human immunodeficiency virus–associated collapsing glomerulopathy (29). Though it is more common in patients with a history of HIV infection and intravenous heroin addiction, there is no history of high risk behavior or serologic evidence of HIV infection in 20% of affected patients.

Clinically this disorder is manifested by severe nephrotic/nephritic syndrome associated with fever, general malaise, resistance to steroids, and rapid advancement to end stage renal disease (ESRD) or death. There are few reports indicating response to immunosuppression with methylprednisolone and intravenous rituximab (30). In general the prognosis is poor. Genetic predisposition to the development of the disease has been linked to MYH9 gene variants and this may predispose African Americans to the disease.

Since the initial observations by Weiss et al., the disease has been noticed to be increasing in frequency, it affects younger children and women, and it is becoming more recognized in other countries (including China and Pakistan) with negative history of HIV infection or drug abuse.

The disease has resulted from the use of certain medications including pamidronate and Interferon-α, β or γ and is typically accompanied by endothelial tubule reticular inclusions. Of interest is the observation that the condition improves following the discontinuation of the interferon treatment or the offending drug. The prognosis is in general poor for long- term renal function; however, there are occasional cases of successful treatment with immunosuppression including rituximab.

Nephrotic syndrome management

Current strategies for the treatment of nephrotic syndrome in these various disorders are continuously evolving and undergoing considerable reassessment. Most specific treatments require the use of high-dose corticosteroids and, frequently, systemic immunosuppressive agents. The potential short and long-term side effects of these agents are considerable. Where eradication or medical control of the underlying disease is not possible, symptomatic treatment is often used. These treatments most often use a combination of modest dietary sodium restriction in conjunction with diuretics to control the degree of edema, while taking care not to compromise the plasma volume. New strategies for the symptomatic medical control of nephrotic edema and the long-term management of intractable proteinuria are currently under investigation (see tables 9 and 11).

Membranoproliferative glomerulonephritis (MPGN)

Membranoproliferative (MPGN) (also known as mesangiocapillary glomerulonephritis) is characterized by histological findings of diffuse proliferative lesions and thickening of the capillary wall and splitting of the glomerular basement membrane by mesangial interposition given the aspect of double contour. Membranoproliferative glomerulonephritis denotes a pattern of glomerular injury, common to different diseases processes. By electron microscopic examination, three types of MPGN have described: Type I, Type II and type III. The frequency of MPGN by type based on EME is listed in table 12.

Table 12. The frequency of the various types of MPGN (18)

Totals	Type I (%)	Type II (%)	Type III (%)
412	213 (52%)	109 (26%)	90 (22%)

Type I MPGN is the classic form of the disease and also the most common, is defined as the presence of immune complexes in the subendothelial space and in the mesangium, and is associated with activation of the classic pathway of complement activation. Type II MPGN is also known as dense deposits disease (DDD) which is the preferred nomenclature at present and is considered to be a complete different clinical and pathological entity from MPGN type I as well as type III. In North America and in Europe, types I and III are the most common forms of MPGN to cause nephrotic syndrome in children, adolescents, and adults. In the United States 1.5% of pediatric and adolescent patients reach end stage renal disease (ESRD). The incidence of MPGN-type I varies significantly with geographic location and is more common in other countries. In Nigeria for example it represent up to 52% of cases of nephrotic syndrome in children and adolescents. The pathogenesis of MPGN Type I and III seems to results from chronic antigenemia expossure in susceptible individuals. The disease is seen more often in adolescents as well as young adults and affects Caucasians more often than African Americans in the U.S. There are three clinical presentations of MPGN type- I and III: nephrotic syndrome, acute nephritis, and asymptomatic hematuria. The known causes of MPGN type-I and III are listed in table 13.

Table 13. Causes of MPGN

MPGN I Primary/Idiopathic Familial Secondary Malignancy Lymphomas Chronic Lymphocytic leukemia Non-Hodgkin's Lymphoma Immunologic Cryoglobulinemia Sjogren's syndrome Complement deficiencies SLE	Infectious Hepatitis C Hepatitis B Schistosoma mansoni HIV malaria Other HIV Malaria
	Other Heroin abuse Partial lipodystrophy
	MPGN Type III Primary/idiopathic Familial
	DDD//MPGN-type II Primary Idiopathic/familial Complement deficiency

Clinical observation indicates that the pathogenesis of Type I MPGN is associated with chronic antigenemia containing IgG antibodies, unknown antigen, and complement C3; there is also activation of the classic pathway.

In patients with active hepatitis C infection, the development of cryoglobulinemia correlates better with the disease and is observed in older individuals. The pathogenesis of the disease in younger children is less clear.

The treatment of MPGN-Type-1 requires the need to investigate the possible cause of the disease. This is especially important in adolescents and in young adults in whom a secondary cause of the disease is more likely. Particular attention is necessary to exclude the presence of active hepatitis C and hepatitis B infections. Treatment of the infection is necessary before immunosuppression is initiated. In children as a general rule, hepatitis B or hepatitis C is of lesser concern.

Membranoproliferative glomerulonephritis type I is the most common form of this disease and it may be primary or secondary. The secondary forms of MPGN type I with immune deposits are associated with infections, autoimmune diseases and dysproteinemias. In other cases as in thrombotic microangiopathies and in chronic liver diseases, immune deposits are absent. Of the MPGN type I associated with infections, those associated with hepatitis C and hepatitis B are of particular relevance. Cryoglobulinemia glomerulonephritis type II has been linked with chronic hepatitis C and the clinical manifestations are those of systemic vasculitis with hypocomplementemia. Interferon –alpha is the treatment of choice for patients with hepatitis C associated cryoglobulinemia. The immunosuppressive therapy for the vasculitis is with methylprednisolone and cyclophosphamide; this management is effective but has the risk of activation of hepatitis C and is reserved for those patients with multiple organ involvement.

A secondary form of MPGN type I due to Hepatitis C is hepatitis C-associated glomerulonephritis in patients with positive serology for hepatitis C that may or not be associated with cryoglobulinemia. Hepatitis C- associated MPGN type I is currently recognized as one of the most important causes of infection-associated glomerulonephritis. The treatment is with long term antiviral medications including interferon-alpha and ribavirin. No immunosuppression is indicated because of the risk of activating the hepatitis C infection.

Chronic hepatitis B infection has also been associated with MPGN type I. The pathogenesis involves deposition immune complexes in the glomeruli and hepatitis B antigen can be demonstrated in the glomeruli. The condition is most common in children. Membranous nephropathy is the most common associated pattern of glomerular injury in hepatitis B. The serologic is positive for hepatitis B surface antigen; the clinical manifestations include nephrotic syndrome and less frequent, cryoglobulinemia with vasculitis. The cornerstone of the treatment is antiviral treatment with interferon-alpha; however, immunosuppressive therapy increases the risk of activation of hepatitis B infection.

Type I and type III usually presents in older children, adolescents and young adults; it affects males and females with equal frequency and is responsible for 5%–20 % causes of the nephrotic syndrome in Europe and North America. The general impression is that the incidence of MPGN is declining in these parts of the world. The presence of persistent circulating immune-complexes, as seen in chronic bacterial, viral or parasitic diseases, immunologic diseases (autoimmune), neoplasia, and paraproteinemias, play an important role in the development of MPGN type I.

The clinical presentation of MPGN may assume several forms that includes nephrotic syndrome in about 30% of cases, persistent microscopic hematuria and proteinuria in 35%, chronic progressive glomerulonephritis in 20%, and rapid progressive glomerulonephritis in 10%. Laboratory abnormalities include depletion of complement C3, total hemolytic complement (CH50), and in some cases, C4. At least three mechanisms have been implicated as responsible for the hypocomplementemia in MPGN: circulating immune complexes activating the classical pathway, NF (an autoantibody directed against complement proteins), and excessive breakdown of C3 by C3 convertase of the alternative pathway.

The clinical course of MPGN is generally progressive and prognosis for renal survival is poor, particularly in adults with MPGN type II. The prognosis is better in younger individuals. Indicators of poor renal prognosis include hypertension, impaired renal function, nephrotic syndrome, more than 20% of crescents present, sclerosis, mesangial deposits, and tubulointerstitial disease. Less strong association is seen with being male and also having macroscopic hematuria; no correlation is seen with serum complement levels.

Treatment of primary MPGN type I

There is no specific therapy for primary MPGN. Children and adolescents with MPGN types I and III were treated by the Cincinnati group with steroids at 2 mg/kg/day, up to 80 mg every other day for up to 2 years; there was dose reduction according to clinical response and they reported improvement in renal survival (31). Similar improvement was also reported by the International Study of Kidney Disease in Children with alternated day use of steroids (32). Long- term alternate-day prednisone treatment demonstrates stabilization and improvement in renal function and proteinuria with the administration of prednisone at a dose of 2 mg/kg to a maximal dose of 60 mg for 1 year (depending on the response), followed by 10-20 mg every other day for 2 to 5 years (31). The side effects of this regimen are considerable including hypertension, growth retardation, obesity, and cataracts. Careful monitoring of the patients is necessary. With this regimen the renal survival rate has increased from 50 percent in previous decades to between 60 to 85 percent in this decade. Adult nephrologists are using similar regimens to patients with active disease. Additional therapeutic measures include the use of anticoagulant agents such as dipyridamol, acetyl salicylic acid, and heparin. Other agents for immunosuppression that have been use include calcineurin inhibitor, and mycophenolate mofetil.

Treatment of secondary forms of MPGN type-I

The management of secondary forms of MPGN should be directed to the underlying cause, as for example, α-interferon for hepatitis C and steroids as well as cyclophosphamide for lupus nephritis. Nonspecific treatment, include normalization of blood pressure with the use of ACEs (angiotensin-converting enzyme) inhibitors or angiotensin II receptor blockers (ARBs) to decrease proteinuria, are also indicated.

The treatment of the secondary forms of MPGN type-I is primarily directed to the cause of the disease. Particular consideration is given to those with MPGN-type I induced by hepatitis C and hepatitis B virus infections. In cryoglobulinemia type- 2 vasculitis associated with chronic hepatitis C virus infection, the corner stone of treatment is interferon-alpha and ribavirin; immunosuppressive therapy with pulse methyl prednisolone, followed by oral prednisone and cyclophosphamide is effective in treating the vasculitis; however, the risk of reactivating the hepatitis C infection is high and therefore, this regimen has to be offered with caution only to patients with disseminated vasculitis involving several organ systems. For those with chronic hepatitis C associated MPGN type–I without cryoglobulinemia, the treatment is with antiviral agents interferon-alpha and ribavirin. The use of immunosuppression agents has a high risk of exacerbation of the hepatitis C infection.

In secondary forms of MPGN-type- I associated with chronic hepatitis B infection, the treatment of choice is the administration of antiviral agents interferon-alpha and ribavirin; spontaneous resolution of the glomerulonephritis occurs or may follow the administration of antiviral agents. In general immunosuppression is contraindicated because of the risk of exacerbation of the hepatitis B infection.

In the case of MPGN type I due to lupus (Lupus nephritis class IV), the treatment is based in immunosuppression. The traditional management of these patients includes induction of remission with pulse methyl prednisolone followed by oral prednisone with rapid tapering and cyclophosphamide; maintenance is with cyclophosphamide. Most recently the use of mycophenolate mofetil has been used successfully with induction and maintenance therapy for patients with lupus class IV.

MPGN type II - dense deposit disease (DDD)

DDD is less common than MPGN type I, affecting mostly children and adolescents but adults can also be affected with a frequency is 2-3 cases per one million of population. In DDD, the pattern of glomerular injury as noted by electronic microscopy is characterized by the presence of extremely osmophilic dense deposits in the capillary wall, giving a ribbon-like appearance of electron dense material. The immunofluorescence staining is positive for C3, usually without immunoglobulins or C1q. Extrarenal manifestation may include partial lipodystrophy involving the face and upper body in some patients; there are also abnormalities of the retina (Drusen bodies) resulting in field and color defects and potential deterioration of the retina. Thus, these youth will benefit from ophthalmologic evaluation.

DDD is due to dysregulation of the alternate pathway of complement activation. In 80% of cases there is an association with the presence of C3 nephritic factor (C3NeF) an antibody that stabilizes the enzyme C3 convertase (C3bBbp) resulting in continuous activation of the alternative complement pathway. Defects in other regulatory proteins of this pathway such as factor H, factor I, complement membrane protein (CMP) and other factors, explain familial and acquired case of DDD (33).

With improved understanding of its different causes, the possibilities for the treatment of DDD have improved. A rational treatment of this condition requires careful evaluation of the alternated pathway of the complement by specialized laboratories.

Type III is considered to be a variant of type I and membranous glomerulonephritis, and in some cases with marked membrane thickening with double contours of the GBM that is silver negative. Abundant subendothelial deposits and widespread subepithelial deposits as seen in membranous nephropathy are present.

In MPGN type III the complement activation profile involves both the activation of the alternative pathway with low C3, normal C4 and, and low C5-C9 implicating the presence of low acting nephritic factor properding- dependent stabilizing C5-convertase. Immunofluorescence is positive for IgG, C3, +/- IgM, IgA, C1, with electron dense aggregates diffusely present in subendothelial and subepithelial areas of the membrane. The treatment of MPGN-Type III is similar to the treatment of MPGN-type I.

Treatment of dense deposits disease

Current understanding of the causes of DDD has established a basis for a more rational therapeutic approach for the treatment of these rare and difficult conditions. In general the causes can be divided into three categories: deficiency of complement factor, functional abnormalities of complement factor, and autoantibodies against complement factor. For conditions associated with deficiency of complement factor, the treatment is replacement with plasma infusion or plasma exchange either in an acute form or in a chronic fashion, depending on the nature of the problem. Plasma exchange may be necessary to make room for the volume of plasma infused to avoid fluid overload concentrate. Concentrate of the deficient factor will avoid the need for plasma exchange. Patients with antibodies against complement factor C3 convertase, the most common cause of DDD, are treated by removal of the autoantibody via plasmapheresis, immunomodulation with intravenous immunoglobulins, and/or immunosuppression with steroids or rituximab.

Patients with DDD can also be treated with immunosuppression targeted to C5, the final step in the formation of the membrane attack complex (MAC). The IgG humanized monoclonal antibody *eculizumab* has been used with success in some patients with DDD. All patients with MPGN will benefit from careful monitoring and treatment of hypertension, proteinuria, and renal function. These patients must be under the care of a physician familiar with these complexes disorders.

Membranous nephropathy

Membranous nephropathy is a chronic glomerular disease in which immune deposits of IgG and complement develop mainly in the subepithelial space of the glomerular capillary wall, inducing morphologic and functional changes. Morphologically, there is increasing thickening of the glomerular basement membrane; with silver methenamine staining, there are "spikes" surrounding the intramembranous deposits. Because inflammatory cell infiltration and hypercellularity are not characteristic finding of the disease, the term membranous nephropathy (MN) is preferred.

The incidence of membranous nephropathy in those from 1 to 12 years of age has been reported to be between 1% to 1.5% of nephrotic children; however, this increases to 22% in adolescents between 13 to 19 years of age (34,35). Most cases of membranous nephropathy develop in adults and older individuals. It is more frequent in Caucasian males follow by those from Asia and less frequently in African American and Hispanic-Americans. In the Caucasian adult population, it is responsible for 20%–25% of cases of idiopathic nephrotic syndrome.

Based on histological and ultrastructural features, four stages of the disease are described that give an approximation of the duration, severity, and progression of the disease. The clinical presentation is dominated by proteinuria and microscopic hematuria. The nephrotic syndrome is common but not specific. The diagnosis requires histological examination of the renal tissue. Between 60 to 80 percent of cases are classified as idiopathic while the rest are secondary to a variety of causes including infections, autoimmune, toxic agents, and malignancies (see table 14)

In the child or adolescent the incidence of membranous nephropathy is not well establish, but is uncommon. In contrast to adults in whom primary membranous nephropathy is more frequent, the secondary forms of the disease predominate in the pediatric patients (35%).) The nephrotic syndrome is the most common presentation of the disease, but in 7%, non-nephrotic range proteinuria and/or abnormal urinary sediment may be the presenting findings.

Etiology and pathogenesis of membranous nephropathy

The etiology of primary membranous nephropathy (MN) in humans is unknown; however, previous rat research has elucidated the *in situ* formation of immune-complexes following the deposit of antibodies against locally induced or intrinsic antigens in the glomerular capillary wall membrane (17). The antibodies in rat studies are directed to megaline complex, a glycoprotein located in the sole of the foot processes. In humans these glycoprotein does not manifest in this location. In recent years, substantial advances in the understanding of MN in humans have occurred by the identification of two antigens responsible for the development of MN in humans. *First*, there is identification of neutral endopeptidase (NEP) as the antigen in membranous nephrotic syndrome in the newborn infants resulting from fetomaternal alloimmunization in NEP deficient mothers who are able to transfer IgG antibodies to the fetus via the placenta and induce membranous nephropathy. The disease in the newborn resolves spontaneously within a few months with the disappearance of the circulating maternal antibodies.

Second, the demonstration by the group of Salant DJ et al. of the high proportion of patients with idiopathic membranous nephropathy having circulating antibodies to phospholipases A2 receptor, a transmembrane protein located in podocytes; this also noted that anti-M type -PLA2R-IgG4 subclass is the predominant antibody (36). These new developments will facilitate the diagnosis of patients that until now are classified as primary or idiopathic MN. The recurrence of MN post renal transplantation in association with high levels of anti-PLA2R antibodies, and the remission of the disease with appropriated immunosuppression, correlating with decline in the atni-PLA2R antibodies titer is confirmatory evidence of the role of these antibodies in this formation of MN.

Diagnosis of membraneous nephropathy

There are no specific clinical or laboratory findings that permit the diagnosis of membranous nephropathy. However, some clinical features seem to be relevant. For example, there is a higher tendency for the development of thromboembolic disease (i.e., deep venous thrombosis, renal vein thrombosis, pulmonary embolism).

The diagnosis of membranous nephropathy requires renal biopsy and special histopathologic studies. Histopathologic diagnosis is established by renal biopsy, with special staining techniques (silver-methenamine, PAS), immunofluorescence, and electron microscopy. Plasma C3 is usually normal while terminal complement component C5b-9 is reported to be elevated in urine. Because secondary forms of the disease are more common in the young, a report of the renal biopsy read as membranous nephropathy means it becomes necessary to exclude secondary causes of the disease before starting the patient on potentially toxic immunosuppressive medication. This possibility is particularly relevant in the elderly.

All patients with membranous nephropathy and negative serology for SLE (lupus or systemic lupus erythematosis) will require further evaluation before the disease is considered to be idiopathic. With the present level of understanding of the causes of membranous nephropathy, it is reasonable to look for the presence of M type phospholipase A2 receptor antibodies (36). Complete evaluation for current or previous infection with hepatitis B virus infection and hepatitis C virus infection is also necessary. As serology studies may be negative in the presence of active infection, the most accurate test is DNA- PCR for Hepatitis B virus and RNA- PCR for hepatitis C virus infection.

Because the serious risk of exacerbation of the infection with immunosuppression, it is necessary to treat active hepatitis viral infections before starting immunosuppression; additionally, effective antiviral therapy alone may cause remission of the proteinuria in up to 60% of cases (37).

The goal in HBV infection therapy is control of replication, but the goal for HCV infection is eradication of the virus. As a general rule the treatment of HCV infection is more difficult than the treatment of HBV infection. Hepatitis B virus infection can be treated with interferon-α or pegylated interferon-α. However it cannot be use in advance chronic kidney disease (CKD stage 3) with estimated GFR (eGFR) <30 ml/minute); for that reason nucleotide analog to interferon-α, (such as entecavir or adefovir) are commonly used. In addition, steroids or other immunosuppressive therapy or anti B cell therapy may be indicated.

Table 14. Conditions associated with membranous nephropathy (18,20)

Autoimmune/Collagen vascular disease Autoantibodies against M-type phospholipase A 2 receptor (PLA2R) Autoantibodies against neutral endopeptidase (NEP) Lupus nephritis class V Rheumatoid arthritis Autoimmune thyroiditis Primary biliary cirrhosis Crohn's disease Sjögren' syndrome Ankylosing spondilitis	Medications Penicillamine Gold salts Captopril Mercury Trimethadione
	Neoplasms Carcinomas of colon, lungs, breast stomach, pancreas, kidney, prostate and cervix Melanoma Wilms' tumor Lymphocytic leukemia Hodgkin's disease
Infectious and Parasitic diseases Hepatitis B Hepatitis C Syphilis (congenital syphilis/latent syphilis) Malaria Schistosomiasis Filariasis	Others: renal transplantation, sarcoidosis, sickle cell disease Guillain-Barre syndrome

Accepted therapy for membranous nephropathy and membranoproliferative glomerulonephritis due to hepatitis C virus infection and the duration and the type of therapy is determined by the virus genotype and the glomerular filtration rate (GFR). For patients with eGFR> 30 ml/minute and hepatitis C virus genotype 1, pegylated interferon-α_{2a} with ribavirin is administered for 48 weeks. For Hepatitis C genotypes 2 and 3, the duration is 24 weeks. Steroids, immunosuppression or anti-B cell therapy may also be indicated. For those with eGFR< 30 ml/minute, pegylated interferon-α_{2a} is given as tolerated; steroids, immunosuppression or anti Cell-B therapy may be also indicated. In these patients monitoring of clinical condition, viral load, urine protein to urine creatinine ratio, urinary sediment, eGFR, and cryocrit are necessary.

Treatment of membranous nephropathy

The decision to treat a patient with membranous nephropathy requires consideration of many factors, including the understanding of the natural progression of the disease. The spontaneous remission of the disease is seen in up to 30 percent of cases, particularly younger patients. There is also a correlation with male gender, older age, hypertension, severity of proteinuria at presentation, hypoalbuminemia, and elevated serum creatinine. In secondary forms of membranous nephropathy (i.e., Hashimoto's thyroiditis, membranous lupus nephritis), treatment consists in discontinuation of the offending agent, treatment of viral infection, or the auto-immune disease. Non immune suppressive treatment includes control of blood pressure, with antihypertensive and antiproteinuric medication such as ACEs or ARBs, lipid lowering agents, prophylactic anticoagulation and control of edema.

Immunosuppressive treatment of membranous nephropathy usually includes cytotoxic agents such as cyclophosphamide plus steroids, usually for several months (tables 9 and 11).For those patients that do not respond to traditional immunosuppression therapy, other therapies are currently been evaluated and some have shown encouraging results (38-40)

Auto antibodies to the M-type phospholipase A2 receptor are sensitive and specific for idiopathic membranous nephropathy.

The anti B cell monoclonal antibody, rituximab, is a promising new therapeutic agent for this condition, currently been evaluated. In a group of 25 patients with idiopathic membranous nephropathy, whose M-type phospholipase A2 receptor antibodies titers were known before treatment with rituximab and the titers were repeated after treatment, the auto antibodies disappeared or declined within 12 months after the administration of this agent in 68% of those treated (41). The disappearance or decline of the autoantibodies predicted a positive response to treatment before changes in proteinuria were detected (41)

There is no specific treatment for membranous nephropathy. Additionally, spontaneous remission of membranous nephropathy may occur in up to 40% of the nephrotic syndrome in the child or adolescent. A period of nonspecific treatment with ACE inhibitors, close supervision of renal function, and monitoring of severity of proteinuria, is a reasonable approach for the adolescent with membranous nephropathy. Immunosuppression is indicated if there is deterioration of renal function or if the proteinuria is severe.

Management of Nephrotic Syndrome

General considerations

Current strategies for the treatment of nephrotic syndrome in these various disorders are continuously evolving and undergoing considerable reassessment. Most specific treatments require the use of high-dose corticosteroids and, frequently, systemic immunosuppressive agents. The potential short and long-term side effects of these agents are considerable. Where eradication or medical control of the underlying disease is not possible, symptomatic treatment is often used. These treatments most often use a combination of modest dietary sodium restriction in conjunction with diuretics to control the degree of edema, while taking care not to compromise the plasma volume.

New strategies for the symptomatic medical control of nephrotic edema and the long-term management of intractable proteinuria are currently under investigation. Treatment of associated infections is always important (tables 9 and 11).

Diabetic nephropathy

The incidence of childhood type 1 diabetes has dramatically increased, especially for children below 5 years of age. The development of vascular disease associated with diabetes represent a high risk for the long term complications seen in this disease, resulting in significant decrease in the life expectancy for these individuals (42).

Diabetic nephropathy, one of the serious complications of diabetes, affects up to 40% of patients with diabetes type 1 and is the principal cause of end stage renal disease (ESRD) in the developed and developing countries around the world. The development of microalbuminuria with type I diabetes occurs in pubertal and post pubertal patients and, thus, is an important concern for physicians caring for these populations. The natural evolution of diabetic nephropathy is summarized in table 15 (43).

There are several known risk factors for the progression of diabetes to diabetic nephropathy; some of these factors are amenable to modification and therefore, prevention of progression. Other factors are not modifiable, such as duration of diabetes, genetic factors and puberty. Because the initial morphologic and functional abnormalities develop at puberty and end stage renal disease is seldom seen at this young age there is an opportunity for preventive measures to be implemented to control those factors (table 16). It has been known for a long time that the renin angiotensin aldosterone system plays an important role in the progression of diabetic nephropathy.

The most active component of the angiotensin-II system, is a potent vasoconstrictor that induces hypertension, can induce cell proliferation, matrix expansion and through activation of transforming growth factor beta, induces fibrosis.

Current clinical data indicates that the development of nephropathy can be delayed with excellent glycemic control. Data also suggest that angiotensin-converting-enzyme inhibitors and angiotensin II receptor blockers are not indicated in diabetic patients without microalbuminuria or hypertension (44).

Table 15. Stages of type 1 Diabetic nephropathy structural and functional changes from reference

	Main structural alterations	Albumin excretion	GFR	Blood pressure
Stage 1 at diagnosis hyper function hypertrophy	Increased renal size	May be increase but normalizes after initiation of insulin treatment	Increased by 20-50%	Normal
Stage 2 (after 2 to 5 years) normoalbuminuria, silent phase	Basement membrane thickening	Normal with increased related with poor glycemic control or exercise	Normal or increased by 20 to 50%	Normal
Stage 3 (after 6-15 years): incipient diabetic nephropathy/ microalbuminuria	Further basement membrane thickening and mesangial expansion	Increased :20-200μg/ per minute or 30 to 300 mg/ 24 hours	Normal/ increased	increasing
Stage 4 (after 15 – 25 years) overt diabetic nephropathy, macroalbuminuria	Marked renal abnormalities	Further increased:> 200μg/minute or > 300 mg/ 24 hours	Decreased	Increased
Stage 5 (after 25-30 years	Advanced glomerulopathy	Macroalbuminuria/often decreased due to glomerular occlusion	Marked decreased	Increased

Recommendations for patients with diabetes include vigorous glycemic control. After five years of the onset of diabetes, yearly screening for microalbuminuria is indicated. If microalbuminuria is detected, repeat determination should occur 3 months later; if microalbuminuria is confirmed on three occasions, treatment with angiotensin converting enzyme inhibitors (ACEs) or angiotensin receptor blockers (ARBs) is indicated. Titrate the dose to the therapeutic response. The simultaneous use of both classes of medications has been used in some cases.

Table 16. Strategies for prevention of diabetic nephropathy in children and adolescents (39)

Glycemic control avoiding hypoglycemia
Evaluation and treatment for microalbuminuria starting at 10 years of age if diabetes ≥ 5 years of duration
Treatment of hypertension to bring blood pressure to normal levels using ACE inhibitors
Monitor and treatment of hyperlipidemia. There is no consensus in the use of statins in children and adolescents.
Prevention of obesity, avoid excess of protein intake
Regular moderate exercise
Avoidance of smoking

Table 17. Conditions associated with transient hematuria

Fever
Infections (generalized, urinary, prostatic, and vulvovaginal)
Genitourinary foreign bodies
Cogulation defects
Sickle cell trait or anemia
Posttrauma (both recognized and unrecognized, as may occur in contact sports)
Others

*Used with permission from: Torres AD, Greydanus DE: Genitourinary and renal disorders. In: Essential Adolescent Medicine. Eds: DE Greydanus, DR Patel, HD Pratt. NY: McGraw-Hill, page 568, 2006.

HEMATURIA

Etiology

Gross or microscopic hematuria in an adolescent is a common occurrence. Evaluation of the possibility of red blood cell (RBC) products in the urine requires both dipstick and microscopic analyses. Most dip and read urine stick products are very sensitive, with detection ranges as low as the equivalent of 2–5 RBCs per high power field on microanalysis. Red or red-brown discolored urine or clear urine testing positive for blood on dipstick may indicate the presence of hemoglobinuria or myoglobinuria, rather than hematuria. The absence of RBCs on microanalysis should suggest either of the two former diagnoses, though the possibilities of RBC lysis in a very hypotonic urine (specific gravity <1.007) or a false positive result should also be considered. False positives may occur in the presence of oxidizing contaminants, such as hypochlorite disinfecting solutions and high urinary bacterial contents with release of bacterial peroxidases. False negative results occur in the presence of high urinary ascorbic acid concentrations. Non-RBC products that may give the urine a reddish, smoky, or dark appearance should also be considered when the dipstick fails to be positive for blood. Urate crystals, berries, beets, vegetable dyes, as well as alcaptonuria, tyrosinosis, porphyrin compounds, and bile may all cause factitious hematuria.

The presence of 10 or more RBCs/high power field on a spun urine specimen is considered abnormal in most laboratories. However, borderline RBC counts should be reaffirmed on at least two additional urinalyses, since as many as 80% of cases of microscopic hematuria detected on an initial urinalysis will be transient. Transient hematuria may be encountered in association with various conditions, as noted in table 17. Vigorous exercise or a period of strenuous training can cause hematuria that may be accompanied by proteinuria as well as casts; it typically clears within 24 hours.

Diagnosis

Persistent or recurrent hematuria warrants a thorough investigation for an underlying cause. The initial evaluation should include a carefully focused history, family history, and physical examination, all of which can contribute significantly to the diagnostic evaluation. Table 18 describes general components of the initial clinical evaluation which often prove useful. The diagnostic studies appropriate to the adolescent with hematuria will largely depend upon the suspected site and etiology of the bleeding.

Laboratory studies

Localization of the site of urinary bleeding is often useful in the initial diagnostic evaluation. Hematuria originating in the kidney is often characterized by brown or cola-colored urine. The concomitant presence of >2+ protein by dipstick, or RBC casts, WBC casts, deformed (dysmorphic) RBC, or renal tubular epithelial cells in urine sediment, increases the likelihood of bleeding from the renal parenchyma, especially from glomerular causes. Lower urinary tract bleeding is more often characterized by terminal hematuria, passage of blood clots, and/or normal RBC morphology on microanalysis.

If the cause of the hematuria is not evident from historical and physical findings, the initial empirical evaluation should begin with a urine microanalysis, from which it is determined whether the bleeding is more likely glomerular or extraglomerular (i.e., nonparenchymal). As noted above, the presence of no RBCs and/or pigmented urine casts should raise the possibility of pigmenturia from hemoglobin or myoglobin.

Others to consider in the appropriate setting include intravascular coagulation, mechanical RBC damage (e.g., artificial heart valves), hemolytic anemia (e.g., G6PD deficiency, mismatched blood transfusion), as well as muscle injuries (crush, electrical, post-traumatic compartment syndrome), myositis, and rhabdomyolysis.

A microanalysis showing a dysmorphic RBC subpopulation or RBC casts is indicative of glomerular or renal parenchymal bleeding. In this case, a serum C_3 is often useful to distinguish hypocomplementemic from normocomplementemic causes of renal parenchymal bleeding. In contrast, the absence of urinary casts and the presence of morphologically normal RBCs on microanalysis should suggest extraparenchymal bleeding.

Ultrasound of the kidneys and bladder is a useful and noninvasive tool in the initial evaluation of suspected renal structural abnormalities. Hypercalciuria also appears to be increasingly associated with hematuria and the subsequent risk of urolithiasis. A random daytime urine specimen, in which the ratio of the calcium concentration divided by the creatinine concentration (both expressed in the same units) is greater than 0.21, suggests the presence of hypercalciuria. In the setting of a history or family history suggestive of renal parenchymal disease, or the identification of physical or laboratory findings compatible with underlying glomerulonephritis or renal dysfunction, the decision as to the most appropriate subsequent evaluation (including the possible need for renal biopsy) and/or treatment should be made in conjunction with a specialist in nephrology.

Table 18. Common components of the clinical evaluation of hematuria*

History of:	Suggests:
Dysuria, fever	Upper or lower UTI
Headache, rash, arthralgias, *others*	Systemic infection, vasculitis, collagen vascular diseases, Henoch-Schönlein nephritis
Sinusitis, cough, headache, epistaxis	Wegener's granulomatosis
Flank pain	Renal calculus, acute urinary obstruction, subacute pyelonephritis, cystic diseases
Intermittent gross hematuria	IgA and IgG Nephritis; urethritis, foreign body, hypercalciuria, neoplasm (rare)
Antecedent viral illness	Postinfectious nephritis, IgA nephropathy, other nephritis
Cola-colored urine, edema, hypertension	Glomerulonephritis
Bloody diarrhea	Hemolytic uremic syndrome (serotoxin-producing *E. coli* and others)
Family history of:	
Microhematuria	Thin basal membrane disease, hereditary nephritis, hypercalciuria
Hearing loss	Hereditary nephritis
Renal failure	Hereditary nephritis, cystic kidney disease
Anemia	Sickle cell disease or trait
Physical findings of:	
Hypertension	Acute or chronic glomerulonephritis
Edema, ascots	Glomerulonephritis, membranous nephropathy, focal sclerosis
Bruising	Coagulopathy, collagen vascular disease
Heart murmur, fever	Subacute bacterial endocarditis
Purpura	Systemic infection, Henoch-Schönlein nephritis
Flank mass	Polycystic kidney disease, obstructive uropathy, renal tumor, multicystic dysplastic kidney

*Used with permission from: Torres AD, Greydanus DE: Genitourinary and renal disorders. In: Essential Adolescent Medicine. Eds: DE Greydanus, DR Patel, HD Pratt. NY: McGraw-Hill, page 568, 2006.

Glomerulonephritis (GN)

General

Infection-related glomerulonephritis (table 19) the epidemiology of infection related glomerulonephritis is declining particularly in developed countries; specifically, acute poststreptococcal glomerulonephritis is in decline due to the successful treatment of streptococcal infections. However, because the emergence of antibiotic resistance staphylococcus strains such as methicillin-resistant Staphylococcus aureus (MRSA), the acute of glomerulonephritis of active infection is on the rise. They need to be considered as separated entities, diagnosed, and treated accordingly (45)

In the post infection GN the patients develops an infection and it resolves naturally or with the help of antibiotics. After 2 to 22 days of the initiation of the infection, the first manifestations of GN appear with gross hematuria, hypertension, and proteinuria; usually by this time, the infection has resolved. However, the post infectious GN is just started and the clinical manifestations may be mild or severe. The use of antimicrobial therapy will not modify the disease process at this point.

In the case of GN of active infection (table 20), the patient develops an infection that does not resolve naturally. If the infection is considered superficial, local antibiotics may be applied, and the seriousness of the infection may be missed. The renal involvement will be manifested weeks later with hematuria, proteinuria, hypertension, decreased complement C3 levels, decreased total complement, and elevated serum creatinine. Contrary to what is seen in post- infection GN, in active infection-related GN, antimicrobial agents are necessary to treat and resolve the GN. If the infection is not treated, the GN may progress to chronic GN.

Table 19. Causes and important characteristics of post infectious GN (45)

Name	Site of infection	Organism	Comment
Acute poststreptococcal GN	URI, pharyngitis Tonsillitis, cellulitis	*Streptococcus* group A *(Streptococcus pyogenes)* especially those with specific M types or C *(Streptococcus Zooepidemicus)*	Onset of GN is between 7and 21 days after onset of the infection; GN can be severe; recovery is the rule especially in children.
Acute flare of IgA nephritis	URI, pharyngitis, tonsillitis, gastroenteritis, cystitis, vaginitis	Bacterial or viral pathogens	Onset of the GN is usually 1-3 days after onset of the infection; usually the GN is mild, although gross hematuria may be present
Other acute infection	Pneumonia, gastroenteritis	*Streptococcus pneumonia, Klebsiella, Mycoplasma, Salmonella,* Enterohemorrahgic *Escherichia coli*	The GN appears during the acute infection; the GN is usually mild, manifested by hematuria, but not always, it may be severe in some cases.

Abbreviations: URI, upper respiratory infection, GN, glomerulonephritis.

Table 20. Causes and important characteristics of Active infection related-GN (45)

Name	Site of infection	Organism	Comment
Staphylococcal-related GN	Ischemic limb, cellulitis, endocarditis, osteomyelitis, shunts, central venous catheters (CVC), pneumonia, unknown	Coagulase positive Staphylococcus, often MRSA	Likely the most common cause of GN from chronic bacterial infection
Other bacterial-related GN	Deep-seated visceral abscess (thoracic, abdominal) osteomyelitis, endocarditis, shunts, CVC infection	Gram-positive or gram-negative organisms	Severe acute kidney injury is common
Viral infections	Hepatitis B,C, HIV, CMV, parvovirus	The GN can be mitigated by antimicrobial therapy	
Nonbacterial, nonviral infections	Visceral organs are the usual sites	Parasites, spirochets, fungi, others	These are rare in North America and western Europe

CVC, Central venous catheter; CMV, cytomegalic virus.

Post-streptococcal glomerulonephritis

General

Acute post-streptococcal glomerulonephritis (PSGN) is the most commonly encountered form of postinfectious nephritis in children and younger adolescents. This inflammatory renal disorder results from immune complex formation and localization within the glomerulus associated with specific M-serotype nephritogenic Group A as well as Group C streptococcal infections. Most commonly, the sites of infection are the upper respiratory tract (pharyngitis, otitis, sinusitis) and the skin. The appearance of respiratory tract-associated PSGN is typically 7–14 days after onset of the infection, while onset of pyoderma-associated nephritis may take as long as three weeks. Late treatment (>36 hours after onset of infection) or treatment at the time of appearance of the nephritis does not appear to modify the course of the renal disease. The typical clinical findings of PSGN include the triad of sudden onset of gross hematuria, volume overload (often manifesting as edema or cardiopulmonary congestion), and hypertension. However, many patients may be discovered to have asymptomatic disease, especially during periods of epidemic streptococcal disease.

PSGN: Laboratory studies

The diagnosis of PSGN relies upon the demonstration of the causative organism, though prior empiric therapy may preclude this option. Serological tests for evidence of a preceding streptococcal infection are often useful; however, both chronic asymptomatic streptococcal carriage as well as elevated streptococcal-associated antibody levels is frequently present in unaffected individuals.

Most patients with suspected PSGN are screened with the streptozyme test, which screens for antibodies to several streptococcal antigens. A positive test should be confirmed with specific titers. Approximately 70% of those patients with pharyngitis-associated PSGN will have increased titers of antistreptolysin-O (ASO), though the rise of the ASO titer in pyoderma-associated PSGN is less common. The combination of ASO, antihyaluronidase, and antideoxyribonuclease B (anti-DNAase B) titers should provide evidence of a recent streptococcal infection in almost all patients. Renal biopsy is not routinely indicated; however, it may be required when the presentation is atypical such in rapid progressive renal insufficiency, severe nephrotic syndrome, or persistent hypocomplementemia lasting for more than 8 weeks, suggesting other renal disease. Renal biopsy shows a diffuse mesangioproliferative pattern of injury. In severe cases crescentic lesions may be observed.

Decreased serum C3 levels are detected in approximately 90% of the cases. Therefore, adolescents with acute glomerulonephritis who have normal C3 values at the time of onset should have consideration for other forms of nephritis. In addition, the serum C3 levels almost invariably return to normal within 6–8 weeks of onset of the nephritis. Thus, serial complement measurements are necessary to document the diagnosis. Since other forms of chronic glomerulonephritis may clinically exacerbate in association with an acute viral illness, variation from the typical clinical presentation and course should prompt a more thorough evaluation. Also, other acute bacterial and viral illnesses may be associated with a similar clinical presentation of acute nephritis.

Management

Culture, early diagnosis, and prompt treatment of any residual streptococcal infection may prevent the development of the disease. The antibiotic of choice is penicillin by injection or oral administration. Other suitable antibiotic may be used if penicillin cannot be administered. Prevention antibiotics may be indicated in siblings. Management of the acute nephritis requires evaluation and treatment of the associated hypertension. Long acting calcium channel blockers may be the better antihypertensive medications, particularly in the presence of decreased renal function and/or hyperkalemia. In hypertensive encephalopathy we prefer nicardipine because is easy to administer. ACEs inhibitors can be used if renal function is not compromised and hyperkalemia is not an issue. Low sodium diet and fluid restriction may be necessary. The use of loop diuretics is indicated to treat edema and hypertension when there is intravascular congestion. Renal replacement therapy by peritoneal dialysis or hemodialysis is less frequently needed in the child or adolescent than in the adult. In rapid progressive deterioration of renal function, a renal biopsy may demonstrate crescentic glomerulonephritis and the use of pulse methylprednisolone is then indicated (46).

Prognosis

Current data indicate that the vast majority of patients with PSGN can fully recover if morbidity can be avoided that is associated with the clinical presentation (e.g., hypertensive encephalopathy, congestive heart failure, mineral imbalance associated with acute renal failure, and serious infection). This favorable prognosis excludes that very small percentage of patients with PSGN manifesting as the clinical syndrome of acute oliguric renal failure associated with crescentic glomerulonephritis and in the older population.

Henoch-Schönlein purpura (HSP) nephritis

The European League against Rheumatism/ Pediatric Rheumatology European Society (EULAR/PReS) endorsed criteria for childhood vasculitis criteria for HSP that include the presence of palpable purpura as a mandatory criterion, and any one of the following: diffuse abdominal pain, any biopsy showing IgA deposition arthritis or arthralgias, renal involvement, any hematuria and/or proteinuria (47).

HSP is the most common vasculitis in childhood with an annual incidence of 14 cases in 100,000 children; however, the incidence varies with the geographic area studied. The purpuric/petecchia and palpable rash primarily involves the lower extremities, buttocks, and distal upper extremities. It can also involve the scrotum and mimic torsion of the testicle.

Factors triggering Henoch-Schönlein purpura (HSP) is frequently preceded by an infection in up to 50% of the cases; however, no specific antigen has been identified causing the disease. Bacterial as well as viral infections have been linked to the disease including: Streptococcus β hemolytic group B, yersinia, mycoplasma, toxoplasma, varicella, measles, rubella, adenovirus, and HIV. The HSP clinical manifestations are generally mild, and the treatment is basically supportive with treatment of symptoms.

The arthralgias /arthritis can be treated with the appropriated non-steroidal anti-inflammatory drugs (NSAIDs); the abdominal pain usually responds to small dose of steroids with rapid resolution of the abdominal pain. Recurrent severe abdominal pain and necrotizing skin lesions have been treated by administration of immunoglobulin infusion.

Early steroidal treatment of HSP has been reported that prevents the development of HSP nephritis (48). Renal manifestations of HSP include isolated gross or microscopic hematuria, proteinuria, and occasionally, the nephrotic syndrome.

There is a selection bias in relation with the severity of the renal manifestations of the disease between those patients seen in a general practice as compared to those patients seen by the pediatric or adult nephrologists. Glomerulonephritis occurs in 20%–30% of the patients, though severe nephritis (nephrotic-range proteinuria, hypertension, and azotemia) occurs less than 10% of the time; progression to end stage renal disease occurs in severe cases of HSP affecting adults and children.

Renal biopsy is indicated in patients with deteriorating renal function, persistent proteinuria, and hypertension. The predominant renal lesion is that of a mesangioproliferative disease and characteristically immunofluorence reveals predominant deposition of immunoglobulin A, and co-dominance of C3 in some cases.

There is a good correlation between the severity of the histological lesions and the clinical severity of the disease. Patients with active disease may respond to treatment with corticosteroids and azathioprine (49).

Adolescents with rapid progressive glomerulonephritis and crescents on renal biopsy benefit from aggressive therapy that includes pulse methylprednisolone, cyclophosphamide and plasmapheresis (tables 9 and 11).

Up to 15% of patient with severe HSP nephritis (histology IV-VI) will advance to ESRD. The disease has the tendency to reoccur in the transplanted kidney.

IgA nephropathy

Since the initial description by Jean Berger in 1968, IgA nephropathy is now recognized as the most common pattern of glomerulonephritis around the world, including in those countries that regularly perform renal biopsies in patients with hematuria and proteinuria.

It is known as an important cause of chronic kidney disease and end stage renal disease. The triggering mechanisms for the development of IgA nephropathy are not well-known.

In the case of HSP, infections have been considered important in some cases and the association with systemic diseases is well established, including chronic inflammatory bowel disease, dermatitis, malignancies and chronic liver disease. A particularly severe disease is seen with Staphylococcus aureus infection.

There is a wide range of clinical manifestations of IgA nephropathy that include recurrent macroscopic hematuria, as well as asymptomatic urinary abnormalities (microhematuria and mild proteinuria), nephrotic syndrome, and chronic kidney disease. The renal biopsy most often reveals mesangial proliferation with dominance of immunoglobulin IgA deposition.

The severity of the histological manifestations also correlates with the clinical manifestations. From the histopathologic view point, the lesions seen in IgA nephropathy are very similar to those observe in HSP nephritis. The transformation of IgA nephropathy to HSP has been documented. In IgA nephropathy it is known that abnormal glycosylation of the IgA1 molecule occurs.

It seems that the relationship between HSP and IgA nephropathy is more fundamental than superficial. IgA nephropathy becomes a chronic kidney disease in up to 40 % of adults and leads to ESRD 15 years after renal biopsy.

The treatment of IgA nephropathy includes normalization of blood pressure, reduction of proteinuria, and decreased IgA formation.

Recurrence of IgA nephropathy after related donor transplantation is higher than in those that received a deceased donor renal graft (51).

Hemolytic-uremic syndrome

General

Hemolytic-uremic syndrome (HUS) is not truly a glomerulonephritis. Rather it is a thrombotic microangiopathy affecting the kidney whose causes are multiple and include infections, genetic conditions, and acquired disorders of the alternative pathway of complement activation; other genetic and acquired disorders include Von Willebrand proteinase deficiency (ADAMS13), defects in cobalamine metabolism, cancer chemotherapy, ionizing radiation, calcineurin inhibitors, pregnancy, sclerodermas crisis and unclassified causes.

The most common cause of HUS in the United States is infection by Shiga toxin producing organisms in particular enterohemorrhagic Escherichia Coli (EHEC), especially

0157-H7. Other shigatoxin producing bacteria include Shigella dysenterie type-1, Citrobacter freundii and others. In outbreaks of EHEC HUS, 1 in 10 infected individuals develop diarrhea; between 5%-15% of cases that experience hematochezia will develop HUS. 12.9 % of children < 5 years with bloody diarrhea develop HUS while 6-8% of children 5 years or older with EHEC will develop HUS.

Shigatoxin associated HUS is one of the common causes of acute kidney injury (AKI) in the United States and in the world. It is commonly designated as diarrhea positive HUS (D+HUS), and/or typical HUS. Acute kidney injury (AKI) in children has an average age of onset of 3 years (2–6 years), though it can also affect younger and older individuals. In the United States, it often follows a diarrheal illness due to exotoxin (shigatoxin)-producing E. coli (especially 0157-H7) and other infectious agents, including Salmonella typhi, Shigella, or Campylobacter.

Atypical forms of HUS are usually diarrhea negative or D-HUS and have been associated with such infectious disease agents as Streptococcus pneumonia as well as HIV; other associations include cancer chemotherapy, immunosuppressive drugs (e.g., cyclosporine), pregnancy (including preeclampsia and during the postpartum period), malignant hypertension, and scleroderma. D-HUS has also been reported in families with an autosomal recessive or dominant pattern of inheritance, usually related to abnormal regulation of the alternative pathway of complement activation, the most common of which is abnormalities of factor H (53).

Diagnosis

The clinical manifestation include a prodromal diarrhea illness with cramping abdominal pain and blood in the stool, when the diarrhea subsides the child appears pale; petecchia may be observed as well as gross hematuria and decreased urinary output. The triad of microangiopathic hemolytic anemia (with schistocytes, helmet cell), thrombocytopenia, and AKI establish the clinical diagnosis of HUS. These may be frequently associated with hypertension, seizures, and/or encephalopathy. With the application of the pediatric criteria for the severity of AKI that include risk, injury, failure, loss, and end stage renal disease (pRIFLE), the clinician will be able to assess the severity of renal injury and the need for renal support therapy.

The treatment of EHEC shigatoxin induced HUS is basically supportive and the use of antibiotic is controversial, particularly in case of HEEC infection. Treatment of anemia with pack RBC when needed, control of hypertension, restoration of fluid electrolyte and acid-base homeostasis and careful attention to nutritional needs are the cornerstone of treatment. The use of platelets transfusion is seldom indicated. Renal support should be initiated early, rather than late. Adolescents presenting with features of HUS, in whom central nervous system and hemorrhagic findings predominate, should also be considered to have thrombotic thrombocytopenic purpura (TTP); TTP is a distinct entity from HUS.

Prognosis

With aggressive and early treatment of fluid and electrolyte imbalances (especially potassium imbalance), control of elevated blood pressure, and institution of early dialysis when required, the prognosis associated with the epidemic (D+HUS) form is good; with excellent management, the mortality is less than 5% in young children. Currently the mortality rate for patients with D+HUS in the USA is <5%. However, these individuals compare with controls with negative history of D+HUS, more often have microalbuminuria as well as hypertension, have decreased glomerular filtration rates and in general, higher prevalence of chronic kidney disease and the need for long term follow up (50).

Other infectious causes of HUS (such as those associated with Streptococcus pneumoniae sepsis), require specific therapeutic approach particularly in relation with administration of blood products. There is currently no consensus among nephrologists regarding the use of washed blood products in patients with this disease. Some still use this precaution.

The severity of the HUS is worse in the atypical cases (D-HUS). Important new developments have recently occurred in understanding the diagnosis and therapeutic interventions in atypical cases of hemolytic uremic syndrome (D-HUS), associated with complement dysregulation that occurs in <10% of cases of HUS in the United States (51). In D-HUS, particularly in the familial and recurrent forms of the disease, and in patients with TTP, management includes plasma exchange and plasmapheresis therapy. The short and long term prognosis in these patients is less favorable, and they should be managed in collaboration with a nephrologist.

Lupus nephritis

Systemic lupus erythematosus (SLE) is an autoimmune, chronic inflammatory disease with protean clinical manifestations. In SLE, there is the presence of multiple autoantibodies in the serum reacting to multiple cell components, mainly those of the nucleosome origin (54). It is now known that genetic factors play a significant role in the development of the disease. The prevalence of the disease is ~ 40 in 100,000 of the Caucasian population in Europe and in North America. Populations from Asia have a greater incidence than African-Americans, followed by Hispanics. Females are more frequently affected than males in all populations; the female to male ratio is 2:1 in the prepubertal age, 4.5:1 in adolescence, and increases to 8:1 in adult age group. Twenty percent of SLE cases develop in childhood.

Most frequent clinical manifestations in patients with lupus include fever and weight loss in 100% of cases. Musculoskeletal findings include arthralgias, synovitis, and arthritis. Serosal involvement include pleuritis, pericarditis, and oral ulcers. Skin manifestations consist of butterfly facial rash, photodermatosis, and alopecia. Hematologic manifestations are anemia, leucopenia, thrombocytopenia, and thrombosis associated with antiphospholipid antibodies.

Lupus glomerulonephritis is a common and serious feature of systemic lupus erythematosus. The term denotes the spectrum of immune complexes-mediated renal diseases secondary to SLE. The renal manifestations are extremely heterogeneous and may affect the glomeruli, tubules, interstitium, and blood vessels. Proteinuria is present in 100% of cases with nephrotic range proteinuria occurring between 45 and 65%. Clinical or morphological involvement of the kidneys occurs in 50-80% of lupus patients at any time during the course of their disease. Moreover, renal alterations are found in 90% of patients at autopsy. The lowest 5 year survival has been reported in patients with central nervous system and renal involvement. Abnormal urinary sediment includes granular casts and red cell casts. Microscopic hematuria is seen in up to 80% of cases, and gross hematuria in 1-2% of cases. Reduced renal function at presentation is present in 40-80% of cases. Rapid progressive glomerulonephritis occurs in up to 30% of patients. Acute renal injury with failure occurs at presentation in 1-2% of cases. Hypertension is common, up to 50% of cases. Hyperkalemia is reported in 15% of patients. Tubular abnormalities (distal renal tubular acidosis type IV), are usually asymptomatic and are described in about 60% of patients.

Serology

Anti-dsDNA is noted in 40-90% frequency with a high specificity, and with an association with disease activity. Anti-SSA/Ro is noted in 35% with a low specificity, and no disease activity association. Anti-SSB/La is seen in 15% with no disease activity association, and low specificity. Anti-Sm is noted in 5 to 30% with high specificity, and no disease activity association. Finally, Anti-C1q has a frequency of 80 to 100%, has high specificity, and is associated with disease activity.

Classification

There have been several pathologic classifications of Lupus Nephritis. The current classification of Lupus nephritis according to the in the International society of nephrology/renal pathology society (ISN/PRS) 2004, is depicted in table 21.

Table 21. Lupus neprhitis

Class I Minimal mesangial lupus nephritis – normal by light microscopic, but mesangial deposition by immunofluorescence.
Class II Mesangial proliferative lupus nephritis – mesangial hypercellularity and mesangial deposits by immunofluorescence.
Class III Focal lupus nephritis – IIIA - Purely active lesions – focal proliferative lupus nephritis IIIA/C – Active and chronic lesions – focal proliferative and sclerosing lupus nephritis IIIC – Chronic inactive lesions with glomerular scars – focal sclerosisng lupus nephritis
Class IV Diffuse lupus nephritis – IVA – purely active lesions – diffuse proliferative lupus nephritis IVA/C – active and chronic lesions – diffuse segmental or global proliferative and sclerosisng lupus nephritis IVC – inactive with glomerular scars
Class V Membranous lupus nephritis
Class VI Advanced sclerosisng lupus nephritis – 90% of glomeruli globally sclerosed without residual activity

Treatment of lupus nephritis

Treatment of lupus nephritis depends on the classification of the severity of the disease in the individual patient. Treatment of class I and class II is supportive in nature. The treatment of class III, IV, and V requires, in addition to supportive measures (i.e., treatment of hypertension, pain, hyperlipidemia, and avoidance of sun exposure), immunosuppression is indicated. It is useful to divide the treatment of lupus nephritis class III, IV, and V into two phases: induction therapy and maintenance therapy.

The induction phase of treatment consists of high-dose pulse methyl prednisolone IV, 600-1000 mg/m^2 (maximum 1 g) daily for 3 days. This is followed by oral prednisolone, 1-2 mg/kg/d (maximum 60-80 mg/d) with rapid taper. Concomitant cyclophosphamide monthly pulses for 6 months, 500-1000 mg/m^2. In very severe cases or when the patient doesn't respond to this therapy, plasma exchange daily for 5-10 days has been used, or rituximab may be used in more severe cases following protocol.

Side effects of immunosuppressive therapy for lupus nephritis with methyl prednisolone and cyclophosphamide include amenorrhea, cervical dysplasia, avascular necrosis, herpes zoster, infections, and death. These side effects are more common with cyclophosphamide intravenous (IV) for 6 months, except for vascular necrosis which is more common with the use of IV methylprednisolone.

Due to severe toxicity of the drugs in the above protocol, the Euro-Lupus Nephritis Trial (ELNT) was developed (55). In this trial, 90 patients with diffuse proliferative, focal proliferative nephritis, or membranous nephritis were randomized to receive the 6 month pulse cyclophosphamide followed by either infusion of cyclophosphamide every third month OR a shorter treatment course consistent of 500 mg IV cyclophosphamide every 2 weeks for six total doses and then switch to azothiophrine maintenance therapy for 30 months. Both treatments were equally effective in several renal and extrarenal parameters with fewer infections in the shorter treatment group (55). As this trial was largely performed in a Caucasian population, it is unknown if it will be equally effective in other populations.

Sequence therapies for lupus nephritis using pulse methylprednisolone 500-1000 mg daily x 3 doses are followed by oral prednisone in a rapid taper plus standard dose of IV cyclophosphamide. Maintenance therapy with mycophenolate mofetil was developed in a study involving more than 100 patients; this protocol was proven to be as effective as previously used protocol (57).

Currently mycophenolate mofetil (MMF) and methylprednisolone have been successfully used for induction therapy, followed by MMF for maintenance therapy, without the use of cyclophosphamide. Four randomized control studies involving 268 patients showed significant reduction in the risk for treatment failure for the MMF group as compared with the cyclophosphamide group (58). The risk for death or ESRD may be lower with MMF compared with cyclophosphamide which is an important clinical finding not previously demonstrated. There was no increase in adverse events associated with MMF (58). MMF pediatric dose is based on body surface area. Patients with a BSA 1.25m^2 to 1.5 m2 should receive 750 mg twice a day. Patients with a BSA > 1.5 m^2 should receive 1 g twice a day. Alternatively, 12.5 mg/kg to 18 mg/kg dose twice a day to a daily maximal of 2 g a day for 1-2 years, can be used.

Conclusion

The renal system is a critically important and complex organ system needed for normal growth and health in the adolescent. This paper reviews paramount issues in this regard including urinary tract infections, proteinuria, hematuria, and glomerulonephritis. Concepts of diagnosis and management are presented. Consultation with colleagues in nephrology is recommended for adolescents with complex and refractory renal conditions.

Acknowledgments

This paper is an adapted version of a chapter in the book "Adolescent medicine: Pharmacotherapeutics in medical disorders" edited by Donald E Greydanus, Dilip R Patel, Cynthia Feucht, Hatim A Omar, Joav Merrick and published with permission by Walter de Gruyter, Berlin and New York.

References

[1] Litza JA, Brill JR. Urinary tract infections. Prim Care 2010;37(3):491-507.

[2] Dielubanza EJ, Schaeffer AJ. Urinary tract infectins in women. Med Clin North Am 2011; 95 (1): 27-41.

[3] Bonny AE, Brouhard BH. Urinary tract infections among adolescents. Adolesc Med 2005; 16:149-61.

[4] Meier S, Weber R, Zbinden R. Extended-spectrum β-lactamase-producing Gram-negative pathogens in community-acquired urinary tract infections: an increasing challenge for antimicrobial therapy. Infection 2011 Jun 25. [Epub ahead of print]

[5] Bader MS, Hawboldt J, Brooks A. Management of complicated urinary tract infections in the era of antimicrobial resistance. Postgrad Med 2010;122 (6): 7-15.

[6] Saadeh SA, Mattoo TK. Managing urinary tract infections. Pediatr Nephrol 2011 Mar 16. [EPub ahead of print]

[7] Neuman I, Moore P. Pyelonephritis (acute) in non-pregnant women. Clin Evid (Online) 2011 Jan 13. [EPub ahead of print]

[8] Shields J, Maxwell AP. Acute pyelonephritis can have serious complications. Practitioner 2010;254:19-24.

[9] Vazquez JC, Abalos E. Treatments for symptomatic urinary tract infections during pregnancy. Cochrane Database Syst Rev 2011;19(1):CD002256

[10] Williams G, Craig JC. Long-term antibiotics for preventing urinary tract infection in children. Cochrane Database Sys Rev 2011;16(3):CD001534.

[11] Ejernaes K. Bacterial characteristics of importance for recurrent urinary tract infections caused by Escherichia coli. Dan Med Bull 2011;58(4):B4187.

[12] Epp A, Larochelle A, Lovatsis D, et al. Recurrent urinary tract infection. J Obstet Gynaecol Can 2010;32(11):1082-101.

[13] Kodner CM, Thomas-Gupton EK. Recurrent urinary tract infections in women: diagnosis and management. Am Fam Physician 2010;82(6):638-43.

[14] Damiano R, Quarto G, Bava I. Prevention of recurrent urinary tract infections by intravesical administration of hyaluronic acid and chondroitin sulphate: a placebo-controlled randomized trial. Eur Urol 2011;59(4): 645-51.

[15] Barbosa-Cesnik C, Brown MB, Buxton M, et al. Cranberry juice fails to prevent recurrent urinary tract infection: results from a randomized placebo-controlled trial. Clin Infect Dis 2011;52(1):23-30.

[16] Schnarr J, Smaill F. Asymptomatic bacteriuria and symptomatic urinary tract infections in pregnancy. Eur J Clin Invest 2008;38(Suppl 2):50-7.

[17] Torres AD, Greydanus DE. Orthostatic proteinuria genitourinary and renal disorders. In:

[18] Greydanus DE, Patel DR, Pratt HD, eds. Essential adolescent medicine. New York: McGraw-Hill;2006:335-6.

[19] Fogo A. Renal pathology. In: Avner ED, Harmon WE, Niaudet P, Norishige Y, eds. Pediatric nephrology, 6th edition. Berlin: Springer, 2009:555.

[20] Peter J Lavin PJ, Winn MP. TORcin up the importance of calcium signaling. J Am Soc Nephrol 2011;22:1391-3.

[21] Hildebrandt F, Herringa SF. Specific podocin mutations determine the age of onset of nephrotic syndrome all the way into adult life. Kidney Int 2009;75:669-71.

[22] Peter F. Hoyer PF. Minimal change nephrotic syndrome. In: Floege J, Johnson RJ, Feehally J, eds. Clinical nephrology, 4th ed. St Louis, MO: Elsevier Saunders, 2010:222-45.

[23] Garin EH, Diaz LN, Mu W. Urinary CD80 excretion increases in idiopathic minimal-change disease. J Am Soc Nephrol 2009;20:260-6.

[24] Becker DJ. Minimal change disease. Nephrol Rounds 2008;34:111-34.

[25] Hodson EM, Night JF, Willis NS, Craig JC. Corticosteroid therapy for nephrotic syndrome in children. Cochrane database Syst Rev 2005;1:CD001533.

[26] Hiraoka M, Tsutkahara H, Matsubara K, et al. West Japan Cooperative study Group of Kidney Disease in Children. Am J Kidney Dis 2003;41(6):1155.

[27] Herlitz LC. Markowitz AB. Farris JA. Development of focal segmental glomerulosclerosis after anabolic steroid Abuse. Jam Soc Nephrolo. 2010;21:163-72.

[28] Kambham N, Markowits GS, Valeri AM, et al. Obesity related glomerulopaty: An emerging epidemic. Kidney Int 2001;59(4):1498-509.

[29] Ritz E, Kolgeganova T, Piecha G. Is there an obesity- metabolic syndrome related glomerulopaty? Curr Opin Hypertens 2010;45:222-31.

[30] Winkler CA, Nelson G, Oleski TK, et al. Genetics of focal segmental glomerulosclerosis and human immunodeficiency virus –associated collapsing glomerulopaty: the role of the MYH9 genetic variation Sem Nephrol 2010;30(2):111-25.

[31] Kaito H, Kamel K, Kikuchi E. Successful treatment of collapsing focal segmental glomerulosclerosis with a combination of rituximab, steroids and ciclosporin. Pediatr Nephrol, 2010;25(5):957-9.

[32] McEnery PT, McAdams AJ, West CD. Treatment of mesangiocapillary glomerulonephritis: improved survival with alternated day prednisone therapy. Clin Nephrol 1980;13:117-24.

[33] Tarshis P. Treatment of mesangiocapillary glomerulonephritis with alternate day prednisolone: a report from the international study of kidney diseases in children. Pediatr Nephrol 1992;6:123-30.

[34] Smith RJ. Dense deposit disease focus group, new approaches to the treatment of dense deposit disease. J Am Soc Nephrol 2007;18:2447-56.

[35] International Study of kidney diseases in Children. Nephrotic syndrome in children: Prediction of histopathology from clinical and laboratory characteristic at time of diagnosis. A report of the International study of International Study of Kidney Diseases in Children. Kidney Int 1978;13:159-65.

[36] Moxey-Mims MM, Stapleton FB, Feld LG. Applying decision analysis to management to adolescents with idiopathic nephrotic syndrome. Pediatr Nephrol 1994; 8:660-4.

[37] Beck LH Jr., Bonegio RG, Lambeau G. M-type phospholipases A2 receptor as target antigen in idiopathic membranous nephropathy. N Engl J Med 2009;361(1):11-21.

[38] Duffield JS, Qamar A Advances in the etiology and management of immune-mediated glomerulonephritides Nephrol Rounds 2008;6(10):111-8.

[39] Remuzzi G, Chiurchiu C, Abbate M. Rituximab for idiopathic membranous nephropathy. Lancet 2002;360:923-4.

[40] Flavio V, Cohen SD, Appel G. Novel B cell therapeutic targets in transplantation and immune - mediated glomerular diseases. Clin J Am Soc Nephrol 2010;5:142-51.

[41] Fernando C. Fervenza, Roshini S. Rituximab therapy in idiopathic membranous nephropathy: A 2-year study. Clin J Am Soc Nephrol 2010;5:2188-98.

[42] Beck LH Jr., Fervenza FC, Beck DM et al. Salant Rituximab-induced depletion of anti-PLA2R autoantibodies predicts response in membranous nephropathy J Am Soc Nephrol 2011;22:1543-50.

[43] Narayan KM, Boyle JP, Thompson TJ. Life time risk for diabetes mellitus in the Unites States. JAMA 2003;29:184-89.

[44] Marcovecchio ML, Chiarelli F. Diabetic nephropathy. In: Avner ED, Harmon WE, Niaudet P, Yoshikawa N, eds. Pediatric nephrology, 6th ed. Berlin: Springer, 2009:324-40.

[45] Bilous R, Chatuverdi N, Sjolie AK, et al. Effect of candesartan on microalbuminuria and albumin excretion rate in diabetes: Three randomized trials. Ann Intern Med 2009; 151(1):11-20.

[46] Nadasdy T, Herbert LA. Infection related glomerulonephritis: understanding mechanisms. Sem Nephrol 2011;31:369-75.

[47] Rodriguez-Iturbe B, Burdmann EA, Barsoum RS. Glomerular diseases associated with Infection. In: Floege J, Johnson RJ, Feehally J, eds. Clinical nephrology, 4th edition. St Louis, MO: Elsevier Saunders, 2010:662-7.

[48] Ozen S. Ruperto N Dillon MJ, et al. EULAR/PReS endorsed consensus criteria for the classification of child hood vasculitis. Ann Rheum Dis 2006;65:936-41.

[49] Weiss PF, Feinstein JA, Luan X, et al. Effects of corticosteroids on Henoch-Schoenlein purpura: A systemic review. Pediatrics 2007;120:1079-87.

[50] Shin JI, Park JM, Shin YH. Can Azathioprine and steroids alter the progression of Henoch-Schoenlein purpura nephritis? Pediatr Nephrol 2005;20:1087-92.

[51] Sharma AP, Filler G, Dwight P, Clark WF. Chronic renal disease is more prevalent in patients with hemolytic Uremic Syndrome who had a positive history of diarrhea. Kidney Int 2010;78:598-604.

[52] Waters AM, Licht C. aHUS caused by complement dysregulation: New therapies on the Horizon.Pediatr Nephrol 2011:26:41-57.

[53] Koyama A, Sharmin S, Sakurai H. Staphylococcus aureus cell envelope antigen is a new candidate for the induction of IgA nephropathy, Kidney Int 2004;66:121.

[54] Johnson S, Taylor CM. Hemolytic uremic Syndrome. In: Avner ED, Harmon WE, Niaudet P, Yoshikawa N, eds. Pediatric nephrology, 6th ed. Berlin: Springer, 2009:1156-8.

[55] Van der Vlag J, Berden JHM. Lupus nephritis role of antinucleosome autoantibodies. Sem Nephrol 2011;31:386-9.

[56] Houssiau FA, Vasconcelos C, D'Cruz D. Immunosuppressive therapy in lupus nephritis: the Euro-Lupus Trial, a randomized trial of low-dose versus high-dose intravenous cyclophosphamide. Arthritis Rheum 2002;46(8):2121-31.

[57] Contreras G, Pardo V, Leclercq B. Sequential therapies for proliferative lupus nephritis. N Engl J Med 2004;350(10):971-6.

[58] Appel GB, Contreras G, Dooley MA. Lupus Management Study Group. J Am Soc Nephrol 2009;20(5):1103.

[59] Walsh M,. Mycophenolate mofetil for induction therapy of lupus nephritis: A systemic review and meta-analysis. Clin J Am Soc Nephrol 2007;2:968-75.

Submitted: November 10, 2011. *Revised:* December 15, 2011. *Accepted:* December 22, 2011.

SECTION TWO – HEALTH ISSUES AND RISKS

In: Child and Adolescent Health Yearbook 2013
Editor: Joav Merrick
ISBN: 978-1-63117-658-6

Chapter 7

THE SELF-MANAGEMENT AND TRANSITION TO ADULTHOOD PROGRAM "UNC STAR$_X$": INSTRUMENTS AND LESSONS FROM THE FIELD

Maria E Ferris, MD, MPH, PhD*[*1], *Michael T Ferris, BA*[2], *Carolyn Viall, RN, PhD*[3], *Heather D Stewart, MD*[1], *Nicole Fenton, MS*[1], *Cara Haberman, MD*[4], *Edward A Iglesia, BA*[5], *Lauren E Hancock, PNP*[4], *Donna H Harward*[1], *Donna Gilleskie, PhD*[6], *James O'Neill*[7], *Robert Imperial*[7], *Zion Ko*[1], *Mary H Benton*[1], *May Doan, BA*[1], *Kristi Bickford*[1], *BA, Randy Detwiler, MD*[1], *Kenneth Andreoni, MD*[8], *John D Mahan, MD*[8], *Zachary Smith, MD*[1] *and Keisha Gibson, MD, MPH*[1]

[1]University of North Carolina Kidney Center, Chapel Hill, North Carolina
[2]Script-a-wish and Simione Health Care Consultants, Cincinnati, Ohio
[3]The North Carolina Children's Hospital, Chapel Hill, North Carolina
[4]Victory Junction Campand Wake Forrest University, Winston-Salem, North Carolina,
[5]Robert Wood Johnson Medical School, Piscataway, New Jersey
[6]University of North Carolina School of Economics, Chapel Hill, North Carolina,
[7]University of North Carolina Department of Internal Medicine, Chapel Hill, North Carolina
[8]Nationwide Children's Hospital/The Ohio State University, Columbus, Ohio, United States of America

---

* **Correspondence:** Maria E Ferris, MD, MPH, PhD, Associate Professor of Pediatrics and Medicine, The University of North Carolina at Chapel Hill, Founder and Director, the UNC TR$_x$ANSITION and Self-management Program, Director, Pediatric Dialysis and Kidney Transplant Programs, Chapel Hill, NC 27599-7155 United States. E-mail: maria_ferris@med.unc.edu

Abstract

The University of North Carolina's Self-management and Transition to Adulthood with R_x=therapies Program (UNC $STAR_x$) has gained experience since 2006. This manuscript describes the program's evolution from a nephrology-centric intervention to addressing multiple-conditions in an institution-wide interdisciplinary program. We illustrate the lessons and insight informed by youth with chronic conditions/disabilities, parent, health provider and community partner perspectives across the continuum of health care transition (HCT). Specifically, lessons relate to program sustainability, including the importance of a dedicated program coordinator, inter and intra-institutional collaboration to validate tools that promote and assess patient self-management skills and HCT, strategies to improve youth, provider (pediatric and adult-focused) and parent communication, and the important role for peer volunteers (in person or through social media) are addressed. The UNC $STAR_x$ Program's collaboration has produced IRB-approved tools that promote communication between youth with chronic conditions and providers, while outlining customized interventions based on patient's level of knowledge and skill mastery. Two private foundations provided initial funding and it now has become an institution-wide collaborative funded primarily by the North Carolina Children's Hospital. The UNC STARx partners include youth with chronic conditions and disabilities, families and researchers from several disciplines and institutions in our state, nation and the world. Our innovative program holds great promise and it already appears to improve health outcomes and quality of life for youth and their families (based on participation rate and user satisfaction both at >95%). Our lessons from the field may assist other institutions as they strive to improve adolescents'/young adults' health outcomes through evidence-based and cost-effective interventions.

Keywords: Transition, health care transition, transition program, self-management, adolescence, chronic conditions, social media, parents, disabilities

Introduction

Health care transition (HCT) is a dynamic, patient- and family-centered process that involves the purposeful, planned movement of adolescents and young adults with chronic physical and medical conditions from child-centered to adult-oriented healthcare systems(1-3). The consensus goal of HCT is for adolescents and young adults (youth) to successfully engage the adult healthcare system in order to receive high-quality, developmentally-appropriate health care services, thus maximizing their lifelong functioning, potential, and quality of life (3,4). Toward this end, the HCT process is deliberate and focused, meets the needs of an individual, and prepares an adolescent or young adult with a chronic illness to assume progressive increasing responsibility for the management of their health (3,5-7).

HCT planning ensures a smooth, uninterrupted, and coordinated transfer from pediatric to adult health care providers and services. Ideally, the HCT process is flexible, responsive, continuous, comprehensive, and well-coordinated, and is championed by a transition program and/or care providers that ensure appropriate HCT planning and support are provided (3,4,6,7). The recommended key components of an effective HCT program are: 1) a designated professional responsible for HCT coordination, 2) development of written HCT plans at the onset of adolescence and 3) formulation of a written portable medical summary ready at the time of transfer to adult providers (3,5-7).

Despite consensus recommendations that youth with chronic conditions benefit from HCT programs (3-7), barriers to the establishment of effective HCT programs still persist. Firstly, there is lack of agreement regarding a theoretical model to support transition, despite a few proposals of interest (8,9). By extension, there is lack of agreement about the identified targets of intervention and clinical outcomes to measure transition (10). Secondly, there is no consensus about which individual should serve as the HCT coordinator, the coordinator's level of training, or the coordinator's function. Thirdly, health provider compensation to carry out HCT services also remains a barrier. Additionally, HCT program funding is a critical barrier as most HCT programs are not supported by institutional budgets and thus must rely on external sources of funding.

In this paper, we describe our experience in launching our institution-wide HCT program: called the UNC $STAR_x$ (Self-management and Transition to Adulthood with Rx=treatment). We share the lessons we have learned and the insight we have gained from working with youth, parents, and community partners. We also briefly describe the tools that we have developed, currently utilize, and continue to validate in order to guide youth with chronic medical conditions/disabilities, their families, and the health providers who serve them in the HCT process.

Program organization and sustainability

In 2006, with the enthusiastic support of adolescent/young adults with chronic conditions and their parents, the need for the interdisciplinary self-management and transition program was acknowledged and addressed. The initial impetus for this collaborative effort was triggered by anecdotal experience with survivors of pediatric-onset chronic kidney disease who had poor outcomes (loss of transplant, lost to follow up, or death) subsequent to their transfer to adult-focused health. In preparation for establishing a formal program at UNC, the founder and program director visited the transition programs of Dr. Alan Watson (Nottingham, UK) and Dr. Janet McDonagh (Birmingham, UK) and conducted semi-structured interviews with published experts in the field of transition (see acknowledgments). The purpose of these initial discussions was to explore organizational models, ascertain how programs were funded, determine how multidisciplinary, intra-institutional partners were identified/ recruited, and identify available tools for assessing young adults' progression in achieving readiness for transfer (see acknowledgments). Two distinct lessons derived from these exploratory visits informed our programmatic plans: 1) no validated tools were available for dissemination, and 2) funds to support a targeted transition program were difficult to secure.

It was clear that a distinct organizational advantage at UNC was that pediatric nephrology resides within the internal medicine nephrology group. This embedded model provides pediatric nephrology with greater fiscal stability and shared clinic space, promoting collaboration between pediatric and adult providers. In addition, increased communication between UNC pediatric and adult nephrology providers engendered improved communication between external providers who either referred or received adolescent/young adult patients.

Initial funding for the $STAR_x$ was through a three-year award from the K.B. Reynolds Charitable Trust, and following HCT consensus guidelines a full-time transition coordinator position was established. This position proved critical to achieving timely execution of readiness assessments and was instrumental in achieving patient-centered education and in promoting communication between community partners (teachers, support agencies), the health care provider, the patient and the parent(s). Ms. Kristi Bickford has a BA degree in Psychology and extensive experience working with children and adolescents in the judicial, social service, and mental health fields. She has been the sole transition coordinator since the inception of our program. Following the expiration of the initial grant support, bridge funding was secured from the UNC Departments of Internal Medicine and Pathology.

A grant from the Agency for Healthcare Research and Quality through the UNC Center for Education Research and Therapeutics, partly supported the development one of our tools, the STAR$_x$ Survey; a self-administered questionnaire to assess transition readiness and disease management skills (11).

The UNC Kidney Center and the Department of Pediatrics partially funded the development of our second tool, the TR$_x$ANSITION Scale™. It is a provider-administered survey to measure the adolescent/young adult's self-management skills and disease specific knowledge. The development of a parallel TR$_x$ANSITION Scale-Parent Version™ was partly funded by the Renal Research Institute. Dr. Maria Ferris had previously developed and used a medical passport, which was adapted to be used in the STAR$_x$ Program started, and it is now known as the TR$_x$ANSITION Medical Passport.™

Since 2010, the University of North Carolina Children's Hospital Administration has provided funding for the program's full time transition coordinator, providing important stability. This substantial financial support has facilitated the expansion HCT services to receiving care in other pediatric subspecialties, including: Gastroenterology, Rheumatology, Endocrinology, Hematology, and Pulmonology. Additional research manpower, in the form of a psychology graduate student, two medical students and a coordinator, has been achieved with awards from the Renal Research Institute and the American Society of Nephrology, supporting two one-year funding for two medical students and 20% of Dr. Ferris' salary. In-kind donations from the UNC Kidney Center and the UNC Schools of Arts and Science, Public Health, and Nursing, as well as the Carolina Institute for Developmental Disabilities, the Center for Faculty Development and the Odum Institute are essential sources in our continued effort (administrative support, office space and research program). With a dedicated HCT coordinator and additional research personnel, over 300 are being followed longitudinally, including post-transfer to adult focused health care. For further detail on the program timeline, partners, tools and funding, please see Figure 1.

Patients served and staff/volunteers

Patients: Our program enrolls patients between the ages of 12-24years who have been diagnosed with a chronic health condition for at least 6 months. Additional inclusion criteria include: taking at least one medication daily for the diagnosed chronic condition and the cognitive ability (as deemed by their providers) to understand and answer questions about their medical condition(s) and treatment. All patients that accept our invitation to participate in our program sign an IRB-approved consent permitting access to their medical and pharmacy records for longitudinal data collection. Patients and their parents are enrolled in person during a routinely scheduled clinic visit. During the clinic visit the majority of the tool administration and assessments are completed, followed by phone or online administered surveys when necessary). We currently have a 95% program enrolment rate with an equally high proportion of reported participant satisfaction in the program at 95%).

Program staff and volunteers: By in large, our most influential team members are the youth with chronic medical conditions and their parents who volunteer their time, knowledge, and suggestions, guiding the advancement in our work. The $STAR_x$ team is multi-disciplinary and composed of paid staff, grant funded researchers, and volunteers. The medical director receives 20% salary support via grant funding and a fulltime transition coordinator whose salary is 100% supported by the UNC Children's Hospital.

We collaborate with professionals amongst various disciplines including: nursing (nurses and nurse practitioners), pharmacy, clinical psychology, developmental disabilities, education, social work, public health and recreational therapy. Furthermore, the UNC $STAR_x$ Program is aided by the work of five diligent student researchers (two medical and one psychology graduate student whose positions are funded by research grants provided by the American Society of Nephrology; and two part-time pre-medical students funded by the Renal Research Institute). Our team is also composed of a cohort of diverse student researchers volunteering their time during summer breaks.

TOOLS TO MEASURE TRANSITION READINESS

The $STAR_x$ Transition-Readiness Survey: This questionnaire was a collaborative work utilizing valuable input from adolescents and emerging adults with various chronic medical conditions. The 18-question survey was developed through the use of patient focus groups, focused interviews, and cognitive interviews, including the "concurrent think-aloud" technique in which responses are probed extensively. This tool was created with supplemental input acquired from patient-graduates and existing patients of our pediatric renal program; information obtained from published check lists of transition skills; and interdisciplinary collaboration between students of the UNC School of Public Health (Department of Health Behavior/Health Education). Using the Stages of Change Model, the STARx survey was designed to longitudinally measure self-reported health care transition readiness and disease self-management skills. The STARx Transition-Readiness Survey includes self-reported knowledge of (1) disease diagnosis, (2) medications/treatment, (3) health insurance, (4) ability to make medical appointments, (5) ability to use health resources and (6) disease self-management. This web-based tool is administered every 6-12 months and is undergoing validation in clinical and therapeutic camp settings (11). Most recently, we are comparing the performance of this survey among adolescents with chronic conditions to another self-administered tool (12). (See Figure 1).

The TR_xANSITION Scale™: The TR_xANSITION Scale™ (trademark 2006, University of North Carolina) is a longitudinally designed tool used to assess and monitor the HCT process; and is readily accessible (web-based) and reproducible in clinical practice (Ferris et al. in press Renal Failure). This scale produces a collective score using the following 10 transition related domains: **T**ype of illness, **R**x (medications), **A**dherence, **N**utrition, **S**elf-management, **I**ssues of reproduction, **T**rade/school, **I**nsurance, **O**ngoing support, and **N**ew health providers. The scale has been revised thrice to support and reflect the current structured interview format.

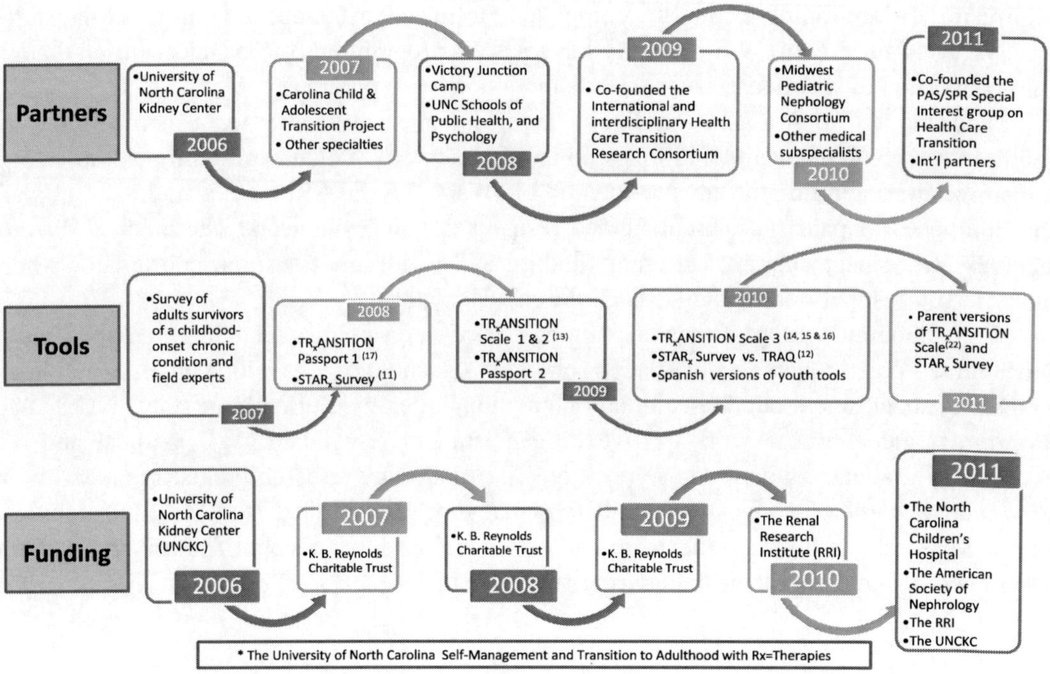

Figure 1. Transition & Self-Management UNC STAR$_x$* Program Timeline.

It should be noted that administration of the scale not limited to health providers. Our program is an example of how people with limited to no medical knowledge or backgrounds can be trained to effectively administer this tool (reproducibility kappa score 0.76). The scale collects information through both, confirmation of attained knowledge and skill mastery claimed (i.e., the patient has to name his/her medication(s) to get credit for the answer) and patient self-report (13-16).

This allows the health provider to commend the youth on their attained knowledge/skills and helps them provide developmentally-appropriate patient-education activities in the areas of low competency. The scale is administered every 6-12 months, monitoring progress in a de-identified web-based format.

Preliminary analysis of a cross-sectional pilot study revealed adolescents younger than 17 years had a significantly lower score than older teens and young adults, with those younger than 14 years having the lowest scores (13,14,16). This may reflect life experiences and time-varying development as the adolescent matures. Validation studies are underway to assess the instruments' effectiveness in a longitudinal study design. Internal medicine and combined internal medicine-pediatrics fellows assume the care of transitioned patients when the youth achieve a TR$_x$ANSITION Scale™ score of > 80%.

The TRxANSITION medical passport™: This tool helps teach youth with chronic medical conditions about their disease and facilitates communication between health care providers in emergency rooms and clinic settings. This laminated, wallet-sized document contains the following patient-specific health information: medical diagnosis, current medication list (type, dosage, frequency, and purpose), drug allergies, and medical provider contact information. The TR$_x$ANSITION Medical Passport™ also includes the patient's name, photograph (if they wish), emergency contacts, and their unique patient ID number. The medical passport is updated every 6-12 months to reflect their most current health and personal information. In an effort to evaluate retention and usability, patients are contacted and asked if they have their medical passport in their possession(17). To confirm that they do in fact have it, they are asked to read their ID number located in the upper right-hand corner of the card. User satisfaction and feedback from providers (in emergency departments and clinics throughout the state) has been enlightening.

Peer-support and on-line Facebook™: Our transition coordinator is the administrator of a Facebook™ page for some of the young adults who participate in our STAR$_x$ program. She monitors communication between the invited members and proposes relevant, age-appropriate topics of discussion. This expansion into a social media forum has led the participants to discuss their challenges to self- manage their conditions, and finding the appropriate support systems.

This platform encourages active communication among members and provides a non-threatening, non-judgmental environment. Youth share stories, coach one another, ask questions, and seek support.

There have been several instances when a group member has been hospitalized and other members coordinate a visit to the hospital. Many of the young adult members of this group have said that they don't feel comfortable posting status updates about their health on their personal Facebook™ pages. In contrast, our HCT Facebook™ page monitored by our transition coordinator provides is an environment where they feel comfortable to post about their feelings (e.g., being different from "healthy" peers, sadness about having a health condition, frustration with taking medications daily), struggles (e.g., medication side effects, special diets, wheel-chair dependence), and triumphs (e.g., hospital discharge, receiving a transplant, medication removed, etc.) related to their health. Table 1 depicts recommendations for health providers that the youth in our program have.

Recurring themes youth have taught us through personal and on-line conversations include:

- The importance that health providers have in their lives and sense of well-being.
- Providers can inspire trust particularly if they express confidence in the youth's ability to manage their condition and lives. On the other hand, providers can also inspire distrust if the youth are treated without respect or their opinions are discounted.
- Youth…
  - like to be included in all conversations that affect their lives
  - actually hear what the health providers advise, but don't necessarily agree at times
  - worry about the burden their diagnosis brings to their parents/siblings and family
  - like to have peer support and the ability to share "war stories" and advice from peers who are experiencing the same struggles they encounter (18)
  - would like having more relaxed communications with their providers as conversations expand to survival and life goals
  - want to be affirmed of their growing autonomy

Table 1. UNC STAR$_x$ Program Youth Recommendations to Health Providers

1. **Customer service**
   In the outpatient setting:
   a. Everyone should have a smile to show they are happy to see you
   b. Good bed-side manners by providers
   c. All signage should be clear and visible (as in an airport) to navigate the system.
   d. Clean environment in the clinic but not smelling like a hospital
   e. A waiting room that is the "Apple™ stores of clinic", airy, nicely designed, not cluttered
   f. Magazines that are up to date and today's news-paper,
   g. Relaxing music in the background at low volume/having a fish tank
   h. Health message in posters, computer screens or TV monitors with nicely designed graphics with colors that are great to look at, almost artistic; surprising the consumer that they are actually health education messages
   i. Email system for staggered appointments with times that are respected.
   j. Paying co-pays up-front to stand in line at the check-in/out counter once
   k. Patient portal to access medical record

   In the in-patient setting:
   l. Hospital gowns are not cool, they are demeaning and revealing
   m. Children's wards prevents the youth from getting sleep (crying babies next door)
   n. Adult wards is also not appropriate and they would prefer an adolescent and young adult unit that caters to their unique needs and morbidities
   o. Being able to eat or drink on a timely basis if a potential procedure is cancelled
2. **Health care providers that**
   a. Direct the conversation to the adolescent and young adult
   b. Ask for the youth's opinion
   c. Ask the parents to leave the room
   d. Reassure the youth that all conversations are private
   e. Inspire confidence and trustworthiness, as a friend. Youth patients often "don't know what we don't know" until they are faced with a question or having to explain it to someone else.
   f. Listen to the youth's concerns
   g. Relates to young-adults interests by being up-to-date in music, movies, sports
   h. Encourage questions by the youth and help navigate the system
   i. Teach how to explain their condition to their peers
   j. Showing the awards the clinic or providers have received or the results of the research
3. **Continuous Quality Improvement**
   a. Individualized patient and parent education, re-education and re-training, particularly those patient who were diagnosed early in life
   b. Counseling about how to successfully self-manage their condition
   c. Meeting older patients serving as mentor/coaches or even examples of what not to do with tangible consequences (i.e., Somebody who lost a transplant due to no-compliance)
4. **Creating a patient health ambassador program:** Using the principle " You see something, you do something ,you teach something"
5. **Getting a Health Care Transition Graduation Certificate**
6. **Ecological Aspects of Health**
   a) Secure individualized education plans and assistance with 504 Educational plans
   b) Participation in therapeutic camp
   c) Involvement in peer-support group

Lessons from the parents of youth with chronic medical conditions

For youth with chronic medical conditions, parents assume a variety of roles that include care coordinator, medical expert, and patient advocate (19). Additionally, as their child develops through adolescence and acquires self-management skills, the role of a parent ideally transitions from that of a manager, to a supervisor, and then finally a consultant (20). Through their monitoring, supervision, coaching, and support of skill-development, parents play a significant role in HCT (8,9,21)

Initially, the UNC TR$_x$ANSITION Scale™ was administered to patients in private, without their parent(s) present. About two years ago, our transition coordinator began to administer the scale to the youth in the presence of their family members, as long as the family members remain silent during the assessment. Due to time constraints and limited clinic space, she recognized that a parent's non-participatory presence during assessment served as an excellent learning and teaching opportunity to both, the youth and the parent. By doing this, our HCT coordinator discovered that many parents did not know the level of skills their children possessed, or, worse yet; parents would mention that they themselves did not know the answer to many of the questions related to their child's medical condition(s) and management. This was a very concerning finding, since parents are important facilitators of their children's acquisition of medical knowledge and disease self-management. We considered this as one of the most valuable lessons from the field as this experience reinforced the need for a targeted educational intervention that is both patient- and family-centered.

As a direct result of this experience, the complement to the UNC TR$_x$ANSITION Scale™ for Adolescents and Young Adults was expanded to include a parent version (22). This parent version serves as an assessment of a parent's disease and medication knowledge of their child's condition and as an additional proxy report for the youths' self-management, medication adherence and other HCT-related skills mastery (23). In table 2 we have summarized the UNC TR$_x$ANSITION Program parent recommendations for health providers.

Community partners and volunteers

We have partnered with Victory Junction, a camp located in Randleman, NC, providing year-round programming for children with chronic and life-threatening conditions and their families. Victory Junction has allowed the UNC STAR$_x$ Program to conduct summer research programs that include the deployment of web-based surveys to children and adolescents with a variety of chronic medical conditions who participate in this therapeutic camp (18,23). In-kind donations by Victory Junction have allowed an expansion of services to organize the annual Young Adult Weekend, serving adolescent and emerging adult patients with chronic medical conditions. During this annual weekend, 16-24 year-old participants are able to engage in camp activities and teambuilding sessions, while learning about health care transition and disease self-management.

The UNC STAR$_x$ Program has attracted the assistance of undergraduate, graduate and medical students from several institutions. Two of our students have received "abstract of the year awards" in international conferences (22,23) and summer students have secured funding from the NIH and private foundations. This year, two of our participating medical students each received a 12-month grant from the American Society of Nephrology to conduct research in the area of health care transition (14,22).

Table 2. UNC STAR$_x$ Program Parent Recommendations to Health Providers

1. **Customer service: Similar to the youth recommendations plus...**

   In the outpatient setting:

   a. Have a care coordinator, particularly if multiple consultants are involved
   b. Psychological services should be offered as soon as the chronic diagnosis is made and presented to the family as an expected referral *for all* patients
   c. Schedule 2-4 appointments in one day to avoid losing work days
   d. Identify parent and patient support groups

   In the inpatient setting

   a. As much as possible be consistent with the rounding time, so that they can rest and are able to talk with the provider every day
   b. Have a multidisciplinary family meeting once per week to improve communication with all involved
   c. Having the same nurse care for their child to allow continuity
   d. Participate in holiday-related decorations or floor activities to be considered part of the team, improve the environment and get respite
   e. Getting blood work at 4:00 AM is not friendly, especially when it has been a rough night
   f. Try to do blood work from peripheral IV when possible to decrease veni-punctures
   g. Admission to the same floor whenever possible
   h. Minimize radiation exposure
   i. Have laundry-related services available for long-term admissions
   j. Being able to have your child use regular clothes and not the hospital gowns
   k. Have a parent tray of food

2. **Their fears**

   a. That their child will not be able to survive
   b. Who will assist their child manage their health conditions and their lives as they age
   c. Financial burden
   d. Strain in their marriage
   e. Losing their jobs
   f. Having enough time for their other children and themselves
   g. Keeping their sanity and optimism

3. **Their need for continuous education on**

   a. Their child's diagnosis, especially if the diagnosis is early in life.
   b. Education material that is literacy- and culturally-appropriate
   c. Guidance on how to find community resources

Partnering with other HCT programs

The UNC STAR$_x$ Program has also collaborated with the North Carolina Health and Transition Project, a grant by the Agency of Healthcare Research in Quality to the North Carolina Department of Health. Following the conclusion of the grant, we continued our state-wide collaboration by contacting other HCT programs and researchers outside of North Carolina. As a result, we co-founded what is now known as the *International and Interdisciplinary Health Care Transition Research Consortium.* This consortium holds monthly telecommunication conferences and has bi-annual face to face meetings, with the purpose of advancing the evidence in the field of HCT (22). This has allowed for formal research collaboration of our proprietary tools with Nationwide Children's Hospital/The Ohio State University (pediatric and adult transplant programs), Carolinas Medical Center, the University of Michigan, Hospital Infantil de Mexico, and Universidad de Puerto Rico.

The (long) road ahead

Our program will continue to provide needed services while collecting longitudinal data and evidence on health care transition readiness and disease self-management. Innovation and program development will continue, driven by our patients' experiences and what they teach us. Generalizability of these innovative tools and applications will come from collaborative studies with our committed present and future partners. Understanding and appreciation of the efforts of other practitioners and investigators in this field will continue to inform us and help us all develop the science of HCT. Of paramount importance will be defining cost-effectiveness of our efforts – the costs of failed transplants and unnecessary medical complications is all too evident to many but need to be assessed systematically and balanced against our HCT efforts and costs. Over time, evidence and best practices will emerge and be defined.

We will continue to recognize and honor the essential input of youth and their families who ultimately define how we can best serve their needs. Interdisciplinary collaboration among pediatric patients, team members and practitioners will further assist in tool refinement to assure general application. Our commitment to collaboration with other programs in North Carolina, the United States and countries around the world will continue to advance the evidence and knowledge in the field of health care transition. In the end, expanding our HCT program to those with varying medical conditions, and linking to innovative programs underway at other centers, will allow us all to develop useful and valid HCT-specific tools and reliable outcome measures to decrease morbidity/mortality of our youth with chronic health conditions/disabilities and to improve their health-related quality of quality of life.

ACKNOWLEDGMENTS

Funding (present and past): The North Carolina Children's Hospital, The Renal Research Institute, The American Society of Nephrology, K.B. Reynolds Charitable Trust, UNC Center for Education Research and Therapeutics, The UNC Departments of Medicine, Pediatrics and Kidney Center.

We would like to thank our adolescent/young adult patients, their parents/families and our team of volunteers. We also would like to thank Ms. Jennifer Hoskins, Ms. Regina Andreoni, Sandra Kim, MD; Maureen Kelly, NP; Patricia Jones, MD; Elisabeth Dellon, MD; Elizabeth Champion, MD; Benjamin Harris, MD, Laura Robinson, MD; Mary Campion, MD; Amanda Cartee, MD; Jim Belsante, MD; Bradley Layton, MPH, PhD; Ahinee Amomoo, PhD; Susan Hogan, PhD; Steve Hooper, PhD; Sohini Sengupta, PhD; Ms. Rebecca Ferris, Alexander Ferris, Mike Ferris; Alan Stiles, MD; Marschall Runge, MD; Alan Stiles, MD, Sue Tolleson-Reinhart, PhD; Ms. Janet Hadar, Heather Ansede, MSW, David Tauer, RN, Carol Ford, MD; Victoria Pham, MD; Sarah Massie, MPH; Sandy Grubbs, RN, CNP; Debbie Gipson, MD, MS; William Primack, MD, William Conley, MD; Clara Neyhart, RN; Lynn McCoy, RN; Caroline Jeannette, MSW; Ms. Trina Pugh, Ms. Jean Brown; Elizabeth Prata, FNP, Ms. Claudia Rojas, Lauren Kerns, RN, Cecily Betz, RN PhD*; Patience White, MD*, David Wood, MD, MPH; Greg Sawicki, MD; Mara Medeiros, MD; Melvin Bonilla-Felix, MD, Mary Carter, PhD; Nathan Levine, MD; Peter Kotanko, MD, PhD; Geri Matsoon, MD, MPH; Monique Winslow, MPH, Irene Jurczyk; Tejas Desai, MD, Susan Massengill, MD, the North Carolina CHAT Program, Lorraine Bell, MD*; John Reiss, PhD*, Nikki Becker, MD*, Betty Presler, RN, PhD*, Roberta Williams, MD*, Megumi Okumura, MD, Peter Scal, MD, Mary Ciccarelli, MD, MPH, Sophie Jan, MD, Jason Woodward, MD, Peter Sim, MD, the UNC Transition Team; the Renal Research Institute, K.B. Reynolds Charitable Trust; the American Society of Nephrology, the Victory Junction Camp Staff; the UNC Kidney Center, Center for Faculty Development and the Odum Institute, the Mountain Area Health Education Center in North Carolina, the Midwest Pediatric Nephrology Consortium and the members of the International and Interdisciplinary Health Care Transition Research Consortium.

***Published/field experts consulted prior to our program's inauguration.**

References

[1] Blum RW, Garell D, Hodgman CH, Jorissen TW, Okinow NA, Orr DP, et al. Transition from child-centered to adult health-care systems for adolescents with chronic conditions. A position paper of the Society for Adolescent Medicine. The Journal of adolescent health : official publication of the Society for Adolescent Medicine. 1993;14(7):570-6.

[2] Ferris ME, Mahan JD. Pediatric chronic kidney disease and the process of health care transition. Seminars in nephrology. 2009;29(4):435-44.

[3] A consensus statement on health care transitions for young adults with special health care needs. Pediatrics. 2002;110(6 Pt 2):1304-6.

[4] Rosen DS, Blum RW, Britto M, Sawyer SM, Siegel DM. Transition to adult health care for adolescents and young adults with chronic conditions: position paper of the Society for Adolescent Medicine. The Journal of adolescent health : official publication of the Society for Adolescent Medicine. 2003;33(4):309-11.

[5] Bell LE, Ferris ME, Fenton N, Hooper SR. Health care transition for adolescents with CKD-the journey from pediatric to adult care. Advances in chronic kidney disease. 2011;18(5):384-90.

[6] Cooley WC, Sagerman PJ. Supporting the health care transition from adolescence to adulthood in the medical home. Pediatrics. 2011;128(1):182-200.

[7] Watson AR, Harden PN, Ferris ME, Kerr PG, Mahan JD, Ramzy MF. Transition from pediatric to adult renal services: a consensus statement by the International Society of Nephrology (ISN) and the International Pediatric Nephrology Association (IPNA). Kidney international. 2011;80(7):704-7.

[8] Wang G, McGrath BB, Watts C. Health care transitions among youth with disabilities or special health care needs: an ecological approach. Journal of pediatric nursing. 2010;25(6):505-50.

[9] Schwartz LA, Tuchman LK, Hobbie WL, Ginsberg JP. A social-ecological model of readiness for transition to adult-oriented care for adolescents and young adults with chronic health conditions. Child: care, health and development. 2011;37(6):883-95.

[10] Betz CL. Transition of adolescents with special health care needs: review and analysis of the literature. Issues in comprehensive pediatric nursing. 2004;27(3):179-241.

[11] Bickford K, Ford C, Bozik K, Tolleson-Rinehart S, Chin H, Gipson D, et al. Measuring readiness for transition in adolescents and young adults with chronic kidney disease [Abstract]. 4th Congress of the International Pediatric Transplant Association; 2007; Cancun, Mexico.

[12] Sawicki GS, Lukens-Bull K, Yin X, Demars N, Huang IC, Livingood W, et al. Measuring the transition readiness of youth with special healthcare needs: validation of the TRAQ--Transition Readiness Assessment Questionnaire. Journal of pediatric psychology. 2011;36(2):160-71.

[13] Ferris M, Ford C, Gipson D, Tolleson-Rinehart S, Bickord K, Chin H. The UNC TR$_x$ANSITION Scale^{TM} among adolescents with chronic kidney disease [Abstract]. American Society of Nephrology Renal Week; 2007; San Francisco, CA.

[14] Doan M, Fenton N, Iglesia E, Bickford K, Ferris M. Baseline TR$_x$ANSITION Scale^{TM} scores across multiple health conditions [Abstract]. Pediatric Academic Societies Annual Meeting; 2012; Boston, MA.

[15] Sengupta S, Bickford K, Ferris M. Psychometric validation of the UNC TRxANSITION Scale^{TM} version 3 to measure health care transition among adolescents and emerging adults with chronic disease [Abstract]. Pediatric Academic Societies Annual Meeting; 2011; Denver, CO.

[16] Ferris M, Harward D, Bickford K, Bradley J, Ferris M, Ford C. The development of the UNC TR$_x$ANSITION Scale^{TM}: a clinical tool to measure the components of health care transition. Renal Failure. 2012(In press).

[17] Ferris M, Kelly M, Martin N, Freeman K, Kim S, Gipson D. Sustained use of a practical tool to assist adolescents with disease self-management [Abstract]. Society for Adolescent Medicine Annual Meeting; 2008.

[18] Ko Z, Fenton N, Benton M, Hancock L, Haberman C, Ferris M. Social media use and adolescents' transition readiness [Abstract]. Pediatric Academic Societies Annual Meeting; 2012; Boston, MA.

[19] Kratz L, Uding N, Trahms CM, Villareale N, Kieckhefer GM. Managing childhood chronic illness: parent perspectives and implications for parent-provider relationships. Families, systems & health : the journal of collaborative family healthcare. 2009;27(4):303-13.

[20] Kieckhefer GM, Trahms CM. Supporting development of children with chronic conditions: from compliance toward shared management. Pediatric nursing. 2000;26(4):354-63.

[21] Modi AC, Pai AL, Hommel KA, Hood KK, Cortina S, Hilliard ME, et al. Pediatric self-management: a framework for research, practice, and policy. Pediatrics. 2012;129(2):e473-85.

[22] Iglesia E, Fenton N, Bickford K, Doan M, Ferris M. Parent and adolescent concordance on transition readiness among adolescents with chronic conditions [Abstract]. Pediatric Academic Societies Annual Meeting; 2012; Boston, MA.

[23] Fenton N, Ferris M, Baucom D, Bickford K, Gibson K, Primack W. How resilience factors influence adjustment in adolescents with chronic kidney disease [Abstract]. 13th International Conference on Dialysis, Advances in CKD 2011; 2011; Miami, FL.

Submitted: January 04, 2012. *Revised:* February 03, 2012. *Accepted:* February 12, 2012.

In: Child and Adolescent Health Yearbook 2013
Editor: Joav Merrick

ISBN: 978-1-63117-658-6

Chapter 8

YOUTH SUICIDE PREVENTION AT GRASSROOTS

Said Shahtahmasebi, PhD*

Centre for Health and Social Practice, Wintec, New Zealand,
The Good Life Research Centre Trust, New Zealand and Division of Adolescent Medicine, Department of Pediatrics, Kentucky Children's Hospital, University of Kentucky, Lexington, Kentucky, United States of America

ABSTRACT

The suicide literature suggests that mental illness and in particular depression are the main causes of suicide. Worldwide government policies of addressing mental illness have been the main focus for suicide prevention, which coupled with a moratorium on reporting and public debate of suicide appears to deliver ineffective services. A prevention scheme that is based on intervention will be ineffective because intervention mainly occurs at or after an outcome such as incidence of an illness. Not everyone suffers from mental illness, and not everyone who suffers from mental illness will commit suicide. However, there is a growing body of literature that challenges the mental illness-suicide link. This paper argues that suicide is the result of a complex decision making process by individuals who live in communities and contribute to society. Therefore any interventions must be holistic and at grassroots level. The application of Kentucky University's 'stop youth suicide' campaign to a New Zealand community is briefly discussed.

Keywords: Adolescence, suicide, prevention, New Zealand

INTRODUCTION

In spite of the large volume of literature on suicide the public health strategy on suicide prevention is still reliant on a medical model that treats suicide as a mental illness. There is

* Correspondence: Said Shahtahmasebi, PhD, Director; The Goodlife Research Centre Trust, 4 Orkney St., Strowan, Christchurch. New Zealand. E-mail: radisolevoo@gmail.com

however, confusion within the literature which is often due to poor study design and methodological flaws associated with human behaviour. Suicide data, in particular those based on psychological autopsy type investigations such as Beautrais (1-3), are often plagued with a high degree of bias. Given the current public mindset, helped by the medical model and the media, that depression causes suicide, the collection of data on suicide cases from friends and relatives after the event of suicide will be highly biased towards mental illness, as is the case with the Canterbury Suicide Project (1-3). Studies that fail to address the methodological issues related to design, data collection and analysis will lead to misleading and conflicting conclusions. For example, Beautrais (1-3) used a psychological autopsy method and collected information about suicide cases from family and friends to conclude that mental illness causes suicide. Khan et al. (4) claimed that antidepressants do not reduce suicide and may increase the risk of suicide, while, Hall et al. (5) claimed that antidepressants reduces suicide rates.

The suicide literature also suggests a link between other health, social and environmental factors with suicide. For example, some studies suggest bereavement, e.g., (6-8), early childhood trauma, e.g., (9), socio-economic group and employment issues, e.g., (6), financial strain and negative life events, e.g., (10, 11) and so on as risk factors for suicide. Although, suicide prevention is very slowly and gradually taking notice of alternative medical models, nevertheless, in terms of policy development suicide prevention is still listed under mental health policy. Despite a move by WHO to increase awareness on mental illness which was taken up by some governments (e.g., UK's no health without mental health policy document (12)), more of the same appears to be the main policy for suicide prevention. In other words, the policy documents recommend more mental health services to be made available to the public (13). In the meantime the suicide rates appear to maintain an overall upward trend with cycles where suicide rate trends may reverse for a short period of time. The response from the authorities has often been to praise mental health services during the cycle(s) when trends appear to be downwards, but when the trends reverse it is claimed that suicide is a very complex public health issue and depends on many social, economic and environmental variables which require further research. The lack of progress in suicide prevention appears to be related to budgeting, developing and carrying out "further research" as policy documents appear to suggest "further research" and further investment is often translated into more of the same, i.e., more investment into mental health services (13).

Furthermore, the problems with suicide prevention are exacerbated with the restrictions in the reporting of suicide in the media and public places such as schools and youth clubs which matter most. One main implication of banning discussions of suicide is for the suicide survivors (e.g., see (14)). The ban on an open discussion of suicide has effectively been to shut survivors out and restrict discussion of suicide with their counsellor, if they had one. It is obvious that there will be further complications such as the availability of skilled and culturally sensitive counsellors. This is an important issue when the suicide case is a young adolescent person survived by parents, siblings and friends.

In this paper we discuss the rationale for adopting a holistic approach to suicide prevention and in order to have an impact on future suicide rates emphasis should be placed on educating the young. The issues of interest will be illustrated through a real life application of a grassroots approach to youth suicide prevention.

RATIONALE

Over the years there has been more discussion in the literature about other non-medical risk factors for suicide (15-24) suggesting that a medical model alone will not be an effective form of treatment and prevention. Over the last decade or so, researchers and governments' strategy policies appear to acknowledge the complexities of suicide, however, their action plans seem to divert from these complexities towards a medical model for both prevention and intervention (e.g., see (25, 26)), in other words governments' action policy only offer more of the same (13).

In New Zealand, like other countries, there has been a long established view of the direction of causality from mental illness (specifically depression) to suicide. This has been achieved by the hasty reporting of so called research and in particular the media's slant and uncritical reporting. In announcing a $6.4 million campaign to reduce the impact of depression, the New Zealand Government claimed "We know that up to 90% of suicides are *caused* by depression and that each year 500 New Zealanders are dying by suicide." The Government further claimed "The World Health Organisation has predicted that by the year 2020, depression will be second only to cardiovascular disease, in contributing to the global burden of disease. We must tackle this problem head on and the National Depression Initiative will go a long way to achieving this objective." [http://www.beehive.govt.nz/release/new-campaign-beatdepression]. This announcement is a reflection of the ineffectiveness of health and social policies in reducing cardiovascular disease.

The New Zealand Government's suicide prevention strategy document (25) is testament to this confusion. The document attempts to demonstrate a move away from the medical model by including almost all other possible factors reported in the literature as potential contributors: from alcohol and drug abuse to bereavement, family break-ups, unemployment, educational and financial failure and so on. The strategy (25) is not clear as to how this wide range of contributory factors may relate to policy and therefore budget allocation. It is imperative that policy makers do not fall in the trap of attempting to achieve a perceived desired effect by symbolic manipulation of an outcome process, e.g., removing the 'fail' as an outcome in school exam. In other words, such a policy unwisely assumes that removing 'fail' from an education outcome will lead to positive adolescents. This is analogous to a policy that encourages people to move from their homes because most accidents happen at home.

The main point of concern that all of us (not just practitioners and researchers) must remember, is that at the centre of this decision making process there is a person. In the case of young adolescents, the individual has already gone through their own process of decision making by which time it is too late for any external influence/intervention. Time is a particularly important factor in preventing adolescent suicide due to the fact that the process of decision making takes place much more rapidly than in adults. In adolescents the risk of a complete suicide is heightened when there is immediate access to quick methods of killing (e.g., guns) following a 'trigger' event/factor. Conversely, this risk can be reduced as quickly when the access to means is denied or made difficult thus providing time for the young individuals to reflect on the trigger event whilst attempting suicide. This is not to say that some teenagers do not take time and plan to end their own lives. Although, these suicides may appear as sudden decisions, this does suggest a wish by the individual to be in the driving seat and is in control.

As reported earlier, most of the suicide cases had no psychiatric records suggesting that for these people the decision making process had been completed and executed before any "intervention" could be actioned. Clearly, in these cases not even a holistic treatment would have been effective because of the choice they made. However, such an approach may be modified and extended to understand individuals through an understanding of the society they live in, in order to influence the individual's process of decision making. In medical treatments a "holistic" approach is often referred to as treating the person and not just the physical or emotional symptoms. Ventegodt and Merrick (27) suggest that we must, as holistic physicians and health practitioners, support and guide our patients through the *dynamics* of suicide. To understand the dynamics of human behaviour in the current age of an advanced information culture, the "holistic" notion must go beyond the individual and accept that decision making processes are influenced by many other processes such as social, economic, environment, media (28). Physicians on their own have little or no control over these dynamic processes.

The Good Life Approach (28) may be adopted to develop social and health policy actions incorporating possible influences from these processes.

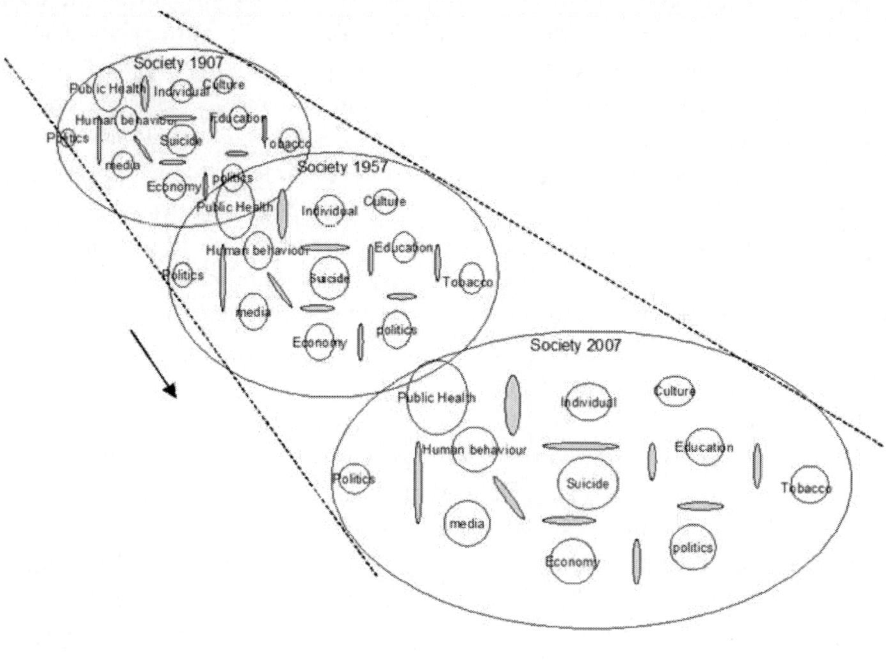

Figure 1. An example of a conceptual holistic model of suicide.

As shown in Figure 1, the Good Life model assumes the individual as well as society are the central processes that are subject to influence from other processes. Some of these processes we know about and are related to human behaviour; politics, economy, education, public health and medicine, whilst others such as the environment are inter-related with human behaviour but we do not have complete control over them. The problem is that the dynamics of human behaviour may influence these processes in a conflicting and diverging direction to contradict and lead to adverse interactions between the processes. Erroneous results and mis-conclusions from a biased and subjective assessment of suicide will have further ramifications for policy and treatment. For example, anti-smoking or anti-violence policies may be ineffective in the light of how politicians behave, and the media's portrayal of a hero as a violent smoker who dabbles in risky behaviour.

The main points being presented here are:

a) the current list of risk factors for suicide and suicidal behaviour (e.g., see (25, 26)) suggests that suicide is a complex health and social issue that can affect anyone. In other words the whole population is at risk of suicide.
b) There are overlaps and conflicts in human behaviour leading to conflicting consequences in behaviour outcomes such as the interaction between entertainment media, social and health policies, and behaviour outcomes such eradicating family and sexual violence, reducing smoking rates, and preventing a suicide.

CONCEPTUALIZATION

It can be visualised from Fig. 1 that prevention actions based on a single model may not have an impact on suicide but will affect the parameters of other processes and can itself be affected by them. Such dynamic interactions may in fact produce outcomes in the opposite direction. For example, the emphasis by the medical model on mental illness may in fact help maintain the taboo status of suicide, and influence other health and social behaviour outcomes, e.g., social attitudes and perceptions of mental illness as the main cause of suicide and a lack of service uptake, see (17, 29). Furthermore, the generally upward trends since World War II in Figure 2 can be interpreted that such an approach of relying on a sustained application of a single model has not worked.

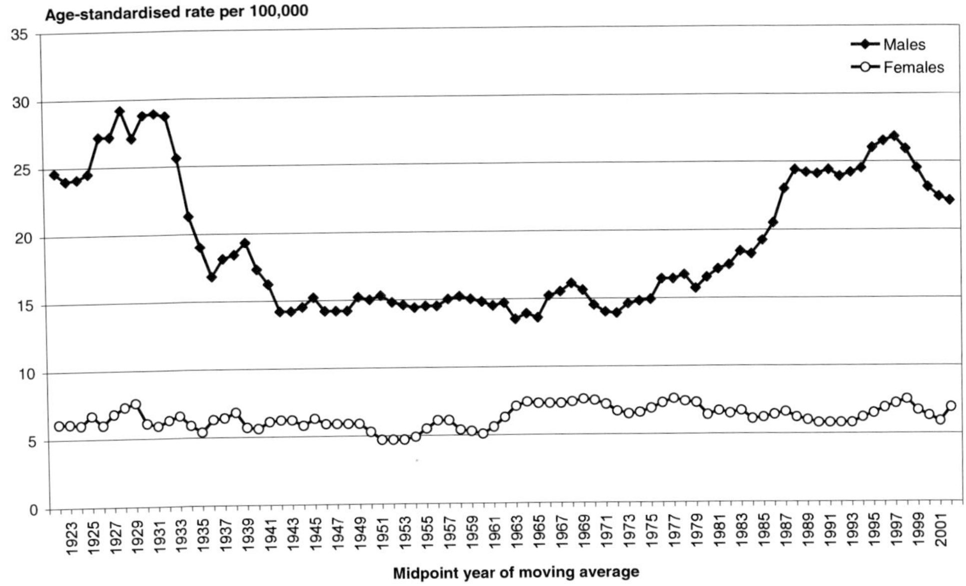

Source: New Zealand Health Information Service (30).

Figure 2. Death from suicide by sex, New Zealand, 1921-2003.

Surely, after so many decades of 'more of the same' it must be time to follow a different direction and adopt a more collaborative approach. However, bearing in mind the conceptual model in Figure 1, we must first try and understand not just suicide but human behaviour. Second, any new direction and approach must take account of the residual effects of health and social policies on behaviour. For example, it will not be easy to reverse the effects on policy development of the well-established view in the public mind set that mental illness causes suicide.

As suggested above, risk factors for suicide are many and cover many aspects of society. The literature on suicide, e.g., (25, 26), suggests a large number of variables from depression to trauma, bereavement, unemployment, marriage break up, poor health, drug and alcohol abuse, poor nutrition, childhood events and so on may cause suicide. A pragmatic translation of the literature is that the general population is at risk of suicide. This interpretation actually makes sense and reinforces that suicide cannot be explained by one discipline or a model. Suicide is a process of decision making.

Suicide prevention policy development should allow a multidisciplinary approach to include input from members of the public. However, in most countries the policy development for suicide prevention and intervention has been a top-down approach where governments develop mental health strategy documents with respective policy action documents in order to allocate and distribute resources. As discussed elsewhere (13), strategy documents and policy actions are often translated into mental services which the public are told they need. In other words there is no input from the public about what they really need and what they really want.

It is evident that suicide prevention and intervention must start with a willingness from the public to take part in (31). In order to achieve this, the direction of policy development must be reversed. That is, prevention and interventional policies must be holistic, and to be holistic they must be developed at the grassroots.

Community-based actions are not new phenomena. The University of Kentucky's "stop youth suicide" Campaign (http://stopyouthsuicide.com) started in 2001 because the coroner was concerned to see so many young suicide cases. His approach was without presumption and simple. He approached the adolescent medicine department at the University of Kentucky and asked the question 'what can we do to reduce youth suicide? The "stop youth suicide" campaign began with the knowledge and understanding of adolescents and therefore their communities. Through such an approach we can then gain insight into the society and communities of these young people. The "stop youth suicide" Campaign has enlisted community workers, politicians, schools, teenagers themselves (32).

The Campaign has been successful in reducing youth suicide rates from around 19 to under 12 per 100,000 and attributes this success to the involvement at grassroots. The Campaign has brought about law changes including gun-safety, public discussion of suicide, and suicide education programmes at schools. Most of these programmes are longitudinal and are an integral part of the curriculum to maintain continuity.

THE NEW ZEALAND EXPERIENCE

As mentioned in the background, New Zealand aligns itself with Western democracies on suicide. Despite acknowledging the multidimensional risk for suicide, the prevention and interventional strategies are top-down and based on a medical model. Internationally, New Zealand's suicide rate is high. In 2010, 522 people died as a result of suicide. The national suicide rate is 11.5 per 100,000 people (http://www.health.govt.nz/publication/suicide-facts-deaths-and-intentional-self-harm-hospitalisations-2010). Youth suicide is of particular concern in New Zealand. Suicide rates for young people are high, with deaths between the ages of 15 and 24 making up 23% of all suicides in the Waikato region. Suicide is the second most common cause of death for young people. Between 2002 and 2006, over a quarter of deaths in the Waikato region for people aged 15-19 were due to suicide.

In New Zealand, Waikato Institute of Technology (Wintec) funded a proposal in 2009/10 to run youth suicide prevention. Wintec is a tertiary education provider with a strong commitment to the community it serves. The workshops were facilitated by the Chair of Kentucky's 'Stop Youth Suicide campaign' (32).

A programme of four workshops targeting communities that had been identified with high rates of youth suicide and a public lecture was put together.

During these workshops the extent of community despair and frustration caused by suicide and its politics became more evident. Despite the high level of frustration with the politics of suicide most front line service providers and those affected by suicide demonstrated a strong passion about suicide prevention and wanted to talk about it. Despite limited publicity the workshops were well attended.

Workshop evaluations were 100% positive and demonstrated a very strong demand for a community-based strategy. The workshop evaluations also suggested a strong demand for more details of workshops providing skills training. At least one community set up a support group made up of volunteers. The media showed interest, too, but the workshops did not get much air time due to an unfortunate major mine disaster with many fatalities in New Zealand around the same time as the workshops. However, one of the key messages was that we cannot keep suicide a secret and must talk about it otherwise our youth could make *un-informed* decisions about their understanding of suicide based on secretive rumours.

Due to the feedback and demand for training, in association with participating communities, and through a Fulbright Specialists Grant, advanced training workshops were offered in 2011. Wintec's community alliance consisted of many frontline health and social services groups including Waahi Whanui, Huntly Community Advice, Raukura Waikato Social Services, mental health awareness forum or the Maori Women's Welfare League, South Waikato District Council, Raukawa Iwi and Te Puna Oranga (Māori Health Service) Waikato District Health Board (DHB), Population Health Service of the Waikato DHB, Safe Kawerau Kids Injury Prevention Project (SKKIPP) and Rangatahi group for Kawerau. The Fulbright grant was supplemented with local communities' financial support and a grant from Trust Waikato to cover expenses. These workshops were run during the latter part of November 2011. There were more communities who had joined the first group of communities which stretched from Thames (North Waikato), central and South Waikato, and an interest group in Christchurch (in the South Island). Although, the workshops were designed for the health professionals (including social workers, counsellors, health promoters,

GPs, psychiatrist and mental health workers), attendance was open to the public with an interest in youth suicide prevention.

The communities that were involved with the workshops have now joined forces and have regular contact with each other to share information and action plans, and to support each other and share scarce resources where there are overlaps. Most of the communities have now set up support groups made up of mostly volunteer parents, concerned individuals, suicide survivors (parents who have lost to suicide). These groups do not see themselves as frontline suicide prevention workers but as a buffering force, to be a 'non-threatening' and approachable resource for young people or anyone to feel comfortable to contact and talk about their issues. The groups have collated a list of resources including emergency phone numbers to crisis, national suicide prevention, mental health services and other local services that may be appropriate.

The groups have no funds nor have they any resources to operate effectively. However, armed with a knowledge of their community and a passion to prevent suicide have adopted a strategy of simple actions that could have a major impact on the outcome. For example, talking about the evils of suicide, providing a cell phone help-number for people to contact, taking a chance and start a conversation with people at any opportunity e.g., at the bus stop or in the park. Simple steps like talking to people have already helped some people in the community who had otherwise been contemplating suicide.

However, without any resources even the simple steps can become a major problem and could take months if not years to organise. As an example, one group recognised a community need for youth to contact the group but found organising a cell phone very difficult. Although, it was relatively easy to get hold of a handset which was donated by a local resident, getting mobile service providers on-board to donate air time has not come to fruition despite its success and local relevance and the cost is being borne by the group. The group has already received calls from local youths seeking help.

Amongst other success it appears that suicide is beginning to lose its taboo stature and is being discussed and debated at a community level. In 2012, Lifeline Aotearoa (www.lifeline.org.nz) launched a three month television campaign on Maori TV called 'start the conversation today- Me timata te korero i tenei ra!'

CONCLUSION

A top-down approach coupled with a lack of communication between support service agencies is often ineffective and has very little effect on the outcomes for which the services are designed in the first place (13, 33). Within a top-down policy formation, the authorities become less receptive to community input. For example, it is reported that the Associate Health Minister was to chair a meeting of media, mental health professionals and researchers early this year to update the guidelines (http://www.stuff.co.nz/the-press/news/4550480/Anger-over-missing-voice). There is no mention of communities or victims/survivors of suicide in this statement of intent. Such groups were mentioned in a non-specific way by a spokesman for the Associate Health Minister that family and friends would be able to participate in the meetings this year, after an uproar by suicide survivors.

Relevant and effective policy actions can be developed through the *depoliticisation* of research and science so that collaboration can occur more fluidly within and between the various agencies in conjunction with the communities at grassroots level. By engaging the community and the public at the beginning of the process of decision making will help make policy actions more relevant and effective. At the time of writing, the author received a report from one of the communities that through engaging the public a young teenager intervened and prevented a potential suicide of another adolescent by turning up at their doorstep.

In the context of a grassroots approach, the role of the experts would be to critique the available research collaboratively and not in competition. It must be remembered that every policy action will have a multi-dimensional reaction on behavioural outcomes (Figure 1). We must avoid a situation where society and communities are defined by individualism, thus, eroding the most intrinsic of human behaviour, which is keeping in contact and looking out for friends and neighbours and other members of the community.

REFERENCES

[1] Beautrais AL. Serious suicide attempts in young people: A case control study. Dissertation. Christchurch: Christchurch School Medicine, 1996.

[2] Beautrais AL. Suicides and serious suicide attempts: Two populations or one? Psychol Med 2001;31:837-45.

[3] Beautrais AL, Joyce PR, Mulder RT. The canterbury suicide project: Aims, overview and progress. Commun Ment Health NZ 1994;8(2):32-9.

[4] Khan A, Warner HA, Brown WA. Symptom reduction and suicide risk in patients treated with placebo in antidepressant clinical trials: An analysis of the food and drug administration database. Arch Gen Psychiatry 2000;57:311-7.

[5] Hall WD, Mant A, Mitchell PB, Rendle VA, Hickie IB, McManus P. Association between antidepressant prescribing and suicide in Australia, 1991-2000: Trend analysis. BMJ 2003;326:1008.

[6] Agerbo E, Nordentoft M, Mortensen PB. Familial, psychiatric, and socioeconomic risk factors for suicide in young peopl: Nested case-control study. BMJ 2002;325(7355):74-7.

[7] Murphy SA, Tapper VJ, Johnson LC, Lohan J. Suicide ideation among parents bereaved by the violent deaths of their children. Issues Ment Health Nurs 2003;24(1):5-25.

[8] Rozenzweig A, Prigerson H, Miller MD, Reynolds CFr. Bereavement and late-life depression: Grief and its complications in the elderly. Annu Rev Med 1997;48:421-8.

[9] van der Kolk BA, Hostetler A, Herron N, Fisler RE. Trauma and the development of borderline personality disorder. Psychiatr Clin North Am 1994;17(4):715-30.

[10] Baumeister RF. Suicide as escape from self. Psychol Rev 1990;97(1):90.

[11] Duberstein PR, Conwell Y, Conner KR, Eberly S, Caine ED. Suicide at 50 years of age and older: Perceived physical illness, family discord and financial strain. Psychol Med 2004;34(1):137-46.

[12] Department of Health. No health without mental health: A cross-government mental health outcomes strategy for people of all ages. HM Government, 2011.

[13] Shahtahmasebi S. A review and critique of mental health policy development. Int J Child Health Hum Dev 2012;5(3):forthcoming.

[14] Shahtahmasebi S, Aupouri-Mclean C. Bereaved by suicide. Primary Health Care: Open Access (http://wwwomicsgrouporg/journals/ArchivePHCOA/currentissuePHCOAphp) 2011:1:101.

[15] Abbar M, Caer Y, Schenk L, Castelnau D. [psychosocial stress factors and suicidal acts]. Encephale 1993;19(Spec No 1):179-85.

[16] Conwell Y, Duberstein PR. Prevention of late life suicide: When, where, why and how. Psychiatr Clin Neurosci 1995;49(Suppl 1):S79-83.

[17] Hamdi E, Price S, Qassem T, Amin Y, Jones D. Suicides not in contact with mental health services: Risk indicators and determinants of referral. J Ment Health 2008;17(4):398-409.

[18] Heikkinen M, Aro H, Lonnqvist J. Life events and social support in suicide. Suicide Life Threat Behav 1993;23(4):343-58.

[19] Heikkinen M, Aro H, Lonnqvist J. Recent life events, social support and suicide. Acta Psychiatr Scand Suppl 1994;377:65-72.

[20] Murphy BM, Puffett A. Pathways to suicide prevention. Br J Hosp Med 1995;54(1):11-4.

[21] Neeleman J. Beyond risk theory: Suicidal behavior in its social and epidemiological context. Crisis 2002;23(3):114-20.

[22] Shahtahmasebi S, Shahtahmasebi R. A holistic view of suicide: Social change and education and training. J Altern Med Res 2010;2(1):115-28.

[23] Ventegodt S, Clausen B, Merrick J. Clinical holistic medicine: The case story of anna. Iii. Rehabilitation of philosophy of life during holistic existential therapy for childhood sexual abuse. ScientificWorldJournal 2006;6:2080-91.

[24] Webb D. Bridging the spiritual gap. Australian e-Journal for the Advancement of Mental Health (AeJAMH): http://wwwauseinetcom/journal/vol4iss1/webbpdf <http://wwwauseinetcom/journal/vol4iss1/webbpdf> 2005;4(1).

[25] Associate Minister of Health. The new zealand suicide prevention strategy 2006-2016. Wellington: Ministry of Health 2006;http://www.moh.govt.nz/moh.nsf/pagesmh/4904/$File/suicide-prevention-strategy-2006-2016.pdf.

[26] Lorant V, Kunst AE, Huisman M, Costa G, Mackenbach J. Socio-economic inequalities in suicide: A european comparative study. Br J Psychiatry 2005;187(1):49.

[27] Ventegodt S, Merrick J. Philosophy of life and suicide: To be or not to be is still the question. In: Merrcik J, Zalsman G, eds. Suicidal behaviour in adolescence: An international perspective. Tel Aviv: Freund, 2005:9-17.

[28] Shahtahmasebi S. The good life: A holistic approach to the health of the population. ScientificWorldJournal 2006;6:2117-32.

[29] Shahtahmasebi S. Suicides by mentally ill people. ScientificWorldJournal 2003;3:684-93.

[30] Ministry of Health. New zealand suicide trends: Mortality 1921-2003, hospitalisations for intentional self-harm 1978-2004. Wellington, NZ: Ministry of Health, 2006.

[31] Shahtahmasebi S. Suicide research and adolescent suicide trends in New Zealand. ScientificWorldJournal 2008;8:287-302.

[32] Omar H. A model program for youth suicide prevention. Int J Adolesc Med Health 2005;17(3):275-8.

[33] Shahtahmasebi S, van den Berg L, Hermann F. What do you do when no health and social agency wants to care for you? Int J Child Health Hum Dev, in press.

Submitted: February 03, 2012. *Revised:* April 05, 2012. *Accepted:* April 23, 2012.

In: Child and Adolescent Health Yearbook 2013
Editor: Joav Merrick
ISBN: 978-1-63117-658-6

Chapter 9

ATTENTION DEFICIT HYPERACTIVITY DISORDER: NEUROPSYCHOLOGIC AND PHARMACOLOGIC ASPECTS

Donald E Greydanus, MD, DrHC (ATHENS)*[*,1], Gabriel Kaplan, MD[2,3] and Kevin M Antshel, PhD[4]

[1]Department of Pediatric and Adolescent Medicine, Western Michigan University School of Medicine, Kalamazoo, Michigan
[2]University of Medicine and Dentistry of New Jersey, Newark, New Jersey
[3]Behavioral Health, Bergen Regional Medical Center, Paramus, New Jersey
[4]Department of Psychiatry and Behavioral Sciences, SUNY – Upstate Medial University, Syracuse, New York, United States of America

ABSTRACT

Attention deficit hyperactivity disorder (ADHD) is noted in 3-9% of children and adolescents by American research, three times more commonly in males than females; it is found in 3%-5% of adults with equal male to female ratios if the diagnostic criteria are based on the DSM. The neuropsychiatric etiology of ADHD was suspected from early on so that significant research was aimed at elucidating its neuropsychological deficits. Impairments in attention, impulse control, and motor activity -the condition's core deficits- are well documented in neuropsychological studies. So are the beneficial effects of medication for ADHD which have been unambiguously supported by hundreds of studies in the expert academic literature. While stimulants are the most effective therapeutic agents, non stimulants also play an important role. Theoretical constructs linking molecular neurotransmitter actions to neuroanatomical macro structures and cognitive and behavioral findings have found solid empirical confirmations. Although medication related cognitive improvements appear to be supported only in short term studies, it is recommended that ADHD be actively treated, as patients with this condition

* Correspondence: Professor Donald E Greydanus, MD, Dr. HC (ATHENS), Pediatric and Adolescent Medicine, Western Michigan University School of Medicine, , 1000 Oakland Drive, Kalamazoo, MI 49008-1284, United States. E-mail: Donald.Greydanus@med.wmich.edu

can show serious long term disabilities that go beyond academic failure, and overall clinical improvements are strong and the agents prescribed relatively safe.

Keywords: Attention deficit hyperactivity disorder, psychiatry, behavior

Introduction

Few conditions in the mental health field have shown a closer link to neuropsychological constructs than the Attentional Disorders. From the word "attention", prominently listed in the current Diagnostic Statistical Manual of Mental Disorders (DSM-IV-TR) (1) nomenclature of "Attention Deficit Hyperactivity Disorder (ADHD)" and recent sophisticated neurotransmitter findings, to previous descriptions such as "minimal brain dysfunction", the disorder has been associated with neuropsychiatric substrates throughout its history (2).

ADHD is noted in 3% to 9% of children and adolescents by American research, three times more commonly in males than females; it is found in 3%-5% of adults with equal male to female ratios if the diagnostic criteria are based on the DSM (3). Clinicians in European countries tend to use criteria based on the International Classification of Diseases in which the condition is called "attention-deficit/hyperkinetic disorder", and estimate a much lower prevalence for ADD/ADHD (4). However, various studies from different countries based on similar diagnostic criteria confirm the widespread prevalence of ADHD (5,6). In 2006, 5 million individuals in the United States were prescribed psychostimulant medications, the most commonly recommended ADHD agents, 3.5 million between ages 3 to 19 years, and 1.5 million between ages 20 and 64 years (3).

ADHD Core Features

The DSM-IV-TR presents a detailed list of symptoms and criteria for arriving at a diagnosis. Core features include attention dysfunction along with variable degrees of hyperactivity and impulsivity that interfere with day to day functioning (1,7). This disorder is a lifelong condition with persistence from childhood and adolescence into adulthood in approximately up to 66% of those diagnosed with ADHD in childhood (2). Sometimes, ADHD is not diagnosed until adolescence or adulthood. Inattention in childhood may evolve into difficulty sustaining attention, paralyzing procrastination, and severe disorganization skills in teens or adults. The impulsivity of childhood may persist manifesting in adults as severe impatience characterized by frequent losing one's temper, quitting or losing jobs, or ending relationships. The classical hyperactivity of childhood is observed less commonly in the older populations and may evolve into an inner restlessness, excessive talking, and/or self-selection of jobs that mask ADHD symptomatology (8).

ADHD is considered a neurobehavioral disorder with abnormalities in various neurotransmitter systems, mainly dopaminergic and noradrenergic (9-11). Neuroimaging (i.e., PET scans) and genetic studies further suggest that dopamine transporter dysfunction (6) appears to be implicated in the pathophysiology of ADHD. Heritability is about 75% with at least seven genes involved in ADHD: DRD4, DRD5, DAT, DBH, 5-HTT, HTR1B, and

SNAP25 (12). Current research is attempting to identify different types of attentional dysfunction based on what areas of the brain are involved and then using specific medication to correct or moderate the identified defects; these areas include the cortex (prefrontal and parietal), brain stem (reticular formation), thalamus, basal ganglia, cingulate gyrus, and limbic structures (amygdala-hippocampus) (13). It is hoped that this brain mapping may allow more specific ADHD medications in the future.

Current psychopharmacologic practices

There are over 70 years of research noting that medication can ameliorate ADHD symptoms in children, adolescents, and adults (9). Drugs used for treatment include US Food and Drug Administration (FDA) approved stimulant and non stimulant agents as well as other various non - FDA approved agents.

FDA approved agents

a. Stimulant agents

Hundreds of research studies on patients with ADHD have established the beneficial effects of stimulant medications in all ages: children, adolescents, and adults (3,14-17). Approximately 75% or more of those with ADHD achieve some benefit (9) and the utilization of medication has become a standard part of management for these patients by many clinicians. A comprehensive study was sponsored by the National Institute of Mental Health (NIHM) in the United States; this research was named the NIMH Collaborative Multisite Multimodal Treatment Study of Children with Attention-Deficit/Hyperactivity Disorder, Combined type (or the MTA study) (18,19). The MTA study posed 3 questions. How do long-term medication and behavioral treatments compare with one another? Are there additional benefits when they are used together? What is the effectiveness of systematic, carefully delivered treatments versus routine community care? In this study, 579 children with ADHD Combined Type, aged 7 to 9.9 years at study entry, were randomly assigned to 14 months of treatment with: rigorous medication management; intensive behavioral treatment; the 2 combined; or standard community care (delivered by community providers who in two thirds of the cases treated patients with medications). Seventy-four percent of the MTA Study subjects in the medication management group received methylphenidate immediate release (MPH IR) 3 times per day with an average dose of approximately 31 mg/d, which was well tolerated overall. Because of ethical concerns about the duration of the trial, a placebo or sham treatment control group was not included; the community care group served as the comparator arm. Although all groups showed considerable reductions in symptoms with time, there were significant differences between the 4 groups. For core ADHD symptoms, children in the combined treatment and medication management groups showed significantly greater improvement than those given intensive behavioral treatment and community care. However, the combined treatment offered no significantly greater benefits than medication management alone for core ADHD symptoms. The MTA results validated the clinical experience that children who largely adhere to a well-titrated regimen of stimulants continue to benefit significantly for at least 14 months.

Methylphenidate preparations

MPH, the stimulant most commonly prescribed for patients with ADHD since its production started in 1957, is a sympathomimetic agent with mild central nervous system (CNS) stimulant properties. Preparations are available for racemic dl-MPH as well as the single d-MPH isomer. Its beneficial effect on attention span dysfunction results from blocking the presynaptic dopamine transporter in the CNS striatal and prefrontal areas, leading to rise in extracellular dopamine (20). It also causes a blockade of the CNS norepinephrine transporter in the norepinephrine system. Stimulant medication therapeutic actions include reduced motor restlessness (i.e., less gross/fine motor movement), reduced impulsivity, reduced hyperarousal, enhanced concentration and less aggressive and/or antisocial behavior. There is no correlation between weight of the patient and optimal MPH dose, and plasma levels of MPH are not useful. A number of tools, some of which are listed in table 1, are used to assess treatment effectiveness and include patient/family interviews, parent ratings, school grades or reports, and others. These instruments are helpful to monitor the efficacy of any type of ADHD therapy.

Various IR or short acting preparations of MPH had been popular until recently, when a number of longer-acting products were developed. All these agents are listed in table 2.

There is only one "head to head" study comparing agents (21), so the absence of comparison data at this time makes the selection of the most appropriate agent truly a veritable blend of art and science (9). The process of identifying the best agent for specific patients is addressed later in this chapter. Reasons for failure of MPH to be effective are listed in table 3 and its side effects in table 4.

Table 1. Most commonly used ADHD rating scales

NAME	MAIN FEATURES
Conners Scales	Available in Parent, Teacher, Adolescent Versions Long, Short, and Abbreviated (10 item) Forms www.mhs.com
ADHD Rating Scale-IV	Based on the DSM-IV 18 symptoms, School and Home versions available. www.guilford.com
Brown ADD Scales	Available in Parent, Teacher, and Adolescent self report versions. Assess executive functions psychcorp.pearsonassessments.com
SKAMP	Brief 10 item version for Teacher or Observer www.adhd.net
CBCL	Not ADHD specific but one of the oldest and most studied tool. Multiple informant versions www.aseba.org

Table 2. Methylphenidate Preparations

Brand name (in USA)	Dosage form	Dosing regimen			Duration of effect in hours
		Start	Titrate weekly	Maximum per day	
Active ingredient: d,l,methylphenidate					
Ritalin; Generic form available	Scored tablets: 5,10,20 mg	5 mg 2-3 times/day; 1 dose before breakfast, 1 before lunch	5-10 mg; Give a third dose in the afternoon if needed	Not to exceed 20 mg/dose; 60 mg/day	3-4
Methylin	Scored tablets: 5,10,20 mg; chewable tablets: 2.5,5,10 mg; oral solution: 5mg/ml, 10 mg/10 ml	5 mg 2-3 times/day; 1 dose before breakfast, 1 before lunch	5-10 mg; Give a third dose in the afternoon if needed	Not to exceed 20 mg/dose; 60 mg/day	4-8
Ritalin SR	Sustained release tablets: 20 mg	20 mg before breakfast	20 mg; Give a second dose in afternoon if needed; for desired dose and duration, short acting form may be used	60 mg	6-8
Metadate ER	Extended release tablets: 10, 20 mg	10 mg before breakfast	10 mg; Give a second dose in afternoon if needed	60 mg	4-8
Methylin ER	Extended release tablets: 10, 20 mg	10 mg before breakfast	10 mg; Give a second dose in afternoon if needed	60 mg	4-8
Metadate CD	Extended release capsules: 10, 20, 30 mg. Can be sprinkled	20 mg before breakfast	20 mg; Give a second dose in the afternoon if needed	60 mg	4-8
Ritalin LA	Long acting capsules: 10,20,30,40 mg; can be sprinkled	10 mg before breakfast	5-10 mg; Use short acting form (Ritalin) to titrate if needed	60 mg	4-8
Concerta	Capsules: 18,27,36,54 mg; do not split or chew or crush	18 mg before breakfast	18 mg	72 mg	8-12
Daytrana	Transdermal patch: 10,15,20,30 mg	10 mg patch applied 2 hour before desired effect; remove 9 hours later	10 mg	30 mg	12
Active ingredient: d, methylphenidate					
Focalin	Scored tablets: 2.5, 5, 10 mg	2.5 mg 1 to 2 times a day	2.5 mg; Give a third dose in afternoon if needed.	30 mg	4-5
Focalin XR	Extended release capsules: 5, 10 mg; can be sprinkled	5 mg before breakfast	5 mg; Give a second dose in afternoon if needed; for desired dose and duration short acting form (Focalin) may be used	30 mg	8-12

Table 3. Reasons for failure of Methylphenidate

- Inaccurate diagnosis
- Comorbid disorders that overshadow the ADHD
- Medication doses that are too high or not high enough
- Medication is diverted to others in or outside the family
- Intolerable medication side effects
- Medication is used as a drug of abuse for its euphoric effects
- Patient and/or family not accepting of medication
- Patient does not respond to MPH but does to other stimulants or alternative medications
- Patient does not respond to medications of any kind

Source: Modified with permission from: Greydanus DE, Pratt HD et al: Psychopharmacology of ADHD in adolescents. Adolesc Med 2002;13:604.

Table 4. Potential side effects of stimulant drugs

Headache*
Nausea/vomiting*
Anorexia*
Insomnia (delayed onset of sleep)

Weight loss*
Moodiness (irritability)

Tachycardia
Palpitations
Sudden cardiac death
Increase in blood pressure
"Unmasking" of Tourette Syndrome
Rebound phenomenon

Reduced seizure threshold
Irritability/ restlessness
Emotional lability
Appearance of psychosis or psychotic features

Growth retardation (at higher doses, over longer times, in those with short stature or slow axial growth)
Skin rash (rare)

***Commonly seen side effects**

Source: Modified with permission from: Greydanus DE, Pratt HD et al: Psychopharmacology of ADHD in adolescents. Adolesc Med 2002;13:607.

Amphetamine preparations

Table 5. AMP preparations

NAME/FORMULATION	DOSE	STARTING	MAXIMUM DOSE
DURATION	FORMS	DOSE	(May increase as per MD judgment)
SHORT ACTING			
Adderall	5, 7.5, 10, 12.5, 15,	3-5y: 2.5 mg q.d	40mg.
(Mixed AMP salts)	20, 30 mg tab	>6y: 5 mg q.d.	

NAME/FORMULATION	DOSE	STARTING	MAXIMUM DOSE
DURATION	FORMS	DOSE	(May increase as per MD judgment)
SHORT ACTING			
Dexedrine	5 mg cap	3-5y: 2.5 mg q.d	40mg.
(d-AMP)		>6y: 5 mg q.d.	
LONG ACTING			
Dexedrine Spansule	5, 10, 15 mg cap	>6y: 5-10mg q.d.	40mg.
Adderall XR	5, 10, 15, 20, 25,	>6y: 10 mg q.d.	30mg;
(Mixed AMP salts XR)	30 mg cap	contents can be sprinkled	
PRODRUG			
Vyvanse	20, 30, 40, 50, 60,	>6y: 20mg q.d.	70 mg
(LDX)	70 mg cap	contents can be dissolved in liquid	

The description of beneficial effects of amphetamine (AMP) on hyperactivity and inattention date back to 1937 (22). The amphetamines are non-catecholamine, sympathomimetic amines that act as CNS stimulants. Their putative mechanism of action involves reuptake blockade of neurotransmitters (dopamine and norepinephrine) into presynaptic neurons, as well as an increased release of those neurotransmitters into the synaptic cleft (20). Amphetamines are available as dextroamphetamine sulfate (the dextro isomer of d, l amphetamine sulfate) or as mixed amphetamine salts (dextroamphetamine plus levoamphetamine) as well as lysdexamfetamine, a prodrug formulation of d-amphetamine. The potential adverse effects of amphetamines are the same as of MPH (see table 4). Available amphetamine products are listed in table 5.

Contraindications for stimulant use

Unless stated otherwise, it is assumed that any medication will have as a contraindication sensitivity to that medication or any of its ingredients. Patients with significant levels of anxiety, inner tension, or psychomotor agitation should generally not be on psychostimulants. Other contraindications include glaucoma, psychosis, and hyperthyroidism. Due to significant comorbidity with substance abuse disorders, the field has taken a fresh look at the traditional contraindication of drug and alcohol dependence although it is still present on the labels (9). Because of potential cardiovascular side effects, stimulants should not be used in patients with uncontrolled hypertension, symptomatic cardiovascular disorder (i.e., angina, heart failure), serious structural cardiac abnormalities, cardiomyopathy, and serious heart rhythm abnormalities.

The use of stimulants in the presence of motor tic disorder or Tourette's syndrome is relatively contraindicated along with a history of epilepsy. Stimulants should not be combined with monoamine oxidase inhibitors since this combination can lead to a hypertensive crisis. Therefore, two weeks should be allowed between prescribing a stimulant and discontinuing a monoamine oxidase inhibitor. Mixing a stimulant with a tricyclic antidepressant may lead to sudden death from cardiac arrhythmias in rare cases. MPH can interfere with the metabolism of some anticonvulsant drugs, such as phenytoin and phenobarbital.

Side effects of stimulants

Adverse effects of stimulants, some of which are transient, can be reduced if the patient starts with a low dose and slowly increases the dosage to maximize benefit. Nausea or emesis that may occur with stimulants often improves if the medication is taken with meals. Dizziness occurs in some patients and is worse with short-acting stimulants versus long-acting types. If dizziness occurs, dehydration or blood pressure changes may be responsible and need to be treated as necessary. Headaches may develop while taking stimulants and this may be related to peak plasma levels or related to drug withdrawal. A change to a different formulation may provide symptomatic relief. The use of stimulant medication does not appear to increase the risk of substance abuse, although it is important to be cognizant of potential stimulant diversion and prescribe longer acting formulations that are less preferred in patients with drug dependence histories (23).

The phenomenon of stimulant related delayed growth remains controversial and seems to be, in part, related to appetite suppression with decreased caloric intake (24).It appears to be a transient effect, and most children eventually seem to attain expected adult height. However, youth on stimulants who are not growing properly need careful supervision. If the appetite is blunted while on stimulants, a number of measures can be taken, including taking food when the stimulant wears off (as in the evening), using high-caloric foods or nutritional supplements, taking the patient off stimulants when not in school (such as during vacation or on weekends), and trying other non stimulant ADHD medications (9).

Tolerance may develop in some patients receiving high stimulant doses. Management involves tapering off the stimulant and trying a different ADHD medication. Rebound can develop in which increased ADHD symptoms (i.e., irritability, sadness, and excitability) develop as the stimulant effect wears off. This can be managed by giving a smaller immediate-release dose in the afternoon or changing to a sustained release product. Stimulants may interfere with sleep and this side effect tends to diminish with time. In addition to stimulant side effect, the patient with sleep disturbances should be carefully evaluated for other causes of sleep disturbances (25).

Administering the last dose of the day earlier, eliminating or reducing the last dose of the day, or the use of a long-acting preparation are some of the strategies that may help with sleep problems. Pharmacological options for sleep problems in children are limited. Drugs such as tricyclic antidepressants, alpha2 agonists [i.e., clonidine, guanfacine], trazodone, and melatonin have been used. However, potential complications of combination of these drugs with stimulants must be carefully considered, in particular regarding antidepressants. Recent data suggests that combinations with melatonin (26) and guanfacine XR (27) are safe.

ADHD is found in 50% to 75% of patients with Tourette Syndrome (TS) and TS may become apparent in some children or adolescents after starting stimulant drugs. Research does not suggest that stimulant medications cause TS and the presence of tics is a relative, not absolute contraindication to stimulant medication. Patients with both ADHD and TS may be given both stimulant medications (if effective) and anti-tic medication (such as risperidone, haloperidol, or pimozide). If the tics are worsened by the stimulant drugs, other ADHD medications may be tried that do not typically worsen tics such as guanfacine and atomoxetine.

Because of reports of serious cardiovascular adverse events in recent years, the FDA has required that a strong warning be placed on the label of stimulant drugs. Before starting a patient of any age on a stimulant drug a careful cardiovascular screening is recommended with the goal of identifying those at risk for serious underlying cardiovascular disease and adverse events related to stimulant use (28).

How to monitor patients on stimulants

In cases of long term use of stimulants, periodic complete blood count (with differential and platelet count) is recommended. Height and weight should be monitored routinely in pediatric patients, and any significant slowing should prompt further evaluation and possible discontinuation of the stimulant medication.

Blood pressure and pulse should be checked as both values can increase with stimulant treatment. The use of rating scales is recommended to aide in the periodic assessment of therapy efficacy.

b. Non stimulant agents

Atomoxetine

Atomoxetine is a selective inhibitor of norepinephrine reuptake. Its actions include the blockade of the presynaptic norepinephrine and dopamine transporter in the prefrontal cortex (29). The efficacy of atomoxetine has been documented in many short and long term studies in children and adults (30). Full therapeutic effect can take up to 4 weeks to develop. It can be used in those not wishing to take a stimulant, where stimulant or other medications are ineffective, or in patients with anxiety symptoms. Table 6 shows the main features of the preparation. The duration of atomoxetine effect is 18-24 hours.

Table 7 lists potential adverse effects. Atomoxetine has been associated with an increased risk of mydriasis, and should not be used in patients with narrow angle glaucoma. Due to reporting of several cases of severe liver injury, the manufacturer's package insert was modified in December 2004 to recommend baseline liver function tests with periodic monitoring. Patients should be monitored for an increased risk of suicidality due to reports of increased risk of suicidal ideation and behavior as atomoxetine carries an FDA black box warning similar to that for antidepressants. Drug-drug interactions can occur with inhibitors of the cytochrome P450, 2D6 isoenzyme, including selective serotonin reuptake inhibitors.

Table 6. FDA approved non stimulant preparations main features

NAME/FORMULATION	DOSE FORMS	STARTING DOSE	REMARKS
Strattera (Atomoxetine)	10, 18, 25, 40, 60, 80, 100 mg cap	<70 kg: 0.5mg/kg/day. Increase up to 1.2mg/kg/day not faster than every three days. Can be given in 2 divided doses.	Maxdaily dose=100mg or less than1.4mg/kg. Higher doses have not shown greater efficacy. In CYP 2D6 poor metabolizers or with 2D6 potent inhibitors, titrate dose after 4 weeks of initial dose if symptoms fail to improve

Table 6. (Continued)

NAME/FORMULATION	DOSE FORMS	STARTING DOSE	REMARKS
Intuniv (Guanfacine extended release)	1, 2, 3, 4 mg	1mg at bedtime, then increase by 1mg per week up to 4 weeks.	Max daily dose=4mg. However, if tolerated, doses up to 0.12mg/kg may provide additional benefit. Do not crush or chew. Upon d/c, ↓ dose by 1mg every 3-7 days to prevent withdrawal.
Kapvay (Clonidine extended release)	0.1 & 0.2mg	0.1mg at bedtime, may increase by 0.1mg daily at weekly intervals	Max daily dose = 0.4mg. Do not crush or chew. Upon d/c, ↓ by 0.1mg every 3-7 days to prevent withdrawal.

Guanfacine XR

Guanfacine is a selective alpha 2A adrenoreceptor agonist. An extended branded release formulation (GXR), was approved by the FDA in 2009 for the treatment of ADHD in children ages 6-17 years. It appears that guanfacine strengthens pre frontal cortex (PFC) regulation of attention and behavior by directly stimulating postsynaptic alpha 2A adrenocreceptors in that region. Controlled short term studies as well as open label studies of up to 24 months duration concluded that GXR was effective and safe as monotherapy. These studies also found that GXR improves both hyperactive as well as inattentive symptoms (31).

Table 7. Atomoxetine side effects

Anorexia
Constipation
Dry mouth
Nausea
Emesis
Sedation
Fatigue
Headache
Dizziness
Mood swings
Suicidal ideations
Aggressive behavior
Dyspepsia
Stomache
Growth delay
Tachycardia
Hepatotoxicity

The side effect profile is considered mild with a preponderance of sedation which attenuates with continued use. Because guanfacine is a hypotensive agent, researchers followed its cardiovascular effects in detail in both the controlled and open label studies and results were similar across subject populations. Mild decreases in blood pressure and heart rate were noted which tended to normalize with continued treatment.

In clinical settings, it would be prudent to obtain baseline and follow up readings of blood pressure and pulse. Research did not show weight loss or delayed growth and some patients experienced the opposite. Commonly reported side effects include abdominal pain, dizziness, dry mouth, and constipation. GXR does not carry a black box warning. It is contraindicated in patients showing sensitivity to guanfacine. Discontinuation should take place over time because while this was not observed with GXR, there are reports that immediate release a2 agents can cause rebound hypertension. It is recommended that dosing be titrated upwards slowly and based on a mg/kg method. Improvement can be seen in some cases at the second week of treatment (9).

Clonidine XR (Kapvay)

Clonidine is another ά 2 agonist that was approved as an extended release formulation in October 2010 for the treatment of ADHD in those aged 6-17 years. This agent, like guanfacine, was originally approved for the treatment of hypertension and has been used off-label for ADHD for many years. Dosage is initiated at 0.1mg daily at bedtime and can be titrated up to a maximum of 0.4mg daily (two divided doses) at weekly intervals. Side effects most commonly reported include sedation, fatigue, irritability, nightmares, constipation, and dry mouth. Due to the potential for bradycardia/hypotension, patient's heart rate and blood pressure should be monitored at baseline, after dosage increases and periodically thereafter. Due to the risk for rebound hypertension, abrupt withdrawal should be avoided (no more than 0.1mg decrease every 3-7 days).

NON FDA APPROVED AGENTS

Over the years, clinicians have searched for alternatives to the traditional stimulant treatments. A few agents that were found to be effective to some degree have not been approved by the FDA. Due to their effects on central neurotransmission, antidepressant agents were among the first options researched. For instance, multiple controlled and open label studies showed that imipramine and desipramine are effective for ADHD symptoms. However, they appear to improve behavioral problems more than cognitive deficits. Despite their efficacy, they are rarely used today due to concerns regarding cardiovascular toxicity (9). Bupropion considered to be a safer antidepressant from the cardiovascular perspective, has shown efficacy in controlled ADHD studies as well (32) and can be considered a second line agent. It works by inhibiting dopamine and norepinephrine reuptake into the presynaptic neuron. At higher doses, bupropion is associated with an increased seizure risk. In contrast to the tricyclics and bupropion, the SSRI antidepressants have not shown efficacy in ADHD. Modafinil, a wake-promoting agent with actions similar to amphetamine and methylphenidate, showed efficacy in ADHD (33). Nonetheless, the FDA rejected its approval because of concerns regarding Stevens Johnson syndrome, reason for which it is not often recommended. Clonidine is a presynaptic, central-acting alpha2-adrenergic agonist that is used by some clinicians to manage ADHD symptoms, though it may take 4 to 6 weeks to achieve full benefit and is less effective than stimulants (34,35). Abrupt discontinuations can result in severe rebound hypertension, cerebrovascular accidents and sudden death. Blood pressure should be monitored for hypotension and rebound hypertension. Clonidine is used as an alternative or adjunctive medication to MPH. It is often given with MPH to treat the insomnia related to MPH.

Linking psychopharmacologic neurophysiology and pathophysiology

A brief outline of current thinking regarding the pathophysiology of ADHD is helpful in understanding the potential remedial role that pharmacological agents play. The cognitive and behavioral impairments experienced by ADHD patients can be viewed from a unifying neuropsychological perspective as representing deficits in executive functions (EF). These functions encompass higher order cognitive tasks such as organizing, prioritizing, focusing, sustaining effort, managing frustration, utilizing working memory, monitoring and self regulating, as well as certain aspects of behavior and emotion (36). The literature shows that the neuronal substrate for these functions is located in the PFC and its connections to other cortical and subcortical structures and that anatomical as well as neurochemical integrity are instrumental for healthy EF. For instance, dopamine (DA) and noradrenaline (NA) are essential to PFC function and a growing body of evidence suggests that normal PFC activity is attained when NA/DA availability reaches an optimal level. Either too much or too little catecholaminergic presence can result in PFC dysfunction (37). DA and NA appear to exert different actions at the cortical level. While NA strengthens network connections, sometimes referred to as increasing "signal", DA seems to weaken unnecessary connections or decrease "noise". Not surprisingly, all the agents with demonstrated efficacy in improving ADHD symptoms are believed to improve catecholaminergic transmission. As mentioned, stimulants increase synaptic cleft DA and NA by inhibiting their intracellular reuptake; atomoxetine blocks the NA transporter resulting in higher synaptic levels of both NA and DA; and guanfacine selectively blocks post synaptic alpha 2a receptors thus mimicking increased levels of NA (37).

Neuropsychological outcomes: Positive and negative

Because stimulant medications exert a primary effect on the DA system by preventing catecholamine reuptake it is not surprising that the most heavily researched neurological regions in ADHD are those that have inputs and outputs which affect the DA system. These regions are the PFC, basal ganglia, and cerebellum. This is logical given that these same areas are also involved in executive functioning, a core cognitive vulnerability in individuals with ADHD.

The PFC and basal ganglia are the primary targets of two ascending dopamine pathways, the neocortical and nigrostriatal pathways (38). The cerebellum, especially the posterior-inferior lobules of the cerebellar vermis, is also a target of DA projection from the ventral tegmental area (39). There are also reciprocal connections between the PFC, basal ganglia, and cerebellum via the pons, dentate nucleus and thalamus (40). The cerebellar vermis also has projections to the ventral tegmental area and locus ceruleus, affecting the turnover of DA and NA in the basal ganglia (41). In sum, there is much connectivity between these regions, permitting feed-forward and feedback loops.

Stimulant medications reduce unwanted ADHD symptoms (hyperactivity) and increase desired symptoms (attention), in both individuals with ADHD as well as those without ADHD (42,43). Investigators found that non ADHD children who received MPH showed improved response inhibition and memory, and healthy adults who were administered stimulants displayed improved attention, vigilance, and working memory (44). Thus, a positive response to a stimulant medication is not diagnostic of ADHD. These cognitive benefits appear to be mediated not only by DA stimulation but also by NA release (45).

A great deal of research has been centered on studying the cognitive effects of stimulants which has focused more on short-term treatment effects rather than long term effects. The methodologies utilized varied greatly in the doses prescribed, length of treatment, presence of comorbidity, and outcome measures. MPH and AMP salts are thought to increase availability of DA in the striatum. Research shows that increasing striatal DA availability increases the salience of task-relevant stimuli (46), decreases impulsivity (47) and decreases the variability of response patterns (48). Stimulant medications, however, do not appear to reliably improve task motivation (49). A recent exhaustive review of the cognitive effects of MPH in children found that it reliably improved saccadic eye movement, planning/cognitive flexibility, attention/vigilance, and inhibitory control (44). On the other hand, in adults, studies evaluating stimulant effects of cognition in ADHD patients showed consistent effects only in improving attention and less reliable findings in other domains of executive function. (50)

Regarding effects on behavior, stimulant medications have been demonstrated to reduce disruptiveness (51,52) and negative verbalizations (53) as well as increase compliance to rules / expectations (54,55). Motor planning, motor coordination, and motor sequencing have all been demonstrated to be improved with stimulant medications (56-58). Physical aggression, however, does not appear to be as easily decreased by stimulant medications (59).

Atomoxetine and guanfacine both reduce core ADHD symptoms, although their effect size is lower than that of MPH and AMP (9). In contrast to stimulants, atomoxetine and guanfacine have received less neuropsychological research foci. Of the existing data, atomoxetine has been demonstrated to decrease impulsivity on a laboratory measure of inhibition (60), increase visuospatial working memory (61), and improve the memory and learning domains of the NEPSY children's battery (62). Guanfacine was associated with significant decreases in both commission and omission errors on the CPT (63) as well as improved planning and spatial working memory (64).

While there is a large body of literature documenting medication cognitive improvements, clinicians do not measure these routinely in order to determine therapeutic effectiveness and treatment progress. In part, this is due to the absence of user friendly instruments to assess cognitive domains in ADHD beyond inattention. In fact, the most widely utilized rating scales for ADHD (Table 1) preponderantly document behavioral manifestations of inattentiveness.

Despite improvements found in attention, task attractiveness, impulse control, response control, and multiple other domains, research has not been able to demonstrate that medication has an impact on long-term academic achievement (50,65,66). This lack of evidence has been puzzling to clinicians and researchers alike. If ADHD subjects experience acute medication improvements on a number of skills that are necessary for learning, why has this not resulted in verifiable enhancement of academic long term outcomes? The literature explains this contradiction in part by pointing out to methodological research issues. For instance, studies have varied greatly in their use of pharmaceutical formulations, dosage ranges -some perhaps suboptimal-, and times of medication administration. It is also possible that duration of treatment was not sufficient enough to demonstrate change or that patients did not adhere to treatment as prescribed. These issues may have interfered with the power to demonstrate effectiveness for an outcome measure that is very complex and multidetermined to begin with. In addition, one study (67) showed that even in the context of treatment considered optimal, while stimulants significantly improved cognition in ADHD children, they did not normalize it. Ultimately, it is also possible that for long term academic achievement to occur, medication alone may be insufficient and much more comprehensive wraparound modalities may be necessary.

AGENT SELECTION

The selection of a specific starting agent is not guided by its neuropsychological effects because as noted above, all agents improve core ADHD deficits alike. The decision of which agent to use is based on the assessment of individual patient needs and the pharmacodynamic/pharmacokinetic properties of a particular medication (9), as follows. Before beginning pharmacotherapy, it is important to record baseline measures to help determine the safety and feasibility of treatment. More specifically, information should be obtained from a recent physical examination that includes blood pressure, heart rate, and growth rate. Also, parents and teachers can complete pretreatment symptom rating scales or if this is not possible, a clinical estimation of baseline severity can be made. It is essential to discuss target symptoms to determine improvement, and carefully review possible adverse effects with the patient and family. Despite guidance from specialty medical associations, the multiplicity of agents available and the variety of patient clinical presentations call for a true blending of art and science in order to tailor the choice of medication to individual patient circumstances. It is normally recommended that treatment be started with an FDA approved agent but should it be a stimulant or a non stimulant? Unless specific contraindications exist, stimulants are the favored first choice because of their high degree of efficacy for core ADHD symptoms, rapid onset of action, ease of use, and generally benign side effect profile. Non stimulants could be used first if there is patient/caretaker preference, patient/caretaker substance abuse (due to diversion or abuse concerns), comorbidity, prior stimulant failure, or recent intolerance to stimulant side effects.

Longer acting preparations are the best first option for children and adults, for several reasons. First, once daily administration affords the patient full day symptom coverage in school, afterschool activities, homework, and evening family time. In addition, by virtue of the ease of following a once/day regimen, these agents may improve adherence. Unquestionably, they eliminate the need to involve school nurses, and they potentially are less likely to be abused. In general, the longest acting preparation that induces no side effects or side effects that are deemed acceptable to the patient is the one preferred. On the other hand, children under 6 are usually started on short acting preparations because they are more sensitive to dose dependent adverse effects and long acting agents are not available in low enough strengths. However, once a safe dose of an IR formulation has been established, conversion to a longer acting agent maybe considered.

While AMP was the first described agent to treat ADHD, concerns about its illicit use led the way for MPH to become more frequently prescribed. Nonetheless, in the past few years, AMP has regained considerable popularity. There have been several studies comparing AMP with MPH formulations that show differences in effectiveness and side effect profiles but these differences are not clinically meaningful enough to dictate choice of one type over another. It is important to understand that both types of stimulants have demonstrated high efficacy. When one fails, the other kind could be recommended next in order to increase overall treatment effectiveness to 80%. Usually, clinicians tend to become comfortable with one stimulant type they start patients with and use the other if the first trial fails. For example, a clinician may recommend Concerta but switch to Vyvanse if there are problems or vice versa. In special circumstances, such as children who cannot swallow pills, physicians may recommend one of the various preparations described in Tables 2 and 5 that do not require ingesting an intact pill.

For treatment of naive patients, the rule of thumb is to start with the lowest possible stimulant dose and to monitor side effects and efficacy every few days. If parent/teacher rating scales show inadequate improvement and there are few significant side effects, it is reasonable to increase to the next dose level. This strategy can continue until either the desired effect is reached or intolerable side effects appear. In general, doses can be titrated upwards until improvements in rating scale scores of 40-50% are obtained.

In cases where the patient is not improving and has side effects, the first step is to discontinue the initial stimulant and switch to the other type, or switch to a non-stimulant. There are no evidence based data that preferentially support continuation with either strategy after a first treatment fails. If the main issue is intolerance to stimulant side effects, then switching to a non stimulant is preferred. There is evidence that adding a non stimulant to stimulant therapy potentiates the effectiveness of the overall regimen; thus, combination therapy is another accepted strategy. However, if there is no improvement after two ADHD treatments, a diagnostic reassessment is necessary. For instance, is there comorbidity with affective disorder, anxiety disorder, or substance abuse? Can adherence be clearly ascertained? Are there psychosocial stressors that require resolution?

Only a small minority of patients will not respond to FDA approved treatments, either as monotherapy or in combination. Therefore, if there is little or no improvement, a diagnostic reassessment is mandatory. In the absence of diagnostic issues, non FDA approved treatments can be entertained. On the other hand, these have yielded lower effect sizes than approved agents. A trial of behavior therapy for which there are evidenced based data of effectiveness should also be presented to the family. If medication is preferred by caretakers, a trial of bupropion, modafinil, or tricyclics can be entertained as long as appropriate informed consent is obtained.

The need for continued treatment should be reevaluated periodically, as some patients may no longer require pharmacotherapy. In order to avoid disruptions in school function, treatment should generally be maintained through the academic year. On the other hand, it is important to have school input when assessing the need for continued care. Thus, a reasonable strategy is to taper first and finally discontinue treatment near the end of the year. For adolescents, it is important to maintain treatment until final examinations are taken. By the end of the year, teacher input is still available but final grades are not jeopardized as there is time to reinstitute treatment if the patient relapses off medication. Regarding medication use during the summer, for non stimulants, unless the goal is to reassess need for ongoing care, it is not advisable to stop treatment because it may take several weeks to return to therapeutic success. Weekend holidays are impractical for the same reason. With respect to stimulants, if a patient becomes symptomatic without them, routine discontinuation on weekends is not recommended. However, in cases in which there is notable growth delay, drug holidays have been recommended as a strategy to allow for "catch up" growth. Routine summer discontinuations are no longer recommended since symptom relapse often occurs in the absence of medication. On the other hand, if growth delay is a concern or the patient prefers stopping, summer discontinuation should be considered.

Conclusion

The neuropsychiatric etiology of ADHD was suspected from early on so that significant research was aimed at elucidating its neuropsychological deficits. Impairments in attention, impulse control, and motor activity -the condition's core deficits- are well documented in neuropsychological studies. So are the beneficial effects of medication for ADHD which have been unambiguously supported by hundreds of studies in the expert academic literature. While stimulants are the most effective therapeutic agents, non stimulants also play an important role. As described above, theoretical constructs linking molecular neurotransmitter actions to neuroanatomical macro structures and cognitive and behavioral findings, have found solid empirical confirmations. However, medication related improvements appear to support only short term gains (50) and just while patients remain under carefully monitored treatment conditions (68). Plausible reasons exist for the apparent lack of scientific proof in documenting long term academic gains and further research is needed in this respect. Nonetheless, because of the strong beneficial effects in alleviating current symptomatology and the relative safety of the agents used, the clinical psychiatric community strongly recommends that ADHD be appropriately treated, as patients with this condition show very serious long term disabilities that go beyond academic failure (69).

References

[1] American Psychiatric Association. Diagnostic and statistical manual of mental disorders, 4th ed, text revision. Washington, DC: American Psychiatric Association, 2000:85-93.

[2] Barkley R. The nature of ADHD in attention-deficit hyperactivity disorder, third edition: A handbook for diagnosis and treatment. New York: Russell A Guildford, 2006.

[3] Greydanus DE, Pratt HD, Patel DR: Attention deficit hyperactivity disorder across the lifespan. Disease-a-Month 2007;53(2):65-132.

[4] Faraone SV, Sergeant J, Gillberg C, Biederman J. The worldwide prevalence of ADHD: is it an American condition? World Psychiatry 2003;2:104-13.

[5] Katragadda S, Schubiner H. ADHD in children, adolescents, and adults. Prim Care Clin Office Pract 2007;34(4):111.

[6] Biederman J, Farone SV. Attention-deficit/hyperactivity disorder. Lancet 2005;366;237-48.

[7] Barkley RA: Attention-deficit/hyperactivity disorder. Sci Am 1998;3:66–71.

[8] Adler L, Cohen J. Diagnosis and evaluation of adults with attention-deficit/ hyperactivity disorder. Psychiatr Clin North Am 2004;27:187-201.

[9] Kaplan G, Newcorn JH, Ivanov IS. Pharmacologic management of ADHD in children and adolescents. Int J Child Adolesc Health 2010; 3(2):143-61.

[10] Biederman J. Attention-deficit/hyperactivity disorder: A selective overview. Biol Psychiatry 2005;57:1215-20.

[11] Greydanus DE, Pratt HD. Attention deficit/hyperactivity disorder in adolescents. In: Greydanus DE, Patel DR, Pratt HD, eds. Essential adolescent medicine. New York: McGraw-Hill, 2006:751-68.

[12] Faraone SV, Khan SA. Candidate gene studies of attention-deficit/hyperactivity disorder. J Clin Psychiatry 2006;67(Suppl 8):13-20.

[13] Wilens T. Personal Communication, 2007.

[14] Clarke SD. ADHD in adolescence. J Adolesc Health 2000;27:77–78.

[15] Pliszka SR, Crismon ML, Hughes CW, et al. The Texas Children's Medication Algorithm Project: Revision of the algorithm for pharmacology of attenton-deficit/hyperactivity disorder. J Am Acad Child Adolesc Psychiatry 2006;45(6):642-57.

[16] Schubiner H, Robin AL, Young J. Attention-deficit/hyperactivity disorder in adolescent males. Adolesc Med 2003;14:663–76.

[17] Staufer WB, Greydanus DE. Attention-deficit/hyperactivity disorder psychopharmacology for college students. Pediatr Clin North Am 2005;52:71-84.

[18] Jensen PS, Hinshaw SP, Swanson JM, Greenhill LL, Conners CK, et al. Findings from the NIMH Multimodal Treatment Study of ADHD (MTA): Implications and applications for primary care providers. J Dev Behav Pediatr 2001;22:60–73.

[19] National Institute of Mental Health (NIMH): Attention Deficit Hyperactivity Disorder. NIMH, NIH Publication No. 01-4589, 2001. Available at: http://www.nimh.nih.gov/publicat/helpchild.cfm.

[20] Solanto MV, Arnsten AFT, Castellanos FX. The neuroscience of stimulant drug action in ADHD. In: Solanto MV, Arnsten AFT, Castellanos FX, eds. Stimulant drugs and ADHD. London: Oxford University Press, 2001:355-79.

[21] Muniz R, et al. Efficacy and safety of extended-release dexmethylphenidate compared with d,l-methylphenidate and placebo in the treatment of children with attention- deficit/hyperactivity disorder: a 12-hour laboratory classroom study. J Child Adolesc Psychopharmacol 2008;18(3):248-56.

[22] Bradley C. The behavior of children receiving Benzedrine. Am J Psychiatry 1937;94:577-85.

[23] Ivanov I, Pearson A, Kaplan G, Newcorn J. Treatment of adolescent ADHD and comorbid substance abuse. Int J Child Adolesc Health 2010; 3(2):33-40.

[24] Swanson JM and MTA Cooperative Group. National Institute of Mental Health Multimodal Treatment Study of ADHD Follow-up: Changes in effectiveness and growth after the end of treatment. Pediatrics 2004;113:762–9.

[25] Chhangani BS. Sleep disorders in children and adolescents. In: Greydanus DE, Patel DR, Reddy VN, Feinberg AN, Omar HA, eds. Handbook of clinical pediatrics: An update for the ambulatory pediatrician. Singapore: World Scientific, 2010:87-115.

[26] Weiss MD, Wasdell MB, Bomben MM, Rea KJ, Freeman RD. Sleep hygiene and melatonin treatment for children and adolescents with ADHD and initial insomnia. J Am Acad Child Adolesc Psychiatry 2006;45(5):512-9.

[27] Spencer TJ, Greenbaum M, Ginsberg LD, Murphy WR. Safety and effectiveness of coadministration of guanfacine extended release and psychostimulants in children and adolescents with attention-deficit/hyperactivity disorder. J Child Adolesc Psychopharmacol 2009;19(5):501-10.

[28] Vitiello B, Towbin K. Stimulant treatment of ADHD and risk of sudden death in children. Am J Psychiatr 2009;166(9):955-7.

[29] Atomoxetine: Strattera revisited. Med Med Lett 2004;46:65.

[30] Faraone SV, Glatt SJ. A comparison of the efficacy of medications for adult attention-deficit/hyperactivity disorder using meta-analysis of effect sizes. J Clin Psychiatry 2010;71(6):754-63.

[31] Biederman J, Melmed RD, Patel A, McBurnett K, Donahue J, Lyne A. Long-term, open-label extension study of guanfacine extended release in children and adolescents with ADHD. CNS Spectr 2008;13(12):1047-55.

[32] Paykina N and Greenhill L. Attention deficit hyperactivity disorder. In: Findling RL, ed. Clinical manual of child and adolescent psychopharmacology. Washington, DC: APP, 2008:33-87.

[33] Biederman J, Spencer TJ. Psychopharmacological interventions. Child Adolesc Psychiatr Clin North Am 2008;17(2):439-58.

[34] Greydanus DE, Sloane MA, Rappley MD. Psychopharmacology of ADHD in adolescents. Adolesc Med 2002;13:599–624.

[35] Greydanus DE, Pratt HD, Sloane MA, et al. Attention-deficit/hyperactivity disorder in children and adolescents: Interventions for a complex costly clinical conundrum. Pediatr Clin North Am 2003;50:1049–92.

[36] Barkley RA. Behavioral inhibition, sustained attention, and executive functions: Constructing a unifying theory of ADHD. Psychol Bull 1997;121(1):65-94.

[37] Arnsten AF. Toward a new understanding of attention-deficit hyperactivity disorder pathophysiology: an important role for prefrontal cortex dysfunction. CNS Drugs 2009;23(Suppl 1):33-41.

[38] Swanson J, Volkow N. Pharmacokinetic and pharmacodynamic properties of methylphenidate in humans. In: Solanto MV, Arnsten AFT, Castellanos FX, eds. Stimulant drugs and ADHD: Basic and clinical neuroscience. Oxford: Oxford University Press, 2001:259-82.

[39] Ikai Y, Takada M, Mizuno N. Single neurons in the ventral tegmental area that project to both the cerebral and cerebellar cortical areas by way of axon collaterals. Neuroscience 1994;61:925-34.

[40] Middleton FA, Strick PL. Basal ganglia and cerebellar loops: motor and cognitive circuits. Brain Res Brain Res Rev 2000;31:236-50.

[41] Snider RS, Maiti A, Snider SR. Cerebellar pathways to ventral midbrain and nigra. Exp Neurol 1976;53:
714-28.

[42] Berridge CW, Devilbiss DM, Andrzejewski ME, et al. Methylphenidate preferentially increases catecholamine neurotransmission within the prefrontal cortex at low doses that enhance cognitive function. Biol Psychiatry 2006;60(10):1111-20.

[43] Rapoport JL, Inoff-Germain G. Responses to methylphenidate in attention-deficit/hyperactivity disorder and normal children: update 2002. J Atten Disord 2002;6(Suppl 1):S57-60.

[44] Pietrzak R, et al. Cognitive effects of immediate-release methylphenidate in children with attention-deficit/hyperactivity disorder. Neurosci Biobehav Rev 2006;30:1225–45.

[45] Arnsten AF, Dudley AG. Methylphenidate improves prefrontal cortical cognitive function through alpha2 adrenoceptor and dopamine D1 receptor actions: Relevance to therapeutic effects in attention deficit hyperactivity disorder. Behav Brain Funct 2005;1(1):2.

[46] Volkow ND, Wang GJ, Fowler JS, Telang F, Maynard L, Logan J. Evidence that methylphenidate enhances the saliency of a mathematical task by increasing dopamine in the human brain. Am J Psychiatry 2004;161:1173–80.

[47] Scheres A, Oosterlaan J, Swanson J, Morein-Zamir S, Meiran N, Schut H. The effect of methylphenidate on three forms of response inhibition in boys with AD/HD. J Abnorm Child Psychol 2003;31:105–20.

[48] Pliszka SR, Liotti M, Bailey BY, Perez R, Glahn D, Semrud-Clikeman M. Electrophysiological effects of stimulant treatment on inhibitory control in children with attention-deficit/hyperactivity disorder. J Child Adolesc Psychopharmacol 2007;17:356–66.

[49] Groom MJ, Scerif G, Liddle PF, Batty MJ, Liddle EB, Roberts KL. Effects of motivation and medication on electrophysiological markers of response inhibition in children with attention-deficit/hyperactivity disorder. Biol Psychiatry 2010;67(7):624-31.

[50] Advokat C. What are the cognitive effects of stimulant medications? Emphasis on adults with attention-deficit/hyperactivity disorder (ADHD). Neurosci Biobehav Rev 2010;34:1256-66.

[51] Bukstein OG, Kolko DJ. Effects of methylphenidate on aggressive urban children with attention deficit hyperactivity disorder. J Clin Child Psychol 1998;27(3):340-51.

[52] Reitman D, Hupp SD, O'Callaghan PM, Gulley V, Northup J. The influence of a token economy and methylphenidate on attentive and disruptive behavior during sports with ADHD-diagnosed children. Behav Modif 2001;25(2):305-23.

[53] Pelham WE, Gnagy EM, Greiner AR, Hoza B, Hinshaw SP, Swanson JM. Behavioral versus behavioral and pharmacological treatment in ADHD children attending a summer treatment program. J Abnorm Child Psychol 2000;28(6):507-25.

[54] Evans SW, Pelham WE, Smith BH, Bukstein O, Gnagy EM, Greiner AR. Dose-response effects of methyphenidate on ecologically valid measures of academic performance and classroom behavior in adolescents with ADHD. Exp Clin Psychopharmacol 2001;9(2):163-75.

[55] Pelham WE, Gnagy EM, Burrows-Maclean L, Williams A, Fabiano GA, Morrisey SM. Once-a-day Concerta methylphenidate versus three-times-daily methylphenidate in laboratory and natural settings. Pediatrics 2001;107(6): E105.

[56] O'Driscoll GA, Dépatie L, Holahan AL, Savion-Lemieux T, Barr RG, Jolicoeur C. Executive functions and methylphenidate response in subtypes of attention-deficit/hyperactivity disorder. Biol Psychiatry 2005;57(11):1452-60.

[57] Rubia K, Noorloos J, Smith A, Gunning B, Sergeant J. Motor timing deficits in community and clinical boys with hyperactive behavior: the effects of methylphenidate on motor timing. J Abnorm Child Psychol 2003;31(3):301-13.

[58] Sheppard DM, Bradshaw JL, Georgiou N, Bradshaw JA, Lee P. Movement sequencing in children with Tourette's syndrome and attention deficit hyperactivity disorder. Mov Disord 2000;15(6):1184-93.

[59] Matier K, Halperin JM, Sharma V, Newcorn JH, Sathaye N. Methylphenidate response in aggressive and nonaggressive ADHD children: distinctions on laboratory measures of symptoms. J Am Acad Child Adolesc Psyciatry 1992;31(2):219-25.

[60] Chamberlain SR, Del Campo N, Dowson J, Müller U, Clark L, Robbins TW, Sahakian BJ. Atomoxetine improved response inhibition in adults with attention-deficit/hyperactivity disorder. Biol Psychiatry 2007; 62(9):977-84.

[61] de Jong CG, Van De Voorde S, Roeyers H, Raymaekers R, Allen AJ, Knijff S. Differential effects of atomoxetine on executive functioning and lexical decision in attention-deficit/hyperactivity disorder and reading disorder. J Child Adolesc Psychopharmacol 2009;19(6):699-707.

[62] Maziade M, Rouleau N, Lee B, Rogers A, Davis L, Dickson R. Atomoxetine and neuropsychological function in children with attention-deficit/hyperactivity disorder: results of a pilot study. J Child Adolesc Psychopharmacol 2009;19(6):709-18.

[63] Chappell PB, Riddle MA, Scahill L, Lynch KA, Schultz R, Arnsten A. Guanfacine treatment of comorbid attention-deficit hyperactivity disorder and Tourette's syndrome: preliminary clinical experience. J Am Acad Child Adolesc Psychiatry 1995;34(9):1140-6.

[64] Jäkälä P, Riekkinen M, Sirviö J, Koivisto E, Kejonen K, Vanhanen M. Guanfacine, but not clonidine, improves choice reaction time performance in young healthy volunteers. Neuropsychopharmacology 1999;21(4):495-502.

[65] Raggi VL, Chronis AM. Interventions to address the academic impairment of children and adolescents with ADHD. Clin Child Fam Psychol Rev 2006;9:85-111.

[66] Schachar R, Jadad AR, Gauld M, Boyle M, Booker L, Snider A, et al. Attention-deficit / hyperactivity disorder: Critical appraisal of extended treatment studies. Can J Psychiatr 2002;47:337-48.

[67] Gualtieri T, Johnson L. Medications do not necessarily normalize cognition in ADHD patients J Attend Dis 2008;11(4):459-69.

[68] Molina BS, et al. The MTA at 8 years: prospective follow-up of children treated for combined-type ADHD in a multisite study. J Am Acad Child Adolesc Psychiatry 2009;48(5):484-500.

[69] Barkley R. Appendix A. International Consensus Statement on ADHD in attention-deficit hyperactivity disorder, third edition. In: A Russell, ed. A handbook for diagnosis and treatment. New York: Guildford, 2006.

In: Child and Adolescent Health Yearbook 2013
Editor: Joav Merrick
ISBN: 978-1-63117-658-6

Chapter 10

UPPER-AIR OBSERVATION INDICATORS PREDICT OUTBREAKS OF ALLERGIES AMONG ELEMENTARY SCHOOL CHILDREN: INTEGRATION OF DAILY ENVIRONMENTAL AND SCHOOL HEALTH SURVEILLANCE SYSTEMS IN PENNSYLVANIA

Wasantha P Jayawardene, MD*, Ahmed H YoussefAgha, PhD and David K Lohrmann, PhD

Department of Applied Health Science, School of Public Health - Indiana University, Bloomington, Indiana, United States of America

ABSTRACT

Objectives of this study are to determine if a relationship exists between occurrence of allergies among elementary school children and daily upper-air observations (temperature, relative humidity, dew point, mixing ratio) and to derive a mathematical model that predicts allergies. Using an ecological study design, school health records of 168,825 students in elementary schools enrolled in "Health eTools for Schools" within 49 Pennsylvania counties were analyzed. Data representing allergy occurrences were originally recorded by school nurses as the type of treatment given to a student during a clinic visit on a particular day. Daily upper-air measurements from ground level to the 850mb pressure level, covering a radius of 800 kilometers around Pittsburgh, PA, were obtained. Wilcoxon Two-Sample test was used to identify associations. A Generalized Estimating Equation model was used to predict the occurrence of more than 13 cases, the daily mean for 2008-2010. Results showed that the surveillance of allergies among school children in Pennsylvania has increased over these three years. The primary occurrence of allergies among school children was in August-September, followed by December and April, while the lowest was in January and May. Annual averages of

*Correspondence: Wasantha P Jayawardene, MD, Doctoral Student and Associate Instructor, Department of Applied Health Science, Room 116, School of Public Health - Indiana University Bloomington, 1025 E 7th Street, Bloomington, IN 47405, United States. E-mail: wajayawa@indiana.edu

upper-air observations were significantly different between seasons ($p<0.02$). Upper-air temperature, dew point, and mixing ratio above their three-year mean values were significantly associated with occurrence of allergies ($p<0.011$). In conclusion, monitoring of upper-air observation data over time can be a reliable means for predicting outbreaks of allergies among elementary school children. Such predictions could help parents and school nurses implement effective precautionary measures.

Keywords: Temperature, relative humidity, dew point, mixing ratio, allergies, school health records, Pennsylvania

INTRODUCTION

Hay fever, respiratory allergies, food allergies, and skin allergies are the main types of allergies among children in the US. Percent of children with diagnosed hay fever in the past 12 months is 9.5% (7.1 million), while 11.5% (3.4 million) of children reported with respiratory allergies. In addition, 4.6% (9.4 million) of children in the US had food allergies in the past 12 months, while 12.6% of children reported with skin allergies (1). Seasonal allergies are fairly common in children older than five years old. According to the American Academy of Allergy, Asthma, and Immunology, about 10-15% of school-age children have seasonal allergies (2).According to CDC, about 10% of children under 17 years had suffered from hay fever, 12% from respiratory allergies, 5% from food allergies, and 13% from skin allergies in the past 12 months (3). There is some evidence that more than 10% of children were sensitized to pollen and a high proportion of the children sensitized only to pollen were also sensitized to other inhalant allergens later. Technically, an allergen is a non-parasitic antigen capable of stimulating a type-1 hypersensitivity reaction in atopic individuals (4).The most common allergens are pollen, dust, food, insect stings, animal dander, mold, medications, and latex. Most humans mount significant Immunoglobulin E (IgE) responses only as a defense against parasitic infections. However, some individuals mount an IgE response against common environmental antigens (4).

Seasonality of allergies (5,6) and their association with asthma (7) are well-known phenomena. Atopic eczema and allergic rhinitis were found to be higher in the period September–May. Some evidence support that non-summer warmth and urban air pollution (8), probably mediated through exposure to common allergens, such as dust mites, are possible risk factors for allergies in school-aged children (9).The highest frequencies of IgE reactivity to food were found in the group of children sensitized to several types of pollen (10).

Seasonal allergy symptoms are commonly experienced due to pollen in summer, fall, or spring, when certain trees or grasses pollinate. The season of pollination depends on the type of tree or grass. As an example, grasses such as Bermuda, timothy and orchard pollinate in the summer, while some trees such as oak, elm, and maple pollinate in the spring. Grass allergy is generally linked to hay fever because their symptoms and causes are somehow similar to each other. Symptoms include rhinitis, which causes sneezing and a runny nose, as well as allergic conjunctivitis, which includes watering and itchy eyes (2). Also, depending on the season, the symptoms may be more severe. The immune system has strong influence on seasonal allergies, since it reacts differently to diverse allergens like pollen. Meteorological factors are very important for the occurrence of pollen grains in the air. Dry and hot weather speeds up maturation and the loosening of pollen grains from anthers, and the concentration of pollen grains is considerably higher than in cold and wet weather (11). It has been found that the temperature has a positive correlation with pollen count, while relative humidity has an inverse correlation with the pollen count in the atmosphere. The total daily rainfall also has a negative correlation (11). Wind and thunderstorms are also accelerating the process of pollen release, especially in spring and summer months (12).

The current study investigated was undertaken to determine if a relationship exists between occurrence of allergies among school children, based on school health services records and routine upper-air variables, such as mixing ratio, relative humidity, temperature, and dew point. Mixing ratio is the mass of water vapor per unit mass of dry air, while relative humidity is the partial pressure of water vapor in air, given as a percentage of the saturated vapor pressure under the same conditions. Air temperature at which condensation first begins is the dew point, another measure of humidity. Although temperature and relative humidity at ground surface level have been considered in allergy studies, neither dew point nor mixing ratio have been linked with allergies or used for prediction of allergy outbreaks. The concept of relative humidity is complex. The amount of humidity is relative to the temperature available to do the work of evaporation, and can fluctuate even if no change occurs in the actual amount of water vapor per unit mass of dry air (mixing ratio). Therefore, dew point and mixing ratio provide the best assessments of humidity as it relates to allergy outbreaks.

The atmospheric variables examined in this study are upper-air observations. Upper-air observations constitute measurements of atmospheric conditions at higher altitudes, as distinct from surface weather observations, which are evaluations of the state of the atmosphere as observed at a point on the earth's surface and a set of instruments sent by a free-flight balloon (radiosonde), measures atmospheric variables from the surface to a height of 6 to 30 km (troposphere and stratosphere), and transmits the data to a ground receiving system. Radiosondes typically measure temperature, dew point, mixing ratio, relative humidity, and sometimes, pressure and wind speed/direction (13).The US National Weather Service's Upper-Air Observation Program monitors the operation of 92 radiosonde stations in North America and the Pacific islands Observations are updated twice daily. Temperature normally decreases throughout the troposphere as altitude increases. This phenomenon is called the lapse rate which, on average, occurs in the troposphere at a rate of 3.6°F per 1,000 ft. This means that a strong, consistent correlation exists between upper-air temperatures and ground temperatures. None of these daily upper-air observation parameters described above has been utilized in allergy research to date, either to detect associations or for prediction of allergy outbreaks.

School health records have been utilized for allergy-tracking because they are readily accessible through the existing school data collection and storage infrastructure (14). In many Pennsylvania schools student health records are compiled through a web-based software application portal called "Health eTools for Schools" (hereafter referred to as "eTools") that was funded by the Highmark Foundation through its Healthy High Five Initiative (15) and developed by InnerLink, Inc., a private, for-profit company. With the utilitarian purpose of providing data for state and local health planning, eTools is provided free of charge to local public, private and parochial schools. Implemented in approximately 1,100 schools in 49 Pennsylvania counties located in or near the Pittsburgh area, eTools is used by school nurses to routinely collect student health record data. The School Health Services section of eTools allows nurses to efficiently enter and download student health data using a hand-held electronic device and, via computerized programming, compile and submit required annual reports to the Pennsylvania State Health Department. This study involved analysis of existing de-identified student health record information pertaining to allergy occurrences that was routinely collected and aggregated in the eTools data management system by school nurses.

Purpose of the Study

1. To determine whether associations exist between allergies among elementary school students and upper-air observation parameters (relative humidity, dew point, actual mixing ratio, and temperature) in Pennsylvania
2. To determine if a mathematical model can be developed to estimate and predict the daily burden of allergies based on upper-air observations for the purpose of inferring future policy and programmatic initiatives

METHODS

Ecological study design was adopted in order to understand the relationship between daily occurrence of allergies in a "whole population" of elementary school students and daily measurements of upper-air observation parameters (16). In the ecological design, which investigates group-level variables, a geographical region can be analyzed in a cross-sectional manner (once or repetitively) to investigate the variation in a health-related variable (e.g., mean blood pressure, hospitalizations for allergies, and homicide rates) and its associations with regional characteristics (e.g., salt intake, air pollution, handgun laws, and drug policies) (16).

Two categories of group-level variables are found in epidemiological study designs. The first is aggregate variables; summary measures of individual characteristics (e.g., per capita income). These variables demonstrate a distinction between individual-level and group-level characteristics, because the group-level measure is inferior to (is a weaker measure than) the individual-level measure. The second is integral variables; group-level variables that are not summary measures of individual-level variables (e.g., weather, air pollution, and laws). These variables do not have corresponding individual-level values and can only be investigated at the group-level. Since upper-air variables in the current study are integral variables, ecological study design is the most appropriate analytic approach.

An ecological design also has the advantageous ability to control for individual-level variability while at the same time addressing influences at the regional-level. In addition, this study design enables researchers to include all the students of the enrolled elementary schools in the study sample, contrary to a study design in which each student with an allergic condition serves as his/her own control and excludes other students (16). Moreover, extracting daily upper-air data from existing environmental databases and retrieving computerized daily health data from existing repositories, such as eTools, is inherently cost-effective in that it requires a very low level of effort.

Study population

School districts located in 49 of the 67 counties in Pennsylvania participated in eTools. From 2008 to 2010, enrolled school districts received eTools services for 168,825 elementary school students. These students constituted the study population. All eTools services for participating school districts were subsidized by the funders of eTools (the Highmark Foundation) and covered costs of utilizing eTools through a three-year period. School districts that opted into eTools had to meet five requirements in order to receive a fully paid subscription service: (1) Make a three year commitment to use the portal, (2) Increase the amount of instructional time spent on nutrition education to 75 minutes per marking period, (3) Provide increased opportunities for physical education and physical activity through age appropriate instruction, (4) Participate in in-service training and professional development offerings that enhance use of the portal, and (5) Participate in an annual evaluation of eTools effectiveness. Pennsylvania schools that met participation criteria were eligible to be covered under the subsidy program during the three-year period and were considered for participation on a first-come, first-served basis.

Therefore, all students attending the 1,100 schools in participating school districts were represented by eTools. At the individual level, the sole participation eligibility requirement was to be a student with a health record in an elementary school that utilized eTools. Student records from these schools were excluded if they contained incomplete or inaccurately entered health record data. In addition, no race-, ethnicity-, or income-based bias existed in the enrollment of school districts, schools, or students in eTools. All of the above factors are important in respect to generalizability of study results to elementary school students at the state level or beyond the state level (16).

Data collection

Within the 49 Pennsylvania counties, 168,825 records of elementary school students were identified for this study. Data on allergies were originally noted in records maintained by school nurses as the type of treatment given to a student on a particular day. Treatment options for school health nurses were based on the prescribed medication provided for the student. For purposes of this study, having allergy was defined as "any case managed with antihistamines." In fact, school nurses recorded the trade name of all the medications administered, which were then later categorized into functional groups (i.e., antihistamines, analgesics, etc.). It was assumed that the treatment option noted by a school nurse correctly represented the disease.

Data analyzed for this study were provided to the authors by InnerLink, Inc. which had custodial responsibility under a common Statement of Understanding and Service Level Agreement with all participating school systems. Data pertaining to total use of antihistamine medications at the school level was unavailable. Likewise, demographic characteristics of students in each school or school district were not included in the eTools database and, therefore, were unobtainable. The school year in Pennsylvania usually begins in August, ends in June, and typically includes an extended winter break. Therefore, surveillance data were commonly unavailable for the last three weeks of June, all of July, the first three weeks of August, and the second half of December every year.

According to Pennsylvania State regulations, each school entity (e.g., school district) must have a written policy to allow for the possession and self-administration by school-age children of medications and the prescribed medication to be administered thereby in a school setting (17). The policy under this section shall require a child of school age that desires to possess and self-administer medications in a school setting to demonstrate the capability for self-administration and for responsible behavior in the use of medications. The physician, certified registered nurse practitioner, or physician assistant shall state whether the child is qualified and able to self-administer the medication. A written request is also required from the parent or guardian to the effect that the school entity complies with the order of the physician, certified registered nurse practitioner, or physician assistant (17). Because of these regulations, which rely on developmentally-appropriate restrictions, self-administration of medications for allergies, while being allowed on an individual basis at any age, is less likely to occur among elementary school students. The number of visits by middle school and high school students to a school health nurse's office, therefore, may not accurately represent the number of allergy occurrences. Hence, only data from elementary school students' records were included in this study.

All US school districts, including those in Pennsylvania, must collect and maintain all student records, including health records, in accordance with provisions of the federal Family Educational Rights and Privacy Act (FERPA). Regardless of whether a school is in a contractual arrangement with Innerlink, school nurses must maintain proper records safeguards; therefore, participation in eTools created no added burden for nurses in participating schools. FERPA regulations also give states the flexibility to share data for the purpose of ensuring that taxpayer funds are invested wisely in programs as long as students' personal information is properly safeguarded (18). This study involved analysis of existing de-identified student health record information pertaining to allergy attacks that was routinely collected and aggregated in the eTools data management system by school nurses who followed all FERPA safeguards. A common contract with InnerLink holds school districts responsible for maintaining the privacy, confidentiality, and integrity of all data, systems, and intellectual property related to eTools. InnerLink requirements affirmed that all school districts adhere to the FERPA regulations of 1974. Upper-air observation data were utilized for this study, for three reasons: (1) they are closely correlated with surface weather observations; 2) upper-air observations are following the same protocol as common for all locations in Pennsylvania, so a single value can be used for the entire state; 3) no study has tested the association and usefulness of upper-air observations in allergy research. The upper-air data used in this study were downloaded from the Wyoming University web site (13). Measurements were obtained from the ground level to the 1500- meter level (which is equivalent to 850 mb pressure). These upper-air observation values cover an area with a radius of about 800 kilometers, around Pittsburgh, PA (Figure 1).

As the coverage area includes the whole state of Pennsylvania, the geographical distribution of schools within the state did not affect study results. For each day of the three years (2008-2010) the measured values at time 12Z were obtained for analysis. The Z-time is the basis for synoptic meteorology, which requires collection of all measurements at the same time every day and, thereby, produces a snapshot of the state of the atmosphere worldwide. The 12Z time in the United States is 6 a.m. in January (Eastern Standard Time) and 7 a.m. in July (Eastern Daylight Time).

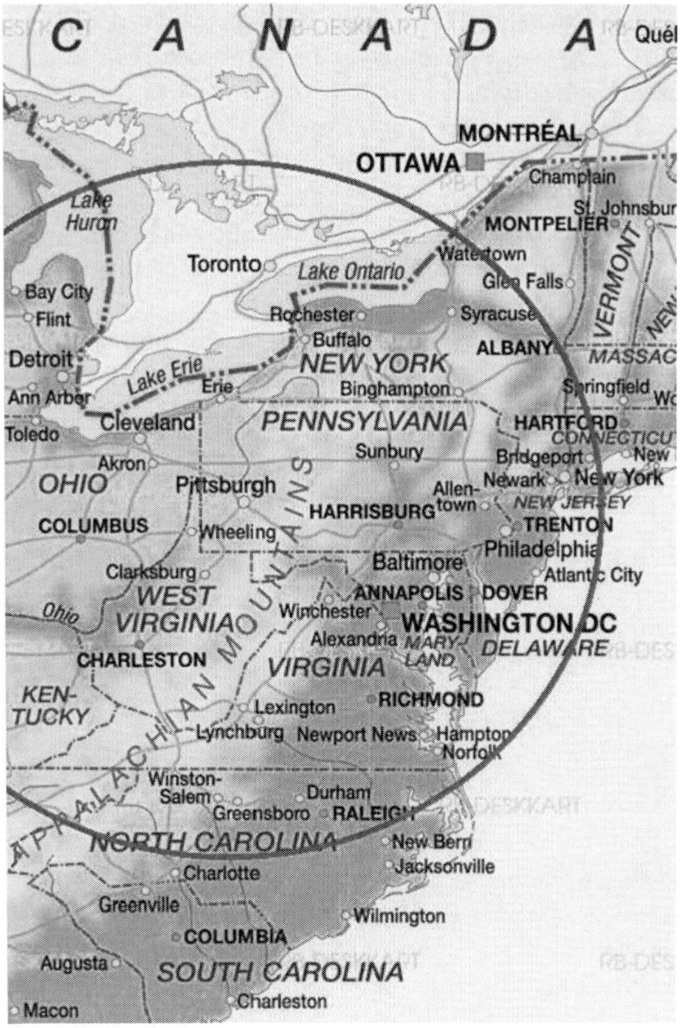

Figure 1. Map of Pennsylvania and Surrounding States Depicting Coverage Area of Upper-Air Observation Data, Which is Equal to a Radius of 800 km Around Pittsburgh.

This particular time was selected because 7 a.m. is closer to the usual time when students travel to school and are exposed to outdoor climatic factors. Due to this, any difference between the outside air temperature and the air temperature in the school is irrelevant. The variation of upper-air measurement values over the day is very small; the range of upper-air temperature over a day is less than 5°F (13).

Analysis

Descriptive statistics were used to summarize the mean changes of allergy cases throughout years. Two ratios were created: (1) daily mean allergy cases to annual average of allergy cases and (2) daily mean of allergy cases to number of schools enrolled. The first ratio was employed to study relationships between upper-air observation factors and allergies, and the second ratio was used to study the pattern of allergy occurrences over years. A nonparametric test, the Wilcoxon Two-Sample test, was used to compare means of first ratio that correspond to low and high groups of upper-air observations (with cutoff at three year median). Chi Square test was used to identify associations between the relative humidity (with cutoff at relative humidity = 50%) and occurrence of allergies.

The Generalized Estimating Equation (GEE) model was used to predict the probability of occurrence of cases greater than or equal to 13 (a cutoff value equal to the 2008-2010 mean). The repeated subject (cluster) in the model is the "matched date." For example, March 8th in 2007, 2008, 2009, and in 2010 is a subject. GEE needs at least 100 clusters to study 5-12 exploratory variables; however, a great deal of confidence is assured with 200 clusters, (19, 20) the circumstance in the current study. "Logit" link function on binary distribution was used on a binary dependent variable. "P" represents Daily Allergy Cases $\geq$ 13 and "1-P" represents Daily Allergy Cases < 13. The independent variables were the upper-air observation variables.

Human subjects approval statement

This study was approved by the Indiana University Bloomington Institutional Review Board, Bloomington, Indiana, United States.

RESULTS

Offices of school health nurses in Pennsylvania had 259,951 visits of elementary school students for various health problems during the three-year period 2008-2010 (Table1). This was equal to 40.9% of total student visits (preK-12) for the period. The treatment option in more than 60% of these occasions was either analgesics (30.7%) or Attention Deficit Hyperactivity Disorder drugs (30.0%). Antihistamines were given in 1.61% of occasions, which reflected the occurrence of this disease or disease exacerbations among students of all grades.

A gradual increase of allergy cases was observed from 2008 to 2010, both in elementary schools and in schools with higher grades (Table 2). This is partially explained by the increase in the number of schools participating in the allergy surveillance system.

The total number of schools (elementary, middle, and high schools) increased from 2008 to 2009, with a slight decrease from 2009 to 2010. However, a boost from 0.85 to 1.77 (208% increase) in the ratio of daily average of allergy cases to number of schools (preK-5) partially explained the real increase in allergy prevalence among school children, because that particular increase is not influenced by an increase in the number of schools participating in the allergy surveillance system. It may, however, be influenced by increased reporting of school nurses, since any surveillance system takes a few years to reach the full functional capacity. Geographical differences in new school enrolment may also have influenced this 208% increase. Differences between daily means of allergy cases reported from elementary schools in each year (2008, 2009, and 2010) were statistically significant (p<0.001; Kruskal-Wallis test). This statistical significance is true for both the daily mean and the ratio of daily cases to annual average (p<0.004).

Table 1. Student visits to offices of school nurses for various types of treatments in Pennsylvania, pre K-12 and pre K-5, during 2008-2010, and daily means for the period

Disease	No. of Visits by preK-12	No. of Visits by preK-5	% of Visits by preK-5	Daily Mean preK-5	Daily Median preK-5	Daily St Dev preK-5
ADHDs	190,992	110,833	58.00%	194	188	99
Analgesics	195,449	38,079	19.50%	67	66	36
Anti-asthmatics	39,185	27,123	69.20%	48	45	27
Anti-diabetics	65,361	26,440	40.50%	46	45	25
Gastrointestinals	60,318	22,601	37.50%	40	40	21
Antibiotics	27,070	15,585	57.60%	27	25	21
Other Psychotropics	22,135	9,121	41.20%	16	16	9
Antihistamines	8,546	4,185	49.00%	7	6	6
Anticonvulsants	8,838	3,461	39.20%	6	6	3
Anti-inflammatories	18,189	2,523	13.90%	4	3	4
Total	636,083	259,951	40.9%			

Table 2. Visits to school health nurses due to allergies as reported by school heath nurses in Pennsylvania, 2007-2010

Year	Number of Schools	Avg. of Allergy Daily Visits (preK-5)	Ratio of [Daily Cases/Schools] for the Year
2008	471	4 (SD=3)	0.85
2009	675	7 (SD=5)	1.04
2010	621	11 (SD=8)	1.77

Use of antihistamines among school children as reported by school health nurses has an almost identical pattern in each year during 2008-2010 (Figure 2). The peak of antihistamine use lies in the period from late August to early September, although there are noticeable increases in December (early winter) and in April (early spring) too. The lowest use of antihistamine use is reported in January and in May (Figure 2). It should be considered that the last three weeks of June, whole month of July, and first three weeks of August have no surveillance due to summer vacation, and the second half of December has no reporting due to winter break. Differences between daily means of allergy cases reported from elementary schools in each season were statistically significant ($p<0.001$) according to the Kruskal-Wallis test. This significance is not only true for the daily mean, but also true for the ratio of daily cases to annual average ($p<0.001$). As winter has the lowest number of cases, it was considered the baseline for number of allergy cases in odds ratio estimates. The summer season compared to winter had 17 times higher tendency of exceeding the daily mean of allergy cases (7 cases), which was followed by fall (2.6 times higher), and spring (2.1 times higher). In other words, 68% of days in summer exceeded the daily mean of allergy cases for three years, followed by fall (38%) and spring (35%). Upper-air temperature peaks in July (hot) and has its minimum in January (cold). None of the annual means of four upper-air observations showed differences between years according to the Kruskal- Wallis test.

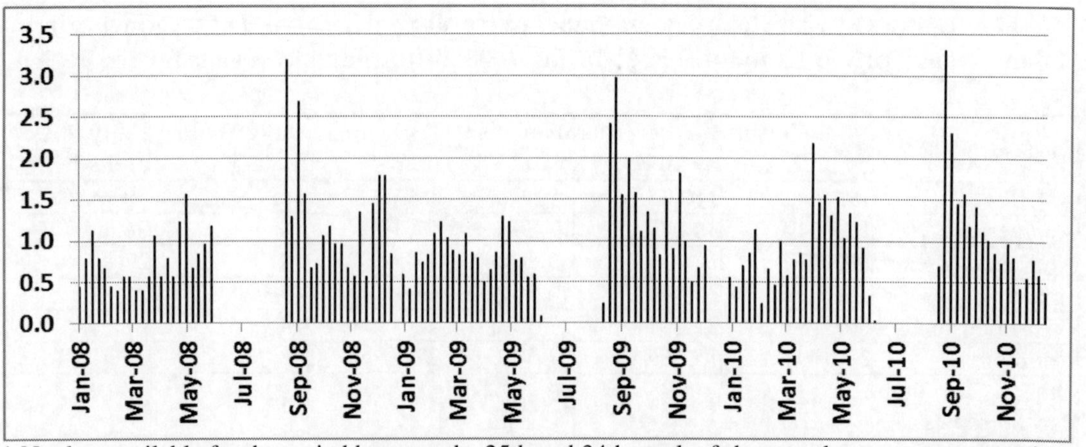

* No data available for the period between the 25th and 34th week of the year due to summer vacation; No data available for the last (52nd) week of the year due to winter break.

Figure 2. Antihistamine Use Among preK-5 Students (Ratio of Weekly Mean to Annual Mean), 2008-2010.*

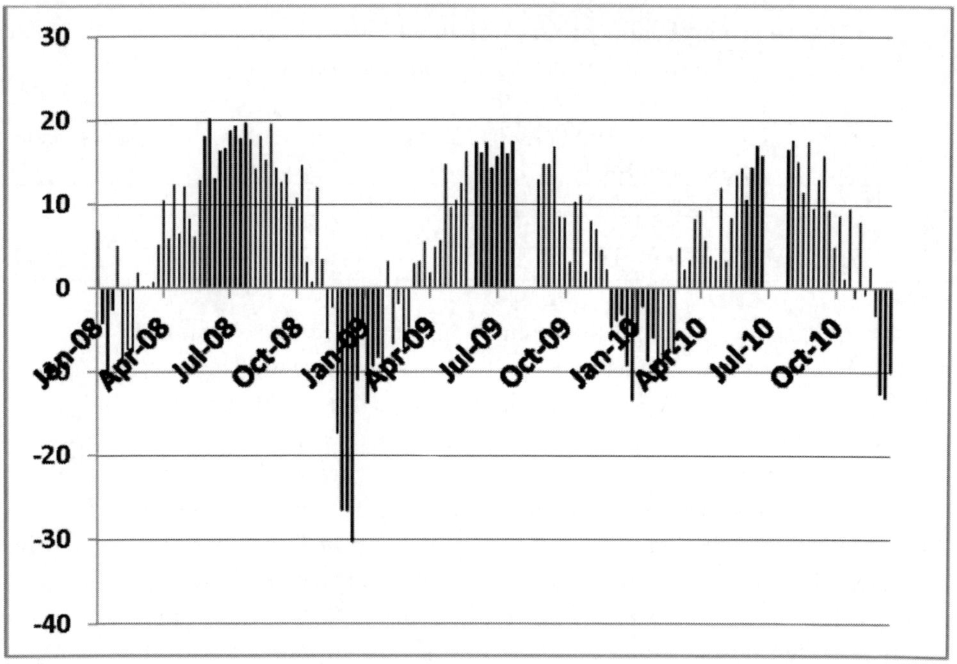

Figure 3. Fluctuation of Weekly Mean of Upper-Air Temperature (Celsius), 2008-2010.

There were significant differences between temperature means for each season ($p<0.001$), with the highest in summer, followed by spring and then fall (Figure 3). Similarly, upper-air dew point peaks in July (wet) and reaches its minimum in January (dry). Significant differences existed between seasons ($p<0.001$), with the highest in summer, followed by spring and then fall (Figure 4). Significant differences between mixing ratio means for each season were also statistically significant ($p<0.001$), with the highest in summer, followed by spring and fall.

Variation in upper-air relative humidity is complex and it's difficult to identify a specific pattern (Figure 5). Differences between relative humidity means for each season were statistically significant ($p<0.02$), with the highest in summer, followed by winter and then fall. The lowest relative humidity was recorded in spring.

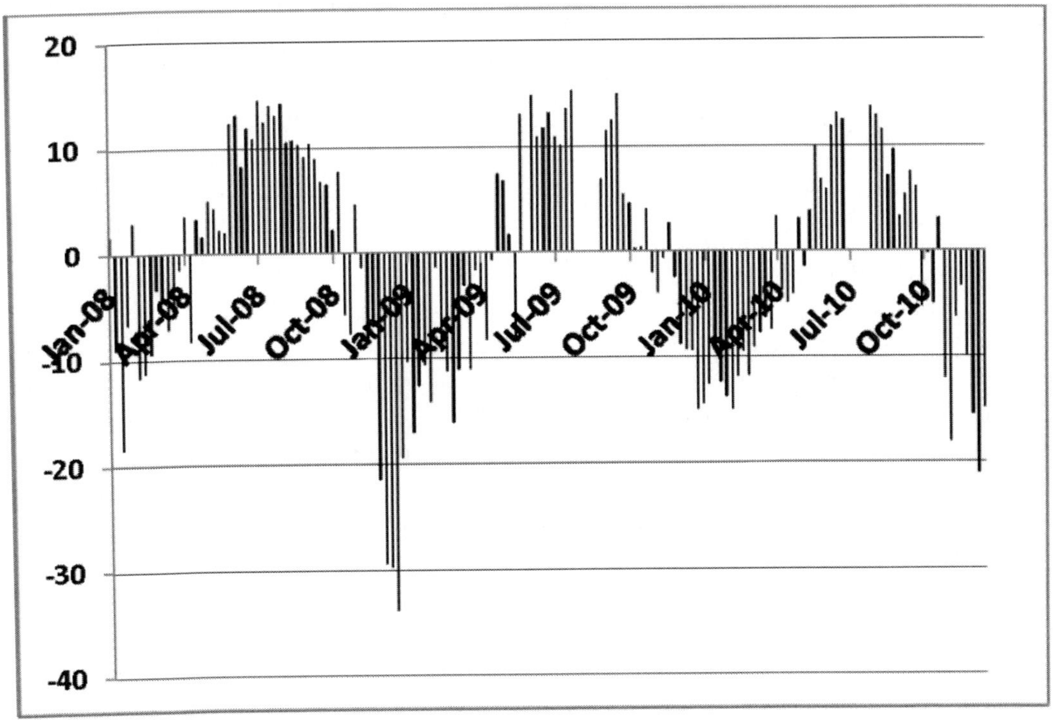

Figure 4. Fluctuation of Weekly Mean of Upper-Air Dew Point (Celsius), 2008-2010.

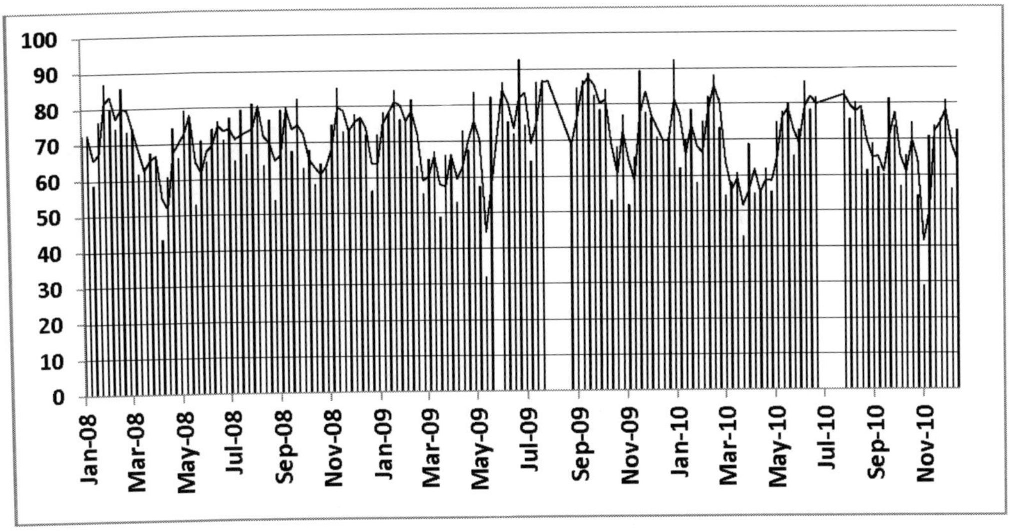

Figure 5. Fluctuation of Weekly Mean of Relative Humidity (Percent), 2008-2010.

Table 3. Comparing means of allergy cases ratio[1] by low/high classes of upper-air observations, 2008-2010

Dew Point § (⁰C)	N	Mean Of Ratio Ψ	SD	Wilcoxon Test
DWPT > -3.42	296	1.125	0.849	Pr< 0.0001
DWPT <= -3.42	272	0.887	0.675	
Mix Ratio § (g/kg)				
MIXR >4.36	236	1.181	0.902	Pr< 0.0001
MIXR<=4.36	332	0.886	0.647	
Temperature § (⁰C)				
Temp >2.92	305	1.130	0.851	Pr< 0.0006
Temp<=2.92	263	0.878	0.666	

Ψ Allergy Cases Ratio = Daily Cases / Annual Average.

§The cutoff values are three-year median values for dew point, mixing ratio, and temperature.

The Wilcoxon two-sample test was used to determine the significance of association between allergy cases reported from elementary schools during three years (2008-2010) and each upper-air observation indicator (Table 3). The ratio of daily allergy cases to annual average was utilized for analysis instead of using the absolute number of daily allergy cases to minimize the effect of increase in allergy reporting over three years. The ratio of allergy occurrence has statistically significant associations with all four upper-air observation indicators. Cut-off points for dew point, temperature, and mixing ratio were considered as the median values (for the three-year period) of each variable: -3.42, 4.36, and 2.92, respectively. When the upper-air dew point was higher than its median value, the occurrence of allergy cases was higher and this difference was statistically significant ($p<0.0001$). Similarly, a higher number of cases reported with a higher value of upper-air mixing ratio ($p<0.0001$). Finally, when the upper-air temperature was higher than its median value, a higher number of allergy cases were reported ($p<0.0006$).

The cut off for relative humidity (50%) was obtained using guidelines from the Mayo Clinic and American College of Allergy, Asthma, and Immunology (ACAAI) (21, 22). The Chi-Square test revealed that relative humidity had no significant association with occurrence of allergy cases. The Chi-Square test revealed that season, mixing ratio, and interaction of temperature with relative humidity are important in determining whether or not the number of allergy cases is greater than the daily mean of allergy cases for the particular year.

Finally, using the GEE model, the following equation was adopted for determining the probability of having ≥ 13 cases (three-year mean + one standard deviation) on a day:

$$y = a_0 + a_1x_1 + a_2x_2 + a_3x_3 + a_4 (x_4{*}x_2)$$

$$\log\frac{P}{1-P} = -4.3212 - 0.2685\,(T) - 2.4288\,(MR) - 0.1012\,(RH) - 0.074\,(DP * MR)$$

log P/(1-P) = Logarithm of odds ratio for the [mean + one standard deviation] cases (=13 cases) on a day

P = Probability of having ≥ 13 allergy cases on a particular day

1 – P = Probability of having allergies on that day

T = Upper-air temperature °C (in Celsius)

MR = Upper-air actual mixing ratio g/kg (in grams per kilogram)

RH = Relative humidity % (in percent)

DP = Upper-air dew point temperature °C (in Celsius)

As an example, if the upper-air temperature, upper-air mixing ratio, upper-air relative humidity, and upper-air dew point temperature are 12°C, 5 g/kg, 55%, and 5°C respectively on a particular day, the probability (P) of having more than 13 cases of allergies within the surveillance system on that day is 64%.

DISCUSSION

The surveillance of allergy among school children in Pennsylvania has improved during the last four years in two aspects: the school enrollment in the surveillance system and the disease reporting by school health nurses, a proven, reliable data source (23). The increased exposure to allergens and changes in other socioeconomic and sociodemographic factors among school children may be the main reasons for an increase in allergies in Pennsylvania. The finding of the current study that peaks (main outbreaks) of allergy occurrence were reported in August-September and in April was compatible with the previously stated evidence from empirical studies. However, having the highest prevalence in the summer months may be associated with characteristics of pollen that cause allergic symptoms (2).

Annual averages of upper-air observations (temperature, relative humidity, dew point, mixing ratio) did not differ between years. As explained previously, a higher temperature (greater than the three-year median) is associated with occurrence of more allergies among Pennsylvania school children. However, this study considered only the upper-air temperature, not the surface-level ambient temperature. Similarly, a higher upper-air dew point was found to be related to the occurrence of more allergies. In addition, a higher upper-air mixing ratio was associated with occurrence of more allergies. The review of literature found no record of these latter two associations. It is important that all three associations were considered in isolation during the analysis, rather than assessing their interaction with each other or with any other variable, such as relative humidity, air pollution, or pollen. The upper-air relative humidity showed no association with occurrence of allergies at its median value cut off, although the upper-air relative humidity ≥ 50% was significantly associated with allergies. As discussed previously, the concept of relative humidity is complex because relative humidity is relative to the amount of energy (measured by temperature) available to do the work of evaporation, and it can be changed without having any change in the actual amount of water vapor in the air (absolute humidity). Therefore, dew point and actual mixing ratio in conjunction with temperature provide a better assessment of humidity, which is more relevant to allergies.

Put another way, the routinely measured and publicly available upper-air indicators provide a good estimate and a reliable tool for forecasting allergy burden on the school health system today or on a future day. This output of analysis with GEE is based on a three-year mean of allergies (13 cases) and does not restrict the utilization of the above equation beyond interpolation. Therefore, the extrapolation for forecasting is also realistic given the current analysis, based on the average of allergies for the 2008-2010 period.

Limitations

Apart from decreased accuracy that results from using group averages and ignoring individual level variations, a risk of "ecological fallacy" occurring also exists, which would be the erroneous interpretation that specific children with allergies in the group share the characteristics of the study sample. In prediction of incidence, it is inappropriate to infer that a specific child with an allergy has an X% probability of experiencing an allergy attack on a particular day. However, it is possible to interpret that there is an X% probability of more than N number of allergy occurrences in the study sample on a particular day (16). In addition, there is a possibility that other allergy triggers, such as pollen, air pollution, and respiratory infections, may confound the relationship between upper-air variables and allergy occurrences.

Allergy surveillance in schools is not being conducted during winter break and summer vacations, as well as during weekends and school holidays. The relatively fewer data available for the summer season due to school vacation may somewhat distort the relationships caused by unequal representativeness across seasons.

In addition, it is difficult to exclude the possibility that some students who experience worsening of symptoms at night or early in the morning did not attend the school so their allergy attacks are not included in school health records. It was also impossible to estimate the number of students with respiratory symptoms who did not receive medications in school or who received medication that was not administered by a nurse as some elementary school students may have taken allergy medications without informing the school nurse. Therefore, we cannot exclude the possibility that use of antihistamine medications as recorded by school nurse somewhat under-represented the occurrence of allergy symptoms at school. Unavailability of antihistamine medications usage data at school level as well as absence of data on demographic characteristics (e.g., ethnicity, income) of students in each school or school district were also limitations.

The number of schools using eTools during 2007 was relatively low and, therefore, student data from that year were not included in some of the analyses. The number of schools using eTools changed each year with some schools dropping off and others joining, causing fluctuations in the total number of available student data records. Additionally, each year some students were leaving their school or school district. Nevertheless, the total number of student data strings provided for any one year was sufficiently robust, as was the number of data strings available for multi-year comparisons, to generate reliable results.

Both respiratory and skin allergies may have an association with upper-air variables and both can also be caused by food allergies. Unfortunately, no mechanism exists for distinguishing respiratory and skin allergies from food allergies, because school nurses did not specify the type of allergy associated with treatments they provided. Therefore, we cannot exclude the possibility that a distortion of the relationship between upper-air indicators and respiratory and skin allergies occurred due to the inclusion of food allergies in the analysis. Most likely, a causal relationship between upper-air observations and occurrence of food allergy symptoms does not exist; however, the seasonality of some food allergies is an observed phenomenon possibly caused by seasonal fluctuations in sunlight and perhaps vitamin D (24).

Finally, as we cannot exclude the confounding effect of pollen on a relationship between climatic factors and allergies, another study will be conducted utilizing the same data sources to evaluate the combined effect of pollen in combination with climatic factors on allergies.

CONCLUSION

The surveillance of allergies among school children in Pennsylvania increased over three years in two aspects: school enrollment in surveillance system and the allergy reporting by school health nurses, a proven reliable source. The primary occurrence of allergies among elementary school children was in August-September, followed by April, although the highest overall prevalence was reported in summer, followed by fall. The lowest incident of allergies was reported in winter. Annual averages of upper-air observations (temperature, relative humidity, dew point, mixing ratio) were significantly different between seasons. Upper-air temperature, dew point, and mixing ratio above their three-year mean values were significantly associated with occurrence of allergies, although upper-air relative humidity $\geq$ 50% was not.

Monitoring of upper-air observation data (temperature, dew point, and actual mixing ratio) over time can serve as a reliable means for predicting increased occurrence of allergies among elementary school children. The new mathematical model derived from statistical integration of routine environmental observations and school health records may be used to scrutinize the complexity of allergic diseases as a dynamic outcome determined by multiple environmental parameters. It is also possible to assess the risk for future allergy outbreaks based on fluctuation analysis of a long time series of atmospheric function.

Prediction of allergy outbreaks is important for children diagnosed as having allergies, and their household members can take more preventive measures to avoid allergic conditions, regardless of the severity of allergic condition. In addition, being informed of a possible allergy outbreak on a particular day or week, teachers will be able to pay more attention to early identification of allergic reactions among children in the classroom. Being informed of a possible allergy outbreak, doctors and nurses in emergency rooms or in family practices can take extra preparations and utilize resources more efficiently to serve an increased number of allergy patients. With accurate prediction, the school health system can also play a major role by effectively reallocating both human and physical resources as well as by notifying teachers and children with allergies to take extra precautions and identify allergic reactions very early. Mass media and local media can also play an important role in all of these aspects. Results of the current study can be used to inform similar programming at the national level and in other states. Monitoring of upper-air observation data over time can serve as a reliable means for predicting outbreaks of allergies among elementary school children and for taking more effective precautionary measures.

ACKNOWLEDGMENTS

Authors thank InnerLink, Inc. for developing eTools and also the Highmark Foundation of Pittsburgh, Pennsylvania for implementing the Highmark Healthy High 5 Initiative. The authors report no conflicts of interest in relation to the current study.

REFERENCES

[1] Centers for Disease Control and Prevention. FastStats: Allergies and Hay Fever. Accessed 2011 Aug 21. URL: http://www.cdc.gov/nchs/fastats/allergies.htm.

[2] American Academy of Allergy, Asthma, and Immunology. Allergies. Accessed 2011 Aug 21. URL: http://www.aaaai.org/conditions-and-treatments/allergies.aspx.

[3] United States Department of Health and Human Services. Summary Health Statistics for U.S. Children: National Health Interview Survey, 2010. Hyattsville, MD: Centers Disease Control Prevention, Nation.

[4] Goldsby RA, et al. Immunology, 5 ed. New York: WH Freeman, 2000.

[5] Ricard N, Sauriol L, Christian S. Burden of care and quality of life amongst parents of children with seasonal allergies. J Allergy ClinImmunol 1999;103(1):S72-S.

[6] Moller C, Elsayed S. Seasonal variation of theconjunctivalprovocation test: Total and specific IGE in children with birch pollen allergy. Int Arch Allergy ApplImmunol 1990;92(3):306-8.

[7] Kurt E, Metintas S, Basyigit I, Bulut I, Coskun E, Dabak S, et al. Prevalence and risk factors of allergies in Turkey: Results of a multicentric cross-sectional study in children. Pediatr Allergy Immunol 2007;18(7):566-74.

[8] Penard-Morand C, Charpin D, Raherison C, Kopferschmitt C, Caillaud D, Lavaud F, et al. Long-term exposure to background air pollution related to respiratory and allergic health in schoolchildren. ClinExp Allergy 2005;35(10):1279-87.

[9] Lee YL, Shaw CK, Su HJ, Lai JS, Ko YC, Huang SL, et al. Climate, traffic-related air pollutants and allergic rhinitis prevalence in middle-school children in Taiwan. EurRespirat J 2003;21(6):964-70.

[10] Ghunaim N, Wickman M, Almqvist C, Soderstrom L, Ahlstedt S, van Hage M. Sensitization to different pollens and allergic disease in 4-year-old Swedish children. ClinExp Allergy 2006;36(6):722-7.

[11] Bartkova-Scevkova J. The influence of temperature, relative humidity and rainfall on the occurrence of pollen allergens (Betula, Poaceae, Ambrosia artemisiifolia) in the atmosphere of Bratislava (Slovakia). Int J Biometeorol 2003;48:1-5.

[12] D'Amato G, Liccardi G, Frenguelli G. Thunderstorm-asthma and pollen allergy. Allergy 2007;62(1):11-6.

[13] Unisys Weather Information Systems. Upper air data. Accessed 2011 Aug 21. URL: http://weather.unisys.com/upper_air/details.php.

[14] Knorr RS, Condon SK, Dwyer FM, Hoffman DF. Tracking Pediatric Asthma: The Massachusetts Experience Using School Health Records. Environ Health Perspect 2004;112(14):1424-7.

[15] Mandate HOPHSCwS. Early Intervent 2008;36.

[16] Schoenbach V, Rosamond W, editors. Understanding the Fundamentals of Epidemiology: an evolving text. Fall 2000 ed. Chapel Hill, NC: University North Carolina, 2000.

[17] House Bill 1113, The General Assembly of of the Commonwealth of Pennsylvania, 2003 Sess, 2003.

[18] United States Department of Education. Family Educational Rights and Privacy Act (FERPA). Family Policy Compliance Office (FPCO). Accessed 2011 Aug 21. URL: http://www2.ed.gov/policy/gen/guid/fpco/ferpa/index.html.

[19] Boos D. On generalized score tests. Am Statistician 1992;46:327-33.

[20] Rotnizky A, Jewell N. Hypothesis testing of regression parameters in semiparametric generalized linear models for cluster correlated data. Biometrika 1990;77:485-97.

[21] Mayo Clinic. Humidifiers and Dehumidifiers. Rotnizky A, Jewell N. Hypothesis testing of regression parameters in semiparametric generalized. http://www.mayoclinic.com/health/humidifiers/HQ00076.

[22] American College of Allergy, Asthma, and Immunology (ACAAI). Make Your Child's Room an Allergy-Free Zone. Rotnizky A, Jewell N. Hypothesis testing of regression parameters in semiparametric generalized. Accessed 2011 Aug 21. URL: http://www.acaai.org/allergist/news/New/Pages/childs-room-allergy-free-zone.aspx.

[23] Logue JN, White MV, Marchetto DJ. Pennsylvania's asthma school project and descriptive pilot investigation: A focus on environmental health tracking. J Environ Health 2007;70(3):21-7.

[24] Vassallo MF, Banerji A, Rudders SA, Clark S, Mullins RJ, Camargo CA. Season of birth and food allergy in children. Ann Allergy Asthma Immunol 2010;104(4):307-13.

In: Child and Adolescent Health Yearbook 2013
Editor: Joav Merrick
ISBN: 978-1-63117-658-6

Chapter 11

HEALTH RISK AND DEVIANT BEHAVIORS AMONG UNDERGRADUATE STUDENTS AT AN ACADEMIC INSTITUTE IN ISRAEL

Liat Korn, PhD* and Hagit Bonny-Noach, PhD
Department of Health Management, School of Health Science, Ariel University, Ariel, Department of Sociology and Anthropology, Department of Criminology, School of Social Sciences, Ariel University, Ariel and Department for Youth Care Work, School of Education, Beit Berl Academic College, Kfar Saba, Israel

ABSTRACT

The purpose of this study was to examine the prevalence of health risk behaviors (such as cigarette and hookah smoking, alcohol consumption and marijuana use), and deviant and delinquent behaviors (such as theft, property damage, drug abuse, cheating on exams and various driving violations) among undergraduate students at an academic institute in Israel. The novelty of this study is its investigation of a broad variety of health risk and deviant behaviors as a whole among undergraduate students, and the understanding of their contribution to predicting cannabis use. This study used a structured, self-reported anonymous questionnaire dealing with health, welfare and risk behaviors. The questionnaire was distributed among 1,574 undergraduate students at a large academic institute in Israel. The mean age of the sample subjects was 27 (SD=6.64). The findings demonstrate that approximately one fourth of the students reported cheating on exams. Additionally, around one fourth reported smoking marijuana and over one third of the drivers reported not stopping at a stop sign. All of these behaviors were found in higher frequency among males. The considerable prevalence of these behaviors among undergraduate students raises the question: In their eyes, are these behaviors considered a social norm or a deviance?

Keywords: Health risk behaviors, deviance, cannabis use, cheating on exams, delinquency, undergraduate students

* Correspondence: Liat Korn, PhD, Researcher, Department of Health Management, School of Health Science, Ariel University , Ariel, Israel. E-mail: kornli@zahav.net.il

INTRODUCTION

Health risk behaviors are voluntary behaviors which lead to negative outcomes from a health perspective. A negative health outcome could be an injury, an illness or death. However, these behaviors could also have negative and problematic social outcomes for their implementer (1). The Problem Behavior Theory (PBT) explains that these behaviors are a product of an integration of risk factors which raise the probability of involvement in risk behaviors by providing a model for problematic behavior, broadening the possibilities of involvement in other risky behaviors, and magnifying the personal vulnerability of problematic behaviors. The model also introduces resilience factors which reduce the probability of involvement in risk behaviors by providing a model of positive social behaviors, by means of social and personal supervision and control, as well as a supportive social environment. Both risk and protective factors are present in all of our social and personal systems (2). According to this theory, health risk behaviors are related to each other and have a clustering effect.

Illegal drug use is a common behavior among young-adults including undergraduate students. Cannabis products (marijuana and hashish) constitute the most common drug in general and among undergraduate students in particular (3). A comprehensive study conducted in Israel on behalf of the Israel Anti Drug and Alcohol Authority (IADA) in 2003 examined undergraduate student's attitudes towards drug use as well as drug use rates in a representative sample (N=6,965) from twelve higher education institutes. Over 40% of the students reported experiencing illegal drug use. Close to one third of the students (30%) reported illegal drug use within the last year. Cannabis was found to be the most common drug used amongst the illegal drugs (4).

Excessive alcohol consumption is a growing phenomenon in the Israeli society. Studies in the field show an increase in excessive alcohol use and an expansion of the phenomenon in the various alcohol dimensions such as binge drinking and drunkenness. Binge drinking is defined as drinking five or more servings of alcohol within a few hours- that is, in one event. In research literature it is considered an extremely dangerous behavior, in which under the influence of such quantity of alcohol, judgment and response capabilities are significantly impaired (1, 5). Epidemiological data from various studies shows a significant increase in this behavior in recent years. Ezrahi, Rosiner, Nirel & Bar-Hamburger (6) reported an increase in beer drinking among young-adults aged 18-40 as well as a rise in reported drunkenness.

Cigarette smoking was also examined among young-adults in several studies, and has proved to be a problematic risk behavior among adolescents (7). More than one third of the sample (37.6%) aged 18-40 reported smoking cigarettes in 2009 (6), a lower incidence in comparison to 2005 (41.0%). Youth aged 18-24 reported smoking cigarettes at a higher frequency than the frequency in both of the older age groups (25-34 and 35-40) examined. The prevalence of male smokers (47.2%) was much higher than the prevalence of female smokers (28.0%). Approximately half of the student sample reported that they did not smoke or have ever smoked in the past. About 38% reported smoking cigarettes, and about a quarter reported smoking regularly (4).

Hookah (water-pipe) smoking is a health risk behavior which has expanded in Israel over the last decade and a half from the prevalence of zero to that which is higher than that of cigarette smoking among adolescents (1, 5, 8). Hookah experiencing prevalence stood at

37.7% of Israeli youth while cigarette experiencing prevalence stood at 27.7%. A study conducted on a representative sample of youth in Israel in 2002 found that those who smoke a hookah have a higher incidence of involvement in other risk behaviors in comparison to those who do not smoke hookahs, such as: suffering injuries, involvement in violence, involvement in risky sexual behaviors, cigarette smoking, alcohol consumption and drug use. The study findings indicate that it is important to view the behavior of hookah smoking among adolescents in Israel as a health risk behavior associated with the consumption of addictive substances and as a gateway for experiencing more serious risk behaviors (8). A different survey conducted in 2008, in the Arab sector, among adolescents in the city of Taybeh found an even higher incidence where 37.1% report smoking a hookah regularly- 55.0% among males and 17.4% among females. The probability of hookah smoking increased among undergraduate students with low academic aspirations and smoking parents (9). A survey conducted by the Anti-Drug and alcohol Authority also found that 27.0% of the adolescents and approximately 17.0% of the adults reported hookah smoking within the past month (6).

Academic dishonesty is an additional risk behavior commonly found among undergraduate students, which is attributed to copying and cheating on examinations, copying homework assignments and plagiarism of academic tasks (see for example: 10, 11). Subjects tend to view academic dishonesty as a normative behavior which is not considered immoral, but stress that this does not mean that students perceive this behavior as appropriate (10). With respect to gender differences, there are no consistent study findings which stand out. Some studies found that males copy on exams at a higher rate than females, while others found no significant gender differences (12).

Driving/moving Violations – the Israeli driver, especially the young driver, drives with a sense of immunity from traffic accidents, despite the high incidence, in practice, of involvement in road Accidents. Although young drivers are at the peak of their physical and mental power, their involvement in accidents is particularly high. The reason for this is most likely a combination of several factors: lack of experience (and therefore limited driving skills), underestimation of risk, overexposure to driving in dangerous situations (night driving, driving in a state of fatigue, driving after drinking alcohol, etc.), and an internal need as well as social pressure to demonstrate "masculinity" by taking risks while driving (13).

In international literature, significant gender differences were found with respect to driving. On average, males more than females, tend to drive faster, pass other cars more often, are more involved in drunken driving offenses and generally take more risks. Males are also more likely than females to be involved in serious car-accidents, especially accidents caused by traffic offenses such as speeding, driving under the influence of alcohol, etc. (13, 14). It was also found that Israeli men spend more hours driving and have a higher self-evaluation and higher self-confidence than women (13).

In summary: In this section we have listed various health risk and deviant behaviors among undergraduate students and young-adults in Israel: Illegal drug use, excessive alcohol consumption, cigarette smoking, hookah smoking, academic dishonesty and driving violations. Some of these behaviors (excluding driving violations and academic dishonesty) have been generally examined, especially among children and adolescents; e.g., in a study of the HBSC in Israel, headed by Dr. Yossi Harel-Fisch et al. (5), but few comprehensive studies have been conducted on these topics among undergraduate students. With respect to hookah smoking, for instance, we have found no studies which have been conducted among undergraduate students. The importance of examining these behaviors, as a whole, is derived from the conclusions of the Problem Behavior Theory mentioned above, which led us to examine the combination of these behaviors since the factors contributing to one risk behavior may also be explanative factors for a different risk behavior.

Study objective

Our research goals of the current study are to examine the prevalence of various risk and deviant behaviors among undergraduate students. The study seeks to answer the following questions with reference to existing literature: Will risk behaviors be found in high frequency among undergraduate students? Are risk and daring behavior patterns more common among male students than among female ones? And, is it possible to predict cannabis use among those who exhibit other risk, daring or deviant behaviors?

Based on the literature review conducted, the hypotheses derived from the research questions are: The prevalence of males involved in risk, daring and deviant behaviors will be higher than the prevalence of females who report it. Additionally, as the PBT theory had determined, various risk behaviors will present in clusters. Risk behaviors will be found in high frequency among the undergraduate students examined, and cannabis use can be predicted by examining use of other health risk and deviant behaviors.

METHODS

Research tools: This study is based on a structured, self-reported anonymous questionnaire which was completed by undergraduate students at a large academic institute in Israel. The study questionnaire was based on two main sources: First, the CU (2003) Personal and Social Development Questionnaire, created by Professor Jessor (15) for the examination of risk and well-being behaviors of college students at the University of Colorado, Boulder, USA; Second, the Israeli Health Behavior in School-aged Children (HBSC) study, the Israeli part of a collaborative Cross-National Study headed by the WHO (1). Our complete questionnaire included questions on different topics as detailed: various socio-demographic questions; self-perceptions; self-esteem and body-image; psychosomatic symptoms; stress; social support; social relationships; academic studies; religion and security; excitement and daring behaviors; nutrition, diet and eating habits; exercise; dental hygiene; sexual behavior; cigarette smoking habits and smoking cessation; hookah smoking; alcohol consumption; reckless driving, and drug abuse. The questionnaire constructed for this study was mainly composed according to the American questionnaire used and was adapted to the student population in Israel. Due to the large quantity of topics presented in the questionnaire and due the desire to not excessively burden the students, the questions were divided into two columns. The most important core questions of each subject were asked in both columns, but different issues were expanded on in each of the columns. Column A expanded on issues of smoking, alcohol, drugs and driving. Column B expanded on issues of education, excitement seeking, eating habits, sexual behavior, religion and security. Each questionnaire column distributed comprised 16 pages.

Population and sample: A total of 1,574 undergraduate students participated in the study, representing 36% of all registered undergraduate students enrolled in an academic institution in Israel. The study was conducted in three faculties (Health, Nature and Social sciences) with their deans' approval. No sampling was, in fact, conducted in this study. Instead, all students present in the classroom who had agreed to complete the questionnaire participated in the study. The surveyors entered all classrooms in the three faculties. The response rate for the questionnaire stood at 93.5%. Of these, 768 completed column A questionnaire, 770 completed column B questionnaire, and 36 students were the pilot group for this study. The sample included 1028 females and 566 males, the average age of the sample was 27 (SD = 6.64). After logic cleaning and cleansing of the data file from significant multiple or missing values, the sample included 1519 subjects.

Research procedure: All students present in the classrooms received the questionnaires within the classroom. Overall the coverage percentage of the sample was 36.3% of students in the sampled departments. The questionnaire was distributed among the students during classes that they attended during April - May, 2009. Overall the surveyors entered approximately 70 classrooms. Questionnaire completion lasted, on average, 20-30 minutes. The three department heads of the faculties participating in the study helped coordinate the classrooms including the number of students attending, the lecturers and the study topic in order to arrange for the most convenient dates for distributing the survey, for the lecturers, the students and the research team. A telephone conversation was conducted between the principal investigator and the various lecturers in order to explain the study and its goals. Considerable cooperation was noted from the lecturers with respect to the completion of the study. Each meeting that was arranged by the principal investigator with a lecturer was followed by an additional reminder telephone call by the surveyor the day before entering the classroom. The surveying team received detailed instructions on how to carry out the questionnaires in the classrooms. Students were told that they do not have to complete the questionnaire if they are not interested in doing so.

Variables: the dependent variables in this study are health risk behaviors, driving violations, deviant behaviors and delinquency. These variables were tested against the independent variables: gender, age, ethnicity, religious background and family income. In addition, in order to examine the odds ratio, indexes were created for driving offenses variables as well as for deviation and delinquency (variable and index details in Appendix 1).

RESULTS

Table 1 presents the dependent variables in the study according to gender. The findings are presented in the table in percentages with standard deviations appearing in parentheses. The table indicates the prevalence of the subject sample according to reports on daring behaviors, health risk behaviors and driving offences. Overall it can be seen that among the deviant behaviors reported, reports on academic dishonesty are highest (25.1%). Of the reported driving offences, reports of speeding are most common (72.9%). With respect to all of the risk and deviant behaviors specified in the table, there is a higher prevalence of males in comparison to females in reporting these behaviors. The biggest gaps between genders were found in the category of binge drinking (42.7% and 17.4% respectively) and in the category of speeding (80.7% and 68.2% respectively).

Table 1. Distribution of study measures by gender (percentages; ±SE)

	Measure list	N	Total	Females	Males
Deviation and Delinquency	Academic dishonesty	1302	25.1 (0.82)	24.1 (0.75)	27.1 (0.94)
	Shop lifting	1308	3.1 (0.34)	2.1 (0.26)	5.0 (0.46)
	Property damage	1308	3.4 (0.33)	1.8 (0.19)	6.6 (0.50)
	Drug sale or practice	1306	3.0 (0.42)	2.3 (0.35)	4.3 (0.53)
	Theft of something valuable	1308	1.3 (0.21)	0.7 (0.14)	2.5 (0.31)
	Hitting someone who said something I did not like	1308	3.7 (0.35)	2.5 (0.21)	6.2 (0.53)
Driving Offences	Not stopping at a stop sign	1107	35.3 (0.87)	33.1 (0.79)	38.7(0.97)
	Failure to keep distance	1102	57.8 (0.98)	54.8 (0.85)	62.6(1.12)
	Driving after drinking alcohol	1102	27.5 (0.84)	20.2 (0.65)	39.1(1.04)
	Speeding	1100	72.9 (1.34)	68.2 (1.22)	80.7(1.42)
	Driving through a red light	1104	8.2 (0.45)	6.9 (0.38)	10.2(0.55)
	Driving after using marijuana	1103	6.4 (0.55)	3.2 (0.36)	11.4(0.75)
	Not always wearing a seatbelt when a friend drives [1]	567	13.6 (0.57)	10.4 (0.44)	18.8(0.74)
	Not always wearing a seatbelt when I drive [1]	563	5.0 (0.41)	3.3 (0.30)	8.0 (0.56)
Health Risk Behaviors	Hookah smoking at least once a week	1192	7.5 (0.70)	4.1 (0.56)	13.3(0.85)
	Regular daily cigarette smoking [2]	341	22.9 (0.83)	19.9 (0.80)	27.3 (0.87)
	Alcohol binge drinking [2]	495	28.5 (1.09)	17.4 (0.69)	42.7(1.38)
	Getting drunk within the last month [2]	525	24.8 (0.91)	20.3 (0.69)	30.5(1.12)
	Any cannabis smoking experience	1265	25.3 (0.78)	22.5 (0.73)	30.5(0.86)
	Smoking cannabis once a week or more in the last month [2]	429	9.1 (1.27)	6.0 (1.11)	13.6(1.45)
	Experiencing ecstasy [1 2]	199	7.5 (0.75)	6.2 (0.29)	9.3 (1.10)
	N	---	---	1000	519

[1]Questions asked only in column A.

[2] filtered questions (from the sample of drivers or from those whom have experienced cannabis).

Table 2 presents the results of predicting the probability of experiencing and regular smoking of cannabis, i.e., what are the chances of, for example, a male to smoke marijuana in comparison to a female. When the safety margin starts at a point greater than 1, the result is significant, and the smaller the range between two points is - the better the result is. Most of the odds ratios values presented in the table are significant (except for deviation and delinquency and ecstasy experiencing – with cannabis experiencing).

The table reveals strong predictors in the areas of: socio-demographic characteristics, driving offenses, deviation and delinquency and health risk behaviors. The table demonstrates that the odds of an undergraduate student to experiment with cannabis are higher if they are males (1.5 times higher) in comparison to females, older (1.9 times higher) in comparison to younger, single (almost twice as high) in comparison to married, and more secular (more than 5 times as high) in comparison to more religious. In addition undergraduate students of Ashkenazi (or Eastern European) decent are more likely to experiment with cannabis (1.72

higher) when compared to students of a Sephardic or Ethiopian decent, and those with a high family income are 1.6 times more likely to experiment with cannabis when compared to those with a low family income. The driving offense index also demonstrates that the probability of experiment with cannabis is 2.5 times higher among students whom have committed driving offenses than among those who have not committed any driving offenses. The examination of all risk behaviors shows that hookah smoking experience raises the probability of a student to experiment with cannabis (by more than 10 times) or use them regularly (more than 11 times).

Table 2. Odds ratios of different variables in predicting experimentation and regular cannabis smoking

	Independent variables	Single experience of smoking cannabis OR (CI)	Regular use of cannabis OR (CI)
Socio-demographic Characteristics	Gender (0-Females, 1-Males)	1.52 (1.17, 1.97)	1.90 (1.42, 2.54)
	Age (0- 25 and younger, 1- 26 and above)	1.89 (1.46 ,2.45)	1.95 (1.46 ,2.60)
	Marital status (0-married, 1- single)	1.96 (1.45, 2.67)	2.37 (1.64, 3.43)
	Religiosity index (α= 0.85) (0-religious, 1- less religious)	5.40 (3.57 ,8.17)	5.09 (3.14 ,8.24)
	Ethnicity (0- Sephardic, Ethiopian 1- Ashkenazi, European decent)	1.72 (1.31, 2.26)	1.63 (1.20, 2.22)
	Family income (0- up to 7000 NIS per month, 1- over 7000 NIS per month)	1.65 (1.18, 2.31)	1.59 (1.09, 2.32)
Driving Offenses 8 items (α =0.61)	Driving offence index (0- none, 1- at least one)	2.50 (1.52, 4.41)	4.06 (1.95, 8.46)
Deviance and Delinquency (α =0.73)	Deviance and delinquency index (0-none, 1- at least one)	1.49 (0.98, 2.26)	1.76 (1.13, 2.76)
Health Risk Behaviors	Hookah smoking experience (0- no, 1-yes)	10.11 (6.53, 15.63)	11.41 (6.55, 19.88)
	Regular cigarette smoking (0- no, 1-yes)	4.69 (3.42, 6.44)	4.34 (3.08, 6.11)
	Alcohol binge drinking (0- no, 1- yes)	2.28 (1.50, 3.46)	2.84 (1.85, 4.36)
	Drunkenness in the last month (0- no, 1- yes)	2.55 (1.67, 3.91)	2.87 (1.85, 4.45)
	Experiencing ecstasy (0- no, 1- yes)	5.68 (0.75, 45.68)	12.69 (1.63, 98.50)

*CI= Confident Interval, OR= Odds Ratio.

While the examination of ecstasy experiencing did not come out significant when compared with experiencing with cannabis (most likely due to the small number of students who reported it), the probability of a person whom has experienced ecstasy to use cannabis regularly is very high (more than 12 times higher) and is clearly significant in comparison to students who have not experienced ecstasy. The findings in the table do show that the essence of drug use in its whole is similar, and that the prospect of students who smoke, drink, get drunk or use ecstasy to experience and use cannabis as well, is high.

The table indicates that the independent variables show a higher probability for regular cannabis use to be preceded by other risk behaviors, than a one-time experience with it. This is especially noticeable with respect to the driving offenses index (2.50 versus 4.06) and ecstasy experiencing (5.68 versus 12.69). In other words, students who commit driving offences and experience cannabis are more likely to be regular cannabis users than those who experience cannabis only once. The table also shows that the deviance and delinquency index does not considerably increase the likelihood of students to experience cannabis.

DISCUSSION

This study examined risk and deviation behavioral patterns among undergraduate students at a large academic institution in Israel. A major query arising, concerns the prevalence of these behaviors, and whether, due to their high frequency, they should be defined as a deviation or whether these behaviors are considered to be a social norm among the students. It was found that cheating on exams was reported by approximately one quarter of the students (25.1%) in comparison to few positive answers to the other questions pertaining to: shoplifting (3.1%), property damage (3.4%), sale of or dealing drugs (3.0%), theft of something valuable (1.3%) and hitting someone for saying something I did not like (3.7%). It may therefore be assumed that cheating on exams is not considered by students as a deviance, but is perceived as a common and legitimate enough behavior in comparison to the other deviant behaviors presented.

An analysis of the driving offenses index shows quite an interesting picture. Of the eight questions in this index, two offenses were answered at a very high rate. These were: Driving at an excessive speed (72.9%) and failure to keep distance (57.6%). It is apparent from this data that these two offenses are perceived as a normative behavior among most students. Two additional questions which were found to be “mainly normative" pertain to not stopping at a stop sign (35.3%) and driving after consuming alcohol (27.5%). It was interesting to see that the lowest prevalence was received in questions about not wearing a seat belt, driving through a red light and the use of marijuana while driving. From this, we can conclude that these behaviors are considered to be a deviation among the students, and the majority of them do refrain from executing them. In other words, it seems that among the students in our sample, not wearing a seat belt in a car is perceived to be more of a deviant behavior than driving after drinking alcohol or speeding. It is possible that the requirement to wear seatbelts, which was implemented in recent years, was internalized and accepted by the Israeli public. Therefore, it seems that it is possible to change deviant behavioral norms if an emphasis is put on preventing these behaviors, along with conducting campaigns for their prevention and using various law enforcement methods against those conducting them.

Another interesting finding pertains to the differences observed between the genders in this study. The study findings showed an unequivocal trend regarding differences in risk and deviant behaviors between the genders. The prevalence of males in all of the behaviors examined in the study was higher than the prevalence of females reporting these behaviors. The greatest disparities between the genders were found in the issues of binge drinking and of speeding. A gap of more than double exists between the genders on the issue of frequent cannabis use (13.6% among males compared to 6.0% among females) and binge drinking (42.7% and 17.4% respectively). The frequency of cannabis use, and these differences between the genders correlates with previous findings presented in the literature with respect to drug use, as shown by Ezrahi et al. (6; 12.3% of the males vs. 5.5% of the females). The large gaps between the genders are also expressed in the issue of alcohol consumption both in our study and in the work of Ezrahi et al., (6; 73.5% of the males vs. 54.9% of the females). Additionally, the frequency of cigarette smoking and gender differences are similar both in the literature examined (4, 6) and in our study. The various daring and deviant behaviors examined also proved to be unfavorable towards the males. With respect to cheating on exams, no consistence stood out in the research literature pertaining to gender differences. Some studies found that males copy on exams more frequently than females, while others found no significant gender differences (12). The findings of this study do not shed new light on the issue and do not show significant differences between the genders in this respect. While, cheating on exams / homework was found to be higher among males in this study, the differences reported were insignificant (27.1% vs. 24.1% respectively). On the issue of driving offenses, however, clear differences emerged between the genders, as found in international literature. Studies have shown that males tend to drive on average faster than females. They also pass cars more often, are involved in more drunk driving offenses and generally take more risks than females. Males are also more likely than females to be involved in serious accidents, especially accidents caused by traffic offenses, such as speeding and driving under the influence of alcohol (13, 14). The current study findings support this data. The prevalence of males was higher than that of females in all driving offense examined (i.e., not stopping at the stop sign, failure to keep a distance, the combination of drinking and driving, cannabis smoking and driving, speeding, driving through a red light and not wearing a seat belt). The price paid by women in a patriarchal society is clear, however even the men pay the price- the price of risk. Males tend to take part in risk behaviors more than females in many fields - as is clearly evident in the present study, among others, in order to prove the superiority of the male gender.

Accordingly, and in order to determine whether a behavior is a deviation, we must examine the practices of a society in a given a time and place. If the behavior violates the practice, rule, law or norm acceptable it is a deviation. Drug use is considered a deviation in the Israeli society, the behavior deviates from the customary rules of conduct in the Israeli culture and by law is defined as illegal. However, students report that drug use is part of the young-adult culture in Israel and that to them, it is not considered a deviance, on the contrary, this is the acceptable norm and those who deviate from it experience peer pressure at times. Cannabis use is illegal in Israel and yet many believe that this law should be changed (16). For example, Bar - Hamburger (4) found that 25% of his sample reported that they are in favor of changing the law pertaining to the legalization of cannabis use, 42% of the students expressed their opinion that the law prohibiting its use should stay as it is, and the rest - 33% were indecisive. Many of the students who reported using drugs in practice favored legalizing their use. In general, young-adults and students do not perceive the use of cannabis products as a deviant or negative behavior (for example: 4, 16), and many of them do not attribute health risk to cannabis (6).

The data obtained in this study helps base the understanding of the reasons for the change observed in the extent of drug abuse among students and also gives a better understanding as to the characteristics of students who use drugs, while relating them to additional risk patterns. In addition, another unique importance of this study is that it presents, in a comprehensive manner, abundant information about various risk behaviors, beyond drug abuse, and in various aspects – behaviors which have a clear and significant relationship between them.

The study findings also try to explain cannabis smoking by means of different variables. The most significant variables for explaining experiencing marijuana are: a religious background, driving offenses, and health risk behaviors - especially hookah smoking. The probability of students experiencing cannabis were 5.4 times higher among the less religious students in comparison to the more religious ones; 2.5 times higher among students who also commit driving offenses; and more than 10 times higher among students who smoke a hookah. The deviance and delinquency index as well as the ethnic origin did not come out significant in the analysis.

The current study adds confirmation the Problem Behavior Theory (2) which shows that relationships exist between the different risk behaviors - cannabis use vs. driving offense, deviation and delinquency, hookah and cigarette smoking, alcohol binge drinking, and experiencing ecstasy. Strong causal and significant relationships were found for all of these in our study. According to the PBT, experiencing and using cannabis are explained by the strengthening of risk factors and the weakening of resilience factors in the personal and social environment. Indeed in our study, as expected, when the risk factors increased, so did the odds of students to experiment and use cannabis regularly. It seems that the content world of smoking and alcohol use considerably affect the likelihood of students to smoke cannabis.

This study has several limitations. First, the study is based on students whom are present in the classroom rather than on all students registered in the various programs. This may have a moderating effect on the degree of their involvement in risk and deviant behaviors. Second, despite the questionnaire being anonymous, the fact that it was distributed in an academic institute may have had a moderating effect on the subjects' responses as they may have feared for impact on their academic record. If these influences exist, it should be presumed that the scope and the severity of risk and deviant behaviors examined in this study are lower than in reality.

Overall, this study is a pioneering study which is meant to be used as a pilot of a larger study which will include a representative sample of students from a number of leading academic institutions in Israel and later, internationally as well.

ACKNOWLEDGMENT

We would like to thank the academic institution where this research was conducted, and to the Israeli Anti-Drugs Authority for the funding assistance and for its support; The students for their willingness to contribute to this research and for their patience in completing the questionnaire; Professor Jessor, from the University of Colorado, Boulder, for his contribution in guidance and theoretical instruction as well as for allowing us to use his research questionnaire and finally we want to thank Mrs. Yael Shaked for her comments and ideas.

APPENDIX 1: VARIABLE DETAILS

The *health risk behaviors* examined in this study are hookah smoking, cigarette smoking, alcohol consumption, marijuana smoking and ecstasy use. The Measure of hookah smoking at least once a week was built from the variable of hookah smoking frequency: "If you smoke a hookah, how often do you smoke a hookah these days?". The answer values to this question were: 1. I do not smoke. 2. Less than once a week. 3. At least once a week but not every day. 4. Every day. This measure included subjects who replied values 3 and 4. For the examination of regular daily cigarette smoking - subjects were asked to indicate whether the statements are applicable for them. This measure was based on the statement: "I smoke regularly and consistently throughout the day". The answer values to this question were: 1. Yes 2. To some extent. 3. No. This measure included subjects who replied value 1. The binge drinking measure was based on the question: "In the last month, how often did you drink five or more alcoholic drinks when drinking?" and the drunkenness measure was based on the question: "In the last month, approximately how many times did you actually get drunk?". The answer values to these questions were: 1. Never 2. Once. 3. Two - three times. 4. Once a week. 5. Five to seven times. 6. Twice a week 7. More than twice a week. Subjects replying values of 2 to 7 were included in these measures. The measure of cannabis smoking experience was based on the question: "Have you ever tried marijuana/ hashish?" Answer values were: 1. No, never. 2. Yes, once. 3. Yes, more than once. This measure included subjects who replied values 2 and 3. Smoking marijuana once a week or more was based on the question: "Over the past month, how often have you used marijuana/ hashish?". The values ranged from 1 never to 7 every day. This measure included values 4-7 from once a week to daily. Ecstasy use experience was based on the question "Have you ever used the following drugs? If so, please indicate how many times you have used each drug during the last month." The values were: 0. No. 1. Yes, and an option of putting down the number of times they had used in the last month.

The *driving offenses indexes* were based on a series of questions as detailed: "Over the past month, how often did you: 1. pass a stop sign without coming to a complete stop? 2. Drive too close to the car in front of you? 3. Drive after drinking at least one whole bear, a glass of wine or something similar? 4. Drive more than 20 kilometers per hour above the speed limit? 5. Drive through a red light? 6. Drive after using marijuana?" The answer values to these questions ranged from 1. Never to 5. Ten times or more. Subjects replying answer values 2 (once or twice) to 5 (ten times or more) were included in these measures. Two additional measures on the use of seat belts were based on the questions: "When you are a passenger in a car that a friend is driving, do you use your seat belt?" And "Do you wear a seat belt when you drive?" The answer values for both questions ranged from 1. Always to 5. Almost never. Subjects replying answer values 2 (almost always) to 5 (almost never) were included in these measures.

Daring, deviant and delinquent behavior indexes were based on a series of questions as detailed: "Over the past month, how often did you: 1. Cheat on exams or homework? 2. Shop lift? 3. Caused damage or marked public or private property on purpose? 4. Sold or dealt drugs? 5. Stole something valuable such as a Palm pilot, a backpack, or a wallet from someone? 6. Hit someone because you did not like what they had to say?". Values for these questions ranged on a scale from 1. Never to 5. 5 times or more. Subjects replying values 2 (once) to 5 (twice or more) were included in these measures.

Independent variables: gender (male, female), The *age* category variable - determined by year of birth (age group distribution was determined by the median value - born in 1984 - distributing the sample to young people – up to age 26, and from age 26 onwards - adults). The variable of *ethnicity* was based on the question: "What ethnic background best describes you?". This question had eight response values as follows: 1. Ashkenazi/ Western Europe; 2. Spain/ Mizrahi. 3. Eastern Europe/ The Soviet Union / Russia. 4. Ethiopia. 5. Arab Israeli 6. Druze. 7. Bedouin. 8. Other. In the construction of the measure, categories were created for Jewish – those who replied values 1 to 4, and non-Jewish – those who replied values 5 to 7. The *marital status* variable included the categories 1. Single, 2. Single living with a partner. 3. Married. 4. Separated. 5. Divorced, 6. Widower. The Analysis included students from the categories 1 + 2 as single, and Category 3 - married. The *family income* variable was based on the question: "What is your family's average monthly income?" Response values were: 1. Less than - 7,000 NIS 2. Between 7,000 NIS and 9000 NIS, 3. Between 9,000 NIS and 13,000 NIS. 4.Between 13,000 NIS and 17,000 NIS. 5. Between 17,000 NIS and 25,000 NIS, and 6. Over 25,000 NIS.

Odds ratio analysis indexes: *Religiosity* index ($\alpha = 0.85$) consisted of five questions as follows: 1. How important is it for you to be able to rely on what religion teaches when you have a problem? 2. How important it for you to believe in God, a higher power or a creator? 3. How important it for you to depend on your religious beliefs as a guide to everyday life? 4. How important it for you to be able to turn to prayer when you deal with personal problems? And Question 5 - How many times did you attend synagogue or other religious services during the last month? In questions 1-4 the students were asked to mark their answer from four values on a scale ranging from "very important" to "not important at all". In the fifth question they were asked to list the number of times from - 1.Never to 7. Eight times or more. For the creation of a secular - religious index, the five questions were put together and their values were divided to two according to the average value.

The *driving offenses* index ($\alpha = 0.61$) consisted of eight questions which asked the respondent to mark frequencies within the last month on a scale of five responses ranging from "never" to "10 times or more", for the questions: 1. Not stopping at a stop sign 2. Not keeping a distance 3. Driving after drinking alcohol. 4. Speeding. 5. Driving through a red light 6. Driving after using marijuana 7. Not wearing a seat belt when a friend drives. 8. Not wearing a seat belt when I drive. For index creation purposes, these eight questions were put together, and the values were divided to 0 - no offense, and 1 - one or more offense.

The *deviation and delinquency* index ($\alpha = 0.73$) consisted of five questions in which the subjects were asked to select, within the past month, how often, on a scale of five responses, ranging from "never" to "5 times or more", have they: 1. Shop lifted. 2. Caused property damage. 3. Sold or dealt drugs 4. Stole something valuable. 5. Hit someone because they did not like what they said. For index creation purposes, these five questions were put together and the values were divided to 0 – none of these behaviors, and 1 – at least one of these behaviors. The "cheating on exams" variable was omitted from the index because it lowered the reliability of items with results of under 0.6.

REFERENCES

[1] Harel Y, Molcho M, Tillinger E. Youth in Israel, health, well-being and risk behavior. Summary of findings from the third national study (2002) and trend analysis (1994-2002). Bar Ilan: Bar-Ilan University, 2003. [Hebrew]

[2] Jessor R, Turbin MS, Costa MF. Adolescent problem behavior in China and United State: A cross-national study of psychosocial protective factors. J Res Adolesc 2003;13(3):329-60.

[3] Bonny-Noach H. Between anti-language, slang and Argo- the Israeli drug users backpackers language. In: Bonny-Noach H, ed. Backpackers and drug abuse: A documentary, research, treatment and prevention perspective. Jerusalem: Bialik Publishers, 2008:260-87. [Hebrew]

[4] Bar-Hamburger R. Survey of attitudes and use of psychoactive drugs among students in institutes of higher learning in Israel. Jerusalem: Israel Anti-Drug Authority, 2003.

[5] Harel-Fisch Y, Korn L, Fogel-Grinvald H, Ben-David Y, Naveh S. Youth in Isreal, health, well-being and risk behavior. Summary of findings from the fifth national study (2006) and trend analysis (1994-2006). Ramat Gan: Bar-Ilan University, 2009. [Hebrew]

[6] Ezrahi Y, Rosiner I, Nirel R, Bar-Hamburger R. Illegal use of drugs and alcohol in Israel, 2009, Seventh national epidemiological survey. Jerusalem: Israel Anti-Drug Authority, 2009. [Hebrew]

[7] Turbin MS, Jessor R, Costa FM. Adolescent cigarette smoking: Health-related behavior or normative transgression? Prev Sci 2000;1(3):115.

[8] Korn L. The nargila smoking phenomenon among teen-agers in Israel: A sociological analysis [Ph.D. thesis]. Ramat Gan: Bar-Ilan University, 2005.

[9] Korn L, Magnezi R. Cigarettes and nargila (water pipe) use among Israeli Arab high school students: Prevalence and determinants of tobacco smoking. ScientificWorldJournal 2008;8:517-25.

[10] Arnett JL, Arnett JJ, Feldman SS, Cauffman E. I'ts wrong, but everybody does it: Academic dishonesty among high school and college students. Contemp Educ Psychol 2002;27:209-28.

[11] Whitley EB. Factors associated with cheating among college students: A review. Res Higher Educ 1998;39(3):235-74.

[12] Jordan EA. College student cheating: The role of motivation, perceived norms, attitudes, and knowledge of institutional policy. Ethics Behav 2001;11(3):233-47.

[13] Taubman-Ben-Ari O, Mikulincer M, Gillath O. From parents to children: Similarity in parents and offspring driving styles. Transport Res Part F Traffic Psychol Behav 2005;8:19-29.

[14] Simon F, Corbett C. Road traffic offending, stress, age, and accident history among male and female drivers. Ergonomics 1996;39:757-80.

[15] CU 2003. Personal and social development wuestionnaire. University of Colorado, Institute of Behavioral Science. Downloaded: August, 2009. Accessed 2012 Mar 12. URL: http://www.colorado.edu/ibs/jessor/questionnaires/questionnaire__guide_spsd2.pdf

[16] Bonny-Noach H. Construction of a social problem among Israeli drug users backpackers. In: Bonny-Noach H, ed. Backpackers and drug abuse: A documentary, research, treatment and prevention perspective. Jerusalem: Bialik Publishers, 2008:13-31. [Hebrew]

In: Child and Adolescent Health Yearbook 2013
Editor: Joav Merrick
ISBN: 978-1-63117-658-6

Chapter 12

ADULT PERCEPTIONS OF YOUTH MENTAL HEALTH ISSUES IN A CANADIAN PROVINCE

Amy Metcalfe, PhD[1], Julius Salegio, MSc[2], Nancy Reynolds, BScOT[2] and Suzanne Tough, PhD*[1,2,3]

[1]University of British Columbia, Department of Obstetrics and Gynecology
[2]Alberta Centre for Child Family and Community Research
[3]University of Calgary, Department of Paediatrics, Calgary, Alberta, Canada

ABSTRACT

Although 15% of Canadian youth experience mental health problems, barriers to disclosure and treatment exist. Objective: This population-based study aimed to assess public opinion about the prevalence of mental illness among youth, treatment for mental illness, and comfort interacting with youth with mental health problems. Study Group: A random sample of adults residing in Alberta Canada. Methods: Chi-square tests and t-tests were used to understand responses by demographics. Logistic regression was used to determine factors predictive of comfort in interacting with youth with moderate mental health problems. Results: Twenty percent were able to correctly identify the prevalence of youth mental health problems. Over 50% stated that they believed that <10% of youth with mental health problems received treatment. Approximately 70% of the sample reported they would be comfortable interacting with youth with moderate mental health problems in work, school, social and community settings. Consistent predictors of comfort interacting with youth with moderate mental health problems included: being between the ages of 18-24, high school completion, Caucasian ethnicity, and annual household income ≥$40,000/year. Conclusions: There are meaningful gaps in Albertans understanding of the prevalence of youth mental health issues, but the majority of adults would be comfortable interacting with youth with moderate mental health problems. Many respondents identified that youth with mental health problems may not be receiving treatment. Increased public awareness about the prevalence and detrimental impact of youth mental health issues may help policy makers allocate resources to effective screening and treatment for youth with mental health concerns.

* Correspondence: Suzanne Tough, Professor and Scientific Director, Child Development Centre, 2888 Shaganappi Trail NW, Calgary, Alberta T3B 6A8, Canada. E-mail: suzanne.tough@albertahealthservices.ca

Keywords: Mental health, children and youth, stigma, literacy, social distance

Introduction

Adequate levels of mental health literacy ('the knowledge and beliefs about mental disorders which aid their recognition, management or prevention'(1)) in the population is important for several reasons. First, it is estimated that in the course of a lifetime, almost everyone will either come into contact with a person with a mental health problem or will develop a mental health problem (1). Second, poor mental health literacy may delay treatment as people are unable to identify the signs and symptoms of mental health problems or be unable to clearly communicate these symptoms to care providers (2). As the majority of mental health problems begin before the age of 24 (3), understanding the public's knowledge of mental health problems in adolescents is crucial as this sets the context in which policy is developed, clinicians are trained and individuals seek care (4). Furthermore, an Australian study found that when dealing with mental health issues, youth (aged 15-25) were most likely to turn to family and friends for assistance before seeking out professional help (3). Therefore, it is important that members of the general public are able to recognize the signs and symptoms of mental health problems and are able to direct individuals to appropriate sources of care.

Poor mental health literacy is believed to contribute to public stigma towards individuals with mental health problems. This in turn can lead to social distancing ('the desire to avoid contact with a particular group of people' (5)) from individuals with mental health problems which can further impact an individual's ability to seek and receive treatment and successfully integrate into society (6). While the desire for social distance from adults with mental health issues has been widely reported on in the literature, the desire for social distance from children and youth afflicted with mental health problems is less clearly understood (5). A 2009 review of social distance from individuals with mental health problems concluded that social distance should routinely be measured as part of national health surveys as an indicator of public stigma and the impact of public health campaigns to reduce stigma towards individuals with mental health problems (5).

This study aimed to assess the mental health literacy of the general population in relation to the prevalence of moderate mental health problems in youth, and to assess their desire for social distance from youth afflicted with moderate mental health problems.

Methods

English-speaking men and women who were at least 18 years of age and were residing in Alberta Canada at the time of contact were involved in this population-based study. Participants were recruited through a random-digit dialling technique targeting landlines and cellular phones. If an individual was contacted on their cellular phone, they were given the opportunity to provide an alternative number for a scheduled call back. Potential participants were contacted up to 10 times at various times of day. Interviews took approximately 30 minutes to complete. Prior to beginning the questionnaire, participants were informed that their participation in this research was completely voluntary, that their individual responses would be kept confidential, and that they could end the interview at any time. An overall response rate of 21.2% (1203/5667) was obtained for this survey and on average it took 3.9 call attempts to complete an interview. This study was approved by the Arts, Science and Law Research Ethics Board at the University of Alberta.

QUESTIONNAIRE

The Alberta Survey is conducted annually by the Population Research Laboratory at the University of Alberta to understand public opinion on issues with relevance to public policy. Community groups, researchers and governmental organizations have the opportunity to add a group of questions to this survey each year.

To understand mental health literacy and a desire for social distance, respondents were asked the following 5 questions regarding their perceptions about youth mental health issues along with questions related to respondent demographics:

1. Generally, what percentage of youth between the ages of 15 to 19 do you think have some kind of mental health problem? (Open Ended)
2. Generally, what percentage of children between the ages of 12 to 14 do you think have some kind of mental health problem? (Open Ended)
3. What percentage of those between the ages of 12 to 19 with a mental health problem receive treatment? (Open Ended)
4. At what age do you think a mental health problem can develop? (Response options: before or after birth (up to 12 months), early childhood (13-59 months), childhood (5-9 years), puberty (10-13 years), teens (14-19 years), early adulthood (20-24 years), adulthood (≥25 years), any age)
5. How comfortable do you think you would feel in the company of a child or youth between the ages of 12-19 who has a moderate mental health problem in the following settings? (Response options: very uncomfortable, uncomfortable, neutral, comfortable, very comfortable)
   a Work
   b School
   c Social setting (i.e., family gathering or party with friends or work colleagues)
   d Community setting (i.e., sports, recreational activities, or church)

The following definition of a moderate mental health problem was provided to survey respondents upon request: An individual with a moderate mental health problem exhibits chronic and pervasive behaviours that interfere with the functioning and safety of the individual and other individuals around him/her. Typically a moderate mental health problem is characterized by a number of maladaptive behaviours, such as: an inability to establish or maintain satisfactory relationships with peers or adults; a general mood of unhappiness or depression; inappropriate behaviour of feelings under ordinary conditions; continued difficulty in coping with the everyday situations in spite of remedial intervention; physical symptoms or fears associated with personal, work or school problems; difficulties in accepting the realities of personal responsibility and accountability; and/or physical violence toward other persons and/or physical destructiveness toward the environment.

Data were collected between May and July 2010 using a computer-assisted telephone interview (Ci3 WINCATI, Sawtooth Software).

Statistical analysis

This analysis was completed using Stata SE version 11 and significance was set at $p<0.05$. Descriptive statistics were used to describe the characteristics of study respondents. Categorical variables were expressed as frequencies and percentages with 95% confidence intervals (CI). Four multivariable logistic regression models were used to determine what demographic variables (marital status, employment, education, age, ethnicity, annual household income) were significantly associated with comfort in interacting with youth with moderate mental health problems in various settings (coded as very comfortable/comfortable vs. neutral/uncomfortable/very uncomfortable). All variables were initially entered into the model, the variable with the highest p-value was purposively removed from the model until all remaining variables had a p-value of <0.05.

RESULTS

This questionnaire was completed by a total of 1203 individuals. Approximately equal numbers of men and women participated in the survey (Table 1). The majority of respondents: lived in a city, were married or in a common law relationship, were employed full-time, had completed post-secondary education, had an annual household income ≥$80,000, were Caucasian, and did not currently have children residing with them in their homes (Table 1).

Respondents are reflective of the Alberta population as captured by the 2006 Canadian census (7) in terms of gender and ethnicity (Table 1). Respondents tended to have completed a higher level of education, have a higher income and be older than the average Albertan (Table 1).

Perceptions regarding the prevalence of youth mental health issues

Approximately 20% of respondents correctly identified that 11-20% of youth between the ages of 12 and 19 years suffer from mental health problems; and many respondents believed that mental health problems influenced fewer than 10% of youth (Table 2). On average, 11% of respondents correctly identified that 21-30% of youth aged 12-19 with mental health problems receive treatment for these issues (Table 2). Slightly over half of respondents believed that no more than 10% of youth with mental health problems received treatment for these problems. Approximately a third of respondents correctly identified that mental health problems can develop at any age, and only 2.0% of respondents believed that mental health problems could not develop until adulthood (Table 2).

Table 1. Respondent characteristics

Variable	Survey Respondents N (%, 95% CI)	2006 Canadian Census: Alberta Population (7) %
Location		
City	774 (64.4, 61.7 to 67.1)	---
Town/Village	238 (19.8, 17.6 to 22.1)	
Rural Area	189 (15.7, 13.7 to 17.8)	
Gender		
Male	598 (49.7, 46.9 to 52.5)	50.0
Female	605 (50.3, 47.5 to 53.1)	50.0
Marital Status*		
Married/Common Law	855 (71.4, 68.8 to 73.9)	64.8
Single/Divorced/Separated/Widowed	343 (28.6, 26.1 to 31.2)	35.2
Employment Status**		
Employed Full-Time	666 (60.1, 57.2 to 62.9)	Employment rate: 70.9%
Employed Part-Time	164 (14.8, 12.7 to 16.9)	---
Retired	227 (20.5, 18.1 to 22.8)	---
Unemployed	52 (4.7, 3.4 to 5.9)	Unemployment Rate: 4.3%
Highest Level of Education Completed***		
Did not complete high school	96 (8.0, 6.5 to 9.6)	23.4
Completed high school	240 (20.1, 17.8 to 22.4)	26.2
Some post-secondary	137 (11.5, 9.7 to 13.3)	---
Completed post-secondary	584 (48.9, 46.0 to 51.7)	45.1
Post-graduate degree	138 (11.5, 9.7 to 13.4)	5.3
Median Age Group***	51.0	36.0
Ethnicity		
Caucasian	1021 (84.9, 82.8 to 86.9)	86.1
Other	182 (15.1, 13.1 to 17.2)	13.9
Median Personal Income	$50,000 to 54,999	$43,964
Children Reside in the Home		
No	805 (67.1, 64.5 to 69.8)	---
Yes	394 (32.9, 30.2 to 35.5)	

* Census results for marital status are for individuals age 20 and older.

** Census results for employment are for individuals age 15 and older.

*** Census results are for all Albertans, while survey participants had to be at least 18 years of age.

Comfort interacting with youth with moderate mental health problems

Approximately two-thirds of respondents reported that they would be comfortable or very comfortable interacting with youth with moderate mental health problems in work, school, social and community settings (Table 3). Only 10% of respondents reported that they would be uncomfortable or very uncomfortable interacting with youth with moderate mental health problems in work, school, social and community settings (Table 3). The proportion of respondents who reported being comfortable/very comfortable interacting with youth with moderate mental health problems was slightly less for social and community settings than it was for work and school settings.

Age and ethnicity were significant predictors in all models examining comfort interacting with youth with moderate mental health problems (Table 4). Consistently, individuals who were 18-24 years old and of Caucasian ethnicity were more likely to report being comfortable or very comfortable interacting with youth with moderate mental health problems. Annual household income was a significant predictor in the models examining comfort in work, social and community settings (Table 4).

Table 2. Respondent beliefs about youth mental health issues (n=1139)

Variable	N	% (95% CI)
What percentage of children between the ages of 12-14 do you think have some kind of mental health problem?		
0-10%	476	46.5% (43.5 to 49.6)
11-20%*	204	19.9% (17.5 to 22.4)
21-30%	151	14.8% (12.6 to 16.9)
31-40%	60	5.9% (4.4 to 7.3)
41-50%	71	6.9% (5.4 to 8.5)
>50%	61	6.0% (4.5 to 7.4)
What percentage of youth between the ages of 15-19 do you think have some kind of mental health problem?		
0-10%	358	34.7% (31.7 to 37.6)
11-20%*	229	22.2% (19.6 to 24.7)
21-30%	149	14.4% (12.2 to 16.6)
31-40%	102	9.9% (8.1 to 11.7)
41-50%	73	7.1% (5.5 to 8.6)
>50%	122	11.8% (9.8 to 13.8)
What percentage of youth between the ages of 12-19 with a mental health problem receive treatment?		
0-10%	495	50.2% (47.0 to 53.3)
11-20%	115	11.7% (9.6 to 13.7)
21-30%*	110	11.1% (9.2 to 13.1)
31-40%	54	5.5% (4.0 to 6.9)
41-50%	114	11.6% (9.6 to 13.5)
>50%	99	10.0% (8.2 to 11.9)
At what age do you think a mental health problem can develop?		
Before or after birth (up to 12 months)	159	14.0 (11.9 to 16.0)
Early childhood (13-59 months)	199	17.5 (15.3 to 19.7)
Childhood (5-9 years)	207	18.2 (15.9 to 20.4)
Puberty (10-13 years)	101	8.9 (7.2 to 10.5)
Teens (14-19 years)	65	5.7 (4.4 to 7.1)
Early adulthood (20-24 years)	12	1.1 (0.5 to 1.6)
Adulthood (25+ years)	10	0.9 (0.3 to 1.4)
Any age*	386	33.9 (31.1 to 36.6)

* correct response.

Table 3. Comfort interacting with youth aged 12-19 with moderate mental health problems in various settings (n=1174)

Variable	Work Setting N (% 95% CI)	School Setting N (% 95% CI)	Social Setting N (% 95% CI)	Community Setting N (% 95% CI)
Very Uncomfortable	55 (5.0, 3.7 to 6.3)	40 (4.1, 2.8 to 5.3)	30 (2.6, 1.7 to 3.5)	30 (2.6, 1.7 to 3.5)
Uncomfortable	66 (6.0, 4.6 to 7.5)	62 (6.3, 4.8 to 7.8)	63 (5.4, 4.1 to 6.7)	55 (4.7, 3.5 to 5.9)
Neutral	214 (19.6, 17.2 to 21.9)	197 (20.0, 17.5 to 22.5)	225 (19.2, 16.9 to 21.4)	222 (18.9, 16.7 to 21.2)
Comfortable	305 (27.9, 25.2 to 30.6)	267 (27.2, 24.4 to 29.9)	352 (30.0, 27.4 to 32.6)	350 (29.9, 27.2 to 32.5)
Very Comfortable	453 (41.4, 38.5 to 44.4)	417 (42.4, 39.3 to 45.5)	504 (42.9, 40.1 to 45.8)	515 (43.9, 41.1 to 46.8)

Table 4. Significant predictors of comfort interacting with youth with moderate mental health problems in various settings

Variable	OR (95% CI)			
	Work Setting (n=828) OR (95% CI)	School Setting (n=730) OR (95% CI)	Social Setting (n=875) OR (95% CI)	Community Setting (n=876) OR (95% CI)
Age Categories				
18-24	Reference	Reference	Reference	Reference
25-34	0.26 (0.08 to 0.80)	0.67 (0.31 to 1.44)	0.31 (0.10 to 0.96)	0.19 (0.05 to 0.68)
35-44	0.31 (0.10 to 0.93)	0.58 (0.28 to 1.21)	0.52 (0.16 to 1.62)	0.26 (0.07 to 0.91)
45-54	0.28 (0.09 to 0.84)	0.48 (0.24 to 0.98)	0.30 (0.10 to 0.90)	0.20 (0.06 to 0.71)
55-64	0.25 (0.08 to 0.76)	0.41 (0.20 to 0.83)	0.28 (0.09 to 0.84)	0.17 (0.05 to 0.61)
65+	0.21 (0.07 to 0.64)	0.29 (0.14 to 0.61)	0.22 (0.07 to 0.69)	0.13 (0.03 to 0.45)
Annual Household Income				
<$39,999	Reference	Not included in final model	Reference	Reference
$40,000-$79,999	2.00 (1.17 to 3.40)		2.27 (1.35 to 3.83)	1.77 (1.03 to 3.03)
≥ $80,000	2.25 (1.36 to 3.71)		2.37 (1.44 to 3.89)	1.85 (1.08 to 3.18)
Ethnicity				
Caucasian	Reference	Reference	Reference	Reference
Other	0.49 (0.32 to 0.76)	0.56 (0.38 to 0.83)	0.48 (0.31 to 0.73)	0.43 (0.27 to 0.66)
Highest Level of Education Completed				
High School Incomplete	Not included in final model	Reference	Reference	Not included in final model
High School Complete		2.25 (1.25 to 4.03)	1.63 (0.85 to 3.13)	
Post-Secondary Incomplete		2.29 (1.22 to 4.29)	1.86 (0.92 to 3.77)	
Post-Secondary Complete		2.27 (1.34 to 3.85)	1.99 (1.09 to 3.63)	
Post-Graduate Degree		2.49 (1.31 to 4.75)	2.02 (1.00 to 4.11)	
Marital Status				
Married/Common Law	Not included in final model	Not included in final model	Not included in final model	Reference
Single/Divorced/Separated/Widowed				0.64 (0.44 to 0.93)

In all models, a positive association was observed whereby the higher the annual household income the more likely individuals were to report that they were comfortable/very comfortable interacting with youth with moderate mental health problems. Education was a significant predictor in the models examining comfort in school and social settings (Table 4). In both scenarios, individuals who had not completed high school were the most likely to report being uncomfortable interacting with youth with moderate mental health problems. Marital status was only a significant predictor in the model examining comfort in a community setting (Table 4), where it was noted that individuals who were single, separated, divorced or widowed were significantly less likely to report being comfortable interacting with youth with moderate mental health issues (OR=0.64, 95% CI: 0.44-0.93).

DISCUSSION

Mental health literacy in this sample appears to be low, as only 20% of respondents were able to correctly identify that 11-20% of youth (aged 12 to 19) suffer from mental health problems and only 11% of respondents were able to correctly identify that 21-30% of youth aged 12-19 with mental health problems receive treatment for these issues. Additionally, only one third of respondents were able to correctly identify that mental health problems can develop at any age. Generally, respondents did not believe that youth with mental health problems were receiving the treatment that they need. This has important implications for government policy as it may indicate public confidence in Alberta's publicly funded health care system in regards to youth with moderate mental health problems could be improved. Most respondents reported that they would be comfortable or very comfortable interacting with youth with moderate mental health problems in work, school, social and community settings indicating a low desire for social distance from youth with moderate mental health problems. Consistent predictors of comfort included: age 18-24, completion of high school, Caucasian ethnicity, and annual household income ≥$40,000/year.

While direct comparison with other studies is difficult due to the differing nature of how questions were asked, respondents in this survey appear to be more willing to interact with individuals with mental health issues. A 2006 US study found that the majority of survey respondents did not want to work or socialize with individuals with mental health problems (4), while only 10% of respondents in this study reported feeling uncomfortable or very uncomfortable interacting with youth in various settings. It is unknown if these large differences are due to methodological differences in how cases were presented and social distance was assessed, or the different population groups (adults vs. youth) that were the focus of the study, or if recent efforts to bring attention to the issue of mental health have influenced public opinion (8-10). Few studies have compared public opinion of child and adult mental health issues. A US study using data from the 1996 and 2002 General Social Surveys found survey respondents were significantly more likely to perceive childhood depression as a serious problem than adult depression and that the problem was unlikely to improve without treatment (11). It is unknown what impact these findings may have on social distance.

The socio-demographic predictors of comfort interacting with youth with moderate mental health problems identified in this study are comparable to that seen in the literature. Other studies that have examined socio-demographic predictors of social distance have consistently found that older individuals are less comfortable interacting with individuals with mental health problems (5, 6, 12, 13) and that gender is not associated with a desire for social distance (5).

This work is not without limitations. Respondents were asked broad questions about mental illness and not presented with specific case examples. While some survey researchers argue that generic questions are less likely to extract discriminating public responses (14), due to the nature of the survey we were not able to ask a series of questions based on case studies. Additionally, while case vignettes are a typical way public opinion has been gathered in similar studies, the public's ability to categorize each case as a mental illness is context dependent (15). A national US study found that while 88% of survey respondents were able to classify a case vignette describing a person with DSM-IV diagnosis of schizophrenia as having a mental illness, less than half of respondents classified individuals with alcohol dependence (49%) or drug addiction (44%) as having a mental illness (15). Furthermore, while we presume that individual responses to questions reflect actual behaviours, we did not assess behaviours directly. A social desirability bias may partially explain the low desire for social distance that is reported in this study in contrast to other studies of this nature; however, this could also be because these questions specifically pertained to youth where there may be less need concern about social distance. Additionally, a low response rate was obtained for this study; however, those that chose to participate are reflective of Alberta population (7), thus increasing the generalizability of these findings.

In conclusion, these results indicate strong public support for social inclusion and connectedness to youth with mental health conditions, while also highlighting gaps in knowledge about the prevalence of youth mental health conditions. Finally, the public correctly identified that it is only the minority of youth who receive treatment for these conditions. Additional treatment or intervention options for youth with mental health conditions would address a gap already identified by the public, and may improve outcomes for youth and their families.

ACKNOWLEDGMENTS

Funding for this study was received from the Alberta Centre for Child, Family and Community Research. The authors would like to thank the Population Research Laboratory at the University of Alberta for their assistance with survey design and data collection. This manuscript was previously presented at the World Congress of Epidemiology meeting which was held in Edinburgh Scotland from August 7-11, 2011. None of the authors have any conflicts of interest to disclose.

REFERENCES

[1] Jorm AF, Korten AE, Jacomb PA, Christensen H, Rodgers B, Pollitt P. Mental health literacy: A survey of the public's ability to recognise mental disorders and their beliefs about the effectiveness of treatment. Med J Aust 1997;166:182-6.

[2] Cotton SM, Wright A, Harris MG, Jorm AF, McGorry PD. Influence of gender on mental health literacy in young Australians. Aust NZ J Psychiatry 2006;40(9):790-6.

[3] Reavley NJ, Jorm AF. Young people's recognition of mental disorders and beliefs about treatment and outcome: findings from an Australian national survey. Aust NZ J Psychiatr 2011;45(10):890-8.

[4] Pescosolido B, Martin J, Long J, Medina T, Phelan J, Link B. A disease like any other? A decade of change in public reactions to schizophrenia, depression, and alcohol dependence. Am J Psychiatr 2010;167(11):1321-30.

[5] Jorm AF, Oh E. Desire for social distance from people with mental disorders. Aust NZ J Psychiatr 2009;43(3):183-200.

[6] Gaebel W, Baumann A, Witte A, Zaeske H. Public attitudes towards people with mental illness in six German cities: results of a public survey under special consideration of schizophrenia. Eur Arch Psychiatry Clin Neurosci 2002;252:278-87.

[7] Statistics Canada. 2006 Census of Population. Ottawa, ON: Statistics Canada catalogue no. 97-560-XCB2006008.

[8] World Health Organization. Atlas: Child and adolescent mental health resources: Global concerns, implications for the future. Geneva: WHO, 2005.

[9] Mental Health Commission of Canada. Toward recovery and well-being: A framework for a mental health strategy for Canada. Calgary, AB: Mental Health Commission Canada, 2009.

[10] Kirby M, Keon W. Out of the shadows at last: Transforming mental health, mental illness and addiction services in Canada. Ottawa: Standing Senate Committee Social Affairs Science Technology, 2006.

[11] Perry B, Pescosolido B, Martin J, McLeod J, Jensen P. Comparison of public attributions, attitudes, and stigma in regard to depression among children and adults. Psychiatr Serv 2007;58(5):632-5.

[12] Stuart H, Arboleda-Florez J. Community attitudes toward people with schizophrenia. Can J Psychiatr 2001;46:245-52.

[13] van't Veer J, Kraan H, Drosseart S, Modde J. Determinants that shape public attitudes towards the mentally ill: a Dutch public study. Soc Psychiatry Psychiatr Epidemiol 2006;41:310-7.

[14] Pescosolido B, Monahan J, Link B, Stueve A, Kikuzawa S. The public's view of the competence, dangerousness, and need for legal coercion of persons with mental health problems. Am J Public Health 1999;89(9):1339-45.

[15] Link B, Phelan J, Bresnahan M, Stueve A, Pescosolido B. Public conceptions of mental illness: labels, causes, dangerousness, and social distance. Am J Public Health 1999;89(9):1328-33.

In: Child and Adolescent Health Yearbook 2013
Editor: Joav Merrick
ISBN: 978-1-63117-658-6

Chapter 13

ACCEPTABILITY OF HPV VACCINE AMONG YOUNG ADOLESCENT GIRLS IN UGANDA: YOUNG PEOPLE'S PERSPECTIVES COUNT

Anne R. Katahoire, PhD[1], John Arube Wani, MPH[1], Daniel Murokora, MD[1], Emmanuel Mugisha, PhD[2] and D Scott LaMontagne, PhD*[2]

[1]Child Health Development Centre, Kampala, Uganda
[2]PATH, Seattle, Washington, United States of America

ABSTRACT

Previous research on human papillomavirus (HPV) vaccine acceptance has focused largely on parental acceptability. Adolescents are the target population and adolescence is a phase associated with increased independence. Understanding adolescents' perspectives regarding vaccine acceptance is therefore critically important. Objective: This paper presents young adolescent girls' perspectives on acceptability of HPV vaccine after a two-year demonstration project. Methods: We explored acceptability of HPV vaccine among girls aged 10 to 15 years during 2008 and 2009. Acceptability was qualitatively defined as the girls' willingness or reluctance to be vaccinated and to complete all three doses. Twenty-seven focus group discussions were conducted with girls who completed all three doses and 17 with those who did not. Girls were purposively sampled from areas where vaccine uptake was either high (greater than 90%) or low (less than 70%). Results: Girls independently made decisions and took actions that resulted in their vaccination or non vaccination. Key influencers of their' acceptability were: their understanding of cancer, concerns about their future as mothers; understanding of the vaccinations; fears of the consequences of being vaccinated or not; their experiences with the first dose; and their understanding of the eligibility criteria for vaccination. Conclusion: Adolescents demonstrate an independent ability in deciding to be vaccinated or not. As this group is the suggested population to receive this vaccine, preparing them for vaccination becomes

* Correspondence: D. Scott LaMontagne, PhD, MPH, FRSPH, PATH, 2201 Westlake Avenue North, Suite 200, Seattle, WA 98144 United States. E-mail. slamontagne@path.org

critical in helping them make informed decisions. Adequate preparation can foster acceptance of HPV vaccine among girls and eventually influence the success of a national HPV vaccination program.

Keywords: Human papillomavirus, HPV vaccine, acceptability, adolescents, girls

INTRODUCTION

Cervical cancer is the third most common cancer in women globally, with an estimated 530,000 new cases in 2008. It is the second most frequent cancer in women between 15 and 44 years of age in developing countries. High-risk regions include Eastern and Western Africa, where the age-standardized rate (ASR) is greater than 30 per 100,000 and it remains the most common cancer in women in Eastern Africa (1).

In Uganda, cervical cancer is the most frequent cancer among women (1). Current estimates indicate that every year 3,577 women are diagnosed with cervical cancer and 2,464 die from the disease. Approximately 74% of invasive cervical cancers are attributed to human papillomavirus (HPV) types 16 and 18 (2). Cost-effectiveness models have suggested that introduction of HPV vaccines could significantly reduce incidence and mortality of cervical cancer in low-resource settings like Uganda (3).

As the World Health Organization (WHO) continues to recommend routine HPV vaccination to be included in national immunization programs (4), acceptability of the vaccines remains key to the success of the program. Generally, factors for considering introducing HPV vaccine include: the country's disease burden; infrastructure, affordability, and cost-effectiveness of vaccination; cultural acceptability of the vaccine; and political will, among others (5).

Previous research on acceptability of HPV vaccine has shown high acceptability of the vaccine by parents for their children, college students, and health workers (6–10). While acceptability of the vaccine by parents for their children is important, there is a dearth of literature on the perspectives of younger adolescents with regards to HPV vaccination (11). Given that young adolescents are the population targeted by HPV vaccine (4), more attention should be paid to their acceptance of the vaccine.

The Ministry of Health in Uganda and PATH, an international nonprofit organization, implemented an HPV vaccination demonstration project to assess vaccine coverage, feasibility, cost, and acceptability of HPV vaccine among key stakeholders, including adolescent girls eligible for the vaccinations (12). The project was implemented from 2008 to 2009 through the Uganda National Expanded Programme on Immunization (UNEPI), in partnership with local government authorities of the two districts of Ibanda and Nakasongola. Approximately 10,000 girls were vaccinated in the two districts.

This paper presents results on an assessment of acceptability of HPV vaccine among young adolescent girls in Uganda. The findings can inform our understanding of younger adolescents' acceptability of the vaccine and the factors underlying their acceptance, which will be important for the future rollout of the program in Uganda and elsewhere in Africa.

METHODS

A cross-sectional qualitative study design was adopted that included fully, partially, and non-vaccinated girls aged 10 to 15 years. Using data from UNEPI on HPV vaccine uptake in 17 sub-counties in the two districts, three sub-counties with high coverage of 90% and above and two others with lower coverage of 70% and less were purposively sampled. In each of the sub-counties sampled, two schools were randomly selected. In each school, one focus group discussion was conducted with 10 to 12 girls who were eligible for HPV vaccination. In the sub-counties that had high coverage, the focus group discussions involved fully vaccinated girls. In the sub-counties with lower coverage, the focus group discussions were with partially or non-vaccinated girls. Due to the high coverage in both districts, it was difficult to convene the same number of focus group discussions of fully vaccinated as those with partially and non-vaccinated girls. In the end, 27 focus group discussions were held with fully vaccinated girls and 17 focus group discussions with partially and non-vaccinated girls (Table 1).

In all, a total of 44 focus group discussions were conducted over a period of two years involving 422 girls drawn from the two districts of Ibanda and Nakasongola that participated in the demonstration project. The focus group discussions with the girls explored vaccine acceptability and reasons for being fully, partially, or not vaccinated at all; their preparation for the vaccinations; their experiences with the vaccination exercise; and their role in deciding whether to be vaccinated or not. Acceptability of the vaccine was qualitatively defined as the girls' willingness and/or reluctance to be vaccinated and to complete all three doses.

Table 1. Study populations and sample sizes for HPV vaccine acceptability study, Uganda

Study population	Sample, year 1	Sample, year 2	Total
Girls fully vaccinated	7 focus group discussions	20 focus group discussions	27 focus group discussions
Girls partially or not vaccinated	2 focus group discussions	15 focus group discussions	17 focus group discussions
	Total number of girls participated		442

As a secondary outcome, we were also interested in the girls' perspectives and the extent to which they portrayed their agency. Agency was defined as the adolescents' capacity or ability to decide and act on what they consider to be in their interest. In analysis, we extracted the children's voices that we have included in the text. In some measure, this portrays the girls as social actors and attributes competence rather than incompetence to them (13). Girls were encouraged to discuss their experiences in the language that they were most comfortable expressing themselves in. The discussions were recorded and later transcribed and translated into English. Key themes and sub themes were identified through textual data analysis and a coding scheme was constructed (14, 15). Atlas.ti software was used to facilitate data management and analysis.

Parental written consent was obtained for girls to participate in the study. Verbal assent was taken from the girls at the time of data collection. The study was approved by ethics committees in Uganda and the United States.

RESULTS

Girls in the focus group discussions explained their reasons for acceptance and/or reluctance to be vaccinated and the actions that they took as individuals to ensure that they were fully vaccinated or not. In the sections that follow, we present the reasons given by the fully vaccinated girls for accepting to be vaccinated and those given by the partially or non-vaccinated girls for refusing to complete their doses or be vaccinated at all.

Reasons for vaccination

Discussions with the fully vaccinated girls revealed that the majority understood HPV vaccine as a prevention of cancer. According to the girls, cancer is a disease that is very painful, has no cure, and kills. A few mentioned cases of people whom they knew who had died of cancer as the following extracts illustrate:

> My uncle died of cancer, they tried everything but there was no cure…
> My aunt who had cancer died a very painful death.

According to the fully vaccinated girls, the idea that cancer could be prevented was a relief, especially because prior to this, the only thing they knew about cancer was that it killed. This influenced their willingness to be vaccinated as illustrated by the following:

> People say that cancer has no cure but the health worker told us that this cancer which they were vaccinating against could be prevented, so I was very happy because it meant that if I got vaccinated I would not die of cancer.

Girls perceived the vaccinations as a way to protect themselves against a disease that had no cure. To them this was an opportunity which they did not want to miss:

> When you get a chance you use it.
> If you do not use an opportunity you may not get another one.

The majority of the fully vaccinated girls also reported that they had decided to complete all three doses because they feared that if they were not fully vaccinated they would not get the full protection, which meant they could still get cancer and die a painful death. The idea that those that got the cancer died a painful death was a recurrent theme in both districts and emerged as an important consideration for the girls:

> The disease is very painful and it kills, that is why I decided to get all three doses. I was told that if you got only one or two it was useless.
> If you get the cancer you stay with it and keep crying till you die and I do not want that…my auntie suffered for a long time.

In nearly all focus groups, the fully vaccinated girls admitted that they were initially reluctant to be vaccinated fearing that the three injections would be painful. When they discussed why they changed their minds, they explained that they realized that the pain arising from the vaccination was likely to be short lived compared to the pain that they could potentially suffer if they got cancer:

> I normally fear injections but when I thought about the pain that I could suffer if I got cancer I decided to be vaccinated no matter what.
> I have had injections before and I know the pain lasts a short time but I feared that the pain from cancer can last forever…

Fully vaccinated girls reported that their experience with the initial dose of HPV vaccine helped them to overcome some of their fears and anxieties and motivated them to get the other doses. The majority also reported that they had initially feared possible side effects; but when they did not experience any after the first dose, they willingly went ahead to get the rest of the doses:

> The first time I had feared but the injection was not painful… so I was ready for the second…
> I didn't have any pain when I was given any of the injections; but I was better prepared for the second injection than I was for the first.

The majority of the fully vaccinated girls understood vaccinations as protection for their uterus. The distinction between the cervix and the uterus was not fully understood by the majority of girls. This was partly because the local term used for the cervix is the opening of the uterus. During the focus group discussions, fully vaccinated girls explained that the vaccine was a means of protecting their uteruses against cancer and highlighted this as one of the important reasons for their willingness to be vaccinated:

> I know that if a woman gets that cancer she cannot bear children and that is very sad.
> I was fully vaccinated because I want to have children without any problems.
> The cancer destroys your uterus and you can never have children. I do not want to die childless so I had to make sure that I got all three doses.
> I wanted to protect my uterus; that is why I was vaccinated.
> I know that if I get cancer I will not give birth and I do not want to be like that; that is why I decided to be vaccinated.

Most of the vaccinations in the two districts took place at school and absenteeism was relatively high in both districts. In cases where girls were absent from school on the day of vaccination, they were often advised to go to the nearest health unit for the missed dose. Fully vaccinated girls reported how they made sure that they attended school on the days of vaccination to ensure that they did not miss any of the doses. Even in cases where their parents or guardians tried to prevent them from attending school for different reasons, they insisted on going. Discussions with fully vaccinated girls revealed that they as individuals were convinced of the importance of being vaccinated and they made sure that they were vaccinated and that they completed all three doses.

Reasons for partial or non-vaccination

Discussions with partially and non-vaccinated girls revealed that their reluctance to be vaccinated was due to lack of understanding of what the vaccinations were for or the disease the vaccinations were protecting against, not knowing the importance of completing all three doses, fear of possible side effects, not understanding the benefit of the vaccine (to protect their uteruses), and lack of understanding of the eligibility criteria.

The majority of the partially and non-vaccinated girls, unlike those fully vaccinated, reported that they had not understood the disease that the vaccine protected against let alone the importance of being vaccinated and completing all the three doses, as illustrated by the following extracts:

> I was not told what diseases I was being vaccinated against… the teacher just told us to go under the mango tree so the next time when they came I hid in the toilet…
> I thought that I was only supposed to receive one injection so when I was told to go for a second one I refused …

It was evident from the discussions with the partially and non-vaccinated girls that they had genuinely not understood what the vaccinations were about. A few reported that they were absent from school when the health worker explained to the others about the vaccinations. Others reported that they were taken by surprise when they were told to go and line up for vaccinations without any explanation:

> The teacher just told us to go quickly and line up outside and be vaccinated but she did not explain against what we were being vaccinated.
> I missed school when the health worker came to explain. When I asked the other girls they did not explain properly; they just told me the teacher said we should line up.
> I was injected the first time at school but when they came the next time I hid because I did not know what the vaccine was for so I did not want to be injected again….

This situation was not helped by the girls lack of understanding of the eligibility criteria, especially in the district where girls were vaccinated based on their age rather than their grade/class in school. It was not clear to the girls why only 10-year-old girls were being vaccinated. Partially and non-vaccinated girls explained that they were suspicious as to why only some girls were being vaccinated and not others:

> I did not understand why we were being told to have three injections when others in the class were not being injected so the next time when the teacher told us not to miss school because the health workers were coming again I missed school on that day and told the teacher that I was sick ….
> The teacher came the first time and told all of us who were 10 years to put up our hands and I did, so they injected me but when they came the second time I hid behind the toilet. I wanted to know why only those who are 10 years were being vaccinated and what the vaccine was for.

The fear of possible side effects was another reason given by the girls for their partial vaccination status. Nearly half of the partially vaccinated girls reported that they received their first dose when the others were receiving their second doses.

When asked why, they explained that they had waited to see if anything happened to those that were vaccinated first before deciding to be vaccinated as well. When they realized that those who received the first dose had not experienced excessive pain or any side effects, they decided that the vaccine was safe for them.

A few partially or non-vaccinated girls reported that they feared that the vaccinations would reduce their chances of giving birth to children later on in life:

> I heard women in the village saying that girls that were vaccinated may not have babies in the future. At the time I had already received the first dose so I decided not to receive the other two.
> I did not understand why they were vaccinating only girls, the boys were laughing at us saying the injection would burn our eggs and we would not be able to give birth in the future so I decided not to go for the vaccinations, I told the teacher that I was nine years.
> At first I agreed to be vaccinated but when I heard that the vaccinations could prevent me from having children I decided not to receive the other doses.

The majority of the partially vaccinated girls reported that they had not understood the dose schedule and when they were told to go to the nearest health unit for their missed doses some decided not to go there:

> I was told by my teacher to go to the health unit and get the missed dose but I decided not to go because I thought one dose was enough.
> When the teacher announced in class that those who missed their doses at school should go to the health unit, I thought they meant those who had not been vaccinated at all.

It was evident from the discussions with the partially and non-vaccinated girls that their reasons were directly related to inadequate preparation for the vaccinations.

Agency

Fully, partially, and non-vaccinated girls explained the different strategies that they devised to ensure that they were fully vaccinated or not vaccinated depending on what they had decided to do. Fully vaccinated girls explained how they made extra efforts to make sure that they attended school on the days of vaccination to ensure that they did not miss any of the doses. Even in cases where their parents or guardians tried to prevent them from attending school for different reasons they insisted on going:

> My mother almost made me miss one of the doses by asking me to accompany her to the hospital on the day of vaccination. I explained to her that I could not miss school on that day because I would miss being vaccinated…
> My grandmother tried to stop me from going to school, I refused. I told her that those who miss school and the vaccinations will have to go to the health centre which was far away from home, and she agreed.

Those who were absent from school reported that they had followed up with the health workers to ensure that they completed all three doses:

> There was a day when I fell sick and missed being vaccinated at school. When I got better I went to the health centre and was injected….
> The teacher told me I missed vaccinations yesterday so you have to go to the health centre, so I went there after school and the health worker injected me…

Others reported that they had made more than one visit to the health unit just to ensure that they were fully vaccinated:

> I went to the health centre the first time and the health worker was not there, so I went again the following day and she was there and she injected me. I had to make sure that I did not miss any of the doses.
> When I missed the vaccination at school the first time I was told to go to the health centre. I went the first time, the health worker was busy and she sent me away; the next time I went back she was not there, then I went the third time and found her and she injected me…

These text extracts from the focus group discussions illustrate girls' conviction and determination as individuals to ensure that they were fully vaccinated.

Partially and non-vaccinated girls also explained the strategies they devised to ensure that they were not vaccinated or that they did not complete all three doses. A few, for example, admitted that they had deliberately lied about their age to avoid being vaccinated:

> When I knew that those who were 10 were the ones to be vaccinated I told the teacher that my mother said that I was 11…
> I told the teacher that I was 9 years so that I could miss the vaccinations and she believed me because I am small…

Others reported that they had hidden or absented themselves from school on vaccination day, so as to not be vaccinated:

> I could not lie about my age to the teacher because she already knew that I was 10, so when they sent us out to be vaccinated I quickly went towards the toilets and hid. I thought that perhaps they wanted to kill us or prevent us from having children.
> When the teacher announced that we should not miss school tomorrow because of the vaccinations, I deliberately stayed at home and pretended to be sick.
> The day when I knew that the vaccinations were going to take place at school I left home and then hid on the way until I was sure the health workers had left, then I went to school.

There is a growing body of literature that argues that young people are social actors with agency, meaning they are able or capable of making decisions on their own, in their own interest, without reference to their parents. A number of fully vaccinated girls reported that their parents or guardians and peers had tried to discourage them from being vaccinated. They reported that they reflected on the advice given in light of the information that they had received and then made their own personal decisions and acted on them. The majority of fully vaccinated girls perceived their decisions to be vaccinated and to complete all three doses among other things as a way of protecting themselves from cancer and as a means of securing their future as mothers. Statements such as 'I decided,' were repeated in many of the comments made by the girls, both fully vaccinated and those partially or not vaccinated.

Partially and non-vaccinated girls also perceived the decisions that they made as protecting themselves from future infertility and pain. These data suggest an agency of these young adolescents which cannot be ignored. School-based programs sometimes assume that young people will more or less fall into line based on what they are told by their teachers or parents, but this obviously is not always the case.

DISCUSSION

Published studies of HPV vaccine acceptability have been primarily cross sectional surveys with adults conducted before the prophylactic vaccines were more widely introduced or available in the public health system (6–9,16,17). Furthermore, most measured knowledge, general attitudes about HPV vaccination, and willingness to vaccinate one's daughter (16,18). Earlier reviews showed that research on adolescent attitudes regarding vaccination, separately from parental attitudes, were very limited in scope, reflecting the dominant role of parents in the vaccination decision. A study from Manchester, UK and another from Australia—two developed countries that have national HPV vaccination programs—have made some contributions in our understanding by exploring with adolescents themselves their experience with HPV vaccination (11,19).

In our study, the majority of the fully vaccinated girls reported that they chose to be vaccinated because they perceived the vaccine as preventing cancer, protecting them from a potentially painful death, and a means of protecting their uteruses. These perceptions of the disease and of the vaccine as protection were key influencers of their willingness to be vaccinated. The reasons girls mentioned for getting vaccinated were strikingly similar to reasons that parents from these same communities mentioned in a survey assessing vaccine coverage – protection against cancer and protection against disease (12). HPV vaccine as prevention was also a concept echoed in the findings from Australia and the UK as a motivator for acceptance by adolescents (14, 19). Over 90% of girls in Manchester, UK said they were vaccinated for protection against cervical cancer.

Concerns regarding the safety of the vaccine mentioned by girls in our study concur with the findings from research conducted elsewhere (18), but surprisingly few parents of girls in Uganda mentioned safety as a concern in a survey of vaccine coverage (12). All girls, regardless of their vaccination status, were concerned about their future as mothers and needed assurances of the safety of the vaccine. Fully vaccinated girls reflected not only on the benefits of being vaccinated but also on the possible consequences of not being vaccinated for their future as mothers. Furthermore, the fully vaccinated girls in our study noted their positive experience with the first dose where they experienced minimal pain and no serious side effects which influenced them to complete all three doses and served as affirmation for them that the vaccine was safe, and they could go ahead to receive the second and third dose. Those not vaccinated or partially vaccinated reflected on possible negative consequences of being vaccinated such as infertility. It was evident from the discussions that the girls did reflect on the vaccinations and made choices based on the information that they had or did not have and on their understanding of the benefits and likely consequences of their choices. Safety has also been a common concern mentioned by adolescents vaccinated in other countries (19), suggesting this concept resonates universally.

For girls that decided not to complete all three doses or those that did not get vaccinated at all, the lack of understanding of the benefits of the vaccine and of the criteria for vaccinating a particular age group and not others resulted in reluctance or unwillingness on the part of some girls to be vaccinated in our study. Consequently, some girls deliberately missed school on the days of vaccination, hid when the vaccinators came to their school, or lied about their ages so as to avoid being vaccinated. Because the majority of vaccinations took place at school, the influence of parents' acceptance of the vaccine on the girls' acceptance was reduced. Discussions with the girls revealed that being vaccinated at school accorded them more space within which they themselves could decide whether to be vaccinated or not. Teachers were responsible for mobilizing the girls at school for vaccination, but this did not seem to have prevented girls from devising ways to avoid vaccinations.

Agency was also a key theme in our findings. Our results show that adolescent girls were actively involved in decision-making and taking action regarding whether to be vaccinated against HPV or not and whether to complete all three doses. They were not passive receivers. About a third of the fully vaccinated girls reported that their parents, and in some cases guardians, tried to discourage and/or prevent them from being vaccinated. Because they were convinced that the vaccine was good for them, they went ahead and got vaccinated. Their independence in making this decision, even when parents were discouraging, suggests a degree of independence girls of this age feel regarding their own health. Brabin et al. also suggested a degree of independence in the vaccine decision from their study of adolescents vaccinated in Manchester, UK. They found that the majority of girls (77%) reported that they had shared in the vaccine decision. A total of 42% of girls whose parents refused vaccination stated that they wanted the vaccine and 70% of those vaccinated thought that girls of their age should be able to agree to have the vaccine without parental consent (11). Independent agency was also noted in the study by Cooper Robbins et al., where there was discordance between the wishes of the girl to receive the vaccine and the parental decision to not provide written consent for their daughter (19). Adolescents often contribute to the familial decision-making and their attitudes were found to be similar to those of their parents regarding vaccine efficacy, the influence of recommendations by health care professionals, and consideration of vaccine cost (20,21). Taken together, these results provide strong evidence for policymakers and program planners to understand the dynamics of decision-making for HPV vaccination and the participation of girls of this age in choices that affect their personal health.

The new sociology of childhood emphasizes the competence of children as 'social actors' and as informants about their lives. With an emphasis on agency and a move away from the assumption of children as passive recipients of action, has come a parallel and consistent move away from relying on statements by adults about children's worlds and experiences and instead toward considering as equally reliable, statements by children themselves. There is emphasis on the need for children's voices in understanding children's experiences (13). Listening to what children had to say about their experiences with the vaccinations enables us to act on their understanding in relation to vaccinations. Policymakers can and should appreciate that children, while 'governed' as objects, are also active subjects who can speak to their lives, their experiences, and their futures as knowing and informed agents (22). What children need is knowledge and information that enables them to make the decision.

Conclusion

Providing full and accurate information to young adolescents enables them to make choices to accept (or not accept) HPV vaccination and to act on the choices they make regarding their lives. The converse is also true, indicating that the girls who did not get full information on why they were being vaccinated or the reasons for a particular age group did choose to avoid the vaccination. This particular age group is not routinely targeted by health programs, and policy and program design needs to take into account the fact that they can receive information independently, make choices, and act on the choices they make.

Acknowledgments

We wish to acknowledge the team of competent researchers who conducted the focus group discussions in the two districts. Special thanks go to Phoebe Kajubi and Eunice Kyomugisha who led the teams in the two districts. Special thanks also go to the District Health Officers, Dr. Julius Bamwine (Ibanda) and Dr. Gerald Ssekitto (Nakasongola), together with the entire District Health Team for their support.

References

[1] Ferlay J, Shin HR, Bray F, Forman D, Mathers C, Parkin DM. GLOBOCAN 2008, Cancer Incidence and Mortality Worldwide. IARC CancerBase No. 10. Lyon, France: International Agency for Research on Cancer; 2010. Available at http://globocan.iarc.fr/.

[2] Who.org [Internet]. Geneva:WHO/ICO Information Centre on HPV and Cervical Cancer; c2011; cited 2011 Dec 21]. Available from: www.who.int/hpvcentre/en/

[3] Goldie SJ, O'Shea M, Campos NG, Diaz M, Sweet S, Kim SY. Health and economic outcomes of HPV 16, 18 vaccination in 72 GAVI-eligible countries. Vaccine 2008;26(32):4080-93.

[4] World Health Organization. Human papillomavirus vaccines, WHO position paper. Wkly Epidemiol Rec. 2009;15(84):117-32. Available from: http://www.who.int/wer/2009/wer8415.pdf

[5] Agosti JM, Goldie SJ. Introducing HPV Vaccine in Developing Countries – Key Challenges and Issues. N Engl J Med 2007;356(19):1908-10.

[6] Breitkopf CR, Pearson HC, Dinh TA, Tran BC, Vu T, Phan GA, et al. Human papillomavirus vaccine decision-making in Da Nang, Vietnam: Perceived spousal and adolescent-parent concordance. Vaccine 2009;27(17):2367-71.

[7] Harries J, Moodley J, Barone MA, Mall S, Sinanovic E. Preparing for HPV vaccination in South Africa: Key challenges and opinions. Vaccine 2009;27(1):38-44.

[8] Coleman MA, Levison J, Sangi-Haghpeykar H. HPV vaccine acceptability in Ghana, West Africa. Vaccine 2011;29(23):3945-50.

[9] Katahoire RA, Jitta J, Kivumbi G, Murokora D, Arube WJ, Siu G, et al.

[10] An assessment of the readiness for introduction of the HPV vaccine in Uganda. Afr J Reprod Health 2008;12:159-72.

[11] Kwan TTC, Chan KKL, Yip AMW, Tam KF, Cheung ANY, Young PMC, et al. Barriers and facilitators to human papillomavirus vaccination among Chinese adolescent girls in Hong Kong: a qualitative study. Sex Transm Infect 2008;84(3):227-32.

[12] Brabin L, Roberts SA, Stretch R, Baxter D, Elton P, Kitchener H, et al. A survey of adolescent experiences of human papillomavirus vaccination in the Manchester study. Br J Cancer 2009;101(9):1502-4.

[13] LaMontagne DS, Barge S, Le NT, Mugisha E, Penny ME, Gandhi S, et al. Delivery strategies for HPV Vaccination programs that achieved high coverage in low and middle-income countries. Bull World Health Organ 2011;89:821¬-30B.

[14] James A. Giving Voice to Children's Voices: Practices and Problems, Pitfalls and Potentials. Am Anthropol 2007;109:261-72.

[15] Miles MB, Huberman AM. Qualitative data analysis: An expanded sourcebook. Thousand Oaks, CA: Sage, 1994.

[16] MacQueen KM, McLellan-Lemal E, Barthalow K, Milstein B. Team-based codebook development: Structure, process, and agreement. New York: Altamira Press, 2008.

[17] Allen, JD, Coronado GD, Williams RS, Glen B, Escoffery C, Fernandez M, et al. A systematic review of measures used in studies of human papillomavirus (HPV) vaccine acceptability. Vaccine 2010;28(24):4027-37.

[18] Young A. HPV vaccine acceptance among women in the Asian Pacific: a systematic review of the literature. Asian Pacific J Cancer Prev 2010;11:641-9.

[19] Brewer NT, Fazekas KI. Predictors of HPV vaccine acceptability: A theory-informed, systematic review. Prev Med 2007;45(2-3):107-14.

[20] Cooper Robbins SC, Bernard D, McCaffery K, Brotherton JML, Skinner SR. I Just Signed. Factors Influencing Decision-Making for School-Based HPV Vaccination of Adolescent Girls. Health Psychol 2010;29(6):618-25.

[21] Zimet GD, Mays RM, Winston Y, Kee R, Dickes J, Su L. Acceptability of human papillomavirus immunization. J Womens Health Gend Based Med 2000;9(1):47-50.

[22] Gamble HL, Klosky JL, Parra GR, Randolph ME. Factors influencing familial decision-making regarding human papillomavirus vaccination. J Pediatr Psychol 2010;35(7):704-15.

[23] Macdonald C. The importance of identity in policy: The case for and of children. Seen and heard: Children as active agents in families, communities and research. SPRC Workshop UNSW; Oct 2007.

In: Child and Adolescent Health Yearbook 2013
Editor: Joav Merrick

ISBN: 978-1-63117-658-6

Chapter 14

MENARCHEAL AGE OF NIGERIAN URBAN SECONDARY SCHOOL GIRLS IN BENIN CITY

Alphonsus N Onyiriuka*, Philip O Abiodun, Rita C Onyiriuka, Frances A Ehirim and Eucharia PA Onyiriuka

Department of Child Health, University of Benin Teaching Hospital, Benin City, Nigeria

ABSTRACT

Age at menarche varies with time and the influence of social factors depends on the population under consideration. Objective: To determine the mean age at menarche among secondary school girls in Benin City and examine some social factors that might influence it. Methods: In this cross-sectional study in Benin City, Nigeria information on age at menarche was obtained from 1,640 menstruating secondary school girls (aged between 10 and 20 years) using the status quo method. Information sought in the structured questionnaire used included date of birth, date of menarche, educational attainment of parents, occupation of parents, birth position, family size and state of origin. Data was analyzed using SPSS (Statistical Package for Social Sciences), version 15.0. Results: The mean age at menarche was 13.44±1.32 years (95% Confidence Interval, CI= 13.36-13.50). Of the 1,640 girls who have attained menarche, 31(1.9%) were below the age of 12 years (early menarche). Socioeconomic status, birth position and family size had significant bearing with mean menarcheal age at $p < 0.001$, $p < 0.01$ and $p < 0.01$ respectively. Conclusion: The current mean age at menarche among secondary school girls in Benin City is 13.44 years and it is influenced by socioeconomic status, birth position and family size.

Keywords: Adolescence, menarche, health, Nigeria

* Correspondence: Alphonsus N Onyiriuka, Department of Child Health, University of Benin Teaching Hospital, PMB 1111, Benin City, Nigeria. E-mail: alpndiony@yahoo.com; didiruka@gmail.com

INTRODUCTION

Menarche (the first menstrual bleeding of a female) (1) represents the endpoint of a complex sequence of events that characterize sexual maturation and puberty in girls (2). It is unique, and probably, the most accurately recallable indicator of puberty among girls and a widely used indicator of adolescence sexual maturation (3,4). Variations in age at menarche between individuals and populations have been documented (5-7). It is influenced by social, environmental and genetic factors (5-9).

The mean age at menarche varies from one population to another. For instance, the reported mean age at menarche were as follows: Iran 12.91+1.23 years (10). South Africa 12.75+1.32 years (8), India 13.18+1.08 years (9), Kenyan 12.5+2.8 years (11). Even within Nigeria, similar variations in age at menarche have been observed; 13.98+1.30 years in the West (12), 13.03+1.02 years in the East (13) and 13.50+1.33 years in the North (14). A study involving one secondary school in Benin City, Nigeria reported a mean age at menarche of 13.16+1.22 years (15). In both developing and developed countries, some studies have reported a decline in the average age at menarche (16-19). This trend towards a reduction in the average age of menarche has been attributed to improvement in living standard and nutrition (1). On the other hand, in some countries, this downward trend seems to have come to a halt (20). In view of the reported secular trend, there is a need to monitor the age at menarche. Data on age at menarche are useful in health planning, establishment of adolescent health centres and improvement in health promotion services for girls (21). In addition, contemporary issues such as introduction of sex education in Nigerian schools require knowledge of the age at menarche as well as the sequence of events of puberty; menarche being the last in this sequence.

An early age at menarche is associated with an increased risk of some clinical conditions, such as breast cancer (22), obesity (23), endometrial cancer (24) and uterine leiomyomata (25). Some studies have indicated that women who attained menarche at the age of 11 years and below have a higher risk of development of breast cancer than those who attained menarche at the age of 12 years and above (26,27). Late menarcheal age is thought to protect, at least to some extent, women in Sub-Saharan Africa from breast cancer (28). In this regard, the observed trend towards a reduction in the average age at menarche in West African countries (Nigeria inclusive) portends some danger as it relates to occurrence of breast cancer (13,14). In addition, there are indications in the literature that the age at menarche might be related to subsequent reproductive performance, such as the age at first intercourse, the age at first pregnancy and risk of subsequent miscarriage (29). From the foregoing, it is obvious that there is a need to monitor closely the average age at menarche in Nigeria. Majority of the Nigerian studies that focused on age at menarche were conducted some decades ago (12-14).

The purpose of the present study was to determine, in this new decade, the age at menarche among secondary school girls in Benin City, Nigeria and identify some social factors that might influence it.

METHODS

This cross-sectional study was conducted in two public secondary schools for female students in Oredo Local Government Area (OLGA), Edo State, Nigeria. According to Edo State Ministry of Education Statistics, there are nine public secondary schools in the LGA comprising 4 females-only, 3 co-educational and 2 males-only (30). Consent for the study was obtained from the school authorities. Of the four girls' secondary schools, two were randomly selected by ballot. The total population of students in the two schools selected were school A 1,394 and school B 772, giving a grand total of 2,166 which was the target study population. The survey was designed to include all the student in the two schools (schools A and B). The principal of each of the two schools introduced the authors during the morning assembly. Subsequently, we addressed the students on the relevance of the study and how to accurately fill the questionnaire. We also emphasized to the students that the questionnaires were anonymous and that their participation was voluntary. Data was collected between October and November, 2011, using a structured-anonymous questionnaire. Information sought in the questionnaire included: date of birth, date of onset of first menstrual bleeding, birth position among their siblings, family size (number of siblings), state of origin, level of education and occupation of both parents/guardian. The family size was categorized into small size (no sibling or one or 2 siblings); medium size (3 or 4 siblings); large size (5 or more siblings). The socio-economic status of the parents was determined using the classification suggested by Ogunlesi et al. (31). This was analyzed via combining the highest educational attainment, occupation and income of the parents (based on the mean income of each educational qualification and occupation). In this Social Classification System, classes I and II represent high social class, class III represents middle social class while classes IV and V represent low social class. In this way, the girls were categorized into high, middle and low socio-economic groups. The data was analyzed using the SPSS (Statistical Package for Social Sciences), version 15.0.

RESULTS

At the time of this survey, a total of 2,166 female students (1,394 in school A and 772 in school B) were attending the two public girls' secondary schools in the LGA (randomly selected by ballot). Seven students (5 from school A and 2 from school B) declined to participate. The response rates were 99.4% in school A and 99.7% in school B. Overall response rate was 99.7%. The questionnaires of 9 students were excluded from the analysis because they were incompletely filled, thereby leaving a total of 2,150 questionnaires (respondents) for data analysis. Students in both schools had similar socio-demographic characteristics, thus further analysis of data was carried out for the combined group of students.

Of the 2,150 respondents, 1,640 (76.3%) have attained menarche while the remaining 510 (23.7%) have not. Analysis of the questionnaire of the 1,640 girls who have attained menarche showed that the mean age at menarche for both schools combined was 13.44±1.32 years (95% Confidence Interval, CI= 13.38-13.50) while it was 13.25±1.23 years (95% CI= 13.19-13.31) for school A and 13.50±1.36 years (95% CI= 13.40-13.60) for school B. Of the

1,640 girls who have attained menarche, 1(0.06%) were before the age of 12 years (early menarche); (Table 1). The mean age at menarche was significantly higher in low socioeconomic group compared to high socioeconomic group (Table 2). Girls belonging to high socioeconomic class attained menarche 8.0 and 9.0 months earlier than girls belonging to middle and low socioeconomic classes respectively (Table 2). As shown in Table 3, first-born children attained menarche earlier than latter-born children with first-born children attaining menarche 8.0 months earlier than eight-born children. Of the 1,640 girls who have attained menarche, 8(0.5%) were the only child in their family and the mean age at menarche was 12.80±1.11 years (95% CI= 12.03-13.57). Table 4 shows the mean age at menarche according to family size. As shown in Table 4, girls from small-size families attained menarche 4.0 and 7.0 months earlier than their counterparts from medium-size and large-size families respectively. Based on state of origin, the mean age at menarche did not differ.

Table 1. Distribution of age at menarche

Age in years	Total number of girls (respondents)	Number (%) who have attained menarche
10	2	0(0)
11	13	1(7.7)
12	109	16(15.1)
13	296	95(32.4)
14	356	218(61.2)
15	380	337(88.7)
16	490	471(96.1)
17	315	313(99.4)
18	112	112(100.0)
19	62	62(100.0)
20	15	15(100.0)
Total	2150	1640(100.0)

Table 2. Socioeconomic status (SES)and mean age at menarche

Age (years) at menarche	Total no of girls who have attained menarche	Socioeconomic status (SES) High Middle		Low
		No(%)	No(%)	No(%)
10	0	0 (0.0)	0(0.0)	0(0.0)
11	1	1(9.1)	0(0.0)	0(0.0)
12	16	10(62.5)	6(37.5)	0(0.0)
13	95	47(49.5)	38(40.0)	10(10.5)
14	218	106(48.6)	95(43.6)	17(7.8)
15	337	31(9.2)	176(52.2)	130(61.4)
16	471	8(1.7)	143(30.4)	320(67.9)
17	313	2(6.5)	16(5.1)	295(88.4)
18	112	0(0.0)	13(11.6)	99(88.4)
19	62	0(0.0)	57(91.9)	5(8.1)
20	15	0(0.0)	12(80.0)	3(20.0)
Total	1640	205(12.5)	548(33.4)	887(54.1)
Mean age at menarche	13.44±1.32	12.78±1.21a	13.42±1.18b	13.56±1.29c
(95% CI)	(13.38-13.50)	(12.61-12.95)	(13.32-13.52)	(13.42-13.59)
t-statistic	a vs b=4.41		b vs c=2.08	a vs c=7.95
(p-value)	(<0.01)		(>0.05)	(<0.001)

Table 3. Birth position and mean age at menarche

Birth position	Total no of girls who have attained menarche	Mean age at menarche	95% Confidence Interval, CI
1st	437	13.02±1.22	12.91-13.13
2nd	333	13.04±1.09	12.92-13.16
3rd	323	13.14±1.12	13.02-13.26
4th	164	13.30±1.23	13.11-13.49
5th	77	13.52±1.19	13.25-13.79
6th	33	13.53±1.38	13.06-14.00
7th	38	13.65±1.40	13.21-14.10
8th	27	13.68±1.43	13.14-14.23
Total	1640	13.44±1.32	13.38-13.50

Table 4. Family size and mean age at menarche

Family size	Total no (%) of girls who have attained menarche	Mean age at menarche	95% Confidence Interval, CI	t-statistic (p value)
Small size	221(13.5)	13.09±1.31a	12.91-13.26	a vs c: t= 4.82 (<0.01)
Medium size	1063(64.8)	13.41±1.28b	13.33-13.49	a vs b: t= 3.32 (<0.05)
Large size	356(21.7)	13.64±1.37c	13.50-13.78	b vs c: t= 2.79 (<0.05)
Total	1640(100.0)	13.44±1.32	13.38-13.50	

DISCUSSION

The mean age (13.44 years) at menarche observed in the present study in Edo State was comparable to 13.43 years reported from Port Harcourt among urban school girls (32), but lower than 14.22 years reported among rural school girls in Etche (both in Rivers State, Nigeria) (33). The lower mean menarcheal age observed in the present study might be explained by differences in socio-demographic factors. For instance, in the present study the subjects were urban school girls while in the study in Etche the subjects were rural school girls. The report of a study in Plateau State, Nigeria indicated that rural school girls tend to achieve menarche at an older age than urban school girls (14). In contrast, Goon et al. (34) reported that the age at menarche was comparable between urban and rural girls. They attributed this parity to improved living conditions among their rural population. It must be noted that the methods of collecting and analyzing data vary from one study to another, indicating the need to exercise caution when comparing age at menarche in different studies.

Data from the present study showed that 0.06% of the girls attained menarche early (below the age of 12 years). A similar prevalence of early menarche was reported from Wannune, Benue State, Nigeria (34). A previous study in Benin City alluded to occurrence of early menarche in their series but failed to report the prevalence (15). The clinical implication is that this small group of girls with early menarche might be at increased risk of breast cancer, obesity, endometrial cancer and uterine leiomyomata (22-25) and require a close follow up. In addition, Schor (29) reported that the age at menarche might be related to the age at first sexual intercourse, which may result in an unwanted teenage pregnancy. Such a pregnancy may be catastrophic for the teenager. The practical implication is that sex education in Nigerian schools should be started early, well before the age of 12 years.

As in previous studies in Nigeria (12-15) socioeconomic status (SES) of the parents influenced their daughters' age at menarche. In the present study it was observed that girls belonging to high socioeconomic class attained menarche 9 months earlier than their counterparts in the low socioeconomic class. This is comparable to the 8.5 months difference reported in a previous study in Nigeria (13). On the other hand, the observed difference in the present study is lower than the 11 and 12 months respectively reported in two previous studies in Nigeria (15,35). The reason for the smaller difference found in the present is not clear but it might mean that the effect of SES is becoming less prominent with time.

In the present study it was observed that first and early born girls tend to attain menarche at an earlier age than their counterparts who were born latter or were last born. A similar observation has been reported in a previous study (15). There is no readily available explanation for this observation. However, it has been speculated that there is usually more pressure and expectation on first-born children to achieve, forcing them to mature faster that latter-born children. It is, therefore, thought that this early attainment of maturity in first-born children, make them attain menarche at an earlier age compared to their latter- born siblings.

Data from the present study indicated that girls from small-size families tend to attain menarche at a younger age than girls from large-size families. A previous study has reported a similar finding (36). Family size may exert its effect on age at menarche through concealed poverty because the larger the family size the lower the income per capita. This effect is likely to be more pronounced in societies with low socioeconomic status.

In conclusion, the current mean age at menarche in Benin City is 13.44 years and it is influenced by social factors such as socioeconomic status, birth position and family size.

REFERENCES

[1] Vaughan VC, Litt IF. Child and adolescent development: Clinical implications. Philadelphia, PA: WB Saunders, 1990:229-91.

[2] Garibaldi L. Physiology of puberty. In: Kliegman RM, Behrman RE, Jenson HB, Stanton BF, eds. Nelson textbook of pediatrics, 18th ed. Philadelphia, PA: Saunders Elsevier, 2007:2308.

[3] Ayatollahi SMT, Dowlatabadi E, Ayotollahi SAR. Age at menarche and its correlates in Shuraxz, southern Iran. Iranian J Med Sci 1999;24:20-5.

[4] Cole TJ. The secular trend in human physical growth: a biological view. Econ Hum Biol 2003;1:161-8.

[5] Thomas F, Renaud F, Benefice E, de Meeus T, Guegan JF. International variability of ages at menarche and menopause: patterns and main determinants. Hum Biol 2001;73:271-90.

[6] Katunori F, Shinichi D. Relationship between change in BMI with age and delayed menarche in female athletes. J Physiol Anthropol 2003;22: 97-104.

[7] Chumlea WC, Schubert CM, Roche AF, Kulin HE, Lee PA, Himes JH, Sun SS. Age at menarche and racial comparison in US girls. Pediatrics 2003;111:110-1.

[8] Henneberg M, Louw GJ. Average menarcheal age of higher socioeconomic status in urban Cape coloured girls assessed by means of status quo and recall methods. Am J Phys Anthropol 1995;96(1):1-5.

[9] Bagga A, Kulkarni S. Age at menarche and secular trend in Maharashtrian (India) girls. Acta Biologica Szegediensis 2000;44(1-4): 53-7.

[10] Ayatollahi SM, Dowlatabidi E, Ayatollahi SA. Age at menarche in Iran. Ann Hum Biol 2002;29(4):355-62.

[11] Ogeng'o DN, Obimbo MM, Ogeng'o JA. Menarcheal age among urban Kenyan primary school girls. Acta Paediatrica 2011;100(5):758-61.

[12] Dare FO, Ogunniyi SO, Makinde OO. Biosocial factors affecting menarche in a mixed Nigerian population. Orient J Med 1994;6(1):45-48.

[13] Ikechebelu JI. The age of menarche in Nigerian schools: its relationship to socio-economic status with comment on secular trend. Orient J Med 1990;2(4):182-4.

[14] Wright EA. Menarche in Plateau State of Nigeria. West Afr J Med 1990; 9(3):204-7.

[15] Momoh MI, Okonkwo C. Age at menarche of school girls in urban Benin City. Ann Biomed Sci 2008;7(1-2):37-43.

[16] Anderson SE, Dallai GE, Must A. Relative weght and race influence average age at menarche: results from two nationally representative surveys of US girls studied 25 years apart. Pediatrics 2003;111:844-50.

[17] Biro FM, Huang B, Crawford PB, Lucky AW, Striegel-Moore R, Barton BA, Daniels S. Pubertal correlates in black and white girls. J Pediatr 2006;148:234-40.

[18] Hosny LA, El-Ruby MO, Zaki ME, Again MS, Zaki MS, El Gammal MA, Mazen IM. Assessment of pubertal development in Egyptian girls. J Paediatr Endocrinol Metab 2005;18:577-84.

[19] Hwang JY, Shin C, Frongillo EA, Shin KR, Jo I. Secular trend in age at menarche for South Korean women born between 1920 and 1986: The Ansan Study. Ann Hum Biol 2003;30:434-42.

[20] Whincup PH, Gilg JA, Odoki K, Taylor SJC, Cook DG. Age at menarche in comtemporary British teenagers: survey of girls born between 1982 and 1986. BMJ 2001;322:1095-6.

[21] Ekerbicer HC, Celik M, Kiran H, Kiran G. Age at menarche in Turkish adolescents in Kahramanmaras, eastern Mediterranean region of Turkey. Eur J Contraceptive Reprod Health Care 2007;12:289-93.

[22] Braithwaite D, Moore DH, Lustig RH, Epel ES, Ong KK, Rehkopf DH, Wang MC, Miller SM, Hiatt RA. Socioeconomic status in relation to early menarche among black and white girls. Cancer Causes Control 2009;20:713-20.

[23] Van Lenthe FJ, Kemper CG, van Mechelen W. Rapid maturation in adolescence results in greater obesity in adulthood: The Amsterdam Growth and Health Study. Am J Clin Nutr 1996;64:18-24.

[24] McPherson CP, Sellrs TA, Potter JD, Bostick RM, Folsom AR. Reproductive factors and risk of endometrial cancer: The Iowa Women's Health Study. Am J Epidemiol 1996;143(1195):202.

[25] Marshall LM, Splegelman D, Goldman MB, Manson JE, Colditz GA, Barbieri RL, Stampfer MJ, Hunter DJ. A prospective study of reproductive factors and oral contraceptive use in relation to the risk of uterine leiomyomata. Fertility Sterility 1998;70:432-9.

[26] Toniolo PG. Endogenous oestrogens and breast cancer risk: the case perspective cohort studies. Environ Health Prospect 1997;105:587-92.

[27] Peeters PHN, Verbeek ALM, Krol A, Matthyssen MMM, de Waard F. Age at menarche and breast cancer risk in nulliparous women. Breast Cancer Res Treatment 1995;33(1):55-61.

[28] Fregene A, Newman LA. Breast cancer in sub-Saharan Africa: how does it relate to breast cancer in African-American women? Cancer 2005; 103(8):1540-50.

[29] Schor N. Abortion and adolescence: relation between the menarche and sexual activity. Int J Adolesc Med Health 1993;6:225-240.

[30] Ministry of Education, Benin City. Department of Planning, Research and Statistics. Directory of Pre-primary, Primary, Junior and Senior Secondary Institutions in Edo State. Benin City: Ministry Education, 2006.

[31] Ogunlesi TA, Dedeke IOF, Kuponiyi OT. Socio-economic classification of children attending Specialist Paediatric Centres in Ogun State, Nigeria. Nig Med Pract 2008;54(1):21-5.

[32] Ofuya MZ. The age at menarche in Nigerian adolescents from two different socioeconomic classes. Online J Health Allied Sci 2007;6:1-4.

[33] Ikaraoha CI, Mbadiwe IC, Igwe CU, Allagua DO, Mezie O, Iwo GTO, Ofori PI. Menarcheal age of secondary school girls in urban and rural areas of Rivers State, Nigeria. Online J Health Allied Sci 2005;4:1-4.

[34] Goon DT, Toriola AL, Uever J, Wuam S, Toriola OM. Growth status and menarcheal age among adolescent school girls in Wannune, Benue State, Nigeria. BMC Pediatrics 2010;10:60-4.
[35] Abioye-Kuteyi EA, Ojofeitimi EO, Aina OI, Kio F, Aluko Y, Mosuro O. The influence of socioeconomic and nutritional status on menarche in Nigerian school girls. Nutr Health 1997;11:185-95.
[36] Cameron N, Nagdee I. Menarcheal age in two generations of South African Indians. Ann Human Biol 1996;23(2):113-9.

In: Child and Adolescent Health Yearbook 2013
Editor: Joav Merrick

ISBN: 978-1-63117-658-6

Chapter 15

NUTRITIONAL STATUS OF NIGERIAN CHILDREN WITH SICKLE CELL ANAEMIA IN STABLE STATE

***Barakat A Animasahun*[*,1], MBBS, MPH, FACC, FWACP, FMCPaed, *Urowoli P Nwodo*[2], MBBS, DPH, MWACP, *Adaobi N Izuora*[3], MBBS, MPH, FMCPaed and *Olisamedua F Njokanma*[a], MBBS, FWACP, FMCPaed**

[1]Department of Paediatrics and Child Health,
Lagos State University College of Medicine, Ikeja, Lagos
[2]Department of Paediatrics and Child Health, Premier Specialist Hospital, Ikeja, Lagos,
[3]Department of Paediatrics and Child health, Isolo General Hospital, Isolo, Lagos

ABSTRACT

Sickle cell anaemia has multi-systemic manifestations and is associated with severe morbidity and high mortality. It commonly affects growth leading to wasting and stunting. The study aimed to determine the nutritional status using anthropometry, of children with homozygous sickle cell anaemia (SCA), aged one year to ten years in steady state at the Lagos University Teaching Hospital (LUTH). Methods: A cross-sectional study involving 100 children with sickle cell anaemia and 100 age, sex, and social class matched controls that fulfilled the inclusion criteria. Height and weight were measured while Weight-for- age, Height- for- age and Weight-for-height and their z scores were derived from NCHS standard while Body mass index was calculated using the formula Weight in kg/ Height in m2 in Kg/m2 . Results: The study demonstrated a significantly lower mean weight and weight-for-height in the SCA patients than those of controls ($p < 0.001$) irrespective of gender, however, female SCA patients were shorter than their healthy controls. There was no significant difference with respect to BMI. The z score analysis revealed that SCA patients had significantly lower z scores for height-for-age, and weight-for-age compared with controls ($p< 0.02$). Further analysis by sex

* Correspondence: Barakat A Animasahun, MBBS, MPH, FACC, FWACP, FMCPaed, Senior lecturer, Department of Paediatrics and Child Health, Lagos State University College of Medicine, Ikeja, Lagos, Nigeria. E-mail: deoladebo@yahoo.com

revealed that the difference was more marked in males than in the females. Conclusion: The study revealed age related poor nutritional status in children with sickle cell anaemia compared with contemporary healthy controls and there was no association between anthropometry of subjects and haemoglobin concentration.

Keywords: Sickle cell anaemia, anthropometry, nutritional status

INTRODUCTION

Sickle cell anaemia (SCA) is a chronic haemolytic disorder caused by homozygous inheritance of abnormal haemoglobin called 'haemoglobin S' (HbS). It is an example of a single point mutation resulting in a qualitative defect in haemoglobin synthesis. (1) It is structurally different from the normal haemoglobin, due to replacement of the glutamic acid by valine in the sixth position of the β Globin. (2)

About 25% of Nigerians are heterozygous carriers of genes for sickle haemoglobin while the incidence of its homozygous state is about 2 - 3%. (1)

Sickle cell anaemia is the commonest haemoglobinopathy affecting people of the Negroid race. (3,4) It has multisystemic manifestations and commonly affects growth leading to wasting and stunting. (5) Assessment of the growth and nutritional status can be done using anthropometry. (6) The present study aimed to determine the nutritional status using anthropometry, of children with homozygous sickle cell anaemia (SCA), aged one year to ten years in steady state at the Lagos University Teaching Hospital.

METHODS

This was a prospective, cross sectional and analytical study carried out at the Lagos University Teaching Hospital (LUTH) in Idi-Araba as part of a large study between October 2005 and January 2006. The subjects were 100 paediatric patients attending the Thursday LUTH sickle cell anaemia clinic who were consecutively recruited. They had haemoglobin genotype 'SS' on haemoglobin electrophoresis and were aged one to ten years. They were in steady state at the time of recruitment.

Steady state was defined as absence of any crisis in the preceeding four weeks, no recent drop in the haemoglobin level and absence of any symptoms or sign attributable an acute illness. (7) Patients with any form of acute illness, congenital heart disease or acquired heart disease, renal disease and hypertension were excluded from the study. Healthy controls were of genotype "AA," from the Community Health Outpatient and Well baby clinics and healthy children attending other clinics at the POP department and were matched for age and sex, one for every sickle cell anaemia patient.

Height was measured to the nearest centimeter with the aid of a graduated wooden panel fixed to a vertical wall with the child barefooted, standing erect with the heels together against the wall, and looking straight ahead with the back against the wall. The head was held in such a way that the subject was looking forward with the lower border of the eye sockets in the same horizontal plane as the external auditory meatus. The wooden panel had a perpendicular (horizontal) projection built in to slide up and down which rested on the head of the subject (8). Subjects were weighed to the nearest 0.1kg using a Seca® scale or basinet scale as appropriate for the patients age with the subject standing or sitting respectively, barefoot wearing only their under-wear. The scales were checked for accuracy with standard weights after every 10th measurement, or whenever it was moved from place to place (8). Weight-for- age, Height- for- age and Weight-for-height were derived from NCHS standard while Body mass index was calculated using the formula *Weight in kg/* Height in m^2 in $Kg/m.^2$ Derived measurements were expressed as centiles using NCHS (9) standards and z scores were generated for each measurement (10).

Haemoglobin concentration was determined using the oxy-haemoglobin method. The data were recorded on standard questionnaires and later entered into a standard IBM compatible computer. The data were analyzed using Microsoft Excel Statistical Software supplemented by Mega Stat Statistical Package. The mean, median, standard deviation and other parameters of statistical location were generated as necessary for continuous data. Tests of statistical significance between subjects and controls included Student t-test for continuous data and chi-square analysis for discrete data. Regression and correlation models were set up and analyzed as necessary. Level of significance was set at $p < 0.05$. The Research and Ethical Committee of the Lagos University Teaching Hospital approved this study. Informed consent was sought from parents or caregivers of potential subjects and the controls before enrolment into the study.

RESULTS

A total of 200 children were recruited into the study, this comprise of 100 test subjects in the 12 month to 10 year age bracket confirmed to have haemoglobin genotype SS who were all in steady state and receiving routine drugs consisting of folic acid, Proguanil and multivitamins. The control group consisted of 100 children within the same age bracket who had haemoglobin genotype AA. The mean age was comparable between subjects and controls (75.1 ± 30.3 Vs 74.8 ± 29.4: $t = 1.02$, $p = 0.15$). The male: female ratio in both subjects and controls was 1.9:1. The mean height and body mass index of the subjects were comparable with those of the controls. Controls however were significantly heavier and also had significantly higher mean weight-for-height. ($p = 0.0001$). Further analysis (Table I) showed that irrespective of gender, subjects were smaller than controls in terms of weight and weight-for-height. Female sickle cell anaemia patients were also significantly shorter than their healthy controls. There was no significant difference with respect to BMI. When the analysis was repeated for under-5 children (Table II), subjects showed a fairly consistent trend of being smaller but no significant difference was observed with respect to any of the selected anthropometric values. A similar trend was observed in children older than five years but this time, subjects were significantly smaller than controls in all parameters except BMI (Table III).

Table 1. Gender-specific comparison of anthropometry between subjects and controls

	Males			Females		
	Subjects n =65 Mean± (SD)	Controls n =65 Mean± (SD)	p	Subjects n =35 Mean ±(SD)	Controls n =35 Mean±(SD)	p
Variables						
Height (m)	1.11±1.0	1.28±0.12	0.17	1.16±0.09	1.20±0.01	0.02*
Weight (Kg)	18.3±4.5	20.9±0.6	0.001*	19.8±6.6	22.1±1.1	0.04*
Wt for ht in (kg/m)	15.4±3.3	16.2±0.4	0.049*	18.3±4.13	20.4±0.7	0.002*
BMI (Kg/m ^{2})	14.8±3.5	15.1±0.4	0.43	14.3±2.6	15.1±0.4	0.06

* Statistically significant.
m = meters.
Kg = Kilograms.
Wt for Ht = Weight- for -height in Kilograms per meter.
BMI = body mass index.
Kg/m2 = Kilogram per meter squared.

Table 2. Comparison of anthropometry between under-5 subjects and controls

	Males			Females		
	Subjects n =27 Mean±(SD)	Controls n =27 Mean±(SD)	p	Subjects n =8 Mean±(SD)	Controls n =8 Mean±(SD)	p
Variables						
Height (m)	0.94±1.6	1.26±0.3	0.3	0.98±0.1	0.98±0.0	0.87
Weight (Kg)	13.79±3.4	14.92±0.7	0.08	14.13±2.9	15.00±1.0	0.4
Wt for Ht	14.24±3.9	14.42±0.8	0.81	16.04±2.9	17.84±1.0	0.08
BMI	15.67±4.5	15.42±0.86	0.78	13.03±1.8	14.03±0.6	0.11

m = meters.
Kg = Kilograms.
Wt for Ht = Weight- for -height in Kilograms per meter.
BMI = body mass index.
Kg/m2 = Kilogram per meter squared.

Tables IV and V show the comparison of weight-for-age z scores, height-for-age z scores and body mass index z scores of subjects and controls. They revealed that sickle cell anaemia patients had significantly lower z scores for height-for-age, and weight-for-age compared with controls ($p< 0.02$). Further analysis by sex revealed that the difference was more marked in males than in the females.

There was no statistically significant correlation between nutritional status and haemoglobin concentration in both subjects and controls.

Table 3. Comparison of Anthropometry between subjects and controls older than five years

Variables	Males Subjects n =38 Mean±(SD)	Males Controls n =38 Mean±(SD)	p	Females Subjects n =27 Mean±(SD)	Females Controls n= 27 Mean±(SD)	p
Height (m)	1.22±0.11	1.29±0.01	0.002*	1.22±0.1	1.26±0.01	0.003*
Weight (Kg)	21.5±5.7	25.2±0.9	0.001*	21.42±6.7	24.16±1.3	0.03*
Wt for Ht	16.23±2.8	17.5±0.5	0.007*	19.0±4.5	21.2±0.9	0.009*
BMI	14.2±2.6	14.9±0.4	0.08	14.8±2.8	15.5±0.6	0.17

* Statistically significant.
m = meters.
Kg = Kilograms.
Wt for Ht = Weight- for -height in Kilograms per meter.
BMI = body mass index.
Kg/m2 = Kilogram per meter squared.

Table 4. Comparison of weight-for-age z scores, height-for-age z scores and body mass indices-for-age z scores of subjects and controls

Variables	Subjects n = 100 Mean ±SD	Controls n =100 Mean ±SD	t	p
Height-for-age z scores	-0.46 ± 0.96	-0.11± 0.1	-3.59	0.001*
Weight-for-age z scores	-0.56 ± 0.63	-0.29± 0.1	-4.35	0.001*
BMI z scores	-0.50± 0.79	-0.33± 0.1	-2.02	0.04 *

* Statistically significant.
BMI =Body mass index.

Table 5. Gender-specific comparison of weight-for-age z scores, height-for-age z scores and body mass indices-for-age z scores of subjects and controls

	Males Subjects n =65 Mean SD	Males Controls n =65 p Mean SD	p	Females Subjects n =27 Mean SD	Females Controls n= 27 Mean SD	p
Height-for-age z scores	-0.47±1.0	-0.11± 0.1	0.005*	-0.44± 0.8	-0.12± 0.1	0.03*
Weight-for-age z scores	-0.55± 0.6	-0.25± 0.1	0.001*	-0.58± 0.6	-0.36± 0.1	0.03*
BMI z scores	-0.52± 0.9	-0.31± 0.1	0.17	-0.44± 0.5	-0.37± 0.1	0.36

Figures shown are mean + one standard deviation of the mean.
*Statistically significant.
BMI =Body mass index.

DISCUSSION

The present study was designed to determine the relationship between the steady state haemoglobin, nutritional status using anthropometry measurements of SCA aged one year to ten years at the LUTH. It was partly based on the premise that repeated and/or severe illness may manifest as sub-optimal growth detectable by anthropometry. Also, steady state haemoglobin level of any index patient may potentially impact on growth because of its direct relationship with oxygen delivery to tissues.

The study revealed poor nutritional status in children with sickle cell anaemia compared with contemporary healthy controls. Sickle cell anemia patients had a significantly smaller mean weight compared with controls ($p<0.001$). A similar finding was recorded by earlier authors (11-14). This is because weight can be affected by acute and chronic stress[15] like sickle cell anaemia which is a chronic disease. On the other hand, in the present study there was no statistically significant difference between the mean heights of sickle cell anemia patients and controls. This agrees with the findings of Scott et al. (16) in a study with a similar age cohort. Deficiency in height is a reflection of chronicity and severity of nutritional insult. It is plausible that the degree of nutritional insult in the sickle cell anaemia subjects was not severe enough to produce a significant difference. On the other hand, some workers demonstrated significant reduction in height among patient with sickle cell anaemia compared to healthy controls (12-14,16-17). The explanation for the discrepancy in findings is not immediately clear. Whitten (13) and Ebomoyi et al. (14) studied children of comparable age (2 years to 13 years) so it is not easy to explain the difference in findings on the grounds of age alone. It may be speculated that other factors like severity of illness, which may not be readily comparable across studies might account for the disparity. However, some of the cited studies (12, 17-18) included much older subjects (16 to 20 years) than the current one. It is attractive to argue that the height of older patients would be more adversely affected because they have had the disease for a longer period. This may not be entirely applicable as some other report[19] observed that sickle cell anaemia patients tend to catch up in height in late adolescence. Unfortunately, the studies referred to earlier (12, 17-18) did not stratify subjects by age to enable further comments. On the contrary, when height was related to age using z scores, subjects were found to be significantly further away from the mean than the controls.

The Z score is a more specific way of commenting on the anthropometry. Most other studies (12-14,17-18) did not reduce anthropometry to z scores and so it was not possible to make comparisons and draw conclusions. The significantly lower height-for-age z score obtained in the subjects can be explained by chronic ill-health, increased susceptibility to infections, high metabolic rate leading to energy wastage, chronic anaemia and relative tissue hypoxia that characterize sickle cell anaemia. The same explanation can be offered for the significantly lower z scores for weight-for-age found among sickle cell anaemia patients. The trend was worse among the males who also had significantly lower BMI z scores.

The weight-for-height of patients with sickle cell anaemia was significantly lower than the controls in this study ($p<0.001$). This is in agreement with the findings of Ebomoyi et al. (14) in Ilorin. Weight-for-height is an index of wasting. Thus, the difference observed reflects some degree of wasting among patient with sickle cell anaemia. This may be due to the elevated resting energy expenditure and elevated protein turnover in these patients (20).

In the current study there were no statistically significant difference between the body mass indices of subjects and controls. This is contrary to the findings of Emodi and Kaine (8) in Enugu. The differences in the findings might be due to differences in the age groups studied. While the current study involved children aged one to ten years, the Enugu study (8) excluded under-fives and included adolescents up to 16 years old and found a statistically significant difference between the body mass indices of subjects and controls. Another plausible reason for similarity in BMI among subjects and controls in the present study may be that subjects and controls were matched for social class. The potential effects of social class may be indirect to the extent that people in the same social class are likely to have comparable health seeking behavior or access to quality health care.

The subjects had a mean steady state haemoglobin concentration of 76.9±19.5g/l, which was significantly lower than that (118.1±2.0) obtained for the controls (t=-21.1, p=0.000). This is in agreement with the findings in other report (5) and is probably as a result of premature haemolysis and reduced red blood cell lifespan in the subjects. Females subjects were observed to have higher haemoglobin level compared with controls, although this did not reach a level of statistical significance. The reasons advanced for this gender difference include hormonal problems secondary to severe hypogonadism in male sickle cell anaemia subjects, which leads to reduced androgen levels and hence poor growth. Females have also been found to have higher oxygen delivery to the tissues (21) and hence vaso-occlusive destruction of tissues is usually comparatively minimal compared with what happens in males. This has been attributed to the transcription factor for haemoglobin F which has been linked to X chromosome, therefore female sickle cell anaemia patient tend to have a higher mean haemoglobin F value and hence less vaso-occlusion, less destruction of RBC, higher haemoglobin and higher packed cell volume (21).

It was also observed that the mean steady state haemoglobin concentration obtained in the current study was somewhat lower than (78.7g/l to 96g/l) reported in some other studies (5, 22-23). There is no obvious reason for the observed difference.

The current study also attempted to establish an association between anthropometry of subjects and haemoglobin concentration, but no such association was found except with height for age. This observation suggests that haemoglobin concentration is not a reliable index of nutritional status, with specific reference to the sickle cell anaemia subject. This is because steady state haemoglobin does not depend on the nutritional status, but on the severity of the disease which depends on genetic factors.[1]

In conclusion this study revealed age related poor nutritional status in children with sickle cell anaemia compared with contemporary healthy controls; the mean steady state haemoglobin concentration of subjects with sickle cell anaemia was 76. 9 (SD 19.5) g/l which was significantly lower than 118.1 (SD 2.0) g/l obtained in the controls and there was no association between anthropometry of subjects and haemoglobin concentration.

There is a need for another to verify the claims in this study that prolong frequent crises has effect on the nutritional status of SCA patients and growth monitoring should extend beyond five years of age for SCA patients.

ACKNOWLEDGMENT

We specially acknowledge the subjects and controls who participated in this study, including their parents.

REFERENCES

[1] Adekile AD. Haemoglobinopathies. In : Azubuike JC, Nkanginieme KEO, eds. Paediatrics and child health in a tropical region. Owerri: African Educational Services, 1999;194-213.
[2] Ingram VM. Abnormal haemoglobins. The difference between normal and sicklecell haemoglobins. Biochem Biophys Acta 1959;36:402-11.
[3] Omotade OO, Kayode CM, Falade SL, Ikpeme S. Routine screening for sickle cell haemoglobinopathy by electrophoresis in an infant welfare clinic. West Afr J Med 1998;17:91.
[4] Attah EB, Ekere MC. Death pattern in sickle cell anaemia JAMA 1975;233:889-90.
[5] Konotey-Ahulu FID. The sickle cell diseases, Clinical manifestations including the "Sickle Crisis". Arch Intern Med 1974;133:611-9.
[6] Francis JRB, Johnson CS. Vascular occlusion in sickle diseases: Current concepts and unanswered questions. Blood 1991;77:1405-14.
[7] Anotia-Egebo O, Alikor EAO, Nkanginieme KEO. Malaria parasite density and splenic status by ultrasonography in stable sickle cell anaemia (HbSS) children. Nig J Med 2004;13:40-3.
[8] Emodi KJ, Kaine WN. Weights, heights and Quetelet's indices of children with sickle cell anaemia. Nig J Paediatr 1996;23:37-41.
[9] United State department of Health and human services. National Centre for Health Statistics; 2000. www.cdc.gov/nchs.
[10] Dibley MJ, Staehling N, Nieburg P, Trowbridge FL, Interpretation of z-scores anthropometric indicators derived from international growth reference. Am J Clin Nutr 1987b;46:749-62.
[11] Lesi FEA. Anthropometric status of sickle cell anaemia patients in Lagos. Nig Med J 1979;9:337-42.
[12] \Olanrewaju DM, Adekile AD. Anthropometry status of sickle cell anaemia patients in Ile – Ife, Nigeria. Nigerian Medical Practitioner 1989:18;63-66.
[13] Whitten CF. Growth status of children with sickle cell anaemia. Am J Dis Child 1961;102:355-64.
[14] Ebomoyi E, Adedoyin MA, Ogunlesi FO. A comparative study of the growth status of children with or without sickle cell disease at Ilorin, Kwara State, Nigeria. Afr J Med Sci 1989:18;69-74
[15] Tanner JM. Physical growth and development. In: Forfar JC and Arneil GC, eds. Textbook of Paediatrics. London: Churchill Livingstone,1984:26-56.
[16] Scott RB, Ferguson AD, Jerkins ME, and Clarke HM. Studies in sickle cell anaemia. VIII. Further observation on the clinical manifestation of sickle cell anaemia in children. Am J Dis Child 1965;90: 683-91.
[17] Osinusi K, Oyejide CO. Secular trends in Nutritional status of children from a low socio-economic background. Nig J Paediatr 1987;14(1):7-12.
[18] Phebus CK, Gloninger MF, Maciak BJ. Growth pattern by age and sex in children with sickle cell disease. J Pediatr 1984;105:28-33.
[19] Henry HB, Kenneth K, Mary EF, Ronald LN. The percentage of dense red cell does not predict incidence of sickle cell painful crisis. Blood 1985;68:301-3.
[20] Barden EM, Kawchak DA, Ohene-Frempong K, Starlings VA, and Zemel BS. Body composition in children with sickle cell disease. Am J Nutr 2002;76:218-25.
[21] Wang WC. Sickle cell anaemia and other sickling syndromes.In: Green JP, Forester J, Lukens JN et al. (eds) Wintrobes clinical haematology, Philadephia, PA: Lippinkott William Wilkison 2004;1263-1311.

[22] Ozigbo CJ, Nkanginieme KEO. Body mass index and sexual maturation in adolescent patients with sickle cell anaemia. Nig J Paediatr 2003;30:39-44.

[23] Batra AS, Acherman RJ, Wong W, Wood JC, chan LS, Ramicone E Ebrahimi M, and Wong PC. Cardiac Abnormalities in Children With Sickle Cell Anaemia. Am J Haematol 2002;70:306-12.

In: Child and Adolescent Health Yearbook 2013
Editor: Joav Merrick

ISBN: 978-1-63117-658-6

Chapter 16

PARENTAL SATISFACTION AND TREATMENT OUTCOME: A 3-YEAR STUDY IN CHILDREN'S MENTAL HEALTH SERVICES

***Stephanie Rosso, PhD**[*1] **and Diomaris E Jurecska, PsyD**[1, 2]*
[1]Children's Hospital and Research Center Oakland, California
[2]Graduate Department of clinical psychology, George Fox University, Newberg, Oregon

ABSTRACT

Our objective was to explore the relationship between customer satisfaction and symptom reduction at a hospital-based behavioral pediatrics clinic for children from low socioeconomic and diverse backgrounds. Parental/customer satisfaction and levels of functioning were assessed by a modified version of the Family Satisfaction Questionnaire (FSQ). Methods: Over a 3-year period, data were collected regarding overall parental satisfaction, access to service, symptom reduction, and increase in functioning. Results: Clinician/staff ability and access to service were the stronger predictors of parental satisfaction. Cultural sensitivity and service ability were strongly associated with overall satisfaction. Conclusion: These results suggest that accessibility to services and cultural sensitivity are vital to the therapeutic relationship and treatment success when working with diverse populations.

Keywords: Cultural competency, parental satisfaction, children mental health services

INTRODUCTION

In the United States alone, one in every four to five youth meets criteria for a psychiatric diagnosis (1). An extensive body of literature supports the indication that most psychiatric

---

* Correspondence: Stephanie Rosso, PhD, Clinical Director of the Behavioral Pediatrics Clinic, Children's Hospital and Research Center Oakland, 747 52nd Street, Oakland, California 94609, United States. E-mail: srosso@mail.cho.org

disorders emerge during childhood or adolescence, making early intervention and prevention vital to future youth's life outcomes (1-4). Recent trends show that externalizing disorders such as Attention Deficit and Hyperactivity Disorder (ADHD) have the highest national prevalence rates when compared to internalized childhood disorders (1). Current studies indicate that the presence of untreated psychiatric disorders leads to comorbidity and predicts severe impairment at the individual level (5). Barriers to mental health access for children are based on epidemiological, cultural, as well as economic factors (6-8).

In terms of demographics, both Hispanic and African American children are significantly less likely to access mental health services when compared to their Caucasian counterparts (1). Current statistics also show an unequal distribution between the genders regarding behavioral diagnoses with male rates being significantly higher than female (5). Fortunately, statistics indicate that some externalizing behaviors, such as ADHD, have the highest service rates 59.8% (1). Although externalizing childhood behaviors are present in a broad range of families; they are more prominent in families where risks outnumber protective factors (6). Barriers to mental health services, specifically for children, are strongly associated with poverty, culture, and being from minority groups (6-8).

Studies in adult services show that patient feedback is a key predictor of treatment efficacy. However; perception of quality of care in child and family services are not part of the current methods of treatment outcome evaluations (9). A lack of effective interventions has been associated with children's mental health services. Therefore, providing evidence-based treatment (EBT) has been identified as one of the key components for moving forward in efficacy research with this population (10). Efforts to promulgate best practices or EBT without including patient's perspective can be counterproductive to treatment. Specifically, when working with families, parental satisfaction needs to be identified as one of the key predictors of treatment success (11-16).

Despite this knowledge, customer satisfaction has often been neglected when evaluating outcomes of mental health services for children. A comprehensive review of the literature revealed less than a dozen studies asking how parents perceive the quality of psychiatric care for their children. Therefore, the aim of the study was to explore the relationship between overall satisfaction and treatment outcomes in children's mental health services.

METHODS

The Developmental and Behavioral Pediatrics Clinic (BPC) at Children's Hospital and Research Center Oakland provides psychological evaluations and behavioral interventions to children ages 3 to 12 who are experiencing difficulties with behavioral regulation, attention, learning, and developmental issues. We value a multidisciplinary viewpoint and collaborate as a team with developmental behavioral pediatricians, and nurse practitioners who have had specialized training. We work from an integrative model of therapy, borrowing from psychodynamic, family systems, attachment theory, and cognitive behavioral therapy. As a teaching hospital, our services are provided by licensed clinical psychologists, pre-doctoral interns, and occupational therapists.

Participants

The total sample consisted of 72 survey parental responses, of which 70% were male and 30% were female. In terms of ethnic makeup, 38 were African American (52.8%), 17 were Hispanic American (23.6 %), 8 were European American (11.1%), 2 were Asian American (2.8%), and 1 was Native American (1.4%). The age reflects a range from 4 to 14 years with $M = 8.97$ ($SD = 2.5$). The entire sample had documented mental health diagnoses, while some of the most common diagnoses were: ADHD, Asperger Spectrum Syndrome (ASD), Mood disorder NOS, and Adjustment Disorder NOS. Inclusion criteria were having a child in treatment at BPC for at least three months.

Instruments

An adaptation of the Family Satisfaction Questionnaire used with the Center for Mental Health Services (CMHS) Comprehensive Community Mental Services for Children and their Families Program Consumer Survey was used to assess parental satisfaction (16). Our modified version contained 15 Likert-type scale questions, and with five-ordered response levels ranging from *strongly disagree*, to *strongly agree*. Items in the questionnaire were aimed at providing insight into the following areas:

1. Overall satisfaction with services received;
2. Changes in the patients levels of functioning at school and home (symptoms reduction);
3. Cultural sensitivity from both the staff and providers;
4. Effectiveness of treatment; and
5. Access to services.

Procedure

Questionnaires were given to parents while they were in the waiting room. They were invited to provide feedback to the clinic for the purpose of improving our services. Parents were asked to complete this questionnaire at their own convenience; the questionnaire included a verbal explanation that participation was voluntary, that participants could discontinue involvement at anytime without penalty, and that only aggregate data would be reported. All surveys were collected during the month of May for a period of up to four weeks. Completed surveys were received (48% response rate) from 72 parents of a potential 150 children. This study followed the American Psychological Association's ethical guidelines to protect the confidentiality of participants' records, including de-identification of data. The Institutional Review Board of Children Hospital and Research Center Oakland authorized this project. The data were analyzed using SPSS for Macintosh to produce descriptive statistics (means and standard deviations) and to calculate Pearson product-moment correlation and multiple linear regressions.

RESULTS

Table 1. Descriptive statistics

Variables	*N*	*M*	*SD*
Overall Satisfaction	72	4.67	.628
Clinician & staff availability	71	4.65	.657
Access to services	72	4.65	.632
Communication with staff	71	4.76	.430
Spirituality/ religion	69	4.67	.533
Effectiveness of interventions	70	4.53	.717
Respect from staff	72	4.75	.524
Cultural/ethnic sensitivity	69	4.68	.469
Overall functioning	71	4.03	.820
Active participation in treatment	70	4.59	.597
School functioning	70	3.87	.910
Coping skills	71	3.83	.910

Table 2. Summary of intercorrelations

	1	2	3	4	5	6	7	8	9	10	11	12
1. Overall Satisfaction	----	.915**	.876**	.749**	.654**	.807**	.813**	.692**	.579**	.533*	.447**	.446**
2. Availability/Response	.915**	----	.795**	.675**	.614**	.807**	.770**	.762**	.737**	.499**	.465**	.452**
3. Access to Services	.876**	.795**	----	.793**	.684**	.768**	.840**	.696**	.602**	.504**	.366**	.316**
4.Communication w/ Staff	.749**	.675**	.793**	----	.847**	.635**	.922**	.836**	.466**	.332**	.193	.151
5. Spirituality & Religion	.654**	.614**	.684**	.847**	----	.601**	.797**	.802**	.506**	.365**	.168	.086
6. Effectiveness	.807**	.807**	.768**	.635**	.601**	----	.745**	.582**	.640**	.554**	.476**	.454**
7. Respect from Staff	.813**	.770**	.840**	.922**	.797**	.745**	----	.770**	.522**	.450**	.394**	.326**
8. Cultural Sensitivity	.692**	.762**	.696**	.836**	.802**	.582**	.770**	----	.553**	.275*	.165	.132
9. Participation	.579**	.737**	.602**	.566**	.506**	.640**	.522**	.553**	----	.271*	.158	.158
10. Overall Functioning	.533**	.499**	.504**	.332**	.365**	.554**	.450**	.275*	.271*	----	.723**	.735**
11. School Functioning	.447**	.465**	.366**	.193	.168	.476**	.394**	.165	.158	.723**	----	.815**
12. Coping Skills	.446**	.452**	.316**	.151	.086	.454**	.326**	.132	.158	.735**	.815**	----

Note. Intercorrelations for pertinent variables **Correlation is significant at the 0.01 level (2-tailed). *Correlation is significant at the 0.05 level (2-tailed).

Our main goal was to assess the relationship between consumer satisfaction and the perception of improvement in the BPC (see descriptive of all the pertinent variables in table 1). To examine this association, we first conducted simple correlations among the primary variables (overall satisfaction, clinician and staff availability, access to services, communication with staff, spirituality and religion, effectiveness of interventions, respect from staff, cultural/ethnicity sensitivity, active participation in treatment, overall functioning, school functioning, and coping skills; see Table 2). Overall parental satisfaction with services was generally positive: the item mean ± *SD* was 4.67 ± .68 on a scale of 1 to 5, with higher scores indicating greater satisfaction. Overall satisfaction was significantly associated with clinician and staff availability, access to services, effectiveness of interventions, and respect from staff. Additionally, respect from staff was strongly associated with sensitivity to cultural and religious (spiritual) beliefs. Effectiveness of interventions was strongly correlated with respect from staff, and moderately associated with overall satisfaction, overall functioning, school functioning, and increase of coping skills. Lastly, we performed a multiple regression analysis for the overall satisfaction score. In this analysis, we treated the overall score as the dependent variable and entered the clinical availability, access to services, effectiveness of interventions, and respect from staff scores as independent variables.

The other variable that also explained a significant proportion of variance in overall satisfaction was access to services, $b = .328$, $t(65) = 3.785$, $p < .001$ in overall satisfaction $R^2 = .899$, $F(4,65) = 144.958$, $p < .001$. This procedure allowed us to determine the strength of the association among the variables. Results indicated that clinician and staff availability significantly predicted overall satisfaction, $b = .546$, $t(65) = 6.078$, $p < .001$.

Discussion

Findings from the current study corroborate those of previous investigations noting a significant association between patient's relationships with providers and staff as an indicator of customer satisfaction (13,17). An unexpected finding in our study was that changes in levels of functioning were not strongly associated with overall customer satisfaction. These results are inconsistent with other outcome evaluation studies (18,19).

For example, Barber, Tischler, Healy (19) found that the highest predictor of consumer satisfaction of parents regarding their children's mental health services was the reduction of symptoms. An explanation for this inconsistent finding may be the wide range of treatment length observed in the sample. Consistent with our philosophy, cultural sensitivity was strongly associated with parent's satisfaction.

It appears that when delivering family services to diverse groups, cultural competence is vital for treatment success. Cultural context is an important consideration in studies of mental health services and customer satisfaction as some cultures might value their connection with the clinicians and the staff even higher than the goals of treatment (15,20). On a comprehensive literature review, Hernandez, et al. (21) provided an institutional model for cultural competence. Their model states that "cultural competence occurs when there is compatibility among four important factors: community context, cultural characteristics of local populations, organizational infrastructure, and direct service support" (12).

Limitations and suggestions for future research

In examining the effectiveness of children's mental health services provided by the BPC, several limitations to this study emerged. First, although all the treatments provided at BPC have elements of EBT modalities, they were significant differences among provider's approaches. It is also important to note that the diversity and needs of this population makes it difficult to have each child receive the same treatment. Our sample presents with significant differences in cognitive, and language abilities, which make treatment standarization a challenge. Although these results contribute to the literature on the effectiveness of mental health services provided to children, parents were the responders of the survey, and our findings do not provide information on the children's satisfaction (22). Finally, the design and analyses make it impossible to infer causality.

The results of the current study point to a number of future directions. First, consistent with the US Public Health Service report (23) more research exploring predictors of success in mental health services delivered to children, adolescent, and families is needed (22). Perhaps, a start is establishing criteria of specific treatments modalities, and settings as best practices for specific disorders. Second, researches would also benefit from an understanding of the role that culture has on the development of the therapeutic relationship and treatment success with diverse patients. Finally, further research is needed to address the various forms of research methodology to access specialized populations. A combination of qualitative, quantitative, and longitudinal methods may be best suited for studying these populations.

References

[1] Merikangas KR, He JP, Brody D, Fisher PW, Bourdon K, et al. Prevalence and treatment of mental disorders among US children in the 2001-2004 NHANES. Pediatrics 2010;125:75-81.

[2] Merikangas KR, He JP, Burstein M, Swendsen J, Avenevoli S, Case B, et al. Service utilization for lifetime mental health disorders in U.S. Adolescents: Results of the national comorbidity survey-adolescent supplement (NCS-A). J Am Acad Child Adolesc Psychiatry, 2011;50(1):980-9.

[3] Osofsky JD, Lieberman AF. A call for integrating a mental health perspective into systems of care for abused and neglected infants and young children. Am Psychol 2011; 66(2):120-8.

[4] Simpson GA, Cohen RA, Pastor PN, Reuben CA. Use of mental health services in the past 12 months by children aged 4-17 years: United States, 2005-2006. NCHS Data Brief 2008;8.

[5] Swendsen J, Conway KP, Degenhardt L, Glantz M, Jin R, Merikangas KR, et al. Mental disorders as risk factors for substance use, abuse, and dependence: results from the 10-year follow-up of the national comorbidity survey. Journal of Addiction, 2010:105(6):1117-28.

[6] Copeland VC, Snyder K. Barriers to mental health treatment services for low-income African American women whose children receive behavioral health services: an ethnographic investigation. Soc Work Public Health 2011;26(1):78-95.

[7] Lopez C, Bergren MD. Latino disparities in child mental health services. J Child Adolesc Psychiatr Nurs 2008;21(3):137-45.

[8] Merikangas KR, Nakamura EF, Kessler RC. Epidemiology of mental disorders in children and adolescents. Dialogues Clin Neurosci 2009;11(1):7-20.

[9] Higa-McMillan CK, Powell C, Daleiden EL, Mueller CW. Pursuing an evidence-based culture through contextualized feedback: Aligning youth outcomes and practices. Prof Psychol Res Pract 2011;42(2):137-44.

[10] La Greca AM, Silverman WK, Lochman JE. Moving beyond efficacy and effectiveness in child and adolescent intervention research. J Consult Clin Psych 2010;77(3): 373-82. .

[11] Biering P, Jensen VH. The Concept of Patient Satisfaction in Adolescent Psychiatric Care: A Qualitative Study. J Child Adolesc Psychiatr Nurs 2011;24(1):3–10.

[12] Buston K. Adolescents with mental health problems: What do they say about health services? J Adolesc 2002;25(2):231-42.

[13] Garland AF, Saltzman MD, Aarons GA. Adolescent satisfaction with mental health services: Development of a multidimensional scale. J Eval Prog Plan 2000;23(2):165–75.

[14] Hart A, Saunders A, Thomas H. Attuned practice; a service user study of specialist child and adolescent mental health. Epid Psich Soc 2005;14(1):22–31.

[15] Kazak AE, Hoagwood K, Weisz JR, Hood K, Kratochwill TR, Vargas LA, Banez, GA. A meta-systems approach to evidence-based practice for children and adolescents. American Psychologist 2010;65(2):85-97.

[16] Brunk M, Koch JR, McCall B. Report on parent satisfaction with services at Community Services Boards. Richmond, VA: Virginia Department Mental Health Mental Retardation Substance Abuse Services, 2000.

[17] Kaplan S, Busner J, Chibnall J, Kang G. Consumer satisfaction at a child and adolescent state psychiatric hospital, J Psych Serv 2001;52(2):202-6.

[18] Godley SH, Fiedler EM, Funk RR. Consumer satisfaction of parents and their children with child/adolescent mental health services. J Eval Prog Plan 1999; 21(1):31-45.

[19] Barber AJ, Tischler V, Healy E. Consumer satisfaction and child behavior problems in child and adolescent mental health services, J Child Health Care 2006;10(1):9-21.

[20] Biever JL, Gómez JP, González CG, Patrizio N. Psychological services to Spanish-speaking populations: A model curriculum for training competent professionals. Training Educ Prof Psychol 2011;5(2):81-7.

[21] Hernandez M, Nesman T, Mowery D, Acevedo-Polakovich ID, Callejas LM. Cultural competence: A literature review and conceptual model for mental health services. Psychol Serv 2009;60(8):1046-50.

[22] Steele RG, Roberts MC, eds. Handbook of mental health services for children, adolescents, and families. New York: Springer, 2005.

[23] Satcher D. Report of the Surgeon General's conference on children's mental health: A national action agenda; Washington, DC: Department Health Human Services, 2001.

SECTION THREE – FROM FRIENDSHIP TO UNDERNOURISHMENT

In: Child and Adolescent Health Yearbook 2013
Editor: Joav Merrick

ISBN: 978-1-63117-658-6

Chapter 17

THE INFLUENCE OF FRIENDSHIP GROUPS AND MEDIA ON EATING BEHAVIOR AND PHYSICAL ACTIVITY IN ADOLESCENTS

Eveline JM Wouters[*] and Rinie Geenen

Department of Allied Health Professions, Fontys University of Applied Sciences, Eindhoven and Department of Clinical and Health Psychology, Utrecht University, Utrecht, Netherlands

ABSTRACT

The worldwide obesity epidemic is a complex problem, resulting from the interaction of individual metabolic, genetic, and psychological factors with meso- and macro environmental factors. Adolescents, with their rapid changes in body composition, together with their shift in orientation from the direct family to the peer-related environment, are particularly vulnerable to unhealthy changes in lifestyle and peers seem to play an important role in shaping the behavior of adolescents. Adolescents tend to mimic their peers' behavior related to both food choices as well as to physical activity. This influence of peers depends on environmental circumstances such as availability of snacks, and it is affected by individual psychological and demographic factors as well as by macro-environmental factors such as cultural and social norms, legislation, food distribution, and media and advertising. Rapidly expanding sources of influence on health behavior are media such as television, the internet, and smartphones. These media may enhance overweight and a sedentary lifestyle. However, potentially these media could be used to monitor and influence snacking behavior and physical activity for the better. An example of the use of new technology to enhance health behavior is the 'Wii' home video game. Using insights from social psychology, thoughtful choice architecture can be established to nudge adolescents to choose what is best for them without restricting freedom of choice and to help them with really implementing healthy intentions. A challenge for the coming decade is to develop 'Apps' aimed to decrease adolescent obesity while making use of social networks.

[*] Correspondence: Eveline JM Wouters, PhD, MD, MSc. Department of Allied Health Professions, Fontys University of Applied Sciences, Th. Fliednerstraat 2, 5631 BN, room 0.214, Eindhoven, The Netherlands. E-mail: e.wouters@fontys.nl.

Keywords: Adolescence, peer influence, friendship groups, eating behavior, physical activity, environment

INTRODUCTION

The obesity epidemic is a major and complex problem, resulting from the interaction of environmental, metabolic, genetic and psychological factors (1). To date, 17% of children and adolescents in the US are diagnosed to be obese (2). This high prevalence in obesity has already been observed since 2007, but notably, within the group of obese children and adolescents, there is a relative increase in prevalence of obesity in the subgroup of adolescents (12-19 years) (2,3).

Many adolescents have unhealthy diets and sedentary behavior (4). This not only bears implications at this age, but many of these behaviors are maintained during later periods of life. What was learned during adolescence has often become a habit in adult life (5). Dieting as a single intervention in adolescence, hardly ever leads to successful weight loss. Moreover, unhealthy dieting during adolescence (both in boys and girls), leads to weight gain and obesity later in life, as well as to substantially enhanced risk of developing eating disorders (6). Therefore, the recognition and prevention of these behaviors and their determinants is very important.

Adolescents, with their rapid changes in body composition, together with their shift in orientation from the direct family to the peer-related environment, are particularly vulnerable to unfavorable changes in life style. Food and exercise habits tend to change substantially in this period, as compared to earlier childhood. Besides their parents, also peers come to play an important role in what they do or what they like. Adolescents, compared to other age groups, have a stronger need to belong to a group and to be accepted by their peers (7).

In this paper, the literature on the influences of peers on eating- and exercise behavior is reviewed and the specific role of modern media in this context is discussed.

INFLUENCE OF SOCIAL NETWORKS IN ADOLESCENCE

Social networks are of great importance in adolescence (7). Many parents perceive with some anxiety that the peers of their youngsters can become very important and influential in developing all kinds of maladaptive or unhealthy behavior. Social learning theory specifies that peers may influence each other by observing, modeling, and imitating individuals in their environment (8). General learning theory suggests that behavior can be shaped by selective reinforcement and punishment by peers.

With respect to unhealthy behavior, there is convincing evidence for peer influence on smoking behavior (9). Having friends who smoke or friends who approve of smoking predicts the probability of adolescents to start smoking (9). Also other unhealthy habits, such as alcohol and drug abuse, are influenced by peers (10,11). The better the perceived quality of the friendship, the more adolescents are apt to conform to the substance use of their peers (10).

Smoking and substance use represent addictions that, after having acquired the habit, are difficult to stop. Behavior that is less related to specific substances but that shares the compulsive nature of addictions and that can be related to the onset of obesity (in a direct or indirect way), is disordered eating such as bulimia. In bulimia, peers (both girls and boys) select each other for personality traits (related to self-esteem and perfectionism), and the socialization process influences the development of similar bulimic symptoms (12). Especially the maintenance of the bulimic behavior appears influenced by peers, because after loosening up of the friendships, bulimia symptoms tend to diminish. Also in anorexia, mostly studied in girls, peers are influential and both peers and media play an important role in the thin beauty ideal of many girls (13).

Thus, unhealthy, harmful habits can be partly attributed to the influence of peers in adolescence. Considering the increase of adolescent obesity, it is useful to gain knowledge on comparable peer influences on the development and persistence of obesity. In adults, obesity has been found to spread in social networks (14). As adolescents tend to create new and strong social networks, it is an obvious assumption that peers are important for the development of overweight and obesity.

INFLUENCE OF SOCIAL NETWORKS ON EATING BEHAVIOR IN ADOLESCENTS

Both observational and experimental studies indicate that children and adolescents model their peers' behavior related to both healthy and unhealthy food choices as well as to physical activity and sports participation (15). In this section the factors that influence eating behavior will be discussed.

Peers and parents

In research of obesity, common eating behavior is measured with variables such as daily fruit- and vegetable intake, regular consumption of breakfast, frequency of fast food restaurant visits, and calorie dense snack intake. The influence of peers varies between these variables. For instance, breakfast consumption, as compared to calorie dense snack intake, is more strongly associated with parental behavior than with peer influence. However, several food-related habits tend to run in friendship groups. For instance, peers influence each other more strongly with respect to eating in fast food restaurants (15). Moreover, snacking, defined as the intake of high caloric food and high energy soft drinks, is rather similar within peer groups of adolescents (16). Also, while hanging out with friends, the tendency to snack is stronger than without friends (17).

Moderators of peer influence on eating behavior

The relation between snacking and friends' influence is not one-to-one. Multiple factors determine snacking in interaction. First of all, the physical environment affects the influence of peers on eating behavior. If snacks are easily available in the environment, for instance, in the shops near school (18) or within school itself (16), the influence of peers is stronger.

Second, individual factors play a role. In the adult population, personality factors such as low conscientiousness (19), high impulsivity and low self-control (20) are associated with unhealthy snacking. Likely, similar personality factors influence snacking in young people.

Third, demographic factors should be taken account of. The influence of friendship groups on snacking is not similar for girls and boys. In boys, peer group snacking is somewhat stronger than in girl peer groups (16), whereas in girls, dieting within peer groups during adolescence, which is related to higher risk for developing obesity in later life, is more common (21,22). There is also a difference between adolescents related to education level. Peer group effects on snacking are stronger in adolescents with lower education levels (16). Besides reinforcement by peers, punishment may affect eating behavior. In girls, more than in boys, peer group teasing and comments about the body appearance of overweight and obese adolescents, influence unhealthy dieting in an unfavorable manner, strengthening the effect in girls already overweight (23).

Environmental influence

There is no single determinant of unhealthy behavior. Just like other health behavior, unhealthy eating is determined by individual (personal) factors, meso-environmental factors, which can be divided into social environmental (family and peers) and physical environmental components (like availability in the community such as shops and school canteens). In addition, macro-environmental factors play a role. Cultural and social norms, legislation, food distribution as well as media and advertising, are amongst these latter factors (24). This framework that summarizes several levels of influence, and that positions individual influences central, and environmental (interpersonal and physical factors) next is illustrated in figure 1.

Up till now, many of the efforts to reduce the obesity epidemic have been directed at the individual level. Individual therapy, preferably multidisciplinary interventions including diet and physical exercise, combined with psychological support, are now common treatment. The observation that also the direct physical environment plays a role, has additionally led to interventions in communities, especially school-based interventions (25).

None of these interventions paid much intention to the role of friendship groups as a risk factor for developing and maintaining unhealthy eating habits. Comparable to the relatively late addition of psychological support to dieting and exercise in the individual treatment of overweight, this is a treatment direction that is, at the moment, still largely underdeveloped. There is ample evidence that groups of school friends have rather similar body mass indices, fast food consumption patterns and body image concerns, dieting habits, and eating disorders (26). This indicates the potential effectiveness of school based interventions addressing the role of these friendships.

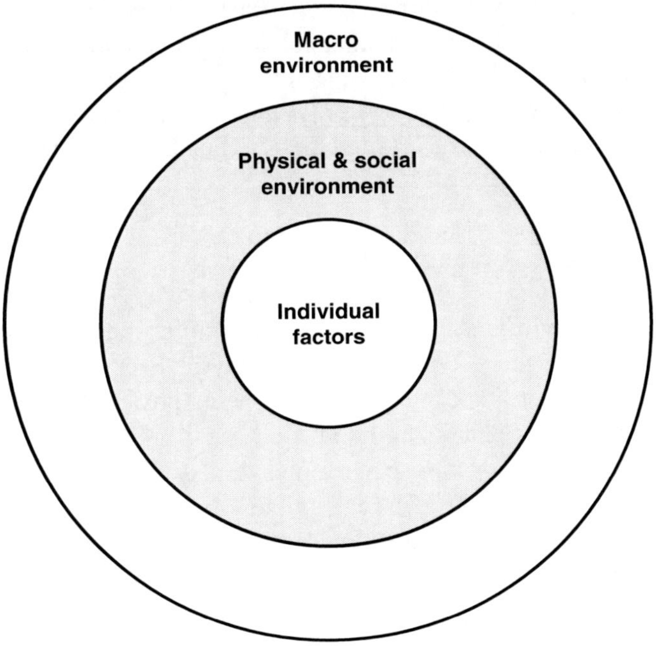

Figure 1. Factors influencing obesity-related behavior.

Future interventions should pay more attention to this opportunity to restrict the obesity epidemic.

INFLUENCE OF SOCIAL NETWORKS ON EXERCISE BEHAVIOR IN ADOLESCENTS

Physical activity and exercise are, next to healthy diets, important in the onset and maintenance of weight loss in obesity treatment (27-29). Moreover, physical activity improves physical and mental health (30-33). Physical exercise as a means to reduce overweight and obesity could be especially indicated in people for whom exercising is easier than stopping superfluous eating (34).

Exercise behavior

Exercise has positive effects for physical and mental health in adolescents and the reversed effect is observed for sedentary behavior (35,36). For adolescents, the effects of exercise can generalize to multiple dimensions of functioning. For instance adolescents who are physically active achieve better results at school (37). Despite all these favorable effects, many adolescents, even after having been physically active in childhood, stop exercising in adolescence (38,39).

Comparable to the change in eating behavior (figure 1), reasons for the decrease of physical activity in puberty have been sought in individual factors (physical changes and maturation) and social and physical environmental factors (38). As an example of individual factors, the decrease in physical activity among adolescents is more prominent in girls (40,41) and in lower income families (42). Physical activity of individuals is closely linked to physical activity patterns of their peers (43). Possibly, self-esteem is a mediator of the association between physical activity of individuals and their peers (42).

Environmental influence on exercise behavior

Regarding the physical environment, the lack of possibilities and opportunities to exercise, and lack of safety in the neighborhood may hamper physical activity (44-46). Comparable to the availability of healthy instead of unhealthy food, being physically active at a regular basis needs appropriate facilities in the neighborhood.

As for eating behavior, peers have been found to play a prominent role in the physical activity patterns of adolescents. Adolescents more often befriend with adolescents with comparable amounts of physical activities and, consecutively, mimic each other's activities (47). By participation in sport activities, adolescents improve self-esteem and get positive social feedback (48). Peers represent role models who may reinforce being physically active by giving encouragement and social support. Therefore, interventions to improve physical activities in adolescents should include and optimize peer support for being successful (49). Preferably, these interventions should start before the onset of puberty, because the effect of friends is counteracted by the effect of age: in case of low baseline physical activity at the start of puberty, the net activity is generally also low during later years.

THE ROLE OF MEDIA

An influence of social networks in children and adolescents not only occurs through face-to-face contacts, but also through media such as television, the internet (e.g., Facebook, twitter), and smartphones. To date, over 900 million persons use Facebook worldwide (50). The rapidly expanding new media may impact on overweight for the worse by reinforcing a sedentary life. However, potentially these media could be used to monitor and influence snacking behavior and physical activity for the better.

Regarding the impact of media, children and youth are a special audience, because they are developmentally vulnerable and because they have always been among the earliest adopters and heaviest users of entertainment technology (51). As in face-to-face contacts, media play a role in the macro environment as well as in the more proximal social environment of adolescents, and media may influence factors related to eating and dieting, as well as energy expenditure and physical exercise.

Media and eating behavior

The role of the media in childhood overweight and obesity as a push factor has been well studied. Especially the influence of commercials of food products on children watching television has been widely established. It has, for instance, been shown that exposure to television food commercials increases the preference for energy-dense foods, particularly in children who watch more television (52). Such an impact appears stronger for boys than for girls (53).

Food markets often advertise unhealthy products specifically directed at youth. Adolescents are such an important group for industry, because people tend to use the brands they used in adolescence lifelong. The psychological mechanisms by which the influence of marketing works is widely accepted as well as the favorable results of interventions aimed at prohibition on food advertisements during daytime, pointing at the importance of governmental policies and strategies (54,55). In some countries bans on “unhealthy” advertisements have now been established (56,57).

The association between media use and obesity is small, but consistent (58,59). Thus, media use is clearly one of several factors that may impact on obesity. The American Academy of Pediatrics policy statement regarding the prevention of pediatric overweight and obesity identifies limiting television and videogame use to no more than 2 hours per day as an important strategy for preventing obesity among children and adolescents (60). However, in order to decrease the total of screen hours, especially the role of the meso-environment appears important. More clearly than policy makers, parents, peers and teachers can play a role in restricting the amount of hours that adolescents watch a screen.

Media and physical exercise

For physical exercise, the influence of media as part of the macro environment is also twofold, but slightly different from the role of media with respect to food. Watching television (or other screens) is directly and importantly related to sedentary behavior and lack of physical activity, and the number of spent hours of television watching is an important predictor of overweight and obesity (36).

Physical exercise can also be enhanced by modern media. Home video games like ‘Wii’ are so popular in adolescents, because they do not experience it as physical effort, but because the game is fun (61). In overweight and obese adolescents, playing ‘exergames’ in a cooperative way is more effective in being physically active and losing weight, than playing competitive exercises (62-65). Playing together and being with peers, is part of the success of these games.

Next to these games, there is a growing availability of Apps about weight-related behavior in electronic phones and tablets. In 2011, already over 2000 Apps about health and fitness were available, most of them assisting the user in logging their calorie intake and physical activity (58). However, most of the Apps are not developed for adolescents, and the effectiveness of these interventions is not yet evaluated (58).

Current and future media use

There is popular and scholarly consensus that today’s adolescents, in particular, have widely adopted the use of digital media for daily life activities (58). Thus, to have an impact on daily activities of adolescents, digital media could be used. Indeed, apart from the potentially unfavorable role of mass media toward eating behavior in children and adolescents, there is also growing evidence that media can be used to prevent unhealthy behavior or to encourage or support positive changes in health behaviors (66). To create a supportive environment against obesity, policy with respect to control of unhealthy advertisement is needed along with promotion of health education.

Policymakers, employers, insurance companies, researchers, and health care providers have developed an increasing interest in using principles from behavioral economics and psychology to persuade people to change their health-related behaviors, lifestyles, and habits (67). For instance, subtle techniques have been developed to "nudge" people toward particular decisions or behaviors. Thoughtful "choice architecture" can be established to nudge adolescents to choose what is best for themselves without restricting freedom of choice (68). An example of a nudge is the development of piano stairs that make music when climbing the stairs as an alternative to using a moving staircases (69). Another nudge is the tough image that was chosen for Coca-Cola Zero to tempt youth to drink this light drink instead of the calorie-dense cola. Thus, commercial techniques that have been shown to be successful to promote unhealthy products in children and adolescents can also be used to promote healthy behavior. The new media offer the opportunity to nudge children and adolescents towards healthy eating behavior and physical activity.

A new challenge is also to develop Apps to help adolescents to translate intentions in implementation intentions or action plans specifying where, with whom, and at what time, what particular health behavior will be performed. Such action plans contribute to really acting on one's intentions (70,71). In complex behavior, it is also important to specify why a habitual, unhealthy response should be replaced with an alternative healthy response in a critical situation. In a study of the efficacy of implementation intentions to replace unhealthy snacks with healthy snacks by linking different types of cues for unhealthy snacking (if-part) to healthy snacking (then-part), implementation intentions specifying motivational (why) cues decreased unhealthy snack consumption whereas the classic specification of where and when did not (72).

Media and social interaction

Thus, media play a role in the meso- and macro environment of adolescents both as a threat and an opportunity to influence health behavior. The popularity amongst adolescents of social media such as Facebook is most easily understood in the light of social processes. Social media offer the possibility to connect to friends in an easy way, and to be together with friends almost all the time. Presence with friends is very important in weight-related behavior (73). The potential of social media in the intervention or prevention of weight-related behavior (eating and exercise), has not yet been subject of study. For alcohol consumption in adolescents, more research results are available. Social norms and adolescents' beliefs about their friends' alcohol consumption are important determinants of alcohol consumption (74). Profiles and pictures showing alcohol drinking peers influence the attitudes towards alcohol use in friends on Facebook (75). Likewise, it can be expected that social interaction on Facebook can influence other more or less harmful health behavior. Knowing that peer influence and social media play an important role in health (including weight-related) behavior is a first step in prevention and intervention. The next, most difficult step is to offering solutions or opportunities to use these networks to promote health.

A future area of research and intervention for health care workers is to use social networks in order to influence the health behavior of adolescents. Apart from Facebook, there are many other local social network media. An example of patient social networks is PatientsLikeMe. These networks offer an opportunity to give health messages and to integrate patient-healthcare interaction within more general social networks. One of the problems of web users is the effort it takes to manage different sources (that is, to have profiles and to keep records), if one is using different social media. Recently, this problem has been addressed for patients, resulting in easier communication between patients and physicians (76). Future research should evaluate the benefits of social networks and effort should be put in linking up and translating lifestyle sites to popular social networks.

CONCLUSION

The global epidemic of overweight and obesity results from individual factors and from meso- and macro environmental factors. Adolescents are especially vulnerable to unhealthy changes in life style. One major influence on health behavior in this age group is represented by friends in peer groups. Young people tend to select and mimic each other with respect to both eating behavior and physical exercise. Peer groups are a close and important source of influence on health behavior and social media strengthens this influence. New research and interventions should take account of the influence of the peer group and social media.

REFERENCES

[1] Wadden TA, Stunkard AJ. Handbook of obesity treatment. New York: Guilford, 2004.

[2] Ogden CL, Carroll MD, Kit BK, Flegal KM. Prevalence of obesity and trends in body mass index among US children and adolescents, 1999-2010. JAMA 2012;307(5):483-90.

[3] Whittle CR, Yarnell JW, Stevenson M, McCay N, Gaffney BP, Shields MD, et al. Is dieting behaviour decreasing in young adolescents? Public Health Nutr 2013;16(5):841-7.

[4] Eaton DK, Kann L, Kinchen S, Shanklin S, Flint KH, Hawkins J, et al. Youth risk behavior surveillance - United States, 2011. MMWR Surveill Summ 2012;61(4):1-162.

[5] Larson NI, Neumark-Sztainer DR, Story MT, Wall MM, Harnack LJ, Eisenberg ME. Fast food intake: longitudinal trends during the transition to young adulthood and correlates of intake. J Adolesc Health 2008;43(1):79-86.

[6] Neumark-Sztainer D, Wall M, Guo J, Story M, Haines J, Eisenberg M. Obesity, disordered eating, and eating disorders in a longitudinal study of adolescents: how do dieters fare 5 years later? J Am Diet Assoc 2006;106(4):559-68.

[7] Coleman JC. Friendship and the peer group in adolescence. New York: Wiley, 1980.

[8] Bandura A. Social foundations of thought and action: a social cognitive theory. Englewood Cliffs, NJ, US: Prentice Hall, 1986.

[9] Gritz ER, Prokhorov AV, Hudmon KS, Mullin Jones M, Rosenblum C, Chang CC, et al. Predictors of susceptibility to smoking and ever smoking: a longitudinal study in a triethnic sample of adolescents. Nicotine Tob Res 2003;5(4):493-506.

[10] Urberg KA, Degirmencioglu SM, Pilgrim C. Close friend and group influence on adolescent cigarette smoking and alcohol use. Dev Psychol 1997;33(5):834-44.

[11] Urberg KA, Luo Q, Pilgrim C, Degirmencioglu SM. A two-stage model of peer influence in adolescent substance use: individual and relationship-specific differences in susceptibility to influence. Addict Behav 2003;28(7):1243-56.

[12] Zalta AK, Keel PK. Peer influence on bulimic symptoms in college students. J Abnorm Psychol 2006;115(1):185-9.

[13] Bell C, Cooper MJ. Socio-cultural and cognitive predictors of eating disorder symptoms in young girls. Eat Weight Disord 2005;10(4):e97-e100.

[14] Christakis NA, Fowler JH. The spread of obesity in a large social network over 32 years. N Engl J Med 2007;357(4):370-9.

[15] Ali MM, Amialchuk A, Heiland FW. Weight-related behavior among adolescents: the role of peer effects. PloS One 2011;6(6):e21179.

[16] Wouters EJ, Larsen JK, Kremers SP, Dagnelie PC, Geenen R. Peer influence on snacking behavior in adolescence. Appetite 2010;55(1):11-7.

[17] Savige G, Macfarlane A, Ball K, Worsley A, Crawford D. Snacking behaviours of adolescents and their association with skipping meals. Int J Behav Nutr Phys Act 2007;4:36.

[18] Bibeau WS, Saksvig BI, Gittelsohn J, Williams S, Jones L, Young DR. Perceptions of the food marketing environment among African American teen girls and adults. Appetite 2012;58(1):396-9.

[19] O'Connor DB, Conner M, Jones F, McMillan B, Ferguson E. Exploring the benefits of conscientiousness: an investigation of the role of daily stressors and health behaviors. Ann Behav Med 2009;37(2):184-96.

[20] Churchill S, Jessop DC. Reflective and non-reflective antecedents of health-related behaviour: exploring the relative contributions of impulsivity and implicit self-control to the prediction of dietary behaviour. Br J Health Psychol 2011;16(2):257-72.

[21] Schutz HK, Paxton SJ. Friendship quality, body dissatisfaction, dieting and disordered eating in adolescent girls. Br J Clin Psychol 2007;46(1):67-83.

[22] Hutchinson DM, Rapee RM. Do friends share similar body image and eating problems? The role of social networks and peer influences in early adolescence. Behav Res Ther 2007;45(7):1557-77.

[23] Thompson JK, Shroff H, Herbozo S, Cafri G, Rodriguez J, Rodriguez M. Relations among multiple peer influences, body dissatisfaction, eating disturbance, and self-esteem: a comparison of average weight, at risk of overweight, and overweight adolescent girls. J Pediatr Psychol 2007;32(1):24-9.

[24] Story M, Neumark-Sztainer D, French S. Individual and environmental influences on adolescent eating behaviors. J Am Diet Assoc 2002;102(3 Suppl):S40-51.

[25] Verstraeten R, Roberfroid D, Lachat C, Leroy JL, Holdsworth M, Maes L, et al. Effectiveness of preventive school-based obesity interventions in low- and middle-income countries: a systematic review. Am J Clin Nutr 2012;96(2):415-38.

[26] Fletcher A, Bonell C, Sorhaindo A. You are what your friends eat: systematic review of social network analyses of young people's eating behaviours and bodyweight. J Epidemiol Community Health 2011;65(6):548-55.

[27] Catenacci VA, Wyatt HR. The role of physical activity in producing and maintaining weight loss. Nat Clin Pract Endocrinol Metab 2007;3(7):518-29.

[28] Ross R, Janssen I, Dawson J, Kungl AM, Kuk JL, Wong SL, et al. Exercise-induced reduction in obesity and insulin resistance in women: a randomized controlled trial. Obes Res 2004;12(5):789-98.

[29] Villanova N, Pasqui F, Burzacchini S, Forlani G, Manini R, Suppini A, et al. A physical activity program to reinforce weight maintenance following a behavior program in overweight/obese subjects. Int J Obes (Lond) 2006;30(4):697-703.

[30] Annesi JJ, Whitaker AC. Weight loss and psychologic gain in obese women-participants in a supported exercise intervention. Perm J 2008;12(3):36-45.

[31] Mathus-Vliegen EM, Basdevant A, Finer N, Hainer V, Hauner H, Micic D, et al. Prevalence, pathophysiology, health consequences and treatment options of obesity in the elderly: a guideline. Obes Facts 2012;5(3):460-83.

[32] Taylor CB, Sallis JF, Needle R. The relation of physical activity and exercise to mental health. Public Health Rep 1985;100(2):195-202.

[33] Khan KM, Thompson AM, Blair SN, Sallis JF, Powell KE, Bull FC, et al. Sport and exercise as contributors to the health of nations. Lancet 2012;380(9836):59-64.

[34] Skender ML, Goodrick GK, Del Junco DJ, Reeves RS, Darnell L, Gotto AM, et al. Comparison of 2-year weight loss trends in behavioral treatments of obesity: diet, exercise, and combination interventions. J Am Diet Assoc1996;96(4):342-6.

[35] Biddle SJ, Asare M. Physical activity and mental health in children and adolescents: a review of reviews. Br J Sports Med 2011;45(11):886-95.

[36] Tremblay MS, LeBlanc AG, Kho ME, Saunders TJ, Larouche R, Colley RC, et al. Systematic review of sedentary behaviour and health indicators in school-aged children and youth. Int J Behav Nutr Phys Act 2011;8:98.

[37] Rasberry CN, Lee SM, Robin L, Laris BA, Russell LA, Coyle KK, et al. The association between school-based physical activity, including physical education, and academic performance: a systematic review of the literature. Prev Med 2011;52 Suppl 1:S10-20.

[38] Duncan SC, Duncan TE, Strycker LA, Chaumeton NR. A cohort-sequential latent growth model of physical activity from ages 12 to 17 years. Ann Behav Med 2007;33(1):80-9..

[39] Kimm SY, Glynn NW, Kriska AM, Fitzgerald SL, Aaron DJ, Similo SL, et al. Longitudinal changes in physical activity in a biracial cohort during adolescence. Med Sci Sports Exerc 2000;32(8):1445-54.

[40] Chung AE, Skinner AC, Steiner MJ, Perrin EM. Physical activity and BMI in a nationally representative sample of children and adolescents. Clin Pediatr (Phila) 2012;51(2):122-9.

[41] Slater A, Tiggemann M. Gender differences in adolescent sport participation, teasing, self-objectification and body image concerns. J Adolesc 2011;34(3):455-63.

[42] Veselska Z, Madarasova Geckova A, Reijneveld SA, van Dijk JP. Socio-economic status and physical activity among adolescents: the mediating role of self-esteem. Public Health 2011;125(11):763-8.

[43] Frisen A, Bjarnelind S. Health-related quality of life and bullying in adolescence. Acta Paediatr 2010;99(4):597-603.

[44] Heath GW, Parra DC, Sarmiento OL, Andersen LB, Owen N, Goenka S, et al. Evidence-based intervention in physical activity: lessons from around the world. Lancet 2012;380(9838):272-81.

[45] Gordon-Larsen P, Nelson MC, Page P, Popkin BM. Inequality in the built environment underlies key health disparities in physical activity and obesity. Pediatrics 2006;117(2):417-24.

[46] Cohen DA, Ashwood JS, Scott MM, Overton A, Evenson KR, Staten LK, et al. Public parks and physical activity among adolescent girls. Pediatrics 2006;118(5):e1381-9.

[47] de la Haye K, Robins G, Mohr P, Wilson C. How physical activity shapes, and is shaped by, adolescent friendships. Soc Sci Med. 2011;73(5):719-28.

[48] Kahn JA, Huang B, Gillman MW, Field AE, Austin SB, Colditz GA, et al. Patterns and determinants of physical activity in U.S. adolescents. J Adolesc Health 2008;42(4):369-77.

[49] Garcia AW, Pender NJ, Antonakos CL, Ronis DL. Changes in physical activity beliefs and behaviors of boys and girls across the transition to junior high school. J Adolesc Health 1998;22(5):394-402.

[50] Facebook statistics 2012 Accessed Aug 29 2012 URL: http://www.socialbakers.com/countries/continents.

[51] Schmidt ME, Anderson DR. The impact of television on cognitive development and educational achievement. N. Pecora JPM, E.A. Wartella, editor. Mahaw (NJ): Lawrence Erlbaum Associates, 2006.

[52] Boyland EJ, Harrold JA, Kirkham TC, Corker C, Cuddy J, Evans D, et al. Food commercials increase preference for energy-dense foods, particularly in children who watch more television. Pediatrics 2011;128(1):e93-100.

[53] Chernin A. Overweight and obesity in America's children: causes, consequences, solutions: section two: media and culture: The effects of food marketing on children's preferences: testing the moderating roles of age and gender. Ann Am Acad Pol Soc Sci 2008;615:102-18.

[54] Harris JL, Pomeranz JL, Lobstein T, Brownell KD. A crisis in the marketplace: how food marketing contributes to childhood obesity and what can be done. Annu Rev Public Health 2009;30:211-25.

[55] Jones SC, Mannino N, Green J. 'Like me, want me, buy me, eat me': relationship-building marketing communications in children's magazines. Public Health Nutr 2010;13(12):2111-8.

[56] Ben-Sefer E, Ben-Natan M, Ehrenfeld M. Childhood obesity: current literature, policy and implications for practice. Int Nurs Rev 2009;56(2):166-73.

[57] Strasburger VC. Children, adolescents, obesity, and the media. Pediatrics 2011;128(1):201-8.

[58] Vandewater EA, Denis LM. Media, social networking and pediatric obesity. Pediatr Clin North Am 2011;58:1509-19.

[59] Marshall SJ, Biddle SJ, Gorely T, Cameron N, Murdey I. Relationships between media use, body fatness and physical activity in children and youth: a meta-analysis. Int J Obes Relat Metab Disord 2004;28(10):1238-46.

[60] Krebs NF, Jacobson MS. Prevention of pediatric overweight and obesity. Pediatrics 2003;112(2):424-30.

[61] Lyons EJ, Tate DF, Komoski SE, Carr PM, Ward DS. Novel approaches to obesity prevention: effects of game enjoyment and game type on energy expenditure in active video games. J Diabetes Sci Technol 2012;6(4):839-48.

[62] Staiano AE, Abraham AA, Calvert SL. Motivating effects of cooperative exergame play for overweight and obese adolescents. J Diabetes Sci Technol 2012;6(4):812-9.

[63] Staiano AE, Abraham AA, Calvert SL. Adolescent exergame play for weight loss and psychosocial improvement: a controlled physical activity intervention. Obesity (Silver Spring) 2013;21(3):598-601.

[64] Staiano AE, Abraham AA, Calvert SL. Competitive versus cooperative exergame play for African American adolescents' executive function skills: short-term effects in a long-term training intervention. Dev Psychol 2012;48(2):337-42.

[65] Johnston JD, Massey AP, Marker-Hoffman RL. Using an alternate reality game to increase physical activity and decrease obesity risk of college students. J Diabetes Sci Technol 2012;6(4):828-38.

[66] Wakefield MA, Loken B, Hornik RC. Use of mass media campaigns to change health behaviour. Lancet 2010;376(9748):1261-71.

[67] Blumenthal-Barby JS, Burroughs H. Seeking better health care outcomes: the ethics of using the "nudge". Am J Bioeth 2012;12(2):1-10.

[68] Thaler RH, Sunstein CR. Nudge: Improving decisions about health, wealth, and happiness. New York: Penguin Books, 2009.

[69] TheFunTheory.com. Piano stairs 2009. Accessed Sept 7 2012. URL: http://www.youtube.com/watch?v=2lXh2n0aPyw.

[70] Gollwitzer PM. Implementation intentions: Strong effects of simple plans. Am Psychol 1999;54:493-503.

[71] Hommel B, Musseler J, Aschersleben G, Prinz W. The Theory of Event Coding (TEC): a framework for perception and action planning. Behav Brain Sci 2001;24(5):849-78; discussion 878-937.

[72] Adriaanse MA, de Ridder DT, de Wit JB. Finding the critical cue: implementation intentions to change one's diet work best when tailored to personally relevant reasons for unhealthy eating. Pers Soc Psychol Bull 2009;35(1):60-71.

[73] Salvy SJ, Roemmich JN, Bowker JC, Romero ND, Stadler PJ, Epstein LH. Effect of peers and friends on youth physical activity and motivation to be physically active. J Pediatr Psychol 2009;34(2):217-25.

[74] Lewis MA, Neighbors C. Social norms approaches using descriptive drinking norms education: a review of the research on personalized normative feedback. J Am Coll Health 2006;54(4):213-8.

[75] Litt DM, Stock ML. Adolescent alcohol-related risk cognitions: the roles of social norms and social networking sites. Psychol Addict Behav 2011;25(4):708-13.

[76] Sahama T, Liang J, Iannella R. Impact of the social networking applications for health information management for patients and physicians. Stud Health Technol Inform 2012;180:803-7.

Submitted: August 14, 2012 *Revised:* September 30, 2012. *Accepted:* October 01, 2012.

In: Child and Adolescent Health Yearbook 2013
Editor: Joav Merrick

ISBN: 978-1-63117-658-6

Chapter 18

CORRELATES OF BULLYING VICTIMIZATION AMONG IN-SCHOOL ADOLESCENTS IN THE 2005 BOTSWANA GLOBAL SCHOOL-BASED HEALTH SURVEY

Patti Herring, PhD[1], Seter Siziya, BA (Ed), MSc, PhD*[*2], Sricharan Pasupulati, MD, MPH[3], Emmanuel Rudatsikira, MD, MPH, Dr PH[4] and Adamson S Muula, MBBS, MPH, PhD[5]

[1]School of Public Health, Loma Linda University, Loma Linda, California, United States of America
[2]School of Medicine, The Copperbelt University, Ndola, Zambia
[3]School of Community and Environmental Health, Old Dominion University, Norfolk, Virginia, United States of America
[4]School of Health Professions, Andrews University, Berrien Springs, Michigan, United States of America
[5]Department of Community Health, University of Malawi, Blantyre, Malawi

ABSTRACT

Bullying victimization is a major public health problem among adolescents. It is associated with poor academic performance, anxiety, depression and suicidal behaviors. There are limited reports on victimization from bullying among Batswana adolescents. The purpose of this study was to determine the correlates for bullying victimization among school-going adolescents in Botswana. The 2005 Botswana Global School-based Health Survey (GSHS) data were obtained from the World Health Organization. A weighted analysis was conducted using statistical software (SPSS version 15.0). We estimated the prevalence of bullying victimization and conducted logistic regression analysis to estimate associations between the outcome (bullying victimization) and selected explanatory variables. Out of 2,165 in-school adolescents who participated in the

* Correspondence: Professor Seter Siziya, BA (Ed), MSc, PhD, The Copperbelt University, School of Medicine, Department of Clinical Sciences, Public Health Unit, Box 71191, Ndola, Zambia. E-mail: ssiziya@gmail.com.

study, 53.1% (54.2% males and 52.2% females; p=0.086) reported having been bullied in the last 30 days. In multivariate analysis, bullying victimization was positively associated with physical fighting (OR=2.17; 95% CI [1.73, 2.73]), truancy (OR=1.84; 95% CI [1.35, 2.50]), and alcohol drinking (OR=1.41; 95% CI [1.04, 1.91]).Victimization is prevalent among in-school adolescents in Botswana. Efforts to prevent and control bullying should take into consideration the factors identified in this study.

Keywords: Bullying victimization, physical fighting, truancy, alcohol, Botswana

Introduction

Where data are available, bullying victimization is prevalent globally with significant regional variations in the rates of victimization (1-2). In a study on bully victimization among in-school adolescents from five continents, Due et al. (2) reported the highest 30 day prevalence for bullying victimization among boys was in Zimbabwe (70.2%), while Zambia had the highest prevalence for girls (67%). Adverse conditions positively associated with victimization from bullying include serious injuries (3), alcohol and drug use (4), truancy (5), depression (6) and suicidal behaviors (7).

Bullying victimization is common in Botswana among school going adolescents. Fleming and Jacobsen (4) report 30 day rates of being bullied as high as 53.0% with no sex difference (52.2% of females and 54.2% of males). They also considered factors (age, sex, symptoms of depression) associated with being bullied in their study but in their analysis they used the relative risk as a measure of the magnitude of association. Unfortunately the relative risk is not an appropriate measure of association in cross sectional studies. The purpose of this study was to re-analyze the data on correlates for bullying victimization among school-going adolescents in Botswana so that we may provide public health officers, school health and administration officials and other stakeholders with correct results for use in interventions.

Methods

This study was based on a secondary analysis of data from the Botswana Global School-based Student Health Survey (GSHS) that was conducted in 2005. The 2005 Botswana GSHS was a school-based survey which included students in classes with the majority ages of 13-15 years. A two-stage cluster sampling design was used to produce data that were representative of students in the country. At the first stage, schools were selected with probability proportional to enrolment size. At the second stage, classes were randomly selected and all students in selected classes were eligible to participate. There was no replacement of students who were not available despite being in the selected schools. Students self-completed the questionnaires and the responses to questions were indicated on a computer scannable answer sheet.

In order to assess history of victimization from bullying, the question that was asked was: During the past 30 days, on how many days were you bullied? Possible responses included 0 days or any number of days. In terms of involvement in a physical fight, students were asked the question: During the past 12 months, how many times were you in a physical fight? Options included 0 times, one up to 12 or more times.

Ethical considerations

These data were obtained from the World Health Organization. The study was approved by the Botswana Ministry of Health. Parents were informed of the study through a letter, and students gave verbal consent to participate in the survey. To preserve individual confidentiality, the questionnaire was anonymously self-reported by the students.

Data analysis

Cases with missing values were not considered in the analysis. A weighting factor was used in the analysis to account for differences in the probability of selecting a school and classroom, and to account for differences in non response rates for various strata.

Data were first analyzed using SPSS version 11.5. Unweighted frequencies and their weighted percentages are reported. For the main outcome (bullying victimization), we recoded the responses in two categories: 0 for not having been victimized in the past 30 days, and 1 for having been victimized in the past 30 days. We conducted bivariate and multivariate logistic regression analyses in order to estimate associations between independent factors and the outcome variable. The hypotheses were "There were no significant associations between socio-demographic factors and bullying victimization". We report prevalence of bullying victimization within the past 30 days of the survey as well as the unadjusted odds ratios (OR) and adjusted odds ratios (AOR) together with their 95% confidence intervals (CI).

RESULTS

A total of 2,165 students participated in the 2005 Botswana GSHS; and 1829 had information on whether they were bullied or not. Overall, 42.4% were depressed; 22.5% consumed alcohol; and 8.7% had used illicit drugs. More than 1 in five (22.5%) participants reported having missed classes without permission. Altogether, 53.1% (54.2% of male and 52.2% of female) participants reported having been bullied in the previous 30 days to the survey. Further description of the sample by gender is shown in Table 1.

Table 2 reports associations between being bullied and selected factors. Being bullied was positively associated with having engaged in physical fighting (OR=2.17; 95% CI [1.73, 2.73]), self reported feelings of depression (OR=1.40; 95% CI [1.16, 1.77]); truancy (OR=1.84; 95% CI [1.35, 2.50]); and alcohol drinking (OR=1.41; 95% CI [1.04, 1.91]).

DISCUSSION

In a study of bullying victimization among in-school adolescents in Botswana, we found that 53.1% of the respondents were bullied in the last month. This prevalence is higher than the average (32%) for 66 countries and territories from five continents (2). In Africa, that prevalence is lower than 62.8% reported in Zambia (9), but higher than 40.1% in Ghana (8) and 39.6% in neighboring Swaziland (5).

Table 1. Socio-demographic characteristics and bullying victimization of the Botswana study sample, 2005

Factor	Male n (%)	Female n (%)	Total (%)
Age (years)			
< 14	78 (8.0)	131 (11.0)	209 (9.7)
14	190 (19.5)	302 (25.3)	492 (22.7)
15	319 (32.8)	372 (31.2)	6 (1.9)
16 +	385 (39.6)	388 (32.5)	773 (35.7)
Physical fight			
No	458 (47.1)	691 (58.3)	1149 (53.3)
Yes	514 (52.9)	494 (41.7)	1008 (46.7)
Parental supervision			
No	326 (34.5)	348 (30)	674 (32)
Yes	618 (65.5)	811 (70)	1429 (68)
Depression			
No	569 (59.6)	651 (55.7)	1220 (57.5)
Yes	385 (40.4)	518 (44.3)	903 (42.5)
Cigarette smoking			
No	817 (89)	1083 (95.2)	1900 (92.4)
Yes	101 (11)	55 (4.8)	156 (7.6)
Alcohol drinking			
No	596 (75.9)	795 (78.8)	1391 (77.5)
Yes	189 (24.1)	214 (21.2)	403 (22.5)
Drug use			
No	840 (86.3)	1138 (95.4)	1978 (91.3)
Yes	133 (13.7)	55 (4.6)	188 (8.7)
Truancy			
No	665 (70.2)	950 (80.3)	1615 (75.8)
Yes	282 (29.8)	233 (19.7)	515 (24.2)
Bullied			
No	377 (45.8)	481 (47.8)	858 (46.9)
Yes	446 (54.2)	525 (52.2)	971 (53.1)

We found that bullying victimization was positively associated with reported depression, having engaged in physical fighting, truancy, and alcohol drinking. In a study of the association between bullying and psychological health among senior high school students in Ghana, Owuso et al. found that bullying victimization was positively associated with depression, suicide ideation, and loneliness (8).The association between bullying victimization and physical fighting was reported previously in other settings such as Zambia (9), Philippines (10) and China (11). In a study of the association between physical bullying victimization and physical fighting among Filipino school going adolescents, Rudatsikira et al. reported a dose-response relationship between the two (10). Previous studies have reported the relationship between bullying victimization and alcohol use and other substances (12,13).

In this study, there was no significant gender difference in bullying victimization. Some studies have reported similar findings (8,10) while others have reported that males were more likely to be bullied than females (9,11). What is consistent in the literature is the gender difference in the types of bullying victimization; males are more at risk for physical victimization while females are more at risk of relational or emotional victimization (14-15).

Table 2. Factors associated with being bullied among in-school adolescents in Botswana, 2005

Factor	Bullied n (%)	OR[1] (95% CI[3])	AOR[2] (95% CI)
Age (years)			
< 14	89 (9.2)	0.95 (0.67-1.35)	1.12 (0.76-1.67)
14	216 (22.3)	0.83 (0.59-1.16)	1.06 (0.79-1.43)
15	309 (31.9)	0.82 (0.59-1.14)	0.97 (0.74-1.28)
16+	355 (36.6)	1	1
Sex			
Male	446 (45.5)	1.08 (0.90-1.30)	0.92 (0.73-1.16)
Female	525 (54.5)	1	1
Physical fight			
No	409 (42.3)	1	1
Yes	557 (57.7)	2.89 (2.38-3.50)	2.17 (1.73-2.73)
Depression			
No	495 (52.2)	1	1
Yes	454 (47.8)	1.74 (1.44 - 2.10)	1.40 (1.16-1.77)
Cigarette smoking			
No	807 (88.8)	1	1
Yes	102 (11.2)	3.54 (2.31 - 5.40)	1.36 (0.77-2.40)
Drug use			
No	853 (88.1)	1	1
Yes	115 (11.9)	3.01 (2.06 - 4.42)	1.26 (0.7-2.26)
Truancy			
No	666 (69.1)	1	1
Yes	287 (30.1)	2.63 (2.10 - 3.33)	1.84 (1.35-2.5)
Parental supervision			
No	314 (33.1)	1	1
Yes	634 (66.9)	0.87 (0.70 - 1.10)	0.80 (0.85-1.37)
Alcohol drinking			
No	538 (69.7)	1	1
Yes	238 (30.7)	2.44 (1.90-3.13)	1.41 (1.04-1.91)

[1] OR Unadjusted odds ratio.
[2] AOR Adjusted odds ratio.
[3] CI confidence interval.

Limitations and strengths of the study

The present study has several limitations and strengths. Data were collected through self-reports. To the extent that study participants mis-reported, intentionally or not, our findings may be biased. The study design was cross sectional which limits us from ascribing causation between the outcome and explanatory variables. It is also important to note that different studies have defined bullying differently. For instance, Sourander et al. (16) defined bullying as "an aggressive act embodying an imbalance of power in which the victims cannot defend themselves accompanied by an element of repetition." Our study only asked whether students had been bullied. However, the sample size was large thus improving precision of the effect measure estimates. That this study is a secondary analysis of existing data can be both a strength and a weakness. A strength in that the subjects' responses could be accurate as study participants may not have anticipated any links between outcome variable and explanatory variables, hence truthful reporting; and a weakness in that there are likely to be several unmeasured confounders that a primary study could have planned to measure.

Conclusion

In this study, we found that bullying victimization was prevalent among school-going adolescents in Botswana. Efforts to prevent and control bullying should take into consideration the factors identified in this study.

Acknowledgments

We thank the World Health Organization for availing the data for further analysis and the students for their participation in the survey.

References

[1] Craig W, Harel-Fisch Y, Fogel-Grinvald H, Dostaler S, Hetland J, Simons-Morton B, et al. A cross-national profile of bullying and victimization among adolescents in 40 countries. Int J Public Health 2009;54(Suppl 2):216-24.

[2] Due P, Holstein BE, Soc MS. Bullying victimization among 13 to 15-year old school children: results from two comparative studies in 66 countries and regions. Int J Adolesc Med Health 2008;20:209-21.

[3] Muula AS, Siziya S, Rudatsikira E. Prevalence and socio-demographic correlates of serious injuries among adolescents participating in the Djibouti 2007 Global School-based Health Survey. BMC Research Notes 2011;4:372.

[4] Fleming LC, Jacobsen KH. Bullying among middle-school students in low and middle income countries. Health PromotInt 2010;25:73-84.

[5] Siziya S, Muula AS, Rudatsikira E. Prevalence and correlates of truancy among adolescents in Swaziland: findings from the Global School-based Health Survey. Child Adolesc Psychiatr Ment Health 2007;1:15.

[6] Fleming LC, Jacobsen KH. Bullying and symptoms of depression in Chilean middle school students. J Sch Health 2009;79:130-7.

[7] Klomek AB, Sourander A, Niemela S, Kumpulainen H, Piha J, Tamminen T, et al. Childhoold bullying behavior as a risk for suicide attempts and complete suicides: a population-based birth cohort study. J Am Acad Child Adolesc Psychiatry 2009;48:254-61.

[8] Owusu A, Hart P, Oliver B, Kang M. The association between bullying and psychological health among senior high school students in Ghana, West Africa. J Sch Health 2011;81:231-8.

[9] Siziya S, Rudatsikira E, Muula AS. Victimization from bullying among school-attending adolescents in grades 7 to 10 in Zambia. J Inj Violence Res 2012;4:30-5.

[10] Rudatsikira E, Mataya RH, Siziya S, Muula AS. Association between bullying victimization and physical fighting among Filipino adolescents: results from the Global School-Based Health Survey. Indian J Pediatr 2008;75:1243-7.

[11] Hazemba A, Siziya S, Muula AS, Rudatsikira E. Prevalence and correlates of being bullied among in-school adolescents in Beijing: results from the 2003 Beijing Global School-Based Health Survey. Ann Gen Psychiatry 2008;7:6.

[12] Swahn MH, Topalli V, Strasser SM, Ashby JS, Meyers J. Pre-teen alcohol use as a risk factor for victimization and perpetration of bullying among middle and high school students in Georgia. West J Emerg Med 2011;12:305-9.

[13] Radliff KM, Wheaton JE, Robinson K, Morris J. Illuminating the relationship between bullying and substance use among middle and high school youth. Addict Behav 2012;37:569-72.

[14] Hampel P. Direct and relational bullying among children and adolescents: coping and psychological adjustment. SchPsycholInt 2009;30:474-90.

[15] Frisen A, Jonsson A, Persson C. Adolescents's perception of bullying: who is the victim? Who is the bully? What can be done to stop bullying? Adolescence 2007;42:749-61.

[16] Sourander A, Ronning J, Brunstein-Klomek A, Gyllenberg D, Kumpulainen K, Niemelä S, Helenius H, Sillanmäki L, Ristkari T, Tamminen T, Moilanen I, Piha J, Almqvist F. Childhood bullying behavior and later psychiatric hospital and psychopharmacologic treatment: findings from the Finnish 1981 birth cohort study. Arch Gen Psychiatry 2009;66:1005-12.

Submitted: April 25, 2012. *Revised:* June 15, 2012. *Accepted:* June 21, 2012.

In: Child and Adolescent Health Yearbook 2013
Editor: Joav Merrick

ISBN: 978-1-63117-658-6

Chapter 19

AGGRESSION AMONG CHANDIGARH HIGH SCHOOL STUDENTS: TO KNOW THE PREVALENCE AND LEVEL OF AGGRESSION IN TERMS OF GENDER

Manmeet Kaur Reen, BSC, MSC, APGDCGFC *
and Deepali Sharma, PhD
Department of Human Development and Family Relations, Government Home Science College, Panjab University, Chandigarh, India

ABSTRACT

A comparative study was carried out on a sample of 140 school going adolescents from class IX. A standardized questionnaire was administered to determine the prevalence of aggression in adolescents of private and government schools of Chandigarh . The results were analyzed using t-test. Regarding the school type, there were no significant differences between adolescents coming from government schools and those studying in private schools. Related to the sub scales of aggression, there was no gender difference except for the Anger scale (AngS) in which female respondents showed significantly higher scores as compared to their male counterparts. The findings highlighted the need of intervention aimed at anger management. Workshops and seminars can also be organized for parents, teachers and adolescents on adolescents' aggressive behavior.

Keywords: Adolescence, aggression, gender, school type

* **Correspondence**: Manmeet Kaur Reen, BSC, MSC,APGDCGFC, Department of Human Development and Family Relations, Government Home Science College, Panjab University, Chandigarh, Chandigarh, India. E-mail: manmeetreen@ymail.com

INTRODUCTION

Adolescence is viewed as a period during which biological, cognitive, emotional and social changes and development takes place. Because of reorganization in all of the developmental areas, young children face various behavioral of adjustment problems (1). It is often assumed that this is a difficult period of life, with the adolescents being at risk of high stress, since they have to cope with enormous changes. Some of these changes are in the physical and sexual behavior following puberty, some of the social and financial area, and some relate to decisions about the future .Thus, this period is certainly a period of change in which the adolescents are burdened by various pressures (2).

It is very important that adolescents pass through this stage successful otherwise problems may occur which may further lead to the formation of various kinds of deviant behavior like aggression, drug and alcohol use. Erikson (3) further argues that adolescents typically experience diffusion, a strong sense of uncertainty and need to achieve a sense of identity. But at this phase of life they find it hard to do this and are always perturbed about who they are and what their future will be? Such unanswered questions might lead to frustration and aggressive behavior among the adolescents (4,5).

Further, biological or hormonal changes in adolescents (increased level of androgen and testosterone) are also associated with behavioral problems like rebelliousness, talking back to adults, and fighting with classmates (6).

Thus, emphasizing upon the critical nature of adolescent stage, it is apparent that adolescence and aggression cannot be separated. Many studies tracing the problems of adolescence over several decades have shown an increase in the rate of aggression among the adolescents (7).

Aggression is defined as physical or verbal behavior intended to harm. Aggression can either be directed inward by self mutilation, or directed outwardly at another person. Aggressive behavior is often used to claim status, precedents or access to an object or territory (8). According to Eysenck (2), two kinds of aggression are identified namely, person oriented and instrumental aggression. Person oriented aggression is designed to hurt someone else were causing harm in the main goal. In contrast, instrumental aggression has its main goal in obtaining some desired reward with aggression. Another category of aggression is based on the initiator of the aggression.

Proactive aggression is aggressive behavior that is initiated by the individual to achieve some desired outcomes whereas reactive aggression in an individual reaction to someone else aggression.

These distinctions clearly revealed that aggression is not simple but a complicated aspect .It is not a single idea but it is of various types such as physical or verbal aggression.

Physical aggression

As the word indicates physical aggression is any response that produces or is intended to produce physical injury or physical pain in the victim or damage to an object. It involves the acts of hitting and kicking (9). The large body mass or higher physical development among the early adolescents is also an important predictor of the growing physical aggression among them. This is particularly supported by Trembley (10) who studied the association among the testosterone, physical development, and social behavior during early adolescence. He suggests that adolescents with larger body masses are more likely to be physically aggressive or socially dominant and tend to have higher testosterone levels, when provoked; adolescents tend to show physical aggressive behavior; like they would hit the person who irritates them.

Verbal aggression

Burbank (11) reports that children are involved in violence and physical aggression until they have attained the verbal skills but when these are developed, physical aggression is replaced by verbal aggression up to some extent. Infante (12) reveals that verbal aggression is a message behavior, which harms the self esteem of a person and thus produces psychological pain. Broadly speaking, verbal aggression is any response that produces psychological or social harm to the victim, hurt feelings, and damage to one's reputation, devaluation that could result in loss of prize, a job, and so forth. Nasty remarks, name calling are the active and verbal forms of verbal aggression whereas stony silence or sulking form a part of passive and non verbal aggression. In general terms verbal aggression is confined to yelling and screaming at others. Verbal aggression is a softer part than the physical aggression and is generally done for betterment. As Burbank (11) reports that verbal aggression is used for escape from demanding or difficult situations, and relief from stress. In the highly competitive world of today's adolescents feel a threat to their identity, so in this process of getting the attention they always try to make others agree with their viewpoints. But when others disagree, they get into conflicts, indulge in heated arguments, and show verbal aggression.

Anger

Good enough and Gesell (13, 14) report that infants and young children respond in anger in a direct and primitive manner, but as they develop the responses become less violent and more symbolic. In the early school years anger reactions become more directed toward a single person and take the form of attempts to hurt the feeling rather than to injure the body of the offender. In the middle school years, the anger is shown more on verbal plane. Anger reaction is displaced on others rather than on the person himself. The study also suggested that children think themselves as bosses if they shout or show violent reaction towards their peers.

Indirect aggression

Indirect aggression means telling untruth behind the back, starts being somebody else's friend in revenge, abuses, argues, sulks, take revenge in play (9).

Theoretical orientation

The study of aggression is a perfect example of nature-nurture debate, which is of central concern in many psychological arguments. The question being asked is whether aggression, as a characteristic of human being, is biologically determined or product of learning and environmental influences.

At this stage the aggression is shown mainly due to the situation or environmental conditions. So, frustration aggression theory and the negative affect theory explain the behavior of the individual during early adolescent periods.

- ***Frustration aggression theory***

Frustration always causes aggression and aggression is always the result of frustration. Aggression is therefore, triggered by frustrating situations and events. Therefore, people are driven to aggression in order to reduce frustration and thus to maintain a balanced internal state (15). Berkowitz (16) modified this original hypothesis to suggest that frustration actually produces a state of readiness for aggression, but that causes the situation are also important. The key concept to grasp this theory is that an external stimulus leads to behavioral response. In this particular topic frustration is the stimulus which leads to an aggressive response.

- ***Negative affect theory***

It states that negative feelings and experiments are the main cause of anger and angry aggression. Sources of anger include: - pain, frustration, loud noises, foul odors, crowding, sadness and depression (16).

The likelihood that an angry person will act aggressively depends on his or her interpretation of the motives of the people involved. It is most applicable to adolescents and adults, who think well and already know lots about the world.

Various other important theories that explain the aggression are:

- ***Psychoanalytical theory***

Freud theorized that human are born with an instinct towards life (which he called Eros) and an instinct towards death (called Thanatos). The death instinct, Freud argued needs to be released through aggression. Freud also stated that there is a conflict between Eros and Thanatos, some of the negative energy of the Thanatos is directed towards others, to prevent the self destruction of the individual. Thus, Freud claimed that the displacement of negative energy of the Thanatos onto others is the basis of aggression (17).

- ***Evolutionary theory or ethnological and socio-biological views***

It states that humans are born with fighting instinct and aggression is built into our nature. Lorenz looked at instinctual aggressiveness as a product of evolution. In essence, he combined Freud's theory of aggression with Charles Darwin's natural selection theory (18).

- ***Social learning theory***

The theory is interested in observational learning and modeling. In this theory, aggression is initially learned from social behavior and it is maintained by operant conditioning (19, 20).

RATIONALE

Adolescence is a crucial stage that involves going through varied physical and emotional changes. One of the most important behavior aspects during adolescence is aggression which is likely to be influenced by gender, and school type. Limited work is available in this area thus suggesting the crucial need to understand the influence of these independent variables on the aggressive behavior of the adolescents.

Are boys more physically aggressive than girls? Are girls more verbally aggressive? How does school environment effect aggressive behavior? Based on study it will hopefully be possible to identify the areas of intervention further promotes the well being of the adolescent.

The following were the objectives of the study:

- To assess the prevalence and level of aggression among high school students.
- To examine gender differences among the respondents related to aggression.

METHODS

The present research was planned as a comparative study on aggression carried out on a sample of 140 school going adolescents (70 Government and 70 from Private schools in Chandigarh. For the present study, aggression was the independent variable and gender and type of school were the dependent variables.

Sample

This study was conducted in Chandigarh and purposive sampling was done when it came to the selection of the school and participants. In total four schools were selected which represented the government and private schools. Care was taken that these four schools represented in the four geographical zones of Chandigarh. Within the government and private schools, the respondents were randomly selected. The sample was further segregated into the sub-category of gender i.e., boys and girls.

Assessment measures

- ***Background information***

A personal information sheet was prepared to collect the background information of the adolescents (Appendix A). It contained questions related to demographic factors such as age, school, gender, class, family type and birth order.

- ***The Aggression Questionnaire (2000)***

A standardized questionnaire was administered to determine the prevalence of aggression in adolescents (Appendix A). The questionnaire had 34 items with the following areas: (i) general information (for example: name, age, gender, type of family, etc.); (ii) physical aggression (for example: I have threatened people I know, I get into fights more than most people); (iii) Verbal aggression (for example: my friends say that I argue a lot, I cannot help getting into arguments when people disagree with me); (iv) Anger (for example: some of my friends think I am short tempered, I have trouble controlling my temper); (v) Hostility (for example: I know that friends talk about me behind my back, I wonder what people want when they are nice to me); (vi) Indirect aggression (for example: I have been angry enough to bang a door when leaving someone behind in the room, I sometimes spread gossip about people I do not like).

The application of the test was discussed among the investigative team and accordingly changes were made. Certain statements or words in the tool that were not applicable in the Indian context were reworded.

The calculation of the level of aggression was done by converting raw scores into T scores by applying the formula given below:

$$T = 50 + 10(X - Y)/Z$$

Where,

X=Raw scores of the students
Y=Average score of the whole cohort
Z=Standard deviation

The previous reports of reliability (coefficient alpha) suggest good to moderate reliability: Physical Aggression ($r = .88$), Verbal Aggression ($r = .76$), Anger ($r = .78$), Hostility ($r = .82$), Indirect Aggression ($r = .71$), and the Total scale ($r = .94$) (Buss & Warren, 2000).

Procedure

The students were contacted by taking an appointment from the school authorities and permission letters were granted by the Principal to conduct the tests. During the meeting with the Principals, the purpose of the study was also explained to them.

Class visits were made to meet the students and build rapport with them. The significance of the study was also explained. Their consent was taken and background information was collected from the students. Questionnaires were administered on both boys and girls and the doubts were clarified. The instructions about the questionnaire were given to students that for each statement they have to select the most preferred option amongst the given options.

- ***Coding***

The coding format was established and worked out by the team of investigators. The data were organized through coding. The purpose was to make it easier to tabulate the information and analyze the data for quantitative analysis. The coded data were entered using SPSS 16.0 version, which is standard statistical software, used for the purpose of analysis in the field of social sciences.

- ***Plan of analysis***

The data were analyzed by computing frequencies and percentages with the help of SPSS software to compare the responses of girls and boys from different government and private school. For analyzing the significant differences in the mean scores, t-test was employed.

RESULTS

The study was conducted on boys and girls of different schools of Chandigarh. It aimed at studying aggression among adolescent: to know the prevalence and level of aggression in terms of gender.

- ***Demographic characteristics***

There was a total sample of 140 students. Amongst them 77 were males and 63 were females. Most of the students constituting the sample were in the age group of 14 years. Most of them were from the nuclear family and the birth order was 1st or 2nd in majority of the sample. The study followed objectives: 1. To assess the prevalence and level of aggression among high school students. 2. To examine gender differences among the respondents related to aggression. Adolescents displayed average scores on aggression. There was no significant difference between the mean scores of the males and the females, on the overall aggression scores (see Table 1).Related to the sub scales of anger there were no gender differences noted on any of the sub scales except for the Anger scale (AngS) which had items like; "I get angry easily, but get over my anger quickly.", "At times I feel like a bomb ready to explode." etc. Female respondents showed significantly higher scores as compared to the males (see Table 2 and Figure 1).

DISCUSSION

The purpose of the study was to assess the prevalence and level of aggression among Chandigarh high school students and to examine gender differences among the respondents related to aggression. The data were gathered using the standardized questionnaire.

The average score on aggression and no significant difference between the mean scores of the males and the females are evident from the results of the present study.

Table 1. Mean aggression scores

Gender	N	Mean	Standard deviation	T scores
Female	63	49.52	9.65	.05
Male	77	49.62	10.05	

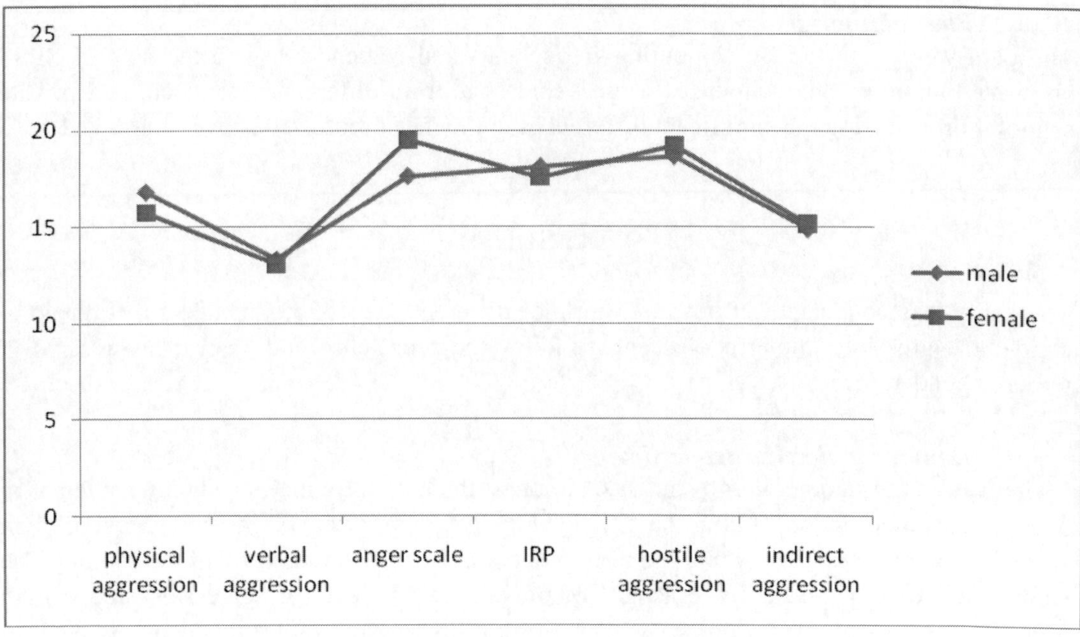

Figure 1. Mean aggression according to different sub scales of male and female respondents.

Table 2. Mean aggression according to different sub scales

Sub Scale	Gender	N	Mean	Standard deviation	t score
Physical Aggression	Female	63	15.74	5.79	1.06
	Male	77	16.83	6.18	
Verbal Aggression	Female	63	13.09	3.82	.37
	Male	77	13.33	3.77	
Anger Scale	Female	63	19.50	4.70	2.17
	Male	77	17.64	5.28	
IRP	Female	63	17.57	5.65	.55
	Male	77	18.12	6.22	
Hostile reaction	Female	63	19.19	5.57	.54
	Male	77	18.67	5.52	
Indirect Anger	Female	63	15.17	4.47	.34
	Male	77	14.90	4.61	

There were no gender differences found on any of the sub scales except the Anger Scale (AngS) for which many reasons can be attributed, which are as follows:

- ***Changing role of society***

Garg (21) attributes significantly higher score of the female respondents' to change in the pattern of Indian society in which appropriate sex role for females are being and replaced by more gender balanced behavior. Research has determined the anger is an important correlate of student aggression, and that there is a clear link between high levels of anger and problem behavior in school, poor academic performance, peer rejection, and psychosomatic complaints (22). Moreover, uncontrolled anger is cited as one of the factors linked to serious violence.

- ***Early Maturation***

The age of beginning of pubertal changes is gradually coming down and due to which adolescents go through varied physical and emotional changes. One of the most important behavior aspect during adolescence is aggression. As adolescence is a high stressful age, because of these adolescents become frustrated and thus show aggression (2).

- ***Exposure to Mass Media***

One of the reasons for no significant difference in the level of aggression in males and females could be exposure to mass media. Huesmann & Eron found increasing rates of aggression for both boys and girls who are exposed to media (23). A high percentage of females prefer to watch a family drama in comparison, to males, who prefer to watch action based programs.

- ***Maternal employment***

Maternal Employment could also be one of the reasons as there is a lack of supervision and parent–child interaction due to maternal employment, the child might indulge in experimentation, risky behavior and delinquent acts (21).

- ***Consumption of junk food***

Due to the change in the life style pattern and westernization the children are consuming more of junk food, which are high in carbohydrates. This results in a high body mass index that lead to attainment of puberty at an early age due to which hormonal changes take place, which may lead to aggression (24).

IMPLICATIONS

These findings can be useful for providing information to the school teachers about the average level of aggression among adolescents. Necessary interventions can be provided on the basis of this research. Physical aggression (as well as property violation) uniquely contributes to each of the health risk behaviors from preschool onwards. This suggests that preventive interventions aimed at physical aggression could be initiated in early childhood in an effort to reduce the risk of each of these outcomes (25). The psychologist and educators should be aware of the peer group interactions that reinforce aggressive behaviors. The intervention programs should extend beyond aggressive children to address the attitude and norms of the peer group that may support aggression and antisocial behaviors (26).

The intervention measures that include parents, peers and individual adolescents may help decrease the aggressive and conduct problems (27). Some workshops can also be organized for parents, teachers and adolescents on anger management. Follow up activities focused on learning and practicing accepting alternatives to aggression. The focus may need to be placed on a child's ability to maintain productive relationships with authority .It may also include opportunities to learn and practice constructive alternatives to non productive arguments and verbal assaults (28, 29).

LIMITATION OF THE STUDY

The participants were only school going adolescents and therefore, it cannot be applied to the same age children who do not go to school.

ACKNOWLEDGMENTS

For the successful completion of this paper, I express my deep gratification to Dr. Deepali Sharma, Assistant Professor, Department of Human Development and Family Relations, Government Home Science College, sector 10, Chandigarh, under whose guidance the present work was carried out. I am grateful for her whole hearted help, keen interest, constructive criticism and valuable suggestions. A special thanks to Dr. Suman Verma, Head of Department of Human Development and Family Relations, Government Home Science College, sector 10, Chandigarh, for her guidance and help. I find it hard to verbalize my deepest sense of gratitude and reverence to my parents Col. Manjeet Singh Reen (Retd.) and Mrs. Satwant Kaur Reen as well as brother Maj. Sarabjeet Singh Reen and sister Dt. Ravleen Kaur Reen for their boundless, support, care, understanding and patience that really helped me to accomplish this work.

I thank the following people whose assistance made this study possible Vandana Vohra, Rashi, Tarneet, Harleen, Renu, Vandana, Kanika, Rishya, Sukhwinder, Kamaldeep, Sofina, Navdeep and Nriti. A word of thanks to all the principals of respective schools, for giving their kind permission to proceed with my research study. I will be failing in my duty if I do not pay my regards to all our respondents for giving me their precious time and cooperation.

(APPENDIX A)

Dear Students,

You are being provided with a battery of self report tests that will assist you gain greater insights into yourself. The goal of these tests is not to provide you with new information about yourself, but rather to help you achieve a better understanding of the barriers that might be standing in your way of a more satisfying and effective life .We hope you enjoy this process of self discovery and find information that will help you have a more satisfying and effective life.

Best wishes
Manmeet Kaur Reen

THE AGGRESSION QUESTIONNAIRE

Name: ______________________________Age: ______________
Gender: Male________Female_______ Class: _________ Section: ______________
School: ____
Birth order: 1st born ______________ 2nd born ____________ 3rd born __________
Type of family: Nuclear ____________ Joint __________ Extended ____________
Please ticks mark the appropriate response.

Answer Key:1= Not at all like me; 2= A little like me; 3=Somewhat like me ; 4=Very much like me; 5 = Completely like me

S. No.	Statement	1	2	3	4	5
1.	My friends say that I argue a lot.					
2.	I let my anger show when I do not get what I want.					
3.	I wonder why sometimes I feel so unpleasant about things.					
4.	At times I feel like a bomb ready to explode.					
5.	I have threatened people I know.					
6.	If I am angry enough, I may spoil someone's work.					
7.	I get into fights more than most people.					
8.	I may hit someone if he or she upsets me.					
9.	At times I can't control the feeling to hit someone.					
10.	If somebody hits me, I hit back.					
11.	If I have to use violence to protect myself I will.					
12.	I get into fights more than the most people.					
13.	I have become so angry that I have broken things.					
14.	I can't help getting into arguments when people disagree with me .					
S. No.	Statement	1	2	3	4	5
15.	I often find myself disagreeing with people.					
16.	When people annoy me ,I may tell them what I think of them .					
17.	I tell my friends openly when I am disagree with them.					
18.	I get angry easily, but get over my anger quickly.					
19.	I am a calm person.					
20.	Some of my friends think I am a short tempered.					
21.	At times, I feel that life has been unfair towards me.					
22.	I have trouble controlling my anger.					
23.	I do not trust strangers who are too friendly.					
24.	Other people are luckier than me.					
25.	At times, I feel that life has been unfair towards me.					
26.	I wonder what people want when they are nice to me.					

S. No.	Statement	1	2	3	4	5
27.	I sometimes feel that people are laughing at me behind my back.					
28.	I know that "friends" talk about me behind my back.					
29.	At times, I am so jealous that I cannot think of anything else.					
30.	When people are bossy, I take my time doing what they want, just to show them.					
31.	When someone really irritates me, I might give him or her silent treatment.					
32.	I like to play practical jokes.					
33.	I have been angry enough to bang a door when leaving someone behind in the room.					
34.	I sometimes spread gossip about people I do not like.					

REFERENCES

[1] Suman EJ, Dorn LD, Schiefelblin VL. Puberty, sexuality, and health. In: Lerner RM, Brooks MAE, eds. Handbook of psychology: Developmental psychology. New York: Wiley, 2003:295-324.

[2] Eysenck, Michael W, Keane, Mark T. Cognitive psychology: A student's handbook, 4th ed. New York: Psychology Press, 2000.

[3] Erickson E. School literacy, reasoning, and civility: An anthropologist's perspective. Rev Educ Res 1984;54(4):525-46.

[4] Miller NE, Dollard J. Social learning and imitation. New Haven: Yale University Press, 1941.

[5] Glanz K, Rimer BK, Lewis FM. Health behavior and health education. Theory, research and practice. San Fransisco: Wiley, 2002.

[6] 24. Hendry LB, Patrick H. Adolescents and television. J Youth Adolesc 1972;6(4):325-36.

[7] Zanden J. Human development, 7th ed. Boston: McGraw-Hill Higher Education, 2000.

[8] Muuss A. A concept analysis of relational aggression. J Psychiatr Ment Health Nurs 1995;14(5):510-5.

[9] Davis JQ. Anger, aggression, and adolescents. New York: Pantheon Books, 2004.

[10] Underwood MK. Social aggression among girls. New York: Guilford, 2003.

[11] Tremblay R. Testosterone, physical aggression, dominance, and physical development in early adolescence. Int J Behav Dev 1998;22(4):753-77.

[12] Burbank VK. Cross-cultural perspectives on aggression in women and girls: An introduction. Sex Roles 1994;30:169-76.

[13] Infante DA. Teaching students to understand and control verbal aggression. Commun Educ 1995;44:51-63.

[14] Goodenough FL.Anger in young children. Minnesota: Minnesota Press, 1931.

[15] Gesell A. Youth the years from ten to sixteen. New York: HarperCollins, 1956.

[16] Dollard J. Frustration and aggression. Yale: Yale University Press, 1939.

[17] Berkowitz L. Aggression: Its causes, consequences, and control. New York: McGraw-Hill, 1993.

[18] Freud S. The ego and the mechanisms of defense. London: Hogarth Press, 1937.

[19] Lorenz K. On aggression. London: Methuen, 1996.

[20] Bandura A. Imitation of film-mediated aggressive models. J Abnorm Soc Psychol 1963;66: 3-11.

[21] Bandura A. Transmission of aggression through imitation of aggressive models. J Abnorm Soc Psychol 1961;63:575-82.

[22] Garg R. A comparative study of aggression among adolescents with respect to gender and maternal employment. Dissertation. Panjab: Panjab University Dept Hum Dev Fam Relat, 2002.

[23] 22. Smith DC, Furlong MJ. Correlates of anger, hostility, and aggression in children and adolescents. In: Furlong MJ, Smith DC, eds. Anger, hostility, and aggression: Assessment, prevention, and intervention strategies for youth. New York: Wiley, 1994:15-38.

[24] Huesmann LR, Eron LD, eds. Television and the aggression child: A cross national comparison. Hillsdale, NJ: Erlbaum,1986.

[25] Reen M K: Sexual behavior, Knowledge and attitude towards reproductive health issues of college going girls in Chandigarh. Dissertation. Panjab: Panjab University Dept Hum Dev Fam Relat, 2009.

[26] Timmermans M, Lier P, Koot HM. Which forms of adolescent external behaviors account for late adolescent risky sexual behavior and substance use? J Child Psychol Psychiatr 2008;49(4): 386-94.

[27] Lee E. The relationship of aggression and bullying to social preference: Differences in gender and types of aggression. Int J Behav Dev 2009;33(4):323-30.

[28] Barnow S, Lutch M, Freyberger H-J. Correlates of aggressive and delinquent conduct problems in adolescence. Behavior Problems Adolesc 2005;31:24-39.

[29] Buss AH, Warren WL. The aggression questionnaire. Los Angeles, CA: Western Psychological Services, 2000.

[30] Buss A, Perry M. The aggression questionnaire. J Pers Soc Psychol 1992;63:452–9.

Submitted: April 31, 2012. *Revised:* June 10, 2012. *Accepted:* June 21, 2012.

In: Child and Adolescent Health Yearbook 2013
Editor: Joav Merrick

ISBN: 978-1-63117-658-6

Chapter 20

PREVALENCE OF MALTREATMENT OF ADOLESCENTS AMONG HIGH SCHOOL CHILDREN IN KERALA

Jyothi Manoj, MPhil* and Josmy Thomas, MSc
Kristu Jayanti College, Bangalore, Karnataka and St Joseph's Hospital, Dharmagiri, Kothamangalam, Kerala, India

ABSTRACT

Purpose was to retrospectively analyze the awareness of adolescents about child rights and assess the prevalence of maltreatment. Methods: 300 students from two schools in Calicut district participated in a cross sectional study. The participants were 153(51%) boys and 147(49%) girls with median age 14 and range 3. Results: 53.67% of the children have poor awareness of child rights and maltreatment. The results provide baseline information on the prevalence and types of maltreatment children face. 47% were exposed to physical maltreatment, 47.6% has suffered emotional maltreatment, 16.7% sexual maltreatment, 29.7% neglect. There is no gender difference in exposure to the types of maltreatments (chi square $p > 0.05$) except sexual maltreatment where boys were found more vulnerable. Monthly income of the family and parents educational level has an influence on prevalence of maltreatment. Conclusion: Child maltreatment is highly prevalent among school children. We suggest schools must introduce interventions which incorporate personal safety, prevention of abuse and mental health issues for students and government and NGOs should develop programmes and counseling to create awareness among parents and teachers to build up a healthy generation.

Keywords: Adolescents, maltreatment, child rights, principal component analysis

* Correspondence: Jyothi Manoj, Assistand professor, Department of Statistics, Kristu Jayanti College, Bangalore-77, India. E-mail: jyothimanoj@kristujayanticollege.com.

INTRODUCTION

Child maltreatment is a state of emotional, physical, economic and sexual about meted out to a person below the age of eighteen and is a globally prevalent phenomenon. However, in India, as in many other countries, there has been no understanding of the extent, magnitude and trends of the problem (1). Children are not recognised as subjects of human rights and adults play arbitrary limits on children's fundamental freedom. Teachers and parents have broad discretionary powers and can restrict children freedom with little accountability. Most of the restrictions that children face on a daily basis are not entrenched in law but are part of school or family rules (2). Discipline is something adults do with and for children, rather than to children to stop them from behaving in undesirable ways (3). Child abuse is more than bruises and broken bones. While physical abuse might be the most visible sign, other types of abuse, such as emotional abuse or child neglect, also leave deep, long lasting scars (4). The impact that child maltreatment leaves has long lasting effects throughout life, damaging a child's sense of self, ability to have healthy relationships, and ability to function at home, at work and at school. There is dearth of research done on the broad array of disciplining techniques adopted in schools of India. This study aims to analyze the awareness of high school children about their own rights that Indian Judiciary dictates for them which will help them protect themselves from being abused. The study also attempts to estimate the prevalence of maltreatment.

METHODS

The study was carried out as a cross sectional survey 2 high schools in Calicut district of Kerala. The participants were recruited to in the study via a stratified random sampling technique with age as factor for stratification. A sample of 300 children was selected. A self-report questionnaire developed and piloted in collaboration with the adolescents, elicited information on socioeconomic status, demographic profile, knowledge regarding child rights and adolescent maltreatment and their experience of maltreatment at home and school. The participants were 150 (50%) rural and remaining urban, 153 (51%) were boys and 147 (49%) girls with median age 14 and range 3. After obtaining institutional ethical clearance, data was collected by the investigators. Statistical analysis was carried out by using SPSS version 17.

RESULTS

Reliability test of the tool suggests that the items in the questionnaire are relevant and ensures the randomness of the data. (Chronback Alpha = 0.94). 50% of the children are from rural area and remaining urban. 83.3% (250) of the children have both their parents together while 14% (42) of their parents are abroad and stay with caretakers and 2.3% (8) have single parents. 75.7% (227) of the children come from nuclear family, 15% (45) of them from three generation families and remaining from joint families. 42% (126) of the families have monthly income less than 5000, 22% (66) have monthly income between 5000 – and 10,000 and the rest 36% earn more than 10000 as monthly income. Based on the response to the set of 15 questions on awareness of child rights, children were classified to have poor awareness about child rights if less than 6 answers were right, moderate awareness if 6 -10 answers were right and the rest to have good awareness. The information was elicited in table 1.

Table 1. Distribution of awareness of children about maltreatment and child rights based on gender

	Poor	Average	Good
Male	94(31.67%)	28(9.33%)	27(9%)
Female	63(21%)	35(11.67%)	49(16.33%)
Total	161 (53.67%)	63 (21%)	76(25.33%)

Table 2. Distribution of awareness of children about maltreatment and child rights based on locality

Area of residence	Poor	Average	Good
Urban	69(23%)	22(7.33%)	59(19.67%)
Rural	92(30.67%)	41(13.67%)	17(5.66%)
Total	161 (53.67%)	63 (21%)	76(25.33%)

Percentage of adolescents who have awareness about child rights and various types of maltreatment, by gender (n = 300)

The analysis reveals that 161 (53.67%) of them had poor knowledge about their rights. Boys lack awareness (31.67%) than girls (21%). When urban and rural children were compared, it was found that among the urban children 19.67% (59) had good awareness about child rights while 23% (69) had poor knowledge (see table 2). 30.67% (92) of rural children had poor awareness whereas about 5.66% of responders (17) had good awareness.

It was observed that children of both genders were vulnerable to the four types of maltreatment and gender had an influence in the case of sexual maltreatment (see table 3). (Chi square p value = 0.00 for sexual maltreatment and for all others it is > 0.05). Boys are more in number who had responded of suffering from maltreatment which is against the usual belief that girl children are prone to abuse more than boys (1-4).

The influences of various factors on the four types of maltreatment were analyzed by MANOVA. The result is presented in the table 4. The children's awareness, parent's education level, family's monthly income and type of family they belong showed significant influence in the prevalence of maltreatment.

Table 3. Percentage of adolescents who has experienced the four types of maltreatments, by gender (n = 300)

Types of maltreatment	Male%	Female%	Chi square	p value
Physical	49.02	44.90	4.067	0.254
Sexual	18.30	14.97	23.715	0.000*
Emotional	49.67	45.58	4.732	0.193
Neglect	29.41	29.93	4.05	0.256

Table 4. The factors influencing the four types of maltreatment

	Wilks lambda	p value
Factors affecting maltreatment		
Parents marital status(Single parent or not)	0.961	0.765
Location of residence(urban or rural)	0.988	0.482
Mother's education level	0.935	0.041*
Father's education level	0.894	0.001*
Monthly income of the family	0.898	0.001*
Level of knowledge of the children regarding maltreatment	0.913	0.004*
Type of family (Nuclear, three generation or joint family)	0.946	0.035

DISCUSSION

The repercussions of various types of maltreatment were critically analyzed. Though various types of maltreatment were highly prevalent in Kerala, it was respite that the adolescents were able to cope up with stress. Less than 20% suffers from problems like sleeplessness, aggressive behavior, loneliness and difficulty in educational performance. The psychosocial problems expected to be present in the children exposed to maltreatment was comparatively less, might be due to the potency in the family bond. However, prevalence of maltreatment was correlated significantly with aggressive behavior (R^2 = 0.036, p- 0.001) and difficulty in educational performance (R^2 =0.12, p= 0.00)

The findings in the study highlight the need for more studies on the prevalence of all forms of child maltreatment. Also the authors suggest that schools must introduce interventions which incorporate personal safety, prevention of abuse and mental health issues. Intervention programmes for parents and teacher emphasizing positive child disciplining practices are the need of the hour.

The investigation revealed that 53.67% of children has poor awareness of child rights of which 31.67% are boys. Comparing with rural and urban children, lack of proper awareness is more among rural children. 19.67% of urban children have good awareness where as 5.66% of rural children have good awareness about child rights. There are various factors influencing the prevalence of maltreatment. The results show that monthly income of the family, parent's educational level and the child's awareness of maltreatment makes a significant difference in the prevalence of the four types of maltreatment. Children of parents with higher education reports no maltreatment. Children who knows about their rights have reported seldom or no exposure to maltreatment. Children from low income family and nuclear family have reported more exposures to multiple mal-treatment. MANOVA results show that the above mentioned factors provide an influential role in the prevalence of maltreatment. The significant consequences reported by the children who have suffered maltreatment are aggressive behavior, feeling lonely, sleeplessness and difficulty in academic performance.

References

[1] Study on Child Abuse: India 2007. Accessed 2012 May 15. URL: wcd.nic.in/childabuse.pdf
[2] Derek K. Child social work policy and practice. London: Sage, 2009.
[3] Tiwari J. Child abuse and human rights. New Delhi: Isha Books, 2011.
[4] Child abuse and neglect. Accessed 2012 May 15. URL: www.helpguide.org/index

Submitted: May 22, 2012. *Revised:* June 15, 2012. *Accepted:* June 21, 2012.

In: Child and Adolescent Health Yearbook 2013
Editor: Joav Merrick

ISBN: 978-1-63117-658-6

Chapter 21

SIBLINGS EXPOSED TO INTIMATE PARTNER VIOLENCE: FAMILY PREDICTORS OF CHILD TRAUMA SYMPTOMS

Ashley Stewart-Tufescu, PhD* (candidate) and Caroline C Piotrowski, PhD, MPH

Applied Health Sciences, Faculty of Graduate Studies and Department of Family Social Sciences, University of Manitoba, Winnipeg, Manitoba, Canada

ABSTRACT

The purpose of the present study was to investigate the influence of familial factors on child trauma symptoms in children exposed to intimate partner violence (IPV). Building upon past research, the trauma symptoms of siblings were compared, and the role of these familial factors, maternal stress and the quality of mother-child interactions, in relation to children's trauma symptoms was explored. Results indicated sibling trauma symptoms were significantly related, and that older siblings demonstrated significantly more trauma symptoms than younger siblings. Sibling trauma symptoms, maternal stress and the quality of mother-child interactions accounted for a significant amount of variance in trauma symptoms for both older and younger siblings. An exploration of maternal differential treatment indicated mothers directed significantly more positive behaviours towards older than younger siblings. Findings indicated that sibling trauma symptoms were mutually influential, and that some mothers may have compensated for stressful life circumstances with positive parent-child interactions.

Keywords: Intimate partner violence, trauma symptoms, siblings, mother-child relationships, maternal stress, differential treatment

---

* Correspondence: Ashley Stewart-Tufescu, PhD (candidate), Applied Health Sciences, Faculty of Graduate Studies, 212 Human Ecology Building, University of Manitoba, Winnipeg, Manitoba, R3T 2N2, Canada. E-mail: Ashley.Stewart-Tufescu@umanitoba.ca

INTRODUCTION

It is well documented that exposure to intimate partner violence (IPV) has numerous detrimental effects on children's developmental outcomes (1). In North America, the prevalence and incidence rates of childhood experiences of IPV vary greatly due to definitional, theoretical, and methodological issues (2). Regardless of this variation, IPV remains a serious and underestimated global public health concern affecting upwards of 275 million children worldwide (3). Childhood exposure to IPV may include seeing the consequences of violence, hearing the violence, witnessing the violence and/or becoming directly involved in the violence (4). Exposure to IPV has been linked to a wide variety of consequences, including but not limited to: negative emotional and behavioural functioning, compromised social competence and cognitive functioning, poor school achievement, internalizing and externalizing difficulties and general health concerns (1, 2). Some work has suggested that children exposed to IPV are also more likely to display symptoms consistent with post-traumatic stress disorder (PTSD); unfortunately, trauma symptoms have not been as widely studied as other behavior problems and are not yet well understood (5, 6). The first main goal of the present research was to better understand trauma symptoms in school-aged children exposed to IPV. Recent research has concentrated on better understanding the nature of heterogeneity in children's trauma symptoms, as well as identifying some of the mechanisms that may account for the range of variability in trauma symptomatology across children exposed to IPV (7).

Our research focus on mechanisms that positively or negatively influence children's well-being is consonant with a developmental psychopathology perspective. This theoretical framework is useful for understanding variability in adjustment, as it focuses on the origins and pathways of individual patterns of maladaptation (8). Risk and protective factors are given equal emphasis. Although risk factors that increase the likelihood of negative outcomes have been more widely studied to date, an understanding of protective factors that either reduce or eliminate adjustment difficulties is equally as important (2). Situating these differing risk and protective factors within specific contexts is vital, as the degree and nature of their influence is often context dependent. For example, some protective factors may be relevant only in certain situations, buffering children who face specific stressors but having a neutral or even negative effect in other situations (8). Lastly, the concept of developmental pathways seeks to explain the interaction of risk and protective factors at differing time points and contexts across the life course.

The body of work examining trauma symptoms of children exposed to IPV has identified several important mechanisms to date, including child and family characteristics; however, family relationships are another potentially important influence that are only just beginning to be investigated (9). From a developmental psychopathology perspective, family risk factors play a crucial role in influencing children's developmental trajectories (8). The quality of mother-child relationships are particularly important, in that they can either lessen or amplify child adjustment difficulties. A second main goal of the present research was to explore the association between the quality of mother-child relationships and child trauma symptoms.

Another issue commonly overlooked in the literature is that the majority of violent families have more than one child. Children within the same family can experience IPV quite differently. Unfortunately, the nature of the sibling experience within families is typically not considered. Siblings in violent families may or may not share exposure to the same stressful events. When exposure is shared, they may have quite different perceptions of such events given individual differences between them such as age and gender. An appreciable body of research on siblings with non-violent histories has demonstrated the influence of both shared and non-shared environments within families (10). In brief, shared factors are considered to contribute to sibling similarity on a given characteristic, while non-shared factors are seen as contributing to sibling differences, such as differential treatment by parents. One of the few studies that has addressed siblings exposed to IPV found that younger and older siblings demonstrated similar patterns of adjustment (11). However, given the paucity of work on siblings to date, another important goal of the present study was to investigate similarities and differences in the trauma symptoms of siblings exposed to IPV.

In summary, the overall goals of the present study were to better understand trauma symptoms of school-aged children exposed to IPV, and to investigate a variety of family predictors that may mediate or moderate these symptoms. Several unique features of the present study make a substantial contribution to the literature. First, the trauma symptoms of more than one child within each family were investigated, allowing for a comparison of similarities and differences between siblings. Next, a multi-method approach was taken which included an observational assessment of the quality of mother-child relationships. Finally, other important family predictors such as maternal stress and sibling trauma symptomatology were also explored as potential mediators of trauma symptoms for IPV-exposed children.

Review of the literature

Recent research suggests that children exposed to IPV are at an increased risk for post-traumatic stress disorder (PTSD) (6). They may experience symptoms which include: traumatic re-experiencing, hyper-arousal, numbing, flat affect, dissociation, sleep disturbances, attention difficulties, cognitive problems, impulsivity and risk taking behaviours, and suicidal ideations (6). One study suggested that up to 50% of children exposed to IPV may meet the stringent criteria for clinical diagnosis of PTSD, while another study reported that clinically significant trauma scores among youth exposed to IPV ranged from 10-14% (5). Lang and Stover (12) suggested that the wide variability in rates of traumatic stress symptoms for children and youth exposed to IPV may be due to the fact that these symptoms receive much less research attention than internalizing and externalizing behavioural problems, and therefore may not be as clearly differentiated from other adjustment difficulties.

An additional challenge to understanding post-traumatic stress symptomatology (PTSS) among children exposed to IPV is the difficulty in differentiating between these symptoms and a specific clinical diagnosis of post-traumatic stress disorder (PTSD). Many of the studies that consider PTSD or PTSS in children exposed to IPV use proxy measures rather than the criterion from the Diagnostic and Statistical Manual of Mental Disorders (DSM-IV) (5). Moreover, the DSM criterion has been criticized for not being developmentally sensitive to children of a young age (6). In addition, co-morbid and secondary problems associated with PTSD may exacerbate symptomatology and/or lead to misdiagnoses; co-morbidity of PTSS is common with internalizing and externalizing difficulties (6). However, it is important to interpret these findings within the context of the methodological challenges of accurate measures of trauma symptoms, as well as the likelihood of co-morbidity with other difficulties such as the co-occurrence of witnessing IPV and experiencing child abuse directly. Given the above-mentioned methodological concerns, rates of traumatic stress in IPV-exposed children may be much higher than currently reported.

Similarities and differences in sibling trauma symptoms

The degree of similarity and differences in the adjustment of siblings exposed to IPV is under-studied. One of the few studies to date that has compared siblings from a shelter-based sample found no mean differences between younger and older siblings on internalizing or externalizing difficulties; however reports on child adjustment by differing family members were inter-related (13). More recently, Piotrowski (11) assessed patterns of adjustment in a community-based sample of siblings exposed to IPV, and found that younger and older siblings demonstrated the same five patterns overall, but that very few siblings matched exactly in terms of their patterns of adjustment. We know of no other work to date that has investigated or compared trauma symptoms in siblings exposed to IPV; given the paucity of attention paid to siblings in the literature, an important goal of the present research was to explore similarities and differences in sibling trauma symptoms.

Maternal stress

A variety of family factors have been suggested as potential mediators or moderators of trauma symptoms in children exposed to IPV. Some work has identified maternal stress as one potential influence, although linkages between maternal stress and child trauma symptoms remain unclear. Previous work reported that maternal parenting stress was found to mediate the relationship between IPV exposure and children's emotional and behavioural outcomes among low income, school-aged children (14). Unfortunately, this study did not include a measure of child trauma. More recently, research addressing the influence of maternal parenting practice and maternal stress on child internalizing problems in IPV-affected families concluded that maternal stress and observed parenting were not related, and found no evidence to support indirect effects of maternal stress on child internalizing difficulties (15). Given the limited research that has examined maternal stress and child trauma symptoms, another goal of the present study was to examine the relationship between maternal stress and child trauma symptoms in families exposed to IPV.

Mothers with a history of IPV often experience significantly greater levels of stress than mothers without such a history (16). In addition, their life circumstances are often more difficult, including lower socioeconomic status, less education and less available social support (17). Given these barriers, it is perhaps not surprising that some researchers have found their parenting to be negatively impacted. Maternal parenting stress has been reported to have a direct effect on child outcomes and behaviour problems following IPV-exposure (16). A recent study found that maternal distress was linked to parenting stress in IPV-affected families, and that maternal stress had a negative impact on the quality of the parent-child relationship. Moreover, it was parenting stress and not exposure to IPV that was found to be the strongest predictor of children adjustment in this study, including trauma symptoms (18).

In contrast, other studies have failed to report an association between maternal mental health, stress and parenting in IPV-affected families. These studies suggest that despite high levels of stress, mothers may utilize compensatory strategies to buffer their children's negative experiences (15, 17). Considering the conflicting nature of the current literature on maternal stress, and the lack of findings specific to the maternal stress and child trauma outcomes following IPV exposure, another goal of the present study was to investigate the potential influence of maternal stress on children's trauma symptoms.

The role of mother-child relationships

Mother-child relationships have also been identified as a significant influence on the adjustment of children exposed to IPV; however, there is currently no consensus as to the nature of this influence on children's trauma symptoms (16, 17). Some studies indicate that poor maternal mental health, particularly stress and depression, contributes to less optimal parenting behaviours (19). Other studies have shown that mothers may compensate for stressful circumstances with heightened sensitivity and attunement that may help protect and promote healthy emotional and developmental outcomes for children exposed to IPV (15, 17, 19). The buffering effects of supportive maternal caregiving have been linked with better child outcomes in violent families, including increased self-esteem and less externalizing behaviour. For example, Skopp and colleagues (13) found that higher levels of maternal warmth were associated with an attenuation of the relation between partner-to-mother aggression and children's externalizing problems. Others have found that mothers of asymptomatic children reported greater warmth than mothers of children with adjustment difficulties (9).

Given these findings, it was hypothesized in the present research that more negative mother-child interactions (e.g., characterized by more hostility, rejection and control) would be associated with more child trauma symptoms and greater maternal stress. Complementarily, it was also hypothesized that more positive mother-child interactions (e.g., characterized by more warmth, sensitivity and affection) would be associated with fewer child trauma symptoms and lower maternal life stress.

Clearly, positive mother-child relationships can play an important protective role in children's adjustment; they may be one crucial factor in understanding why some children exposed to intimate partner violence do not demonstrate trauma symptoms. Unfortunately, the quality of the mother-child relationships are often assessed by maternal self-report only, while observations of the quality of mother-child interaction and parenting are rarely conducted in IPV-affected families, with few exceptions (15, 19). The present study addressed this gap in the literature by utilizing observational methodology to assess the quality of mother-child interactions.

In addition, to our knowledge no empirical work to date has addressed the role of differential maternal parenting on trauma symptoms of siblings with a history of IPV. Previous work investigating non-violent families has shown that differential parental treatment of siblings was significantly associated with negative mental health outcomes and behaviour problems in children, such as depressed mood, low self-esteem and conduct disorders (20). Clearly, further investigation into the potential influence of differential parenting on siblings exposed to IPV is needed. Therefore, the final goal of the present study was to describe differential maternal treatment of siblings exposed to IPV, and to explore linkages between differential treatment and children's trauma symptoms.

In summary, the overall goal of the present study was to address gaps in the literature by investigating the trauma symptoms of siblings exposed to IPV utilizing a community-based, multi-method research design. Our first goal was to explore similarities and differences in sibling trauma symptoms. Taking a developmental psychopathology approach, we investigated if family predictors, such as maternal stress, the quality of the mother-child relationship, and sibling trauma symptoms were mediators of child trauma symptoms. The third and final goal of the present study was to explore the potential association between maternal differential treatment of siblings and children's trauma symptoms in IPV-affected families.

METHODS

A community-based sample of families was recruited through newspaper advertising, mail flyers, and posters displayed in counseling and support centres. Inclusion criteria for families consisted of: a) at least two school-aged children between 5-18 years of age, b) fluency in English of all family members, and c) mothers self-identified as having a history of IPV. As required by the Research Ethics Board, all mothers were required to have some prior counseling for their abuse, which ranged from less than one month (9%) to more than one year (49%).

Mothers. Forty-seven mothers agreed to participate. Their average age was 35 years (SD= 5.30). This sample of mothers indicated their ethnic-cultural backgrounds as 62% Euro-Canadian, 30% Aboriginal, and 8% multiracial. The majority of mothers (75%) reported they were lone parents (separated, divorced, widowed or never married). Thirty families (64%) reported an income that fell below the Low-Income Cut-Off (LICO) for families of three members or more, which was $27,000 at the time of data collection (21).

Children. Younger siblings included 27 boys and 20 girls, with an age range from 4 to 14 years of age (M= 7.89, SD= 2.50). Older siblings included 29 boys and 18 girls with an age range from 6 to 17 years of age (M= 10.83, SD= 3.00). Sibling dyads had an average age spacing of 2.8 years (SD= 2.0) and included 18 brothers, 9 sisters, 8 older brother/ younger sister pairs, and 9 older sister/ younger brother pairs. The majority of mothers (62%) reported that their children had received or were currently receiving family counseling at the time of participating in the study.

Procedures

After mothers signed an informed consent form and children provided oral assent, each family member was interviewed separately and privately. When age-appropriate, each family member was given the option of completing questionnaires on his or her own (with a research assistant available to answer questions). All interviewers were female, and whenever possible interviewers were of similar ethno-cultural origin to study participants. All families were provided $75 remuneration and information about local community resources (e.g., crisis hotlines) for participating in the study.

During the observational component of the study, family members were brought into an observation room equipped with a video camera and microphone. The observation room was furnished similarly to a home environment including couches, chairs, and a coffee table. A snack was also provided. Mothers were observed for ten minutes with each sibling separately. These interactions were semi-structured, in that mother-child dyads were provided with an Issues Checklist created by Robin and Foster (22), which consisted of a list of potential conversational topics that were likely to generate conflict. For example, participants may have discussed problems at home, school, or with friends. Each mother-child dyad was asked to choose any items from the checklist that they most wanted to discuss during the observation session. When a child was not participating in the observational session with their mother, they were asked to complete measures with a research assistant in a separate room.

Measures

Child Trauma Symptoms. The Child Behavior Checklist (CBCL) is a widely used tool for assessing externalizing and internalizing difficulties in children aged 4 to 18 years (23). A subset of items from this measure has also been widely used as a measure of post-traumatic stress disorder symptoms in children (24, 25). This subscale consists of 20-items selected to reflect PTSD criteria as defined in the DSM-III-R (25). These items included: difficulties concentrating, obsessive thoughts, feelings of guilt, moodiness, difficulties sleeping, nightmares, irrational fears, clinging to adults, nervousness, anxiety, sadness or depression, withdrawal, secrecy, feelings of persecution, irritability, frequent arguing, and somatic complaints such as, headaches, nausea, stomachaches, and vomiting. Each item was rated on a 3-point scale, ranging from 0 (not true), 1 (somewhat true) to 2 (often true). The CBCL-PTSD subscale has shown predictive power and incremental validity above and beyond the externalizing and internalizing behaviour scales of the CBCL-Total (24). Previous research using the CBCL-PTSD subscale for 4-18 year olds demonstrated good internal consistency, with a coefficient alpha of .87 (24). Similarly, good internal consistency was found for the CBCL-PTSD in the present study; coefficient alpha was .84.

Exposure to Intimate Partner Violence. Mothers were asked to estimate the length of their children's lifetime exposure to intimate partner violence. On average, younger siblings were exposed for 3.9 years (SD= 2.9) while older siblings were exposed for 4.8 years (*SD*= 3.6).

Maternal Violence History. The Physical Aggression scale of the Conflict Tactics Scale (CTS) was completed by mothers (26). The CTS asked about 9 violent behaviours that occurred within the context of a conflict in the past 12 months. Each violent behaviour was rated on a 7-point scale ranging from 0 (never) to 6 (more than 20 times). Mother reported on their own and their partner's behaviours; however, more mothers reported more often about themselves (n=47) than their partner (n=30). This subscale has been widely used to assess aggression in intimate partner relationships and has demonstrated adequate internal consistency, concurrent validity and construct validity (26). Alpha coefficients for this subscale in the present study were .90 and .85 for self-report and report on partner respectively.

Mothers in this sample reported experiencing moderate to high levels of intimate partner violence. Overall, 66% reported an intimate partner had directed violent behaviour towards them in the context of conflict at least once the past year (mild physical violence subscale *M*= 4.46, *SD*= 5.12; severe physical violence subscale *M*= 4.61, *SD*= 5.63; n=30). Examples of these behaviours included: being pushed, grabbed or shoved (66%), kicked, bitten or hit (50%), beaten up (34%) or threatened with a weapon (28%). Sixty-eight percent of mothers also reported directing at least one violent behaviour towards an intimate partner in the context of a conflict during the year prior to the study (mild physical violence subscale *M*= 3.17, *SD*= 3.89; severe physical violence subscale *M*= 2.28, *SD*= 7.61; n=47). Examples of these behaviours included: pushing, shoving or grabbing (62%), kicking, biting or hitting (34%), and threatening with a weapon (15%).

Maternal Stress. Mothers completed the Parenting Stress Index (PSI) which is a 101-item questionnaire designed to assess parent-child relationships and parenting stress (27). The Life Stress subscale was used to assess maternal stress in the present study; it is a 19-item subscale that provided an index of the amount of stress outside of the parent-child relationship experienced by the parent (27). High scores on the Life Stress subscale indicated stressful situational circumstances that were often beyond the control of the parent (e.g., death of a relative or loss of a job). The items of this subscale were scored dichotomously, with higher scores indicating greater stress. Previous work has shown the PSI has acceptable psychometric properties and good test-retest reliability for both clinical and non-clinical populations; coefficient alpha was .55 for this subscale in the present study (27).

Quality of Mother-Child Dyadic Interactions. The Parent-Child Relationship Coding Scheme, developed for the present study, consisted of six content codes (e.g., verbal content, non-verbal content, proximity, physical contact, compliance, and joint attention) designed to capture the quality of mother-child interaction; each content code was coded as positive, negative or neutral. Content codes were applied to the behaviour of each individual rather than to the dyadic interaction, at the end of every 15-second interval. Mother-child dyads were observed for a total of ten minutes. Inter-rater reliability was computed using Cohen's Kappa coefficients, and these were α= .87 for verbal content, α= .88 for non-verbal content, α= .96 for physical contact, α= .97 for proximity, α= .93 for compliance, α= .92 for joint attention, α= .99 for disengagement, α= .99 for uncodeable and α= .89 for emotional tone.

The six content codes of the Parent-Child Coding Scheme were combined into composite variables based on the proportion of positive, negative and neutral codes assigned to each of the six categories for each family member. By calculating proportional frequencies rather than raw frequencies, small differences in the length of observations were controlled. For example, the composite variable of positive interaction (e.g., warmth, affection, attention) consisted of positively coded content codes combined with positively coded emotional tone ratings for each family member. The composite variable for negative interaction was similarly constructed.

Statistical analyses

SPSS version 18 was used to conduct all analyses. Prior to hypotheses testing, descriptive statistics were conducted on all variables, as well as correlations between variables. All variables were normally distributed, and no outliers were detected. Missing data were not replaced or estimated for any analyses. The minimum alpha level used to test significance for all analyses in the present study was set at $p< .05$. Hierarchal regression analyses were conducted separately for older and younger siblings, using child trauma scores as the dependent variable in each of the models. Predictor variables included: sibling trauma scores, maternal life stress, and the quality of the mother-child interaction.

RESULTS

Our analyses addressed the three main goals of our study: 1) to compare the trauma symptoms of siblings exposed to IPV; 2) to investigate family predictors of trauma symptoms of younger and older siblings, including maternal stress, sibling trauma symptoms, length of child exposure to IPV and the quality of mother-child interactions; and 3) to explore differential maternal treatment of siblings, and the linkages between differential treatment and the trauma symptoms of siblings exposed to IPV.

Comparison of sibling trauma symptoms

Younger and older siblings were first compared on several demographic characteristics, including age, sex, and length of exposure to IPV. Results indicated that older siblings were significantly older (younger M= 8.5 years, older M= 11.3 years, $t(46)= -9.98$, $p<.01$), and exposed to IPV longer (younger M= 46.9 months, older M= 57.9 months, $t(46)= -3.28$, $p<.01$) than younger siblings. Younger and older siblings did not differ in terms of the number of boys and girls; however, overall there were more brother dyads (n=18) than sister dyads (n=9) in this sample.

Two types of analyses were used to compare sibling trauma symptoms. First, the degree of association between younger and older sibling trauma symptoms was assessed; because of the significant demographic differences noted above, a partial correlation controlling for differences in sibling age and exposure to IPV was conducted. Results indicated that sibling trauma symptoms were significantly related $r(42) = .51$, $p<. 001$. Next, an analysis of mean differences indicated that older siblings displayed significantly higher CBCL-PTSD trauma scores (M= 13.67, SD= 6.16) than younger siblings (M= 10.75, SD= 5.98) on average, $t(43)=$ -2.98, $p < .01$ controlling for differences in sibling age and length of exposure.

Family predictors of child trauma symptoms

Pearson product moment correlations were first conducted to assess the degree of association between younger and older sibling trauma symptoms with family predictors including maternal stress, length of child exposure to IPV, maternal violence history, and the quality of mother-child interactions. Results are presented separately for each sibling in Tables 1 and 2.

Table 1. Correlations between younger sibling trauma symptoms and family predictors

	1	2	3	4	5	6	7
Younger Siblings							
1. Trauma Score							
2. Child IPV	.03						
3. Mom IPV	.06	.73**					
4. Maternal Stress	.33*	-.12	-.10				
5. M-Y Positive	.04	.49**	.31	.08			
6. M-Y Negative	-.03	-.11	-.08	.17	-.26		
7. Y-M Positive	-.05	.43**	.26	.10	.78**	-.19	
8. Y-M Negative	.27	-.25	-.12	-.01	-.33*	.76**	-.44**

Note. *N*=46. M-Y=Maternal Interactions with Younger Siblings; Y-M= Younger Sibling Interactions with Mothers, *$p < .05$, **$p < .01$ level (2-tailed).

Table 2. Correlations between older sibling trauma symptoms and family predictors

Variable	1	2	3	4	5	6	7
Older Sibling							
1. Trauma Score							
2. Child IPV	.15						
3. Mom IPV	.16	.91**					
4. Maternal Stress	.13	-.06	-.10				
5. M-O Positive	.04	.17	-.01	-.33			
6. M-O Negative	.09	-.22	-.16	.13	-.64**		
7. O-M Positive	-.01	.10	-.09	-.33	.92**	-.59**	
8. O-M Negative	.13	-.26	-.17	.22	-.67**	.88**	-.68**

Note. *N*=44. M-O=Mother Interactions towards Older Siblings; O-M= Older Sibling Interactions with Mothers *$p < .05$, **$p < .01$ level (2-tailed).

For younger siblings, maternal stress was significantly and positively associated with younger sibling trauma symptoms. In addition, younger sibling trauma symptoms were positively and significantly related to the negative interactions mothers directed towards older siblings $r(32) = .43$, $p < .05$ and the negative interactions older siblings directed towards mothers $r(32) = .43$, $p < .05$. Maternal positive behaviour directed towards younger siblings was significantly related to positive behaviour by younger siblings directed towards mothers. Maternal negative behaviour towards younger siblings was also significantly related to negative behaviour by younger siblings directed towards them. Lastly, younger sibling lifetime exposure to IPV was significantly and positively related to positive behaviour by mothers towards them and positively related to their positive behaviour directed towards their mothers.

For older siblings, there were no significant associations between trauma symptoms and family predictor variables. Similar to findings for younger siblings, maternal behaviours directed towards older siblings was significantly related to older siblings behaviour directed towards mothers, for both negative and positive interactions. No other significant associations were found for older siblings.

Next, hierarchical regression analyses were conducted separately for older and younger siblings, testing both main and interaction effects; these results are displayed in Table 3. In both models, the first step included the main effects of sibling trauma symptoms, maternal stress and negative mother-child interactions. The second step included the interaction term combining sibling trauma and maternal stress. All variables were centered prior to analysis as recommended by Aiken and West (28).

Table 3. Summary of hierarchical multiple regression analyses predicting younger and older siblings trauma scores from sibling trauma, maternal stress and mother-child interactions

Younger Sibling Trauma				Older Sibling Trauma		
Predictor	β	R^2	Adjusted R^2	β	R^2	Adjusted R^2
Model 1						
1. Sibling Trauma	.44**	.50	.45	.75*	.34	.27
2. Maternal Life Stress	.60			-.22		
3. Mother-Child Negative Interactions	21.88**			-14.93		
Model 2						
1. Sibling Trauma	.315*	.62	.56	.01*	.39	.30
2. Maternal Life Stress	.84**			.76		
3. Mother-Child Negative Interactions	21.77**			.29		
4. Interaction of Sibling Trauma X Maternal Life Stress	.11**			.16		

Note: N= 94 mother-sibling dyads. *p< .05, ** p< .01. Younger sibling Model 1 F= 9.13 3, 27**, Model 2 F= 10.55 4, 26 **. Older sibling Model 1 F= 4.70 3, 37**, Model 2 F= 4.19 4, 26 **

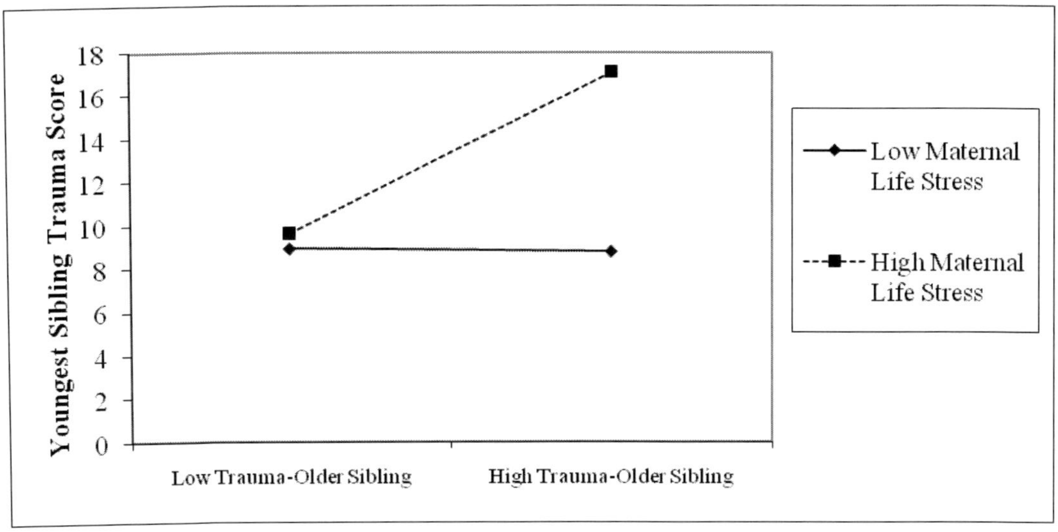

Figure 1. Depiction of interaction between older sibling trauma symptoms (low versus high) and maternal life stress (low versus high) in predicting younger sibling trauma symptoms.

Younger Siblings. The model for younger sibling trauma symptoms accounted for a significant amount of the overall variance (adjusted R^2= .56). The main effects of older sibling trauma symptoms and maternal life stress were both significant, as was the interaction term between these two variables. The interaction was plotted in Figure 1; these results suggest that younger sibling trauma symptoms were more pronounced in the context of higher maternal life stress and higher older sibling trauma symptoms.

Older Siblings. The model for older sibling trauma symptoms also accounted for a significant amount of the overall variance (adjusted R^2= .30). While the main effect of younger sibling trauma symptoms was significant, all other main effects and interaction terms were not significant.

Differential maternal treatment of siblings

The third and final goal of the present study was to explore differential maternal treatment of siblings exposed to IPV. To address this goal, correlational analyses were conducted to determine the degree of association between positive and negative mother-child interactions directed towards younger and older siblings. Results indicated that maternal positive and negative behaviours towards their younger and older children were significantly and negatively related $r(31) = -.58$, $p< .01$. A follow up comparison of mean differences indicated that mothers directed significantly more positive behaviours towards their older children (M = .37, SD = .14), than their younger children (M= .31, SD= .15), $t(32) = 2.96$, $p < .01$. No significant differences were found for negative behaviours mothers directed towards their younger and older children. Similarly, the positive and negative behaviours by siblings directed towards their mothers were also significantly and negatively related, $r(31) = -.64$, $p <$ .01. A follow-up comparison of mean differences revealed that older siblings (M= .37, SD= .16) directed more positive behaviours towards their mothers compared with younger siblings (M= .26, SD= .16), $t(32) = 3.51$, $p< .001$). No significant mean differences were found between siblings concerning negative behaviours directed towards their mothers.

DISCUSSION

The findings of the present study contributed to our understanding of the trauma symptoms of children exposed to IPV in several major ways. First, older siblings demonstrated significantly more trauma symptoms than younger siblings, even when controlling for differences in age and exposure to IPV. Family variables, including maternal stress, the quality of mother-child interactions, and sibling trauma symptoms explained a significant amount of the variance in trauma symptoms for both siblings, but more so for younger siblings. And finally, mothers and older siblings engaged in more positive interactions with each other than mothers and younger siblings. These findings and their implications are discussed below.

Comparison of siblings

Our finding that older siblings demonstrated more trauma symptoms than younger siblings lends some support to the notion of non-shared environment, in that siblings may perceive or respond differently to their experiences within the family (10). Taking into account their differences in age and exposure to IPV, siblings in the present study may have experienced IPV differently; these differences may be attributable to a variety of factors. Exposure to IPV may have begun at a younger age for older siblings than younger siblings, or older siblings may have been aware of more violent events, or had a greater propensity to become involved in the violence while trying to protect/shield their mother and/or their younger sibling (13). It may also be the case that older siblings differed in their appraisal of the threat of IPV, including the degree of self-blame they engaged in (2, 13). Some work has suggested that younger children may be partially protected from the full impact of violence because they may not be as cognizant of their experience and/or the potential risks associated with IPV exposure (29).

Differences in sibling trauma symptoms may also be influenced by the gender composition of the sibling dyad. Some previous work has found sex differences in sibling adjustment, while others have not (30, 31). Although comparison of sex composition of sibling dyads was not possible for the present study due to sample size limitations, it is an important avenue for future research to pursue. Mean differences in sibling trauma symptoms may also be due to other factors not addressed in the present research, such as child temperament or regulatory functioning (32). However, it should be noted that sibling trauma symptoms were highly correlated in the present study, which supports previous work finding similarities between siblings in non-violent families on such characteristics as self-representation (30). This significant association may also reflect shared genetic inheritance between siblings, as shown in other work on externalizing symptoms (33). It may also reflect shared method variance, in that sibling trauma symptoms were measured solely by maternal report using the CBCL. In addition, mothers who have experienced IPV often demonstrate depressive symptoms and previous work has shown that mothers with mental health issues report on their child's behaviour differently from mothers without mental health issues (34).

The potential influence of maternal mental health issues such as depression and post-traumatic stress symptoms on maternal assessment of child trauma symptoms was not taken into account in the present study. A multi-method assessment of child trauma symptoms by a variety of reporters such as clinicians/therapists, teachers, siblings and by the child themselves would provide a more accurate assessment of their trauma symptoms. For example, in one study children exposed to IPV reported on their own trauma-related distress using a developmentally appropriate cartoon-based interview (15). Future research should utilize multi-method assessment from multiple reporters to further delineate the processes that contribute to similarities and differences in trauma symptoms of siblings exposed to IPV, and whether these change over time.

The role of familial factors

The present study is the first to our knowledge to investigate the role of sibling traumatology, maternal stress, and the quality of mother-child interactions on child trauma symptoms.

Interestingly, the quality of observed negative mother-child interactions had a significant influence on trauma symptoms for younger, but not older siblings. This finding suggested that younger siblings may be more sensitive to negative maternal behaviours than their older counterparts. It should be noted that mothers engaged in significantly more positive behaviours with older siblings, which may have further heightened the sensitivity of younger siblings. This association between negative mother-child interactions and trauma symptoms is consistent with previous work, which found mother-child relationships to play an important role in the adjustment of children exposed to IPV (8, 15).

Maternal stress was also a significant influence on trauma symptoms, and was found to interact with sibling trauma symptoms. Consistent with a developmental psychopathology perspective, the trauma symptoms of older siblings had a significant influence on younger siblings in the context of high maternal stress, while this pattern did not occur for older siblings. This finding supports previous work that older siblings bear greater influence on younger siblings than vice versa (31). However, the stronger influence of older siblings does not erase the impact of younger siblings; siblings did mutually influence each other in the present study. Sibling trauma symptoms were a significant predictor for both younger and older siblings, underlining the importance of sibling influence regardless of birth order. Social learning theory suggests that siblings may model or imitate one another. They may also influence each other through the quality of their interactions, whereby more conflictual interactions may exacerbate trauma symptoms, and more affectionate and nurturing interactions may attenuate trauma symptoms. Future research needs to address if the quality of interactions between siblings and their relationship overall influence trauma symptoms in children exposed to IPV.

In the present study, the older sibling trauma symptoms had a greater impact on younger siblings in the context of high maternal stress. It may be the case that children's trauma symptoms were aggravated by the stressful life events reported by their mothers, such as moving to a new location, death of family member, or change in employment status, which directly affected them as well. As noted above, it may also be the case that sibling interactions are more hostile or conflictual under circumstances of high maternal stress, which may further amplify trauma symptoms. Future work that directly considers these questions would be the next step in untangling the role of sibling influence on child trauma symptoms.

Maternal stress was not associated with the quality of the mother-child relationship for either older or younger siblings. These results contradict previous studies reporting adverse impacts of maternal distress on the parent-child relationship, but are consistent with other literature suggesting that despite stressful circumstances, mothers engage in positive interactions with their children and may use compensatory strategies to buffer children from the negative effects of IPV exposure (15, 16). Our findings suggest that parenting can function independently of parental stress, and lend support to the conceptual model in which mothers effectively distinguish their roles as "parent" and as "person" (15). It should also be noted that mothers in the present study directed significantly more positive behaviours as compared to negative behaviours towards both younger and older siblings. It may be the case that this community-based sample of mothers was uniquely resilient in their parenting skills, in that they may have benefited from the prior treatment received concerning their abuse history.

In addition, we found no relation between mother's IPV history and child trauma symptoms, although other studies have documented a significant association between chronicity and severity of maternal IPV history and child adjustment problems (12). Although frequency of violent events were measured in the present study, type and severity of IPV were not, which may account for these differences. In addition, maternal treatment history may also have further attenuated this association. Future research addressing child trauma symptoms needs to address the different characteristics of IPV, as well as the exposure of family members to differing types of violence, such as in the media, in the schools, and in the community.

Lastly, the present study explored the notion of differential maternal treatment of children exposed to IPV. Mothers were observed to direct more positive behaviours towards older siblings than younger siblings, but there were no significant differences in the negative behaviours they directed towards their children. However, since older siblings also directed more positive behaviours towards their mothers than their younger counterparts, it is unclear whether mothers or their older children were driving these positive interactions. These results are particularly interesting considering that older siblings demonstrated significantly more trauma symptoms as compared to younger siblings.

The concept of differential treatment should be distinguished from preferential treatment; differential treatment refers to treating each child within the family differently based on developmentally appropriate characteristics, such as age, gender, personality, etc. This is quite different from preferential treatment that is based on parental favoritism, in which one sibling feels disfavored while the other feels preferred, and which is commonly associated with negative sibling interactions (35). Past research has shown that even young children can understand and detect the difference between the two (36). In the present study, mothers were observed with each of their children separately, rather than with both children together. When alone with older siblings, mothers may have been more attuned to their more serious traumatology, and engaged in more positive interactions to more effectively meet their children's needs.

This notion of maternal attunement and compensatory strategies has been found in other studies primarily with mothers and their infants and younger children, although it clearly also has bearing for families with school-aged and adolescent children (17).

Whether mothers engage in more positive interactions with older siblings when younger siblings are present is an important question for future research that may have important implications for child adjustment in IPV-affected families. It should be noted that the differences in mother-child interaction observed when mothers engaged with younger and older siblings separately in the present study were not associated with child trauma symptoms, lending further support to the notion that their differential treatment of siblings reflected sensitivity in parenting. Overall, these findings provide evidence for positive reciprocal dyadic interaction and mutual influence between mothers and children in families with a history of IPV.

Limitations and future research

The present findings underline the importance of using observational methods to assess the quality of mother-child relationships. While the observed micro-level interactions between mothers and their children were predictive of trauma symptoms for younger siblings, future research should include multi-method assessments of mother-child relationships that incorporate the perspectives of the mothers and children themselves. Future replication with larger heterogeneous samples, compared with samples without a history of IPV, would also strengthen the validity of these findings. Sibling trauma symptoms were found to significantly influence one another; however, this was more pronounced for younger siblings in families with high maternal stress.

Considering these findings from a developmental psychopathology perspective, younger siblings appeared to be more strongly influenced by negative mother-child interactions and older sibling trauma symptoms under these particular conditions.

Unfortunately, older sibling trauma symptoms were not adequately explained in the present study. Future research should explore other potential factors that may contribute to the trauma symptoms of older siblings, including individual characteristics such as temperament, personality, and co-morbidity with other adjustment problems such as depression and anxiety.

Lastly, as noted earlier, future research should also include assessments of maternal functioning, such as post-traumatic stress symptoms, depression or other health issues, which may also impact children's trauma symptoms. In addition, children exposed to IPV are often exposed to violence in their communities and are victims of parental abuse and neglect, as well as the impact of these serious risk factors may significantly influence children's trauma symptoms (37, 38).

In summary, the present study broke new ground by identifying maternal stress, the quality of the mother-child relationship and sibling symptoms as important mechanisms that account for variability in child trauma symptoms.

Our findings lend support to a growing literature that suggests mothers may buffer the detrimental effects of IPV exposure through compensatory strategies including warmth, heightened sensitivity and attunement to their children. The present study should be considered as a first step towards better understanding the influences of familial factors on the trauma symptoms of children exposed to IPV. Next steps should include how mother and sibling trauma symptoms interact to influence the adjustment of these children.

Future work should also take a closer look at the quality of sibling relationships in IPV-affected families. Lastly, a comparison of mother-child interaction that involved both siblings simultaneously would provide a more indepth examination of potential maternal differential treatment, and provide a more complete picture of how these unique relationships may influence child trauma symptoms in families with a history of IPV.

ACKNOWLEDGMENTS

This research was supported by Social Sciences and Humanities Research Council of Canada Grant 410-96-0311 awarded to Caroline C Piotrowski, Principal Investigator. This work also appeared in Dupont M, Renaud J, Eds. *Siblings: Social adjustments, interaction and family dynamics*. New York: Nova Science, 2012. The authors acknowledge the work of Ketan Tailor and Janelle Hoffman, for helping to establish inter-rater reliability. Conflict of interest: None.

REFERENCES

[1] Carpenter GL, Stacks AM. Developmental effects of exposure to intimate partner violence in early childhood: a review of the literature. Child Youth Serv Rev 2009;31(8):831-9.

[2] Evans S, Davies C, DiLillo D. Exposure to domestic violence: A meta-analysis of child and adolescent outcomes. Aggress Violent Behav 2008;13(2):131-40.

[3] Pinheiro PS. World report on violence against children; Secretary-General's study on violence against children. New York: United Nations, 2006:257.

[4] DeBoard-Lucas R, Grych J. Children's perceptions of intimate partner violence: causes, consequences, and coping. J Fam Violence 2011;26: 343-54.

[5] Graham-Bermann SA, De Voe ER, Mattis JS, Lynch S, Thomas SA. Ecological predictors of traumatic stress symptoms in Caucasian and ethnic minority children exposed to intimate partner violence. Violence Against Women 2006;12(7):663-92.

[6] Margolin G, Vickerman K. Posttraumatic stress in children and adolescents exposed to family violence: I. Overview and issues. Professional Psychol Res Pract 2007;38(6):613-9.

[7] Gewirtz AH, Edleson JL. Young children's exposure to intimate partner violence: Towards a developmental risk and resilience framework for research and intervention. J Fam Violence 2007;22(3):151-63.

[8] Cowan P, Cowan C. Developmental Psychopathology from family systems and family risk factors perspectives: implications for family research, practice, and policy. In: Cicchetti D, Cohen, D, eds. Developmental psychopathology, 2nd ed. Hoboken, NJ: Wiley, 2006:530-87.

[9] Graham-Bermann SA, Gruber G, Howell KH, Girz L. Factors discriminating among profiles of resilience and psychopathology in children exposed to intimate partner violence (IPV). Child Abuse Negl 2009;33(9):648-60.

[10] Scarr S, Grajek S. Similarities and differences among siblings. In: Lamb M, Sutton-Smith B, eds. Sibling relationships: their nature and significance across the lifespan. Hillsdale: Erlbaum, 1982:357–81.

[11] Piotrowski CC. Patterns of adjustment among siblings exposed to intimate partner violence. J Fam Psychol 2011;25(1):19-28.

[12] Lang JM, Stover CS. Symptom patterns among youth exposed to intimate partner violence. J Fam Violence 2009;23(3):619-29.

[13] Skopp N, McDonald R, Manke B, Jouriles E. Siblings in domestically violent families: experiences of interparent conflict and adjustment problems. J Fam Psychol 2005;19(2):324-33.

[14] Owen AE, Thompson MP, Kaslow NJ. Family variables that mediate the relations between intimate partner violence (IPV) and child adjustment. J Fam Violence 2006;24:433-45.

[15] Gewirtz AH, DeGarmo DS, Medhanie A. Effects of mother's parenting practices on child internalizing trajectories following partner violence. J Fam Psychol 2011;25(1):29-38.

[16] Huth-Bocks A, Hughes H. Parenting stress, parenting behavior, and children's adjustment in families experiencing intimate partner violence. J Fam Violence 2008;23:243-51.

[17] Letourneau L, Fedick B, Willms D. Mothering and domestic violence: a longitudinal analysis. J Fam Violence 2007;22(8):649-59.

[18] Zerk D, Mertin P, Proeve M. Domestic violence and maternal reports of young children's functioning. J Fam Violence 2009;24(7):423–32.

[19] Levendosky AA, Graham-Bermann SA. Trauma and parenting in battered women. J Aggress Maltreat Trauma 2000;3(1):25-35.

[20] Richmond MK, Stocker CM, Rienks S. Longitudinal associations between sibling relationship quality, parental differential treatment, and children's adjustment. J Fam Psychol 2005;19:550-9.

[21] Statistics Canada. Income in Canada 1998 [internet] Ottawa, Ontario; 1998 [internet]. URL: http://www.statcan.gc.ca/pub/75-202-x/75-202-x1998000-eng.pdf.

[22] Robin AL, Foster SL. Negotiating parent-adolescent conflict: a behavioral-family systems approach. New York: Guilford,1989.

[23] Achenbach TM. Manual for the Child Behavior Checklist 4-18 and 1991 Profile. Burlington: University Vermont, 1991.

[24] Dehon C, Scheeringa MS. Screening for preschool posttraumatic stress disorder with the child behavior checklist. J Pediatr Psychol 2006;31(4):431-5.

[25] Wolfe VV, Gentile C, Wolfe DA. The impact of sexual abuse on children: a PTSD formulation. Behav Ther 1989;20(2):215-28.

[26] Straus MA. Measuring intrafamily conflict and violence: The Conflict Tactics Scales. J Marriage Fam 1979;41(1):75–88.

[27] Abidin R. Parenting Stress Index. New York, NY: Pediatric Psychology Press, 1995.

[28] Aiken LS, West SG. Multiple regression: testing and interpreting interactions. Newbury Park, CA: Sage, 1991.

[29] Osofsky JD. Prevalence of children's exposure to domestic violence and child maltreatment: implications for prevention and intervention. Clin Child Fam Psychol Rev 2003;6(3):161-70.

[30] Gamble WC, Jin Yu J, Card NA. Self-representations in early adolescence: variations in sibling similarity by sex composition and sibling relationship qualities. Soc Dev 2009;19(1):148-69.

[31] Tucker CJ, Updegraff K, Baril ME. Who's the boss? Patterns of control in adolescents' sibling relationships. Fam Relat 2010;59(5):520–32.

[32] Cummings E, El-Sheikh M, Kouros C, Buckhalt J. Children and violence: the role of children's regulation in the marital aggression-child adjustment link. Clin Child Fam Psychol Rev 2009;12(1):3–15.

[33] Natsuaki MN, Ge X, Reiss D, Neiderhiser JM. Aggressive behavior between siblings and the development of externalizing problems: evidence from a genetically sensitive study. Dev Psychol 2009;45(4):1009-18.

[34] Müller JM, Achtergarde S, Furniss T. The influence of maternal psychopathology on ratings of child psychiatric symptoms: an SEM analysis on cross-informant agreement. Eur Child Adolesc Psychiatry 2011;20(5):241-52.

[35] Meunier JC, Roskam I, Stievenart M, van de Moortele G, Browne DT, Kumara A. Externalizing behavior trajectories: the role of parenting, sibling relationships and child personality. J Appl Dev Psychol 2011;32(1):20-33.

[36] Kowal AK, Krull JL, Kramer L. Shared understanding of parental differential treatment in families. Soc Dev 2006;15(2):276–95.

[37] Herrenkohl TI, Sousa C, Tajima EA, Herrenkohl RC, Moylan CA. Intersection of child abuse and children's exposure to domestic violence. Trauma Violence Abuse 2008; 9(84):84-99.

Kennedy A, Bybee D, Sullivan C, Greeson M. The effects of community and family violence exposure on anxiety trajectories during middle childhood: the role of family social support as a moderator. J Clin Chil Adolesc Psychol 2009;38(3):365-79.

In: Child and Adolescent Health Yearbook 2013
Editor: Joav Merrick
ISBN: 978-1-63117-658-6

Chapter 22

RESULTS OF AN HIV STIGMA REDUCTION INTERVENTION ON A UNIVERSITY CAMPUS

***Sara A Millimet*[1], *Beau Miller*[2], *Michael W Ross*[*3], *Pahl Samson*[2] and *Chaitanya Churi*[3]**

[1]School of Health Sciences and Kinesiology,
Rice University, Houston, Texas, United States of America
[2]LIVE Consortium, Houston, Texas, United States of America
[3]School of Public Health, University of Texas, Houston, United States of America

ABSTRACT

We evaluated an HIV anti-stigma campaign at a large liberal arts university in the southern United States using a modified version of the Bogardus and Ross & Hunter Social Distance scale. Data on pre- and post-campaign cross-sectional samples with nearly 50% overlap indicated that the campaign (which included lectures, slogans, t-shirt distribution and chocolates containing slogans) significantly decreased the social distance from (willingness to interact with) people with HIV. Time between pre-test (n=685) and post-test (n=515) was 1 month. Decrease in social distance was uneven, with males changing more than females and white and Hispanic students changing the most. Data suggest that this social distance measure is an effective instrument for measuring a decrease in HIV-associated stigma and that brief anti-stigma campaigns of this nature have an impact short-term on expressed HIV-stigma.

* Correspondence: Professor Michael W Ross, School of Public Health, University of Texas, 7000 Fannin #2622, Houston TX 77030, United States of America., E-mail: Michael.W.Ross@uth.tmc.edu,

Introduction

Stigma against HIV/AIDS has been identified as a barrier to effective diagnosis and treatment of the disease (1). The nature and modes of transmission of HIV/AIDS are taboo in most societies. The unfortunate association of homosexuality with this disease early on additionally attached the stigma that came along with homophobia (2) and has led to a further isolation of patients of this disease, irrespective of sexual orientation. Thus, the disease lends itself to particular scrutiny and discrimination among members of society, as well as health care professionals. It is this stigma, and the opposition borne from it, that prevents many efforts to control and combat the spread of HIV/AIDS from being successful (3).

Researchers have shown the adverse effect of stigma against individuals infected with HIV has on testing, prevention and treatment activities. That stigma prevents and delays individuals from accessing timely diagnostic tests as well as counseling are well documented, especially among those forming the so called "high-risk" groups (4). Further, some have shown that anti-retroviral treatment programs which do not address the issues of stigma, affect treatment seeking behavior (5).

The impact of stigma however, extends beyond these avenues. Stigma against adolescents orphaned by HIV/AIDS has been shown to be associated with fewer positive activities and poorer psychological outcomes (6). Stigma associated with HIV/AIDS creates hostile environments at places of employment, and has been proposed as a predictor of unemployment in people affected with HIV/AIDS (7). In some parts of the world, this stigma even extends to those healthcare providers engaged in caring for HIV/AIDS patients. It may lead to some leaving work related to HIV/AIDS care (8) or burnout (9). It has been noted that even though HIV-related stigma declined from 1991-1999, in 1999, one-third of a population sample in the US still expressed discomfort and negative feelings towards people with AIDS (PWA) (10). In 2009, 87% of US college students did not perceive themselves to be at risk and only 29% had ever been tested for HIV (11).

In this scenario, campaigns looking to address stigma against those affected by HIV/AIDS assume special importance. Experts contend that in order to be successful, campaigns to reduce HIV/AIDS stigma need to be evidence based, and designed after extensive needs-assessment (12). Numerous such campaigns have been developed that look to reduce the stigma around HIV/AIDS in developed as well as developing countries. The WHO developed an international campaign called "Live and Let Live" that looked to eradicate AIDS related stigma through the use of various educational activities including poster campaigns (13).

There is however, a dearth of scientific evidence that examines the impact of such campaigns. It is important to evaluate whether interventions designed to reduce stigma are in fact working. Researchers under the Horizons Program have collated and examined programs regarding stigma prevention. Their report looked at 22 studies on stigma campaigns and their success in reducing stigma and discrimination related to HIV. They found that most studies were lacking in a rigorous evaluation of trends and data. Further, they found that samples were often small and convenience based, and measures of stigma weren't clearly defined. Finally, it was noted that most studies did not look at the long term effects of these campaigns, and whether changes in attitude, if any, persisted for a long duration after the intervention (14).

With this background in mind, in this study, we looked to conduct an educational intervention regarding HIV/AIDS and the stigma attached to it in adolescents (undergraduate college students in a large southern US liberal arts university, Rice University in Houston, Texas), and examine its impact on the study population.

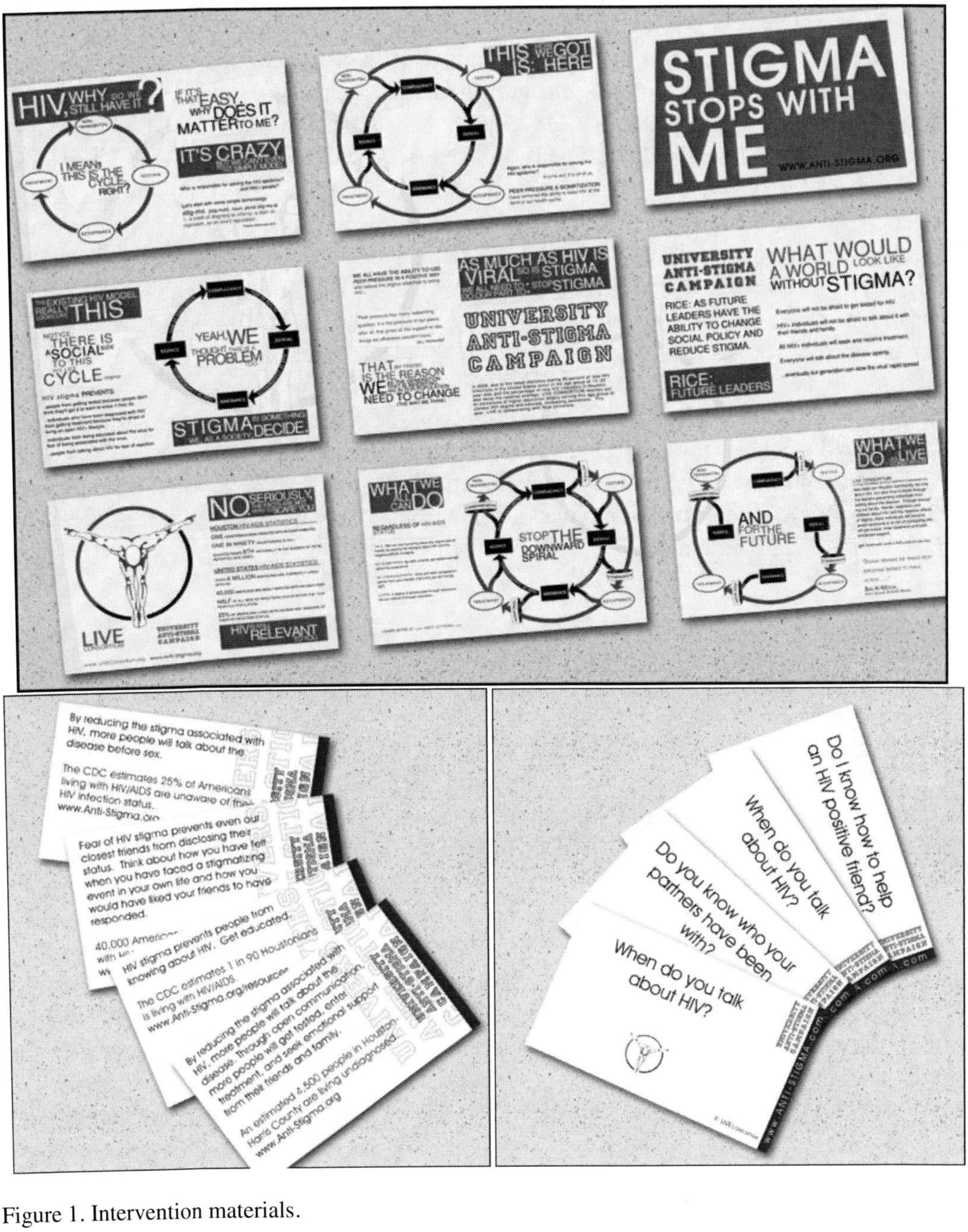
STIGMA STOPS WITH ME
WWW.ANTI-STIGMA.ORG
UNIVERSITY ANTI-STIGMA CAMPAIGN
WHAT WOULD A WORLD LOOK LIKE WITHOUT STIGMA?
RICE: AS FUTURE LEADERS HAVE THE ABILITY TO CHANGE SOCIAL POLICY AND REDUCE STIGMA.
RICE: FUTURE LEADERS
IT'S CRAZY
STOP THE DOWNWARD SPIRAL
AND FOR THE FUTURE
LIVE
HIV RELEVANT
Do I know how to help an HIV positive friend?
When do you talk about HIV?
Do you know who your partners have been with?
When do you talk about HIV?

Figure 1. Intervention materials.

The Intervention

In student focus groups, students crafted interventions based on focus groups which asked the question about HIV/AIDS "what do you and your peers need to hear? "The main message from these groups was that this is a US issue at home and not just an African problem. The campaign took place in Spring 2011 and consisted of: a month long HIV and stigma education marketing campaign in the Rice University student newspaper, the "Thresher"; weekly announcements and emails sent out by the Rice Health Advisors to their respective residential colleges; and Anti-Stigma Day, a day proclaimed by the Mayor of the City of Houston, which included a one thousand t-shirt giveaway (these t-shirts were still being worn a year later on campus) and a lunchtime lecture on stigma, HIV, and homophobia. Fortune chocolates (with a relevant message in the chocolate) were given in return for the student filling out a questionnaire. Business-size cards were handed out across campus with HIV and stigma-related messages (Figure 1) and there was a "viral" campaign in the campus newspaper with black squares containing the same messages, which spread from week to week until they covered almost an entire page. Broad (This is our problem) plus specific (One Houstonian is diagnosed every eight hours with HIV) messages. Each week focused on a particular aspect of the problem, starting with the problem of HIV stigma, what it means to you, what can be done about it, and implementing local and personal solutions.

The intervention was focused on the residential colleges as the effective "communities" of the University, which function much as fraternities or sororities. Illustrations of the intervention messages and media are at www.liveconsortium.org.

Methods

The pre-and post surveys were distributed and collected by the Rice Health Advisors (RHAs). The RHAs are a student run organization at Rice University which seeks to educate and promote both physical and mental well-being among fellow students. They are on hand in the residential colleges to discuss problems, mediate issues, and also provide basic medical supplies such as band-aids, ibuprofen, condoms, and cough drops. Rice has 11 residential colleges on campus, each with a varying number of Rice Health Advisors. The advisors at each residential college were given 100 pre and 100 post surveys per college. The surveys were collected primarily at meal time. Some RHAs took surveys door to door around the college were people were living as well.

The pre survey was completed in return for chocolates containing anti-stigma slogans provided by LIVE and the post-surveys were completed in return for an Anti-Stigma Day t-shirt.

The surveys were attempted to be collected in a 2-5 day period. 685 surveys were collected for the pre-test (62.3% of those provided) and 515 (46.8% of those provided) for the post-test. Once gathered, the data were entered and analyses analyzed using SPSS (version 19). The data were summed for knowledge and for social distance.

The social distance scale items were derived from the Bogardus measure (15) as modified for HIV/AIDS by Hunter and Ross (16). For HIV knowledge, the total number of questions each student got correct was averaged to develop a single mean score and standard deviation for the pre- and post-survey. The questions measuring social distance were scored on a Likert scale of 1 to 7, seven being the most willing to engage in the situation, and scores for each student were summed for all thirteen questions. The increase in the means of social distance implies an increase in willingness to engage in social situations and a consequential decrease in social distance. Questions on sympathy for people with HIV, how much HIV is on one's radar, and how personally one was affected by HIV were also measured on a Likert scale of 1 to 7, and these numbers were averaged individually. Two-sided *t*-tests were run on the on the means from the pre- and post- tests to determine whether changes were statistically significant. Pre-post differences were also run by gender and race/ethnicity. A *p*-value of $\leq .05$ was considered to be statistically significant.

At the start of the survey, students were asked for demographic information, including age, gender and race/ethnicity. The distribution was split fairly equally between male and female students for both the pre- and post-surveys, while race and ethnicity was more distributed predominantly in the White and Asian categories.

This is representative of the overall Rice University population. The study was not longitudinal, in that both the pre- and post-surveys were anonymous, so the surveys could not be linked to individual people before and after. Nearly 50% of the respondents who took the pre-survey also completed the post-survey. The study was approved by the appropriate university committee for the protection of human subjects.

RESULTS

Demographic data appear in Table 1. All participants were undergraduates, with a modal age of 21. Pre-and post-differences for HIV/AIDS salience, social distance, sympathy for people with HIV, the amount HIV was on the student's radar, how personally affected the student felt towards HIV, and how many people a student knew with HIV. These data appear in Table 2. Pre-and post-test differences were significant only for the social distance measure. The *p*-value for the pre- and pre-test results was significant ($p<.008$), indicating an increase in willingness to engage in certain situations with someone who is HIV+ statistically. Measures of HIV/AIDS salience, sympathy for people with HIV, the amount HIV was on the student's radar, how personally affected the student felt toward HIV, and how many people a student knew with HIV were all statistically insignificant.

Table 1. Demographics of sample

	Pre-test	Post-test	Statistic	*p*
Gender: Male	47.5%	48.1%		
Female	52.2%	51.9%	$\chi^2 = 1.77$, df=2	.41
Race/ethnicity: White	51.3%	46.0%		
African American	5.9%	4.5%		
Hispanic	13.3%	15.7%		
Asian/Pacific Isl.	25.9%	29.4%		
Other	3.7%	4.5%	$\chi^2 = 5.64$, df=4	.23

* Post-test respondents who had done pre-test: 49.9%.

All tests 2-tailed.

Table 2. Pre- and Post-test Differences, LIVE HIV anti-stigma Campaign

	Pre-test*	Post-test*	Statistic	*p*
HIV/AIDS knowledge	5.31±1.26	5.30±1.25	*t*=0.27, df=1200	.79
Social Distance	**71.76±15.68**	**73.96±14.74**	***t*=2.65, df=1181**	**.008**
Sympathy for people with HIV	5.95±1.28	5.93±1.20	*t*=0.31, df=1158	.75
HIV "on radar"	3.51±1.69	3.39±1.68	*t*=1.19, df=1157	.23
Feel personally affected	2.00±1.39	2.02±1.36	*t*=0.26, df=1159	.79
People with HIV known personally†	0: 86.0%	0: 85.2%	χ^2 =7.10, df=5	.21
Close friends/family with HIV†	0: 94.5%	0: 93.9%	χ^2 =4.37, df=4	.36
Recognized LIVE logo:		39.1%		
Recognized pseudologo:		14.9%		

* Mean±SD.

† Modal category (0, 1, 2, 3, 4, 5+).

All tests 2-tailed.

Table 3. Pre- and Post-test Differences in Social Distance by Gender: MALE

Pre- and Post-test Differences in Social Distance by Gender: MALE				
	Pre-test*	**Post-test***	**Statistic**	***p***
Social Distance	69.46±17.35	72.41±14.92	t=2.16, df=551	.031
Pre- and Post-test Differences in Social Distance by Gender: FEMALE				
	Pre-test*	**Post-test***	**Statistic**	***p***
Social Distance	73.62±13.46	75.73±13.51	t=1.92, df=557	.056
Pre- and Post-test Differences in Social Distance by Race/Ethnicity				
	Pre-test*	**Post-test***	**Statistic**	***p***
Caucasian	74.0±14.4	76.6±13.3	t=2.25, df=521.6	p=.03
African American	72.6±11.9	71.5±11.6	t=0.35, df=44.4	p=.74
Hispanic	71.7±15.0	76.7±14.0	t=2.21, df=165	p=.03
Asian	66.7±17.9	70.0±15.4	t=1.78, df=321	p=.06
Social Distance based on Recognition of LIVE Logo				
	YES: Recognition	**NO: Recognition**	**Statistic**	***p***
Social Distance	77.16±12.15	71.85±15.74	t=4.22, df=474	.0001

* Mean±SD.

All tests 2-tailed.

In order to examine the difference in the social distance measure in more detail, *t*-tests were run on the pre- and post-test differences in social distance according to gender and race/ethnicity. Complete data can be found in Tables 1-3, and Figures 1 and 2. When analyzing the social distance means for males, the social distance means increased in a manner that was statistically significant. The difference in social distance means for females who took the survey showed a similar trend (p=.056). Therefore, the decrease in social distance demonstrated by the male students likely contributed greatly to the decrease in social distance displayed by the entire student body. All race/ethnicities experienced a decreased social distance, aside from the African Americans, who experienced a slight (non-significant) increase in social distance. The most drastic increase was among Caucasian and Hispanic students, and likely contributed to the overall decrease in social distance among the entire student body. Both these increases in willingness were statistically significant. There was a trend toward decrease in social distance among Asian students, however, it was only borderline statistically significant (p=.06).

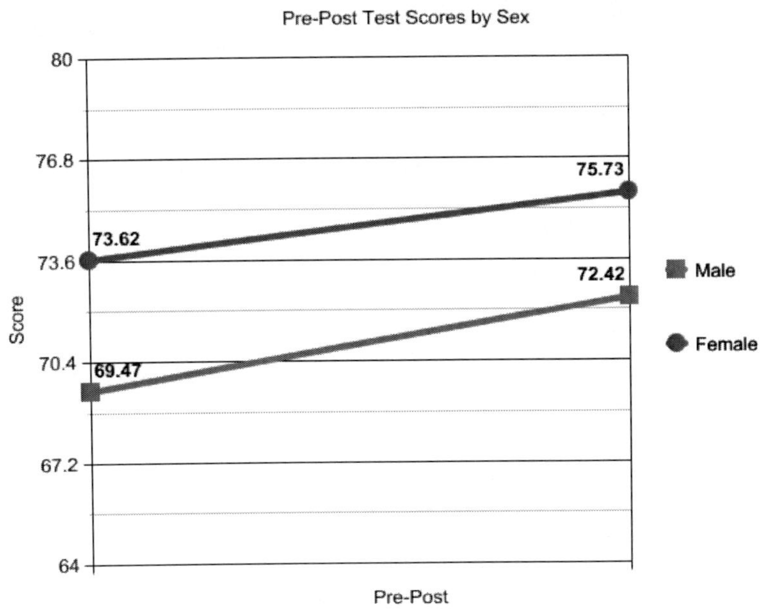

Figure 1. Pre-Post-test scores by Sex.

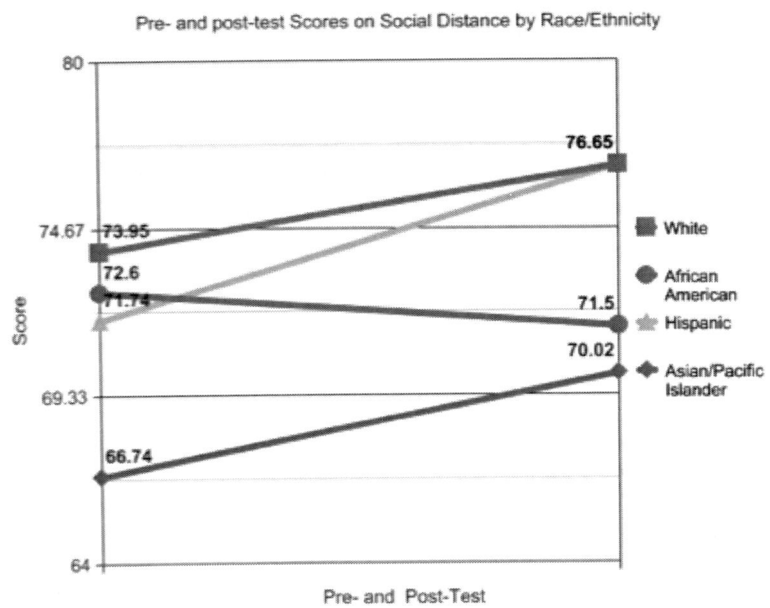

Figure 2. Pre-Post-test scores by Race/Ethnicity.

Finally, a *t*-test was run on only the post-survey data to examine the social distance compared to recognition of the LIVE Consortium logo of a diver, which branded all the stigma week materials, compared with a bogus logo from an unrelated campaign in the northeast US. A total of 39.1% students reported on the post-survey that they recognized the LIVE Consortium logo. Those students who responded that they did recognize the LIVE Consortium logo on the survey had a significantly higher willingness to engage in situations with HIV+ persons, compared to those who did not recognize the logo.

DISCUSSION

These data, while limited by the lack of a longitudinal design and lower power with subsample analyses, indicate that there was a significant decrease in social distance (willingness to interact) with HIV positive individuals on a modification of the Bogardus social distance scale (15). The differences were however uneven, with males changing more than females, and White and Hispanic students changing the most, followed by Asian students. These data suggest that one of the best indicators of an anti-stigma campaign is a measure of social distance from persons with HIV such as that used in the present study.

Breakdown of the data by those who recognized the LIVE logo, while a crude measure of the attention paid to the material, also suggests that those who recognized it (and presumably had recalled more of the content) also had significantly decreased social distance scores toward interaction with people with HIV. This suggests that recognition of the logo meant those respondents paid more attention to LIVE Consortium's educational material, resulting in their increased willingness to interact with people with HIV.

In analyzing the differences in HIV/AIDS salience, social distance, sympathy for people with HIV, the amount HIV was on the student's radar, how personally affected the student felt towards HIV, and how many people a student knew with HIV, before and after differences were only statistically significant for the social distance measure. As explained later, the social distance measure is the most essential data gathered from the survey, as it is directly related to a stigma. However, there were several potential barriers to obtaining significant results on other measures.

First, in regards to students' HIV salience, Rice students' HIV/AIDS knowledge was initially high (students averaged 5.3 out of 7 answers correct), a possible tribute to the highly intellectual nature of Rice students. Therefore, successfully educating students in order to yield a statistically significant increase is difficult to achieve. Nonetheless, in observations made on campus, many students actually complained about never receiving the correct answers after the first survey was distributed. Additionally, it was not necessarily expected that the number of people known with HIV would increase, as the intervention did not address that issue in particular. There were also no significant increases in the sympathy for people with HIV yet, like HIV/AIDS knowledge, sympathy for people with HIV started rather high, at an average of nearly 6 on the Likert scale of 1 to 7. Therefore, due to the ceiling effect, it is difficult to increase students' sympathy in a manner that would yield statistically significant results.

The most important result from the surveys was the significant difference in students' social distance after the intervention's implementation. The results demonstrate that the

University Anti-Stigma Day campaign had a significant impact on the social distance measure indicating Rice students had a greater comfort with people with HIV/AIDS. The social distance scale was the heart of the survey and was the most critical evaluation of whether the campaign effectively reduced stigma. As there is no generally accepted quantitative instrument to measure stigma, stigma reduction is best measured by a reduction in social distance people feel between themselves and others. In his book defining the study of stigma, Goffman (17) described stigma as "an attribute that is deeply discrediting" in social situations and explains that "an attribute that stigmatizes one type of possessor can confirm the usualness for another" (17, page 3-4). Thus, stigma operates by making one less like oneself and creates a social distance between oneself and the other. A greater stigma implies a greater social distance, due to the unwillingness to engage in social situations. Therefore, demonstrating a decrease in social distance likely implies a decrease in stigma towards a person as well. Consequently, the significant reduction in social distance to HIV demonstrates that the University Anti-Stigma campaign was successful in reducing HIV-associated stigma. This university-based campaign indicates that, in terms of short-term impact, the campaign was effective, although it is not possible to know, in this study, whether the difference was maintained in the longer term.

REFERENCES

[1] Machine EM, Ross MW, McCurdy SA. Issues of expressed stigma of HIV/AIDS among professionals in Southern Sudan. Qual Health Res 2011;21:1041-50.

[2] Flowers P, Langdridge D. Offending the other: Deconstructing narratives of deviance and pathology. Br J Soc Psychol 2007;46:679-90.

[3] Miller RL, Reed SJ, Francisco VT, Ellen JM. Conflict Transformation, stigma, and HIV-preventive structural change. Am J Commun Psychol 2011.doi: 10.1007/s10464-011-9465-7.

[4] Dowson L, Kober C, Perry N, Fisher M, Richardson D. Why some MSM present late for HIV testing: a qualitative analysis. AIDS Care 2012;24(2):204-9.

[5] Nattabi B, Li J, Thompson SC, Orach CG, Earnest J. Factors associated with perceived stigma among people living with HIV/AIDS in post-conflict Northern Uganda. AIDS Educ Prev 2011;23:193-205.

[6] Cluver LD, Gardner F, Operario D. Effects of stigma on the mental health of adolescents orphaned by AIDS. J Adolesc Health 2008;42:410-7.

[7] Liu Y, Canada K, Shi K, Corrigan P. HIV-related stigma acting as predictors of unemployment of people living with HIV/AIDS. AIDS Care 2012;21(1):129-35.

[8] Haber DB, Roby JL, High-George LD. Stigma by association: the effects of caring for HIV/AIDS patients in South Africa. Health Soc Care Commun 2011;19:541-9.

[9] Bennett L, Miller D, Ross MW. Health workers and AIDS. Research, intervention and current issues in burnout and response. Chur, Switzerland: Harwood Academic, 1995.

[10] Herek GM, Capitanio JP, Widaman KF. HIV-related stigma and knowledge in the United States: Prevalence and trends, 1991-1999. Am J Public Health 2002;92:371-7.

[11] Inungu J, Mumford V, Younis M, Langford S. HIV knowledge, ttitudes and practices among college students in the United States. J Health Hum Serv Adm 2009;32:259-77.

[12] Bos AE, Schaalma HP, Pryor JB. Reducing AIDS-related stigma in developing countries: the importance of theory- and evidence-based interventions. Psychol Health Med 2008; 13:450-60.

[13] Johnny L, Mitchell C. "Live and let live": An analysis of HIV/AIDS-related stigma and discrimination in international campaign posters. J Health Commun 2006;11:755-67.

[14] Brown L, Macintyre K, Trujillo L. Interventions to reduce HIV/AIDS stigma: what have we learned? AIDS Educ Prev 2003;15:49-69.

[15] Bogardus ES. A social distance scale. Sociol Soc Res 1933;17:265-71.

[16] Hunter CE, Ross MW. Determinants of health care workers' attitudes toward people with AIDS. J Appl Soc Psychol 1991;21:947-56.
[17] Goffman E. Stigma. London: Penguin, 1963.

Submitted: June 17, 2012. *Revised:* August 10, 2012. *Accepted:* August 27, 2012.

In: Child and Adolescent Health Yearbook 2013
Editor: Joav Merrick

ISBN: 978-1-63117-658-6

Chapter 23

MENSTRUAL PRACTICES AMONG ADOLESCENT GIRLS IN A RURAL AREA

Ravish H Shankaraiah**, MBBS, MD,
Sheela P Haveri, MBBS, MD, Katti S Mallappa, MBBS, MD and Wantamutte A Saheb, MBBS, MD
Kempegowda Institute of Medical Sciences, Bangalore, MES Medical college, Mallapuram, Kerala and JN Medical College, Belgaum, India

ABSTRACT

Adolescence is a period of major physical and psychological change with sexual development, as well as great changes in social interactions and relationship· Owing to these normal, rather drastic changes, many have a feeling that they are no longer in control of their body or mind and can develop anxiety and abnormal behavior which can cause long lasting damage to body and personality. The present study was conducted to assess the knowledge and practices regarding menstruation among adolescent girls in rural areas. A cross sectional study was conducted in three rural areas of Belgaum District, India having the cumulative population of 11,886. The data was analyzed using EPI-Info version 6.0 software package. The majority of these adolescent girls had taboos, beliefs or restrictions related to menstruation. The hygienic practices during menstruation of these adolescent girls were not satisfactory. Most adolescent girls had one or more health problems during menstruation. Health education emphasizing on adolescent health in schools as well as through mass media and public health approach is needed especially in conservative and traditional populations. We also should think about educative sessions to the parents especially mothers and other family members, so that they can be trained to impart knowledge on menstruation and related issues to their children.

Keywords: Adolescent girls, menstruation, knowledge, practices, rural area

---

* Correspondence: Ravish H Shankaraiah, Associate Professor of Community Medicine, Kempegowda Institute of Medical Sciences, Banashankari II Stage, Bangalore, 560070, India. E-mail: drravishhs@rediffmail.com

INTRODUCTION

Adolescence is a period of transition from childhood to adulthood. There are an estimated 1.2 billion adolescents, one in every five people in the world today (1). Adolescence is a period of major physical and psychological change with sexual development, as well as great changes in social interactions and relationship· Owing to these normal, rather drastic changes, many have a feeling that they are no longer in control of their body or mind and can develop anxiety and abnormal behavior which can cause long lasting damage to body and personality. This period needs special attention because of the changes the adolescent faces due to development, different needs and diverse problems.

In India, adolescents constitutes to about 23% of the population and adolescent girls constitute to about 10% (2). Adolescent girls in India, have additional problems like menstruation, anemia, early marriages and teenage pregnancy which compounds to the situation (3).

During this phase of growth, the adolescent girl first experiences the menstruation and related problems which is marked by feeling of anxiety and eagerness to know about this natural phenomenon. However, they do not get the appropriate knowledge/advice either in the school due to lack of proper health education programmes or in their house where, in a traditional and conservative Indian society, these matters are hardly discussed and discourage open discussion either in the house or in the school. This leads to culmination in repression of feelings which can intense mental stress. Moreover, the routine health services do not have adequate care about adolescent health problems, which further manifolds the problem. This is more so, in rural areas of our country where majority of them live.

On this background, a study was conducted to assess the knowledge and practices regarding menstruation in adolescent girls, which will help us to know their perception and practices regarding menstruation and help to provide proper health care services for these adolescent girls, so as to promote, protect and maintain her health to meet the demands imposed on her in the future life as a mother and care taker of the whole family especially in rural areas.

METHODS

A cross sectional study was performed up in three rural areas of Belgaum District, India having the cumulative population of 11,886. The study was conducted by the trained post graduate students with the help of medico social workers (female) and health assistants (female).

A pre-designed and pre-tested questionnaire was used during the study after being tested on a pilot project basis. House to house visit in the all the three villages was done and all the adolescent girls in these three villages were interviewed regarding their socio demographic profile, knowledge and practices on menstruation. The data was compiled and analyzed. The data was analyzed using EPI-Info version 6.0 software package.

Results

The present study included 1,071 adolescent girls in the age group of 10-19 years from three rural areas. Among them 18.91 % were illiterates and never went to school because of poverty, gender discrimination and domestic work. 20.61 % of the adolescent girls were already married because of their cultural practice, forced by the family members, peer pressure and ignorance regarding the age at marriage. The mean age at marriage was 16 years. Majority (78.12%) of the married girls were illiterates and from lower socio economic status.

Among the study population, 598 girls had attained menarche and the mean age at menarche was 13.77 years ± 1.17 years with the age range of 11 to 17 years (see table 1). The study showed that, a significantly large proportion (79.39%) of girls were not aware of menstruation, when they first experienced it. Many of these adolescent girls had emotional reactions to first menstrual cycle. These were fear and anxiety in 348 (58.2%), shy and embarrassment in 136 (22.74%) and others (see table 2).

Table 1. Age at menarche among adolescent girls

Age at menarche (in completed years)	Number	Percentage
11	7	1.17 %
12	87	14.55 %
13	138	23.07 %
14	218	36.45 %
15	100	16.74 %
16	46	7.69 %
17	2	0.33 %
Total	598	100.00

Mean ± S.D. = 13.77± 1.17

Range: 11 to 17 years.

Majority of these adolescent girls had taboos, beliefs or restrictions related to menstruation. These were restrictions from prayers and visiting holy places among 510 (85.28%), restrictions to kitchen in 371 (62.04%), restrictions to attend social gathering in 212 (35.45%), going out of the house in 198 (33.11%) and restriction to sleep with others among 118 (19.73%) (see table 3).

Table 2. Emotional reactions to first menstrual cycle

Emotional reactions	Number	Percentage
Fear & Anxiety	344	57.52 %
Shy & embarrassment	136	22.74 %
Nuisance	58	9.70 %
Problem	54	9. 05 %
Confusion	6	0. 99 %
Total	598	100

Table 3. Traditional beliefs and taboos present during menstruation

Taboos	Number	Percentage
Restriction from prayers	510	85.28 %
Restriction to Kitchen	371	62.04 %
Restrictions to social gathering	212	35.45 %
Restriction to going out of the house	198	33.11 %
Restriction to sleep with others	118	19.73 %

Note: Multiple response.

Table 4. Menstrual hygiene practices among adolescent girls

Type of material used	Number	Percentage
Old cloth	440	73.57 %
Sanitary Napkins	72	12.04 %
Both	86	14.39 %
Total	598	100

Table 5. Health problems during menstruation

Health problems	Number	Percentage
Dysmenorrhea	265	44.31 %
Backache	176	29.43 %
Weakness	126	21.07 %
Irritability	75	12.54 %
Headache	48	8.03 %

Note: Multiple response.

Regarding the hygienic practices during menstruation, most of these adolescent girls 440 (73.57%) used old clothes during menstruation and a large proportion of them were reusing the same during subsequent periods after washing and not properly drying. Only about 72 (12.04%) were using sanitary napkins (see table 4). This study also revealed that the literacy status of the mother, socioeconomic status and exposure to media to be important reasons for safe menstrual practices among adolescent girls.

These adolescent girls had one or more health problems during menstruation, they were dysmenorrhea among 265 (44.31%), backache 176 (29.43%), weakness 126 (21.07%), irritability 75 (12.54%) and headache in 48 (8.03%) (see table 5). Among these adolescents, only 19.73% took proper treatment through health care services. The majority managed their problem through self medication and parent or peer advice.

Discussion

The health of adolescent girls is an important issue in public health. They are a vulnerable group for various issues and more so in rural areas as they face multitude of problems.

Our study revealed that, many of the adolescent girls were still illiterates as they do not had the opportunity of going to school because of poverty, household work and gender discrimination, which still exists in our country. Attending school and gaining knowledge is an important factor regarding their own health, normal physiological changes and to discuss their problems with friends and teachers. One of the most important among them is menstruation, which is a normal physiological process that needs to be explained to the adolescent girls.

The adolescent girls in our study attained the menarche at the age of 13.77 years ± 1.17 years, which is similar to the national average age for attaining menarche (4).

Similar findings on age at menarche was observed in a study from rural Haryana, where the average for attaining menarche was 13.6 ± 0.83 years (5). Our study revealed that the majority of the adolescent girls did not have the knowledge on menstruation, until the first period occurred; this shows that school health education is an important approach to educate the adolescent girls regarding menstruation and this topic should be included in the curriculum.

Many of these adolescent girls had emotional problems during the menstrual cycle, which includes fear and anxiety (58.2%), shyness and embarrassment (22.74%). Similarly, in a study from Baroda showed that many (34.66%) of the adolescent girls were embarrassed and repulsed (6). These emotional problems has to be addressed either by the parents or by the school teachers or the elder sisters, which is of utmost importance as it will have an impact on her behavior and health. Therefore, health education to parents is also important to motivate them to discuss these issues with their children to prevent emotional disturbances.

There were many taboos or traditions like restrictions from prayers and visiting holy places (85.28%), restrictions to kitchen (62.04%), restrictions to attend social gathering (35.45%), going out of the house (33.11%) and restriction to sleep with others (19.73%), which were practiced in our study population. Similarly, a study from Pondicherry showed that there were many restrictions during menstruation such as restraining from doing prayers (63.8%) and restricting touching of stored foods (39.6%) (7). These restrictions has to be eliminated through proper health education to both these adolescent girls in school as well as their parents and family members through health education programmes at the village level, as these practices are deep rooted in our society and perhaps the media can play an important role in these aspects.

Menstrual hygiene practices was a major concern as brought about by our study, which showed that even now, the majority (73.57%) used old clothes during menstruation and a large proportion were reusing the same during subsequent periods after washing and not properly drying. These unsafe practices regarding menstruation have serious implications on reproductive and sexual health of these adolescent girls. Similar results were obtained in a study conducted in Rajasthan, India where more than three-forth of the adolescent girls used old clothes during menstruation (8). Therefore, proper health education regarding hygienic practices during menstruation has to be imparted to these adolescent girls through school and mass media and the same has to be reinforced to their parents by health education at the community level.

Health problems during menstruation is also a main concern in these adolescent girls as they experienced dysmenorrhea (44.31%), backache (29.43%), weakness (21.07%), irritability (12.54%) and headache (8.03%) in our study. A similar study from Washington, USA showed that dysmenorrhea is one of the major health problem among adolescent girls which has to addressed properly (9). Therefore, these things has to be included under the school health education, so that these girls must have a prior knowledge regarding the problems, which can occur during menstruation and thereby seek proper health care services through a qualified provider and avoid taking over the counter drugs or approach unqualified people. It is also imperative that health care providers increase their anticipatory guidance regarding normal menstruation, which may aid in the prompt diagnosis and treatment of menstrual disorders, and decrease their associated morbidities. This knowledge must also to be given to all the parents, so that they can encourage their children in times of menstrual related problems to approach proper health care facilities and seek the advice or treatment.

Complementary actions are needed to promote healthy development in adolescents; to prevent health problems or problem behaviors, and to respond to them if and when they arise. They need interventions to decrease and to mitigate their vulnerability. These include: information and skills; a safe and supportive environment; and appropriate and accessible health and counseling services. Health education regarding menstruation & related issues has to be emphasized in schools as well as through mass media and public health approach. We also should think about educative sessions to the parents especially mothers and other family members, so that they can be trained to impart knowledge on menstruation and related issues to their children. Thereby, encourage safe and hygienic practices during menstruation which will help them to maintain proper health.

REFERENCES

[1] World Health Organisation. Programming for adolescent health and development. Geneva: WHO, Technical Report 886, 1999:2-5.

[2] World Health Organisation. Adolescent nutrition: A review of the situation in selected South-East Asian countries. Bali, Indonesia: WHO, 2006:12-5.

[3] RCH Programme. New Delhi: Department Health Family Welfare, 1999:10-2.

[4] Indian Council of Medical Research. Growth and physical development of Indian infants and children. New Delhi: Indian Council Medical Research, Technical Report 18, 1989:61-63.

[5] Singh MM, Devi R, Guptha SS. Awareness and health seeking behavior of rural adolescent girls on menstrual and reproductive health problems, Indian J Med Sci 1999;53:439-43.

[6] Desai P, Hegde K, Hazra M. Adolescents menstruation: Perceptions and practices. J Obstet Gynaecol India 1990;40:259-61.

[7] Narayan KA, Srinivasa DK, Pelto PJ. Puberty rituals, reproductive knowledge and health of adolescent schoolgirls in South India. Asia Pacific Populat J 2001;16(2):228-35

[8] Khanna A, Goyal RS, Bhawsar R. Menstrual practices and reproductive problems. J Health Manage 2005;7(1):91-107.

[9] Houston AM, Abraham A, Huang Z, Angelo LJD. Knowledge, attitudes and consequences of menstrual health in urban adolescent females. J Pediatr Adolesc Gynecol 2006;19(4):271-5.

Submitted: July 14, 2012. *Revised:* August 20, 2012. *Accepted:* August 29, 2012.

In: Child and Adolescent Health Yearbook 2013
Editor: Joav Merrick

ISBN: 978-1-63117-658-6

Chapter 24

SNACK CONSUMPTION PATTERN AMONG ADOLESCENT NIGERIAN URBAN SECONDARY SCHOOL GIRLS

Alphonsus N Onyiriuka*, Eruke E Egbagbe and Eucharia PA Onyiriuka

Department of Child Health, Department of Medicine and Department of Health Education and Human Kinetics, University of Benin Teaching Hospital and Faculty of Education, University of Benin, Benin City, Nigeria

ABSTRACT

The worldwide dramatic increase in the prevalence of obesity in childhood and adolescence has led to a greater public health concerns relating to the dietary and snacking behaviours among the paediatric age group. Objective: To describe the pattern of snack consumption among adolescent Nigerian urban secondary schoolgirls. Methods: In this school-based-cross-sectional study, we assessed the snack consumption pattern of 2,304 adolescent girls (aged 12-19 years) in two urban public girls' only secondary schools selected by balloting. Data was obtained using an anonymous-structured-self-administered questionnaire. All the students were invited to participate. Results: Among the 2,304 participants, 1693 (73.5%) admitted consuming snacks in the last two weeks preceding the survey. The contexts in which adolescent girls most frequently snacked were after school but before dinner (74.8%) and during leisure time while watching television or hanging out with friends (78.3%). The majority (76.4%) of the adolescent girls consumed energy-dense snacks such as meat pie and egg buns along with soft drinks with only 9.4% of them consuming fruits 4-6 days in a week. Taste was the leading factor (88.2%) influencing the choice of type of snack. Among the 1,693 adolescent girls who snacked, 31.6% did so after dinner. Conclusion: The unhealthy snacking behaviours exhibited by adolescent schoolgirls in the present study included low consumption of fruits, consumption of energy-dense snacks along with soft drinks, snacking during

* Correspondence: Alphonsus N Onyiriuka, Department of Child Helath, University of Benin Teaching Hospital, PMB 1111, Benin City, Nigeria. E-mail: alpndiony@yahoo.com or didiruka@gmail.com.

leisure time as well as after dinner. Health education for promotion of healthy snacking behaviours should be given more attention in Nigerian school health programmes.

Keywords: Adolescents, schoolgirls, snacks, Nigeria

INTRODUCTION

A snack is a light food eaten in between the main meals; breakfast, lunch and dinner. Snacking is a key characteristic of the diet of majority of adolescents and it has been estimated to provide one-fourth to one-third of their daily energy intake (1). The choice of snacks in adolescents is based mainly on taste rather than nutrition, resulting in the tendency to choose salty, high-sugar or high-fat foods as snacks instead of healthier alternatives (2). Soft drink is one of the most common snack choices among adolescent schoolgirls (3). Among adolescents, fruits and vegetables are chosen less frequently as snacks (2).The dramatic rise in the prevalence of obesity in the paediatric age group in the past three decades has led to concerns about the dietary pattern of children and adolescents (4,5). In addition, habits acquired during adolescence tend to persist into adulthood. In this context, dietary behaviour developed in adolescence may have a major effect on the risk of chronic disease later in life. It has been emphasized that health-care providers should not only be alert toward unhealthy eating habits and nutrition-related issues among adolescents, but also, provide adequate and timely counselling (6). Health education and promotion in the schools cannot succeed in the absence of a carefully conceived school health programme based on data on snacking pattern. Yet, these data are neither well known nor documented (7).

The prevalence of snacking among adolescents varies widely. The report of one study indicated that 80-90% of adolescent females consumed at least one snack per day, with a range of one to seven snacks daily (1). Different snacking rates have been reported from various countries. For instance, 87-88% in USA (2,8), 62.1% in India (9) and 54.1% in Malaysia (10). A rising trend in the prevalence of snacking among adolescents has been reported (8).Generally speaking, adolescents as a group, is highly receptive to new food products and snack-type meals.

Some undesirable health outcomes that have been linked to snacking include obesity, skipping of meals, unhealthy food choices and poor nutrient intake (11-14). Despite the recognized undesirable health outcome of snacking among adolescents, published studies reporting pattern of snack consumption among Nigerian adolescents is very scarce. A search of the literature indicated that information on the specific contexts in which adolescent Nigerians snack is grossly lacking. The aim of the present study was to describe the pattern of snack consumption among adolescent Nigerian secondary schoolgirls. The knowledge derived from this study will assist those involved in health education and promotion of healthy eating habits among adolescents.

METHODS

This descriptive-cross-sectional study was conducted in two public secondary schools located in Oredo Local Government Area (OLGA), Edo State, Nigeria. The two schools were for girls only. According to Edo State Ministry of Education Statistics, there are nine public secondary schools in the LGA comprising 4 females-only, 3 co-educational and 2 males-only (15). Approval for the study was obtained from the school authorities. The teachers distributed parental consent forms to parents via the students, asking for permission for the child to participate in the study. Of the four girls' secondary schools, two were randomly selected by ballot. The total population of students in the two schools selected were school A 1,605 and school B 772, giving a grand total of 2,377 which was the target study population. The survey was designed to include all the students in the two schools. As a consequence, no sampling was performed. The principal of each of the two schools introduced the authors during the morning assembly. Subsequently, we addressed the students in their classrooms on the objectives of the study as well as on how to accurately fill the questionnaire. We also emphasized to the students that the questionnaires were anonymous and that their participation was voluntary.

Data was collected between October and November, 2011, using a structured-anonymous- self-administered questionnaire. The questionnaire was pre-tested, using 30 schoolgirls of similar age and class in another girls' only secondary school in the same LGA. The questionnaire was divided into two parts: the first part sought information on socio-demographic data, such as age of participants, the number of people in the household, educational status of father and mother, occupation of father and mother, religion and state of origin. The socio-economic status of the parents was determined using the classification suggested by Ogunlesi et al. (16). This was analyzed via combining the highest educational attainment, occupation and income of the parents (based on the mean income of each educational qualification and occupation). In this Social Classification System, classes I and II represent high social class, class III represents middle social class while classes IV and V represent low social class. In this way, the subjects were categorized into high, middle and low socio-economic groups. The second part consisted of questions relating to pattern of consumption of snacks. The questions included frequency of consumption of snacks in the preceding two weeks, type of snacks, context of consumption of snacks, whether or not soft drinks accompanied the snacks, and various factors influencing choice of snacks. In the present study, the recall day was defined as from when the respondent gets up one day until the respondent gets up the next day (17). A snack is defined as a light food and/or a drink that is consumed outside the main meals of breakfast, lunch and dinner. Main meals refer to breakfast, lunch and dinner.

The data were entered directly from the pre-coded questionnaire. Computer printouts of the data were reviewed for any information that was out of range. The statistical analysis was performed using the SPSS software package version 12.0. Descriptive statistics such as frequencies, means, ratios, standard deviations, confidence intervals, percentages were used to describe all the variables.

RESULTS

At the time of this survey, a total of 2,377 female students (1,605 in school A and 772 in school B) were attending the two public, non-boarding girls' secondary schools in the LGA (randomly selected by ballot). Eleven students (8 from school A and 3 from school B) declined to participate. The response rates were 99.5% in school A and 99.6% in school B. The overall response rate was 99.5%. The questionnaires of 62 students were excluded from the final analysis because they were incompletely filled, thereby leaving a total of 2,304 questionnaires (respondents) for data analysis. Students in both schools had similar socio-demographic characteristics, thus further analysis of data was carried out for the combined group of students. Among the 2,304 participants, 81.5%, 15.8% and 2.7% were from Christian, Muslim and Traditional religion families respectively. Based on the state of origin and the religion, the snacking pattern did not differ. Among the 2,304 participants, 1693 (73.5%) admitted consuming snacks at least once in the last two weeks preceding the day of the interview. The socio-demographic characteristics of the participants is depicted in table 1.

Table 1. Socio-demographic characteristics of participants

Socio-demographic parameter	No(%)	Mean ± SD (95% CI)
Age groups		
Below 14 years	560(24.3)	
14-16 years	1281(55.6)	
17-19 years	463(20.1)	
Total	2304(100.0)	14.5 ±2.0 years (14.4-14.6)
Household members		
2-4 persons	286(12.4)	
5-7 persons	1682(73.0)	
8 or more persons	336(14.6)	
Total	2304(100.0)	4.6 ±1.5 (4.5-4.
Socio economic status (SES) of parents		
High SES	302(13.1)	
Middle SES	1260(54.7)	
Low SES	742(32.2)	
Total	2304(100.0)	
Living arrangement		
Living with parents	1890(82.0)	
Living with guardian	414(18.0)	
Total	2304(100.0)	

More than half of the participants (53.8%) were in the age group of 14-16 years. The majority of the participants (84.7%) lived with family members and over two-thirds (70.3%) in households with five to seven members. More than half of the participants were from families in the middle socio-economic status. The family SES did not appear to influence the frequency of snacking among adolescent schoolgirls. The snacking pattern of the participants is displayed in table 2 with ready-to-eat energy-dense snack items (meat pie, egg buns, ice cream and soft drinks) being the most frequently consumed. Among adolescent schoolgirls in this study, fruits was not a popular form of snacks. Less than one in ten of the participants consumed fruits 4-6 days in a week. Over three-quarter (76.4%) of the participants consumed the snacks along with soft drinks. As depicted in table 3, snacking after school but before dinner was the most common context for snacking. Majority of the participants who snacked during school recess time admitted skipping breakfast and they purchased meat pie, egg buns and soft drinks from shops near their schools during recess because they were hungry. Comparing the frequency of snacking during the weekend and during the weekdays, it was 73.2% versus 41.5% OR = 1.8.The three leading factors that influenced choice of type of snack consumed were taste, cost and convenience (table 4).

Table 2. Snack consumption pattern among 1,693 adolescent schoolgirls

Types of snacks	Frequency of consumption per week	
	1-3 times/wk	4-6 times/wk
	No*(%)	No*(%)
Soft drinks	1344(79.4)	867(51.2)
Meat pie	1239(73.2)	720(42.5)
Egg buns	1173(69.3)	571(33.7)
Ice cream	1056(62.4)	538(31.8)
Doughnut	1046(61.8)	503(29.7)
Cake	904(53.4)	466(27.5)
Biscuits (sweetened)	848(50.1)	430(25.4)
Plantain chips	633(37.4)	371(21.9)
Fruits	191(11.3)	154(9.1)

* Some respondents cited more than one type of snack.

Table 3. Mean snacking per week among 1,693 adolescent school girls according to seven snacking contexts

Snacking contexts	No* (%)	Mean ±SD snacking per week	95% Confidence Interval (CI)
During school recess time	254(15.0)	0.4±1.8	0.18 -0.62
After school but before dinner	1266(74.8)	4.2±2.0	4.09-4.31
Leisure time (watching TV and hanging out with friends	1325(78.3)	5.0±1.7	4.91-5.09
On the way to or from school	778(46.0)	1.2±1.5	1.09-1.31
Any time	705(41.7)	1.0±2.0	0.85-1.15
While doing homework or working	579(34.2)	1.0±1.9	0.83-1.17
Snacks after dinner	325(19.2)	0.7±1.1	0.58-0.82

SD= Standard Deviation.

* Some respondents cited more than one snacking contexts.

Table 4. Factors influencing choice of type of snack among 1,693 adolescent school girls

Factors	Respondents (adolescent school girls)	
	Number *	Percentage
Taste of snack	1493	88.2
Convenience	1092	64.5
Cost of snack	953	56.3
Conformity with peers	764	45.1
Nutritive value of snack	637	37.6

* Some respondents cited more than one factor.

Discussion

Data from the present study showed that almost three-quarter of adolescent schoolgirls consumed snacks at least once fortnightly. A similar high prevalence of snacking has been reported among adolescent schoolgirls in Syria, Malaysia and India (9,10,17). This is not surprising as consumption of snacks is a recognized aspect of adolescent eating behaviour (18,19). Although more than half of the participants were from families in the middle socio-economic status (SES), this socio-demographic factor did not appear to influence the frequency of snacking. This finding may be explained by the report of previous studies which proposed that social class gradient may fail to reflect because of the homogenizing effects of school experiences, youth culture and peer-group influence among adolescents (20,21). Consistent with other studies (9,10), the highest frequency of consuming various types of snacks was once to thrice a week.

The major snack items consumed by adolescent girls in this study were meat pie, egg buns, ice cream and soft drinks. This is generally consistent with the reports of previous studies (10). In contrast to the reports of some previous studies (10,22), fruits were not popular as snacks as less than one in ten of the participants consumed fruits 4-6 days in a week in the present study. Indeed, those that consumed fruits in the present study did not regard it as snacks. The finding of low fruit consumption frequency is consistent with the report of previous studies (23-25). The practice of low fruit consumption is worrisome as some studies have reported an inverse association between overweight and fruit consumption (26,28). Given that snacking is a common dietary behavior among adolescent girls, promotion of consumption of nutritious snacks (fruits inclusive) is needed. Soft drinks are known to have a high glycaemic index and are energy dense, consequently are obesity promoting. For instance, in a cluster randomized controlled trial in south west England, a reduction in consumption of soft drinks resulted in a decrease in the number of overweight and obese children over a period of 12 months (29).

In consonance with previous studies (2,30), the present study revealed that the contexts in which adolescent schoolgirls most frequently snacked include after school but before dinner and during their leisure time. Snacking occurred most frequently after school, suggesting that adolescent schoolgirls snack most frequently in the afternoon. This in keeping with the finding in other studies (2,30).The high frequency of snacking after school may be related to the fact that in the Nigerian school system snacking is not permitted during class time, therefore the first opportunity students have to snack is after school. Another noteworthy snacking context in this study was snacking after dinner. The practice of snacking after dinner represents a major threat to both the present and future health of these adolescent girls because it corresponds to the time of the day when physical activity level is at its lowest. A review of the literature revealed that obesity is due to a chronic imbalance between energy intake and energy expenditure which is exemplified by consumption of energy-dense snacks in the face of low physical activity level after dinner (31). Data from the present study revealed a high prevalence of snacking during leisure time among adolescent girls. This eating behaviour is unhealthy. Considering that most of the adolescents spend their leisure time watching television (TV) and home videos, consumption of high-calorie snacks during this sedentary activity will, overtime, results in an imbalance between energy intake and energy expenditure, predisposing to obesity and overweight. This finding linking TV viewing with snacking is not surprising as a previous report has revealed a positive association between TV viewing and snacking (32). In a previous study it was reported that snacking while watching TV is associated with increased overall caloric intake and calories from fat (33). Reports of previous studies indicated that overweight and obesity among school children were directly related to amount of time spent watching TV (34,35).

In the present study, the leading factors in the adolescent girls' environment that influenced her choice of type of snack included taste, cost and convenience. This finding is consistent with the report of previous studies (36). Given that establishment of identity is a key characteristics of the adolescent age group, food (snacks inclusive) choices may convey strong messages about the individual to her family and friends. A pattern of snacking may be adopted as a way of exploring new lifestyles and asserting one's independence. However, the adopted pattern of snacking may affect health adversely. One limitation of the present study is that it involved girls only. Therefore, the results of the study cannot be generalized to include boys.

In conclusion, areas of unhealthy snacking practices among adolescent schoolgirls in the present study include low consumption of fruits, consumption of energy-dense snacks along with soft drinks and snacking after dinner.

ACKNOWLEDGMENT

Competing interest: There is not competing interest.

REFERENCES

[1] Bigler-Doughten S, Jenkins RM. Adolescent snacks: nutrient density and nutritional contribution to total intake. J AmDiet Assoc 1987; 87(12):1678-9.

[2] Cross AT, Babicz D, Cushman LF. Snacking patterns among 1800 adults and children. J Am Diet Assoc 1994;94(12):1398-1403.

[3] Ludwig DS, Peterson KE, Gortmaker SL. Relation between consumption of sugar-sweetened drinks and childhood obesity: a prospective, observational analysis. Lancet 2001;357:505-8.

[4] Lobstein T, Baur L, Uauy R. Obesity in children and young people: a crisis in public health. Obes Rev 2004;5:4-104.

[5] Nicklas TA, Baranwosski T, Cullen KW, Berenson G. Eating patterns, dietary quality and obesity. J Am Coll Nutr 2001;20:599-608.

[6] Mascarenhas MR, Zemel BS, Tershakovec AM, Stallings VA. Adolescence. In: Bowman BA, Rusell RM eds. Present knowledge in nutrition, 8th ed. Washington DC: International Life Institutes Press, 2001:426-38.

[7] Dukes G, Helsing E. Food and drugs: the peril of plenty. World Health Forum 1992;13:218-21.

[8] Jahns L, Siega-Riz AM, Popkin BM. The increasing prevalence of snacking among US children from 1977 to 1996. J Pediatr 2001; 138:493-8.

[9] Shrivastav M, Thomas S. Snack consumption among underprivileged adolescent girls. Indian Pediatr 2010;47:888-90.

[10] Chin YS, Mohd Nasir MT. Eating behaviours among female adolescents in Kuantan District, Pahang, Malaysia. Pak J Nutr 2009;8(4):425-32.

[11] Nicklas TA, Yang SJ, Baranowski T, Zakari I, Berenson G. Eating patterns and obesity in children: The Bogalusa Heart Study. Am J Prev Med 2003;25:9-16.

[12] Cusatis DC, Shannon BM. Influences on adolescent eating behavior. J Adolesc Health 1996;18:27-34.

[13] Haapalahti M, Mykkanen H, Tikkanen S, Kokkonen J. Meal patterns and food use in 10-to-11-year-old Finnish children. Public Health Nutr 2003;6:365-70.

[14] Sjorberg A, Hallberg L,Hoglund D, Huithen L. Meal pattern, food, choice, nutrient intake and life style factors in The Goteborg Adolescent Study. Eur J Clin Nutr 2003;57:1569-78.

[15] Ministry of Education. Directory of pre-primary, primary, junior and senior secondary institutions in Edo State. Benin City: Department Planning Research Statistics, 2006.

[16] Ogunlesi TA, Dedeke IOF, Kuponiyi OT. Socio-economic classification of children attending specialist paediatric centres in Ogun State, Nigeria. Nig Med Pract 2008;54(1):21-5.

[17] Lock K, Pomerleau J, Causer L, Altmann DR, Mckee M. The global burden of disease attributable to low consumption of fruit and vegetables: implication for the global strategy on diet. Bull World Health Organ 2005;83:100-8.

[18] Qotba H, Al-Isa AN. Anthropometric measurements and dietary habits of school children in Qatar. Int J Food Sci Nutr 2007;58:1-5.

[19] Bin Zaal AA, Musaiger AO, D'Souza R. Dietary habits associated with obesity among adolescent in Dubai, United Arab Emirates. Nutr Hosp 2009;24:437-44.

[20] Starfield B, Robertson J, Riley AW. Social class gradients and health in childhood. Ambul Pediatr 2002;2(4):238-46.

[21] Johansen A, Rasmussen S, Madsen M. Health behaviour among adolescents in Denmark: influence of social class and individual risk factors. Scand J Public Health 2006;34(1):32-40.

[22] Liu Y, Zhai F, Popkin BM. Trends in eating behaviours among Chinese children (1991-1997). Asia Pac J Clin Nutr 2006;15:72-80.

[23] Montazerifar F, Karajibani M, Dashipour AR. Evaluation of dietary intake and food patterns of adolescent girls in Sistan and Baluchistan Province, Iran. Functional Foods Health Dis 2012;2 (3):62-71.

[24] Washi SA, Ageib MB. Poor diet quality and food habits are related to impaired nutritional status in13-to-18-year-old adolescents in Jeddah. Nutr Res 2010;30(8):527-34.

[25] Paulus D, Saint-Remy A, Jeanjean M. Dietary habits during adolescence: results of the Belgian Adolux Study. Eur J Clin Nutr 2001; 55(2):130-6.

[26] Hilsen M, Eikemo TA, Bere E. Healthy and unhealthy eating at lower secondary school in Norway. Scand J Public Health 2010;38:7-12.

[27] Bernard L, Lavallee C, GrayDonald K, Dellsle H. Overweight in Cree schoolchildren and adolescents associated with diet, low physical activity and high television viewing. J Am Diet Assoc 1995; 95:800-2.

[28] Kelishadi R, Ardalan G, Gheiratmand R, Gouya MM, Razaghi EM, Deavari A, et al. Association of physical activity and dietary behaviours in relation to the body mass index in a national sample or Iranian children and adolescents: CASPIAN Study. Bull World Health Organ 2007;85(1):19-26.

[29] James J, Thomas P, Cavan D, Kerr D. Preventing childhood obesity by reducing consumption of carbonated drinks: cluster randomised controlled trial. BMJ 2004;328:1237-9.

[30] Anderson AS, Macintyre S, West P. Adolescent meal patterns: grazing habits in the west of Scotland. Health Bull 1993;51:158-65.
[31] Galuska DA, Khan LK. Obesity: A public health perspective. In: Bowman BA, Rusell RM, eds. Present knowledge in nutrition, 8th ed. Washington DC: International Life Sciences Institute Press, 2001:531-41.
[32] Van den Bulck J, Van Mierlo J. Energy intake associated with television viewing in adolescents, a cross-sectional study. Appetite 2004;43:181-4.
[33] Gore SA, Foster JA, DiLillo VG, Kirk K, Smith West D. Television viewing and snacking. Eating Behav 2003;4:399-405.
[34] Ramic E, Kapidzic-Durakovic S, Karic E, Batic-Mujanoric O, Alibasic E, Zildzic M. Influence of lifestyle on overweight and obesity in school-age children. Med Arh 2009;63:280-3.
[35] Robinson TN. Television viewing and childhood obesity. Pediatr Clin North Am 2001;48(4):1017-25.
[36] Shannon C, Story M, Fulkerson JA, French SA. Factors in the school cafeteria influencing food choices by high school students. J Sch Health 2002;72(6):229-34.

Submitted: July 10, 2012. *Revised:* August 22, 2012. *Accepted:* August 29, 2012.

In: Child and Adolescent Health Yearbook 2013
Editor: Joav Merrick
ISBN: 978-1-63117-658-6

Chapter 25

RESIDENTIAL CARE CENTERS FOR PEOPLE WITH INTELLECTUAL DISABILITY IN ISRAEL: TRENDS IN THE NUMBER OF CHILDREN 1999-2007

Ariel Tenenbaum, MD[1,2], Shoshana Aspler, RN, BSci[2], Dan Rorman, MD[2,3], Amanda Sinai, MBChB, MRCPsych[2], Brian Seth Fuchs, MD[2], Mordechai Raskas, MD[2], Meir Lotan, BPT, MScPT, PhD[2,4] and Joav Merrick, MD, MMedSci, DMSc*[1,2,5]

[1]Down Syndrome Center Jerusalem, Department of Pediatrics, Hadassah-Hebrew University Medical Center, Mount Scopus Campus, Jerusalem, Israel
[2]National Institute of Child Health and Human Development, Office of the Medical Director, Division for Intellectual and Developmental Disabilities, Ministry of Social Affairs and Social Services, Jerusalem, Israel
[3]Zur Hadassah Medical Clinic, Zur Hadassah, Israel
[4]Department of Physical Therapy, Ariel University Center of Samaria,Ariel, Israel
[5]Kentucky Children's Hospital, University of Kentucky, Lexington, United States of America

ABSTRACT

In 1997-1998 a questionnaire was developed by the Office of the Medical Director, Ministry of Social Affairs and Social Services. This questionnaire has intended an annual health assessment of the residents with intellectual disability (ID) and the services provided to them by residential care centers within Israel. The present study was conducted in order to examine trends in the number of children with intellectual disability in residential care centers in Israel. We have demonstrated a clear downward trend with

* Correspondence: Professor Joav Merrick, MD, MMedSci, DMSc, Medical Director, Division for Intellectual and Developmental Disabilities, Ministry of Social Affairs ndSocail Affairs, POBox 1260, IL-91012 Jerusalem, Israel. E-mail: jmerrick@zahav.net.il.

regard to the percent of children living in residential care facilities, from 18.1% of the total population in 1999 to 12.6% in 2007. Children living in residential care in 2007 comprised 2.6% of the total population of people with ID serviced by the Ministry of Social Affairs and Social Services.

Keywords: Residential care, intellectual disability, children, long-term-care, Israel

INTRODUCTION

During human history we have in different cultures seen children with severe disability neglected, maltreated or even "mercy" killed, which eventually resulted in the establishment of centers of refuge to protect these children, usually organized by religious or charitable organizations (1). As far as we know, these facilities were first established in Baghdad, Cairo, Damascus and Aleppo to later become introduced in Europe in the 18th century along with schools for deaf and blind children (1). In the 19th century, schools and special residential facilities were established for children with intellectual disability (ID) in Europe and North America (1).

This change was partly the result of the revolutionary work of the French physician Jean-Marc Gaspard Itard (1775-1838) and Phillipe Pinel (1745-1826), the founder of modern psychiatry.

During the 18th and 19th centuries and perhaps as a result of greater social acceptance of individuals with intellectual disability, specialized schools for children and adults were established around the world, specifically in Switzerland, Germany, England, Denmark and the United States (1). This trend continued into the 20th century despite the eugenics movement (1,4), but in the latter half of the 20th century, President John F Kennedy (1917-1963), who had a sister with intellectual disability, made the improvement of conditions for individuals with special needs a personal policy priority. In the late 1960s and 1970 de-institutionalization and normalization, which originated in Scandinavia became widespread, with many large institutions being closed and individuals moved into community settings.

Clinical experience seems to demonstrate that the incidence of intellectual disability (ID) in Israel has not been decreasing due to both religious and cultural factors. However, the dignified and high quality care of this population has remained a pressing concern since the first school for children with ID was established in 1929 in Tel Aviv. Subsequently, residential care facilities for children with ID were opened in 1931 in Jerusalem and in 1945 in Herzliya (5,6). After the establishment of Israel in 1948 the Ministry of Welfare was responsible for providing care to those with ID, but in 1962 the Ministry of Labor and Social Affairs established the Division for Mental Retardation (DMR) to treat and rehabilitate those with ID. The DMR (now called the Division for Intellectual and Developmental Disabilities) is today in contact with approximately 35,000 people throughout Israel, and full-time residential care is provided to about 7,000 of those individuals at 63 residential centers. An additional 2,000 persons receive care through hostels and group homes at another more than 50 locations (7,8). Residential care centers, which in addition to ensuring that their full-time residents receive the appropriate level of support for their daily life, also provide resources to parents, physicians, and other health care professions.

The present study was conducted in order to look at the trends of the number of children with intellectual disability in residential care centers in Israel.

Methods

In 1997-1998 a questionnaire was developed by the Office of the Medical Director, Ministry of Social Affairs and Social Services. This questionnaire has aimed to assess, on a yearly basis, the health of the residents and the services provided to them by ID specific residential care centers within Israel (7). This questionnaire has been useful in evaluating a wide variety of relevant information on the age, gender and level of intellectual disability of the residents. The questionnaire included the following subsections: information on the age, gender and level of intellectual disability of children served at the residential care center in question, status of the population served (educational, treatment, rehabilitation, nursing and challenging behavior), profile (various aspects of the nursing load like number of persons with gastric tubes, catheters, dialysis, oncology, epilepsy, diabetes, hypertension, blindness etc.), nursing, medical and allied professional staff, number of annual examinations, preventive medicine aspects, medications, number of annual cases of infectious disease, annual unintentional injury, number of deaths, number of hospitalizations, internal residential center hospitalization, ambulatory outpatient utilization, utilization of outside laboratory examinations and dental care. Data regarding the number of children in residential care facilities aged 0-19 years from 1999-2007 were analyzed for this study.

Results

The most recent available is from the 2007 National survey (8). The age distribution of 6,872 persons with ID in residential centers from 2007 is presented in table 1, and the level of ID is presented in table 2. There were 9 government, 37 private and 13 public centers with a mean of 116.47 individuals living in each residential center (range 24-341). It is worth noting that government residential centers receive their funding solely from government sources while private and public facilities may receive private philanthropy and have their own administrations but also receive budget support and supervision from the government.

Table 1. The population of people with intellectual disability in residential care centers in Israel 2007

Age in years	Males	Females	Total	Percent
0-9	73	58	131	1.91
10-19	431	304	735	10.69
20-39	1,662	1,115	2,777	40.41
40-49	772	616	1,388	20.20
50-59	637	615	1,252	18.22
> 60	271	318	589	8.57
Total	3,846	3,026	6,872	100.00
%	55.97	44.03	100.00	

Table 2.The level of intellectual disability (ID) in the population of people with intellectual disability in residential care in Israel 2007. Mild MR: IQ 55-70, moderate: IQ 35-54, severe: IQ 20-34 and profound: IQ < 20. Other are 30 persons, who historically were placed in institutions for other reasons and preferred to stay on, because they regarded the institution as their home or persons under observation

Age in years	Mild	Moderate	Severe	Profound	Other	Total	Percent
0-9	2	18	74	35	2	131	1.91
10-19	78	250	286	121	0	735	10.69
20-39	342	1,062	898	452	23	2,777	40.41
40-49	205	631	399	152	1	1,388	20.20
50-59	183	629	335	102	3	1,252	18.22
>60	84	336	139	29	1	589	8.57
Total	894	2,926	2,130	892	30	6,872	100,00
Percent	13.01	42.58	30.99	12.98	0.44	100.00	

Table 3. The population of people with intellectual disability in residential care centers in Israel aged 0-19 during 1999-2007 and their percent of the total population in residential care

Age	1999	2000	2001	2002	2003	2004	2005	2006	2007
0-9 years	209	204	187	169	183	158	159	151	131
0-19 years	897	879	881	847	801	796	787	755	735
Total	1,106	1,083	1,068	1,016	984	954	946	906	866
%	18.07	17.43	16.76	15.99	15.20	14.43	14.02	13.25	12.60

The trend in the number of children and adolescents with intellectual disability in residential care in Israel for the 1999-2007 period has been extracted from the aforementioned national surveys and is shown in table 3. Their percentage of the total residential care population is also presented in table 3.

DISCUSSION

Normalization and de-institutionalization was initiated and promulgated by Niels Erik Bank-Mikkelsen (1919-1990) from Denmark and Bengt Nirje (1925-2006) from Sweden in the late 1960s (9). Over time, this movement has spread widely, resulting in many positive effects for the ID community. Generous government funding in countries such as Denmark and Sweden have ensured that quality care is provided to children with ID in their home environments. This government funding, equivalent to a full time salary at the individual level, has enabled children to remain in their natural environments with their families and receive the support that they need. However, this successful alternative to institutionalization is necessarily costly and has been possible only in select rich countries. Such programs have not been possible in Israel where government welfare support covers a small percentage of the cost associated with caring for a child with ID. As a result, high quality care for children with ID has remained largely within institutional and community oriented settings, where such care can be provided more efficiently.

The purpose of this paper was to examine trends in the number of children with intellectual disability in residential care settings in Israel. Children living in residential care in 2007 comprised 2.6% of the intellectually disabled population serviced by the Ministry of Social Affairs and Social Services, and we have been able to demonstrate a clear downward trend over the years studied.

While it may be ideal for children to remain cared for in their home environments rather than residential care facilities, financial constraints make this an unlikely possibility in the near future for Israel. Furthermore, at present certain medical, mental health and nursing services can be more adequately provided in institutional settings, so the complete de-institutionalization of children with ID may be unlikely for logistical as well as financial reasons.

The annual questionnaire used for this analysis provides limited information about the children living in these facilities and their needs. Thus, we have begun a project under the auspices of the Office of the Medical Director to further study the health and quality of care provided to children living in residential settings.

Public health measures for children with intellectual disability should focus on (10):

- Developing, financing, implementing and monitoring alternative systems of care based on the principles of providing children with a family environment
- Preventing children from being deprived of family care in the first case by fighting discrimination and by supporting appropriate family services
- Resorting to institutional care only as a last resort
- Regulating and monitoring any remaining institutions for children in public care in line with agreed international and national standards
- Restructuring the system of public care in order to diminish the use of large institutions, develop alternative care approaches and strengthen effective community-based preventive and protective services
- Strengthen the legislative framework to ensure the rights of all children deprived of family care
- Adopting standards for public care and develop good monitoring procedures
- Reallocating funds to prioritize preventive and alternative care services
- Strengthening the legislative framework to ensure that the rights of all children deprived of family care are protected.

REFERENCES

[1] Braddock D, ed. Disability at the dawn of the 21st century. Washington, DC: AAMR, 2002.

[2] McDermott DE. Jean Itard: The first child and youth counsellor. J Child Youth Care 1994;9(1):59-71.

[3] Itard JMG. (1962). The wild boy of Aveyron. New York: Appleton-Century-Crofts, 1962. (Original work published 1894)

[4] Black E. War against the weak. Eugenics and America's campaign to create a master race. New York: Thunder's Mouth Press, 2003.

[5] Hovav M, Ramot A. The development of welfare services for the mentally handicapped in Israel. Social Security 1998;5:142-62.
[6] Merrick J, Kandel I. Medical services for persons with intellectual disability in Israel. Public Health Rev 2003;31(1):45-68.
[7] Merrick J. National survey 1998 on medical services for persons with intellectual disability in residential care in Israel. Int J Disabil Hum Dev 2005;4(2):139-46.
[8] Merrick J. Survey of medical clinics, 2007. Jerusalem: Office Med Dir, Min Soc Affairs, 2009.
[9] President's Committee on Mental Retardation. Changing patterns in residential services for the mentally retarded. Washington, DC: President's Committee, 1969.
[10] Stockholm declaration on children and residential care. Stockholm: Second Int Conf Children Residential Care, 2003.

Submitted: January 15, 2012.*Revised:* March 18, 2012.*Accepted:* March 23, 2012.

In: Child and Adolescent Health Yearbook 2013
Editor: Joav Merrick
ISBN: 978-1-63117-658-6

Chapter 26

ADVERSE CHILDHOOD EXPERIENCE AS A RISK FACTOR FOR ADOLESCENT PREGNANCY IN CHINA

***Wei Wei, MD and Xiaoming Yu, MD, MPH*[*2]**

[1]Chinese Center for Health Education, Beijing, China and [2]Institute of Child and Adolescent Health, School of Public Health, Peking University, Beijing, China

ABSTRACT

To determine whether having adverse childhood experience increases the risk of adolescent pregnancy in China. Methods: Using data from 1506 young women between the ages of 15 and 24 who were recruited in the Youth Clinics of 3 maternal care hospitals in three big cities in China. The association between history of adverse childhood experience and adolescent pregnancy was explored using multiple logistic regression analyses. Results: The risk of adolescent pregnancy was significantly higher among subjects with adverse childhood experience. Those who were experienced parents separated or divorced had a 72.0% higher risk of adolescent pregnancy than those without this experience after adjusting for confounding factors. Conclusions: This is the first study in China to demonstrate a relationship between adverse childhood experience and adolescent pregnancy. Greater efforts are needed to increase the awareness about the care of adolescents with adverse childhood experience and expand knowledge as well as relevant life skills about sexual and reproductive health among the vulnerable youth.

Keywords: Adolescence, unwanted pregnancy, adverse childhood experience, China

INTRODUCTION

Adolescent pregnancy is becoming an alarmingly public health problem in China. As the report in 2006 from WHO West Pacific Region Office, the age-specific fertility rate (15-19

* Correspondence: Professor Xiaoming Yu, MD, MPH, Institute of Child and Adolescent Health, School of Public Health, Peking University, No. 38 Xueyuan Road, Haidian District, Beijing 100191, China. E-mail: yxm@bjmu.edu.cn

years) in China mainland was 12 births per 1,000 women (1). The data from the China National Population Sampling Survey in 2009 showed that age-specific fertility rate of 15-19 years and 19 years old in China mainland was 6.2 and 16.7 birth per thousand respectively(2). According to Almanac of China's Health, the number of induced abortions in China has consistently been around 10 million per year for the past decade, with 20-30% provided for unmarried women (3). Some clinic cases analyses from big cities in China also showed that prevalence of pregnancy and abortion was increasing. The study from Guangzhou city in Guangdong Province indicated that the termination rate of pregnancy in 2nd and 3rd trimester among girls aged at 13-19 years was increased from 4.9 to 16.8 percent during 1984-2003 (4). The rate of repeated and multiple abortions among unmarried young women in a number of large cities ranged from 33.0% to 35.8% (5). However, the actual proportion might larger than this statistical data because some girls did not report their true age for some reasons, which may have caused physical and mental suffering and exposed many young people to the risk of STIs and HIV infection.

Adolescent pregnancy and childbearing entail a high risk of maternal death for the adolescent, and the children of young mothers have higher levels of morbidity and mortality (6, 7). These adolescents and their children may experience repercussions in the present, as well as last far into the future. Pregnancy and childbearing may cut short an adolescent's education and threaten her economic prospects, employment opportunities and overall well-being. Adolescent mothers may pass on to their children a legacy of poor health, substandard education and subsistence living, creating a cycle of poverty that is hard to break (8-10).

Understanding the risk factors for adolescent pregnancy is an important step in preventing its occurrence and the associated consequences. Previous research has explored a variety of risk factors for adolescent pregnancy, including the role of adverse childhood experience on the risk of adolescent pregnancy. Adverse childhood experiences in this study were specified that the experiences had to have occurred during the person's first 18 years of life.

With the exception of a study in 2004, in which researchers found that the odds of having an adolescent pregnancy increased with greater exposure to adverse childhood experiences, even after adjusting for ethnicity, education, and age (11). Some studies in teenage mothers on early family life have found that the early family relationships can provide important information in defining the parenting models to which teenage mothers may have been exposed. These studies have reported that parental divorce and separation, domestic violence, and negative parental relationships may be more prevalent in teenage, as compared to older childbearing (12-15).

Meanwhile, drug abuse was a significant problem among the fathers of the teenage antenatal subjects, with half having ever tried drugs and a quarter continuing to use illicit drugs into the pregnancy. Several other studies have also observed this trend. In one U.S. study of 367 teenagers who had fathered a child, 20% of fathers in the setting of teenage pregnancy used drugs compared to 5% of non-father peers (n=997) (16).

What's more, existing theoretical frameworks provide a basis for understanding the mechanisms through which different forms of child abuse can lead to adolescent pregnancy. Some studies of pregnant or parenting adolescents from Washington State have demonstrated high levels of self-reported sexual abuse, from 54% among a sample of rural women, to 66% among a sample of 535 pregnant adolescents in a community program (17,18). Haley et al. examined characteristics of street youth with histories of pregnancy, the results indicated that histories of severe sexual abuse and early injection drug use were extremely frequent in ever pregnant street girls (19). Kenney et al. collected information from over 1900 women aged between 18 and 22 in a population-based study in Arizona. Over 26% were pregnant before the age of 18. Almost 36% reported one or more forms of sexual abuse before age 18, including 20% who had been raped (20).

However, most of the research above has been conducted in the United States and Western Europe, and little evidence is available from China. The study described here makes a unique contribution to the understanding of the association between adverse childhood experience and adolescent pregnancy. Multivariate regression models are used to control for the effect of confounding factors, making this the first study from China, to our knowledge, to do so.

METHODS

Between August 1st to December 31st 2006, a sample of female adolescents who sought medical care or counseling service in the Youth Clinics of three maternal hospitals in each of three cities (Beijing, Guangzhou city and Jinan city) was recruited randomly to participate in the study. All of these girls were unmarried and aged varied from 15 to 24 years (mean=20.45, SD=2.08). The three cities are located in the different regions of China, Beijing, the Capital of China, is located in the north-central part of the country. Guangzhou city, the Capital of Guangdong Province and Jinan city, the Capital of Shandong Province, are bordered to south and eastern coast respectively. They are both typical areas in economic developing fast. And the maternal hospitals selected provide main services for maternal and reproductive health services of women accounting for about 30-40% of total new born cases each year in the city where it located. Therefore, the sample in the sense is representative for type of city in China. A standard questionnaire was used to ask participants about their adverse childhood experiences and other demographic characters. The adverse childhood experiences defined in this study including: 1) Parents separated or divorced; 2) Family member with substance abuse; 3) Father or mother had passed away; 4) Family member with crime; 5) Family member with mental diseases; 6) Language abuse; 7) Sexual abuse before 18 years old; 8) Physical abuse before 18 years old. The questions for the verbal and physical abuse categories were adapted from the Conflict Tactics Scale for which potential responses were never, once or twice, sometimes, often, or very often (21). Questions about contact sexual abuse were adapted from Wyatt (22).

The study was approved by the Biological Medicine Ethics Committee at the Peking University Health Science Center. All participants were informed consent right about the survey procedures so that their voluntary status was ensured.

RESULTS

1,471 women were recruited, the ages of the total group ranged from 15 to 24 (mean age 20.45; SD=2.08), and 66.6% of them were at 20-24 years. The whole subjects were divided into three groups based on whether or not they had sex and pregnancy: a Pregnant Group in which girls had both sex and pregnancy; a Sex Group in which the girls had sex ever but to had pregnancy; a Non-sex Group in which girls had never sex experience. A pregnant group (N = 895, 59.4%) and non-pregnant group including sex group and non-sex group (N = 611, 40.6%). The mean age of the girls in the pregnant group (mean age 20.73; SD=1.88) was significantly higher than the girls in the non-pregnant group (mean age 19.56, SD=2.91; P<0.001). 31.4 percent girls were still school students, and the rest ones had already left school and were mainly employed as waitress, teacher, nurse and so on (see table 1).

Among 895 young girls who had pregnancy, 64.8 percent (580/895) girls reported at the first pregnancy, 3.4 percent (30/895) were having second pregnancy, 24.0 percent (215/895) were having third pregnancy, and the proportion of more than three times was 7.8 percent (70/895). Concerning the pregnant period: 67.6 percent (605/895) girls' pregnant period was less than 49 days, 28.5 percent (196/895) between 2-3 months, while 3.9 percent (35/895) has been over 3 months. Further exploring why the girls with more than 3 months pregnancy did not come to hospital in time, it was found that there were 45.7 percent of girls who reported they did not know get a pregnancy, 28.6 percent of girls were afraid of doing induced abortion.

Table1. Differences in socio-demographic characteristics between pregnant and non-pregnant groups

Characteristics		Total group		Pregnant group	No-pregnant group	
					Sex group	Non-sex group
		N	%	N	N	N
age	15-19	472	32.1	229	66	177
	20-24	999	67.9	666	194	139
	Total	1471	100.0	895	260	351
Educational background	Under junior high school	251	17.1	153	44	54
	Senior high school	603	41.0	379	90	134
	Above collage	617	41.9	363	126	128
	Total	1471	100.0	895	260	316
Occupational status	Students	438	29.8	219	71	148
	Employed	1033	70.2	676	189	168
	Total	1471	100.0	895	260	351
Region	Beijing	297	20.2	150	66	81
	Jinan city	526	35.8	292	91	143
	Guangzhou city	648	44.1	453	103	92
	Total	1471	100.0	895	260	316

The relationship between adverse childhood experience and adolescent pregnancy

Table 2 shows the status of adverse childhood experience. Among the participants with adverse childhood experience, the pregnant group had a significantly higher rate than that of non-pregnancy including sex group and non-sex group (65.8% vs. 18.1% and 16.1%).

Table 2. The description of adolescent adverse childhood experience

		Total group		Pregnant group		No-pregnant group				P-value
						Sex group		Non-sex group		
		N	%	N	%	N	%	N	%	
Having adverse childhood experience	Yes	442	100.0	291	65.8	80	18.1	71	16.1	0.004
	No	1029	100.0	604	58.7	180	17.5	245	23.8	
The type of adverse childhood experience	(1) Parents separated or divorced	187	42.3	131	70.1	34	18.2	22	11.8	0.002
	(2) Family member with substance abuse	182	41.2	120	65.9	31	17.0	31	17.0	0.241
	(3) Father or mother had passed away	113	25.6	78	69.0	22	19.5	13	11.5	0.027
	(4) Family member with crime	47	10.6	29	61.7	8	17.0	10	21.3	0.991
	(5) Family member with mental diseases	48	10.9	27	56.3	11	22.9	10	20.8	0.621
	(6) Language abuse	17	3.8	12	70.6	1	5.9	4	23.5	0.437
	(7) Sexual abuse before 18 years old	15	3.4	11	73.3	4	26.7	0	0	0.114
	(8) Physical abuse before 18 years old	11	2.5	9	81.8	2	18.2	0	0	0.204

The study found many young participants had various types of adverse childhood experience .The types experienced by participants were also shown in table 2. There were significantly more adolescents with the experience of “Parents separated or divorced” and “Father or mother had passed away” in pregnant group and sex group than that in non-sex group (70.1% and 18.2% vs. 11.8%; 69.0% and 19.5% vs. 11.5%).

Eight separate multiple logistic regression models were created, each of them testing the effect of one form of adverse childhood experience in relation to the dependent variable of adolescent pregnancy, while controlling for confounding factors. Besides, a regression model of having adverse childhood experience or not (model 9) was also created and tested the relationship with having pregnancy (see table 3).

The results indicated that having adverse childhood experience increased the risk of adolescent pregnancy by 73.7% after controlling for confounding factors such as age, education, occupational status and region. And having the type of “Parents separated or divorced” increased the risk of adolescent pregnancy by 59.2% after controlling for these same confounding factors.

The association between “Family member with crime”, “Family member with mental diseases” and adolescent pregnancy did not increase a woman’s risk of adolescent pregnancy, and having “Family member with substance abuse”, “Father or mother had passed away”, “Language abuse”, “Sexual abuse”, “Physical abuse” increased a risk but not significantly.

Table 3.Adjusted odds ratios of adolescent pregnancy risk for adolescent adverse childhood experience

	Model 1	Model 2	Model 3	Model 4	Model 5	Model 6	Model 7	Model 8	Model 9
1.Parents separated/divorced	1.592 *P*=0.006								
2.Family member with substance abuse		0.779 *P*=0.133							
3.Father or mother passed away			0.678 *P*=0.065						
4.Family member with crime				1.038 *P*=0.902					
5.Family member with mental diseases					0.822 *P*=0.508				
6.Language abuse						0.644 *P*=0.411			
7.Sexual abuse before 18 years old							0.562 *P*=0.326		
8.Physical abuse before 18 years old								0.343 *P*=0.172	
9.Adverse childhood experience									1.737 *P*=0.010

Note: All models control for age, education, occupational status and region. *Model 1*=Parents separated or divorced; *Model 2*=Family member with substance abuse; *Model 3*=Father or mother had passed away; *Model 4*=Family member with crime; *Model 5*=Family member with mental diseases; *Model 6*=Language abuse; *Model 7*=Sexual abuse before 18 years old; *Model 8*=Physical abuse before 18 years old; *Model 9*=Having adverse childhood experience.

DISCUSSION

The study findings supported for our hypothesis that adverse experience during childhood is associated with an increased risk of adolescent pregnancy. 65.8% of girls having pregnancy reported they had experienced adverse childhood experience, its proportion was much higher than those without pregnancy and sex. Similarly to the study of Adams et al. (23), an interview study was conducted from 100 females between 12 and 24 years of age attending either an adolescent/young adult clinic, or teen obstetrics clinic at an urban academic medical center. It concluded that the frequency of any past abuse was significantly higher in girls who had ever been pregnant compared with "never pregnant" girls (P<0.05).

In addition, our study also found that there were significantly more adolescents with the experience of “Parents separated or divorced” and “Father or mother had passed away” in pregnant group. The results indicated that these two kind of adverse events at early children development were likely to lead to some negative impact on adolescents, even for unwanted pregnancy. Same results could also be concluded in other studies. Spingarn and DuRant demonstrated that the prevalence of teenage parenthood was much higher for adolescents who had lived with only one parent up to 16 years of age than it was for adolescents from 2-parent families. Moreover, those who came from single-parent families due to parental separation were at the highest risk of becoming teenage parents (24). Another retrospective study from the United States also showed that a strong positive relationship of single-parent households with teenage pregnancy was also indicated (25).

Additionally, this study considered multiple logistic regression models to find the correlation between each type of adverse childhood experience and the risk of adolescent pregnancy. The results indicated that having adverse childhood experience increased the risk of adolescent pregnancy by 73.7% after controlling for confounding factors such as age, education, occupational status and region. We especially found that "parents separated or divorced", as an adverse childhood experience, could distinctly increase the risk by 59.2%. The study results of Adams et al., using a regression analysis controlling for the significant age and race differences between the pregnant and non-pregnant groups, revealed that a past history of physical abuse, and the frequency of alcohol use were significantly associated with teen pregnancy (23). Pallitto' study showed that the risk of adolescent pregnancy was significantly higher among women abused as children (26). Our results differed from those studies and only found "parents separated or divorced" as an adverse childhood experience was associated with an earlier age of pregnancy in the multiple logistic regression models. The differences in results may be due to the China traditional culture. From a traditional Chinese perspective, corporal punishment is commonly seen by parents as a legitimate and effective way of discipline, and even though a maltreatment resulting in mild injury is commonly not perceived as abusive (27). Therefore, some adolescents may not perceive that they had adverse childhood experience especially the language or physical abuse.

However, there are still some studies have found that the associations between physical and/or sexual abuse and adolescent pregnancy no longer remained significant after controlling for confounding factors (28), or not controlling for confounding factors (29-31). As a result, further study is needed to explore the relationship between adverse childhood experience and adolescent pregnancy.

Limitations

Some limitations of this study should be mentioned. Firstly, in view of the research targets are still a sensitive and vulnerable group, the study was available in the maternal hospitals where it is a place for related service provision, therefore, the subjects' representative was limited in a sense, and the extending of the results should be considered carefully. Secondly, the cross-sectional nature of the study did not allow us to investigate causal pathways between adolescent adverse childhood experience and pregnancy. For this purpose, longitudinal studies assessing among the young unmarried girls should be conducted in the future.

Conclusion

Adolescent adverse childhood experience, especially the category of Parents separated/divorced was clearly correlated with adolescent pregnancy in China. Efforts to reduce adverse childhood experience and adolescent pregnancy should include the following: awareness rising about the care of adolescents with adverse childhood experience; work with young women to promote self-esteem, learn about sexual and reproductive health, and encourage more healthy negotiation regarding sexual decision making; training of medical personnel to detect adverse childhood experience more proactively and to provide services in a nonjudgmental manner; promotion of multiple mechanisms such as youth clinic or community of support for adolescents.

ACKNOWLEDGMENTS

This study was supported by WHO Western Pacific Region Office/MOH China (grant number ICP/RPH/3.2/001). We are very grateful to all the doctors who provided their contribution in the field study and data collection in Beijing, Jinan City and Guangzhou city, and also would like to thank all the participants in the study for their cooperation and support.

REFERENCES

[1] WHO Regional Office for the Pacific: Demographic tables for the Western Pacific 2005-2010. Manila, Philippine, 2005:7.

[2] Census Office of the State Council.Chinese2010census data. China Statistics Press 2010; 115-7. [Chinese]

[3] Ministry of Health. China Health Statistics Yearbook. Peking Union Medical College press 2010; 207. [Chinese]

[4] Liao GL, Liu HS, Wang YF, et al. The age analysis of termination of pregnancy in 2nd and 3rd trimester among girls during 1984~2003 in gynecological institute in Guangzhou city. Pract Prev Med 2005;12: 1078-80. [Chinese]

[5] Wang JM. The study of unmarried repeat abortion adolescents psychosomatic behavior and reproductive health. Maternal Child Health Care China 2008;15(10):2203-4. [Chinese]

[6] United Nations. World Population Monitoring 2002. Reproductive rights and reproductive health: selected aspects. ESA/P/WP.171, 2002.

[7] Mayor S. Pregnancy and childbirth are leading causes of death in teenage girls in developing countries. BMJ 2004;328:1152.

[8] United Nations. Human Rights Today: A United Nations Priority. E.98.1.22, 1998.

[9] Moore KA, Myers DR, Morrison C, et al. Age at first childbirth and later poverty. J Res Adolesc 1993;3(4):393-422.

[10] Grogger J and Bronars S. The socioeconomic consequences of teenage `childbearing: findings from a natural experiment. Fam Plann Perspect 1993;25(4):156–61.

[11] Hillis SD, Anda RF, Dube SR, et al. The association between adverse childhood experiences and adolescent pregnancy, long-term psychosocial consequences, and fetal death. Pediatrics 2004;113:320-7.

[12] Quinlivan JA, Tan LH, Steele A, Black K. Impact of demographic factors, early family relationships and depressive symptomatology in teenage pregnancy. Aust NZ J Psychiatry 2004;38:197–203.

[13] Palmore S, Millar K. Some common characteristics of pregnant teens who choose childbirth. J SchNurs 1996;12:19-22.

[14] Oz S, Fine M. A comparison of childhood backgrounds of teenage mothers and their non-mother peers: a new formulation. J Adolesc 1988; 11:251-61.

[15] Wellings K, Wadsworth J, Johnson A, et al. Teenage fertility and life chances. Rev Reprod 1999;4:184-90.

[16] Curtis HA, Lawrence CJ, Tripp JH. Teenage sexual intercourse and pregnancy. Arch Dis Child 1988;63:373-9.

[17] Butler JR, and Burton LM. Rethinking teenage childbearing: is sexual abuse a missing link? FamRelat 1990;39:73.

[18] Boyer D, Fine D. Sexual abuse as a factor in adolescent pregnancy and child maltreatment. Fam Plann Perspect 1992;24:4.

[19] N. Haley, E. Roy, P. Leclerc, et al. Characteristics of Adolescent Street Youth with a History of Pregnancy. J Pediatr Adolesc Gynecol 2004; 17:313-20.

[20] Kenney JW, Reinholtz C, and Angelini PJ. Ethnic differences in childhood and adolescent sexual abuse and teenage pregnancy. J Adolesc Health 1997;21:3-10.

[21] Straus M, Gelles RJ. Physical violence in American families: Risk factors and adaptations to violence in 8,145 families. New Brunswick, NJ: Transaction Press, 1990.

[22] Wyatt GE. The sexual abuse of Afro-American and White-American women in childhood. Child Abuse Negl 1985;9:507-19.

[23] Adams JA, East PL. Past physical abuse is significantly correlated with pregnancy as an adolescent. J Pediatr Adolesc Gynecol 1999;12:133-8.

[24] Spingarn RW, DuRant RH. Male adolescents involved in pregnancy: associated health risk and problem behaviors. Pediatrics 1996;98:262-8.

[25] Blake BJ, Bentov L. Geographical mapping of unmarried teen births and selected sociodemographic variables. Public Health Nurs 2001;18:33–9.

[26] Pallitto CC, Murillo V. Childhood abuse as a risk factor for adolescent pregnancy in El Salvador. J Adolesc Health 2008;42:580–6.

[27] Lau JTF, Liu JLY, Yu A, et al. Conceptualization, reporting and underreporting of child abuse in Hong Kong. Child Abuse Negl 1999; 23:1159–74.

[28] Stock JL, Bell MA, Boyer DK, et al. Adolescent pregnancy and sexual risk-taking among sexually abused girls. Fam Plann Perspect 1997; 29(5):200-7.

[29] Rainey DY, Stevens-Simon, Kaplan DW. Are adolescents who report prior sexual abuse at higher risk for pregnancy? Child Abuse Negl 1995; 19(10):1283-8.

[30] Guijarro S, Naranjo J, Padilla M, et al. Family risk factors associated with adolescent pregnancy: study of a group of adolescent girls and their families in Ecuador. J Adolesc Health 1999;25(2):166-72.

[31] Kenney JW, Reinholtz C, Angelini PJ. Ethnic differences in childhood and adolescent sexual abuse and teenage pregnancy. J Adolesc Health1997;21(1):3-10.

Submitted: October 15, 2012.*Revised:* January 04, 2013.*Accepted:* January 05, 2013.

In: Child and Adolescent Health Yearbook 2013
Editor: Joav Merrick

ISBN: 978-1-63117-658-6

Chapter 27

PREVALENCE AND INCIDENCE OF ASYMPTOMATIC BACTERIURIA AMONG NIGERIAN CHILDREN AND ADOLESCENTS WITH TYPE 1 DIABETES MELLITUS

Alphonsus N Onyiriuka * ***and Edirin O Yusuf***
Department of Child Health and Department of Medical Microbiology,
University of Benin Teaching Hospital, Benin City, Nigeria

ABSTRACT

It is commonly believed that patients with diabetes mellitus are at increased risk of urinary tract infection compared with non-diabetic patients. Methods: Bacteriuria was screened for in 34 patients (17 with type 1 diabetes mellitus and 17 with non-diabetic endocrine disorders) at their regular follow-up visits collected every three months for 12 months and cultured. The subjects were matched for age and sex. Results: Among the 34 patients screened, only two (one (5.9%) out of 17 diabetic and one (5.9%) out of 17 non-diabetic) had asymptomatic bacteriuria and the urine culture of each of them yielded a growth of Escherichia coli sensitive to gentamycin. The duration of diabetes in the girl with asymptomatic bacteriuria (ASB) was 7 years. She had a poor glycaemic control and some psychosocial challenges. Her pubertal maturation was delayed (Tanner Stage II at the age of 15 years and has not attained menarche). She weighed 29 Kg, with BMI of 16.0 kg/m2. In addition, she had vaginal candidiasis for which she was appropriately treated, using ketconazole. The other patient with ASB was a 7-year-old girl with precocious puberty due to congenital adrenal hyperplasia diagnosed at the age of 18 months. The two patients with ASB did not progress to symptomatic bacteriuria after a follow-up period of one year. Conclusion: The prevalence and incidence of asymptomatic bacteriuria in diabetic children and adolescents do not differ from those of their non-diabetic counterparts.

Keywords: Asymptomatic bacteriuria, adolescence, childhood, diabetes mellitus, incidence

* Corresponding author: Alphonsus N Onyiriuka, MD, Department of Child Health, University of Benin Teaching Hospital, PMB 1111, Benin City, Nigeria. E-mail: alpndiony@yahoo.com or didiruka@gmail.com.

INTRODUCTION

Asymptomatic bacteriuria refers to the presence of a positive urine culture in an asymptomatic person (1). It is commonly believed that individuals with diabetes mellitus are at increased risk of infection, particularly urinary tract infection (UTI) (2-4). Such an infection in diabetic patients may result in severe complications and death more frequently than would be anticipated among non-diabetics (2,4). Most UTI in diabetic patients are relatively asymptomatic (4). Among diabetic patients, factors presumed to predispose to UTI include age, neurogenic bladder, duration of diabetes and degree of glycaemic control (2,5). Some clinicians consider asymptomatic patients being screened for bacteriuria to be at risk of UTI if two or three consecutive cultures of freshly voided urine reveal more than 105 organisms/ml (6). Whether or not individuals with asymptomatic bacteriuria (ASB) should be treated with antibiotics remains debatable (4). It is recommended that ASB should be treated with antibiotics in pregnant women, children aged 5-6 years and prior to invasive genitourinary procedures (7).

It is not known with certainty whether individuals with diabetes mellitus are at a higher risk of bacteriuria than non-diabetics. Studies on this subject have yielded mixed results. For instance, Lindberg et al. (8) reported that three out of 304 (0.99%) girls and zero out of 337 boys with type 1 diabetes mellitus screened for bacteriuria were positive. They, therefore, concluded that the prevalence of ASB in diabetic children and adolescents did not differ from that of their non-diabetic peers. In contrast, a meta-analysis of published data involving 22 studies revealed that the prevalence of ASB was 12.2% in diabetic children compared with 4.5% in healthy controls (9). Point prevalence was also higher in children and adolescents with diabetes (12.9%) compared with their non-diabetic (2.7%) counterparts (9). A similar increased risk among diabetic children and adolescents was reported from Egypt (10). Some studies have concluded that screening for ASB in diabetic patients is warranted because it has been found to be a risk factor for developing symptomatic urinary tract infection (11). In a survey in Port Harcourt, Nigeria of secondary school students aged 10-17 years the prevalence of ASB was 6.5% and 4.5% in girls and boys respectively (12).

Despite the recognized potential of ASB in diabetic patients to cause renal damage and ultimately, chronic kidney disease, there is a general paucity of information in the literature on its incidence, particularly in developing countries. Besides, it is not known how often ASB progresses to symptomatic bacteriuria. In addition, infection itself can lead to poor diabetic control by increased secretion of counterregulatory hormones (glucagon, cortisol, growth hormone, catecholamines), inhibition of insulin secretion, and insulin resistance of peripheral tissues/increased cytokine secretion (13,14).

The purpose of the present study is to determine the incidence of ASB among children and adolescents with T1DM attending the Paediatric Endocrine-Metabolic Clinic, UBTH and compare the result with those of their non-diabetic peers.

METHODS

The study was conducted in the Paediatric Endocrine-Metabolic Clinic of the University of Benin Teaching Hospital (UBTH), Benin City, Nigeria over a 12-month period for each of the subjects. The study was approved by UBTH Ethical Committee. Consent was obtained from both the patient and their parents. Information sought from the subjects included age, sex, parents educational attainment, parents occupation, antibiotic use and duration of type 1 diabetes mellitus (T1DM). Patients with complaints suggestive of symptomatic urinary tract infection (such as dysuria, frequent micturiction, urgency, pain in the loin or suprapubic region) were excluded from the study. The socio-economic status of the parents of the subjects was determined using the classification suggested by Ogunlesi et al. (15). This was analyzed via combining the highest educational attainment, occupation and income of the parents (based on the mean income of each educational qualification and occupation). In this Social Classification System, classes I and II represent high social class, class III represents middle social class while classes IV and V represent low social class. In this way, the subjects were categorized into high, middle and low socio-economic groups.

A clean catch mid-stream urine specimen was obtained from each of the subjects every three months, over a total period of 12 months, amounting to four urine specimens per subject. In all the subjects, appropriate care was taken before collection of the urine specimen to avoid contamination. Each urine specimen was transported to the Research Laboratory, Department of Child Health, UBTH, where it was refrigerated immediately and cultured within two hours of collection. All the urine samples were cultured on Blood and MacConkey agar plates. The plates were incubated at 37 degree Celcius aerobically for 48 hours. Standard procedure was applied in the handling, staining, microscopy and culture of all the urine specimens (16). Full clinical examination was conducted on each of the patients at every visit. The presence of bacterial growth of 105 colony-forming units/ml was accepted as significant bacteriuria (17). Descriptive statistics such as frequencies, means, ratios, standard deviations, confidence intervals, percentages were used to describe all the variables.

RESULTS

Two (one diabetic and one non-diabetic) out of the 34 patients screened for asymptomatic bacteriuria (ASB) had positive urine culture, giving a prevalence of 5.9% for diabetic and non-diabetic patients respectively. The urine culture of each case with significant asymptomatic yielded a growth of Escherichia coli sensitive to gentamycin. The diabetic patient was a 15-year-old girl diagnosed of type 1 diabetes mellitus 7 years ago. She had a poor glycaemic control and some psychosocial challenges. Her pubertal maturation was delayed (Tanner Stage II at the age of 15 years and has not attained menarche). She weighed 29 Kg, with BMI of 16.0 kg/m2. In addition, she had vaginal candidiasis for which she was appropriately treated, using ketconazole. During the follow-up, appropriate urine samples were collected and screened every 3 months for 12 months for each of the patients but no other patient had significant asymptomatic bacteriuria. Neither of the two patients with significant asymptomatic bacteriuria progressed to symptomatic bacteriuria after two years of follow up. The mean age at presentation of the patients with diabetes was 11.0+4.2 years (95% Confidence Interval, CI=7.7-14.7) for boys; 13.5±1.6 years (95% CI=12.6-14.4) for girls; 12.8±2.9 years (95% CI=11.4-14.1) for both sexes combined. Mean age at presentation: boys versus girls t= 1.28 p>0.05. The age and gender distribution of the subjects is depicted in Table 1.The mean body mass index (BMI) was 18.6±2.5 kg/m^2 (95% CI=17.4-19.8) with 6

(35.3%) having a BMI below 19.0 kg/m^2. None of the subjects had BMI > 25 kg/m^2. Over half of the families (52.9%) of the subjects were in the middle social class. Eleven point eight percent and 35.3% of the families of the subjects were in the high and low social classes respectively.

DISCUSSION

The prevalence (5.9%) of asymptomatic bacteriuria (ASB) found in the present study is two- and 5-fold lower than the 12.2% and 30.0% respectively reported from two different studies, one a meta-analysis of 22 studies and the other among diabetic Egyptian children and adolescents (9,10). Even, prevalence rates lower than that observed in the present study have been reported (8). All reflecting the reported mixed results of prevalence of ASB in children and adolescents, suggesting that some unidentified socio-demographic factors might influence the prevalence of ASB in these subjects. For instance, age, sex, glycaemic control, duration of diabetes and presence of long-term complications have all been variously reported as risk factors (2-4). The method of collection and processing of the urine specimens might have also influenced the different prevalence rates observed. The lower prevalence rate observed in the present study compared to the Egyptian study may partly be because of the differences in the age of the two study populations. Most of the subjects in the Egyptian study were older than 15 years while most the patient in the present study were below 15 years of age. This view is supported by the reports of two studies in Egypt and Hungary which separately showed the prevalence of ASB was higher in girls aged 15 years or older (10,17). In consonance, the only diabetic patient with ASB in the present study was 15 years old. However, the prevalence from our data was within the range (4.5-6.5%) reported from Port Harcourt, Nigeria among non-diabetic secondary school students aged 6 to 15 years(11), suggesting that ASB is not commoner in diabetic compared to non-diabetic children and adolescents. This conclusion is reinforced by the results of the present study which showed that of the two patients with ASB one was diabetic and the other was non-diabetic. Furthermore, as reported by Rozsai et al. (14), the urinary cytokine response to pathogens in both diabetic and non-diabetic children with bacteriuria was comparable.

Table 1. Age and gender distribution of patients with diabetes mellitus

Age group at presentation	Gender		
	Male	**Female**	**Both sexes**
	No(%)	**No(%)**	**No(%)**
Below 10 years	2(33.3)	0(0)	2(11.8)
10-12 years	0(0)	3(27.3)	3(17.6)
13-15 years	3(50.0)	8(72.7)	11(64.7)
Above 15 years	1(16.7)	0(0)	1(5.9)
Total	6(100.0)	11(100.0)	17(100.0)

Consistent with previous reports, the most common bacterial agent in the present study was Escherichia coli (4,10,18). This finding is partly explained by the report of Geerlings et al. (19) which indicated that E coli expressing type 1 fimbrae adhere better to the uroepithelial cells of women with diabetes mellitus compared to the cells of women without diabetes mellitus. The girl with type 1 diabetes and ASB also had vaginal candidiasis which responded satisfactorily to treatment with ketoconazole. The finding of candidial infection in this adolescent with diabetes mellitus is not surprising as other investigators have reported a similar finding (20). The increased frequency of vaginal candidiasis in patients with diabetes mellitus is believed to be due to increase in ambient vaginal glycogen stores in them (20).

In conclusion, prevalence and incidence of asymptomatic bacteriuria do not differ between diabetic and non-diabetic children and adolescents.

REFERENCES

[1] Ooi S, Frazee LA, Gardner WG. Management of asymptomatic bacteriuria in patients with diabetes mellitus. Ann Pharmacotherapy 2004;38(3):490-3.

[2] Guillausseau PJ, Farah R, Laloi-Michelin M, Tielmans A, Rymer R, Warnet R. Urinary tract infections and diabetes mellitus. Rev Prat 2003;53(16):1790-6.

[3] Funftuck R, Nicolle LE, Hanefeld M, Naser KG. Urinary tract infection in patients with diabetes mellitus. Clin Nephrol 2012;77(1):40-8.

[4] Balachandar MS, Pavkovic P, Metelko Z. Kidney infections in diabetes mellitus. Diabetologia Croatica 2002;31(2):95-103.

[5] Keane EH, Boyko EJ, Reller LB, Hamman RF. Prevalence of asymptomatic bacteriuria in subjects with NIDDM in San Luis Valley of Colorado. Diabetes Care 1988;11:708-12.

[6] Rifkin RH. Urinary tract infection in childhood. Pediatrics 1977;60:508.

[7] Raz R. Asymptomatic bacteriuria: Clinical significance and management. Int J Antimicrob Agents 2003;22(Suppl 2):45-7.

[8] Lindberg U, Bergstrom AL, Carlsson E, Dahlquist G, Hermansson G, Larsson Y, et al. Urinary tract infection in children with type 1 diabetes. Acta Pediatr Scand 1985;74:85-8.

[9] Renko M, Tapaainen P, Tossavainen P, Pokka T, Uhari M. Meta-analysis of the significance of asymptomatic bacteriuria in diabetes. Diabetes Care 2011;34(1):230-5.

[10] Salem MA, Matler RM, Abdelmaksond AA, El Masry SA. Prevalence of asymptomatic bacteriuria in Egyptian children and adolescents with type 1 diabetes mellitus. J Egypt Soc Parasitol 2009;39(3):951-62.

[11] Ribera MC, Pascual R, Barbar PC, Pederera V, Gil V. Incidence and risk factors associated with urinary tract infection in diabetic patients with or without asymptomatic bacteriuria. Eur J Clin Microbiol Infect Dis 2006;25:389-93.

[12] Frank-Peterside N, Wokoma EC. Prevalence of asymptomatic bacteriuria in students of University of Port Harcourt Demonstration Secondary School. JASEM 2009;13:55-8.

[13] Leibovici L, Yehehzkelli Y, Porter A et al. Influence of diabetes mellitus and glycaemic control on the characteristics and outcome of common infections. Diabet Med 1996;13:457-463.

[14] Rozsai B, Lanyi E, Berki T, Soltesz G. Urinary cytokine response to asymptomatic bacteriuria in type 1 diabetic children and young adults. Pediatr Diabetes. 2006;7(3):153-8.

[15] Ogunlesi TA, Dedeke IOF, Kuponiyi OT. Socio-economic classification of children attending Specialist Paediatric Centres in Ogun State, Nigeria. Nig Med Pract 2008; 54(1):21-5.

[16] Collee JG, Duguid JP, Frasar AG. Laboratory strategy in the diagnosis of infective syndromes. In: Collee JG, Duguid JP, Frasar AG, Marmion DP, Simmon A eds. Mackie and McCarteney practical medical microbiology, 13 ed. Edinburgh: Churchill Livingstone, 1989:601-49.

[17] Rozsai B, Lanyi E, Soltesz G. Asymptomatic bacteriuria and leucocytouria in type 1 diabetes children and young adults. Diabetes Care 2003;26(7):2209-10.

[18] Makuyana D, Mhlabi D, Chipfupa M, Munyombwe T, Gwanzura L. Asymptomatic bacteriuria among outpatients with diabetes mellitus in urban black population. Cent Afr J Med 2002;48(7-8):78-82.

[19] Geerlings SE, Meiland R, Hoepelman AI. Pathogenesis of bacteriuria in women with diabetes mellitus. Int J Antimicrob Agents 2002;19(6):539-45.

[20] Rein MF, Holmes KK. Non-specific vaginitis, vulvovaginal candidiasis and trichomoniasis. Curr Clin Topics Infect Dis 1983;4:281.

In: Child and Adolescent Health Yearbook 2013
Editor: Joav Merrick

ISBN: 978-1-63117-658-6

Chapter 28

HEALTH CARE SEEKING AVENUES OF PARENTS OF SCHOOL-AGE CHILDREN WITH SEVERE HEALTH PROBLEMS IN A COMMUNITY IN GHANA

Cecilia Obeng, PhD*
Department of Applied Health Science, Indiana University, Bloomington, Indiana, United States of America

ABSTRACT

People living in rural areas in Ghana face impediments to accessing hospitals and clinics. This study examines how culture influences health care–seeking behavior, including the healing processes that participants experience in times of illness, in a Ghana community. The study uses narratives provided by twenty parents about their school-aged children with severe health problems. Results from an analysis of the participants' narratives indicate that participants prefer traditional herbal and/or spiritual 'clinics' to modern clinics/hospitals because of the pleasant relationship established with those healers. Participants also attributed their preference for traditional herbal or spiritual clinics to the low fees charged by the clinics. They noted further that questions about their health problems were always promptly answered at the herbal/spiritual clinics, unlike in modern clinics/hospitals, where they had to wait for hours or days due to delays in releasing laboratory results .However, participants complained about the crowded environment of some of the traditional herbal/spiritual clinics .This study recommends making all traditional clinics patient-friendly in order to expedite healthcare delivery in rural Ghana.

Keywords: Traditional clinics, rural Ghana, parents, children

* Corresponding author: Associate professor Cecilia Obeng, PhD, Department of Applied Health Science, Indiana University, 1025 E 7th Street, HPER 116, Room 296-I, Bloomington, IN 47405 United States. E-mail: cobeng@indiana.edu.

INTRODUCTION

Research on healthcare in Africa indicates that access to healthcare and diagnoses of diseases is difficult on the continent and that many diseases are either misdiagnosed or go untreated (1,2). In spite of the fact that there has been an improvement in healthcare delivery, especially with regard to communicable diseases in the world, communicable diseases are prevalent in Africa (2-4). HIV/AIDS and malaria infection are among the contributing factors associated with a high number of deaths in the region (3,4). It is also true that a number of sub-Saharan African countries still suffer from some of the worst health problems seen in the world.

The healthcare system in some sub-Saharan African countries is in crisis; maternal and prenatal health problems continue to plague the sub-region. Of all the diseases in the world, 24% are in Africa, with only a few healthcare workers caring for individuals who have health problems (5-7). The shortage of health care workers has had a tremendous impact on the continent. Africa has one of the lowest levels of human resources in the world, and out of the 57countries in which there is a shortage of healthcare workers, 36 of them were in Africa (5-7). Mullan et al. (8) and Callaghan et al. (9) attest to these problems and attribute them to a lack of postgraduate education, retention of graduates after their medical education, coordination between the ministries (education and health), and lack of accreditation of the medical schools in sub-Saharan Africa. The above-mentioned problems, the authors state, have led to a shortage of professionals like doctors, especially, in rural Africa (8,9).

Scholarship on the shortage of African healthcare workers indicates further that the problem has led to task-shifting in which jobs that should be done by specific professionals in the appropriate health field are assigned to persons with lower qualifications in the field (6). Furthermore, task-shifting is done in Africa to address the healthcare needs (especially with respect to the HIV pandemic that has affected so many lives) on the continent. Job shifting, scholars indicated, will enable well-trained nurses to be involved in prescribing drugs, counselors to help with testing, and some patients to perform certain tasks in their recovering process (9). The main aim of the above-mentioned care system (task-shifting) has been to provide quality care and relieve some of the pressure on healthcare workers (9). The task-shifting idea was explained by the World Health Organization (WHO) in the guidelines in their 2004 publication Integrated Management of Adult and Adolescent Illness and was extended and formalized by WHO/UNAIDS/PEPFAR in 2008 (9). A report by WHO indicates further that only 1% of the world's funding allocated for health care goes to Africa. It is well known that Africans suffer from high levels of malnutrition (10), the problems of which are attributed to protein energy deficiency (10). Infertility and premature death are also unnecessarily high in some of these regions (11).

Given the unfortunate state of the healthcare situation described above, this study examined 20 narratives of parents in rural Africa (Ghana) in order to understand the healthcare–seeking behavior of the participants. Also examined were the various stages that parents have undergone to find care for their children's health issues.

Methods

This study was approved by the Institutional Review Board of Indiana University's Human Subjects Committee. The population for this study was comprised of 20 participants who visited five traditional clinics in a rural area in Ghana. Participants were interviewed by the principal investigator and two paid research assistants. The research assistants had lived in the school district for over twenty years. The research assistants contacted approximately 30 potential parents for interviews for this study. Four people were not able to participate because of conflicts with their schedules. Twenty out of the 26 qualified for this study because they had children with severe health problems and chronic health diseases, and the parents were also happy to be part of the study. The instrument used in the study consisted of both closed-ended and open-ended questions. The closed-ended questions concerned the demographic information of participants. The open-ended questions were used as the main questions for this qualitative study. The open-ended questions asked participants to narrate their reason(s) for attending herbal/spiritual clinics. Participation was voluntary, and consent was given before parents participated in interviews. In order to verify whether what participants reported was an accurate representation of their views, the researchers returned after 10 days and reviewed with participants what they had reported during the first visit.

Coding and Data Analysis

Two people (the principal investigator and a volunteer colleague) were involved in the coding of the completed questionnaires for this study, Health Care Seeking Avenues of Parents of School-Aged Children with Severe Health Problems in a Community in Ghana. The coding involved an assessment of the narratives and the content of the data (by the coders) with the intent of identifying common themes.

A qualitative analysis was conducted on the responses to the open-ended questions collected during the interviews. Responses were grouped into themes for the purpose of analysis.

Results

The results are organized into and discussed under the following themes: 1) demographic information of participants and 2) participants' narratives about their visits to traditional clinics.

Demographic Information

As drawn from the parents' narratives, their children were aged between seven and seventeen years. Participants' children lived in four different villages approximately eighty-five miles from the capital, Accra, in Ghana. Sixteen of the children whose parents were interviewed lived with both of their biological parents. Four girls lived with their grandparents (mothers' parents). Eight of the children attended school, which was almost two miles away from their homes. The other 12 children were in schools close to their homes at the time of this study. Parents reported their children had asthma, kwashiorkor, epilepsy, and diabetes. The table 1 below details information about the participants.

Table 1. Information about the participants

Participants	Age of Parents	Sex of Parents	No .of Children	School Attended	No .of Visits to a Government Hospital or Clinic	No. of Visits to a Traditional Clinic	Kind of Diseases Reported
Parent 1	50	M	9	Public	2	20 or more	Epilepsy
Parent2	45	F	8	Public	1	Many times	Asthma
Parent 3	43	F	6	Public	2	Over 15 times	Asthma
Parent 4	43	M	7	Pubic	2	Over 15times	Asthma
Parent 5	42	F	7	public	2	Over 10 times	Asthma
Parent 6	41	F	6	Public	0	Over 15 times	Kwashiorkor
Parent 7	41	F	6	Public	0	Over 15 times	Kwashiorkor
Parent 8	40	F	6	Public	1	10	Kwashiorkor
Parent 9	40	F	7	Public	1	Over 15 times	Kwashiorkor
Parent 10	39	F	6	Public	0	Over 15 times	Kwashiorkor
Parent 11	38	F	8	Public	3	Over 20 times	Diabetes
Parent 12	38	M	9	Public	5	Over 15 times	Epilepsy,
Parent 13	35	F	4	Public	3	10	Asthma
Parent 14	25	F	2	Private	4	Over 15 times	Diabetes
Parent 15	23	F	1	Private	2	Over 15 times	Asthma
Parent 16	22	F	1	Public	6	Over 20 times	Asthma
Parent 17	22	F	1	Public	2	Over 15 times	Asthma
Parent 18	21	F	1	Public	1	10	Kwashiorkor
Parent 19	21	F	1	Public	2	Over 15 times	Asthma
Parent 20	20	F	1	Public	1	10	Kwashiorkor

Participants and their narratives

Thematic summaries of participants' narratives are given below. Six participants, one male and five females, reported that a lack of money to send their children to government hospitals/clinics contributed to their decision to send their children to traditional clinics. One participant wrote:

> "We decided to take him to an herbal/spiritual clinic because we had tried several times to save money towards sending him to the hospital but we had not been able to save enough money to afford transportation cost to go to the nearest clinic which is twenty miles away. I think to send him to the hospital, which is about eight-five miles, would have been a lifetime's saving and we couldn't have waited that long given the severity of the illness."

Five of the participants, aged between 21 and 43 years, said that the money that the traditional clinics charge patients motivated them to send their children to traditional clinics. One of the participants who sent his child to a traditional clinic wrote:

> "The day that our family was informed about the herbal clinic was the best day for our family. The money that the healer's clinic charged was just about one-hundredth of what our friends told us it would have cost at the government hospital."

Five participants, all female, said the friendly environment of the traditional clinics motivated them to send their children to the traditional clinic. A participant wrote:

> "Our herbalist/spiritualist doctor was friendly and spent many hours with us. He and his assistant answered all our questions. We understand that in the Western-based clinics the maximum amount of time that the physician can have for you was twenty minutes. The many questions our family had could not have been answered within the twenty-minutes time period let alone the doctors' twenty minutes maximum time frame."

A mother said:

> "The Herbal/ spiritual clinics is the best place for those of us who do not have time to wait for a whole day. I understand some of the tests could take a week or even a whole year for the doctor to tell you the cause of your illness. Also, I understand if you are not lucky they will just say they do not know the cause of your illness. I like the herbal clinic because of their efficient work ethic but the many materials in the herbal clinic made me uncomfortable and added to my stress level."

Four mothers reported that they went to an herbalist clinic because the herbalists were able to answer their questions concerning their children's illnesses. One mother reported:

> "We got all the answers that we suspected were causing the illness from the herbalist and we now know the best place to go when anybody in our family is sick. Our only problem was the many 'materials' that were in the clinic also the place was filthy."

Another mother said:

> "The herbalist and his assistant were patient and answered all our many question but my biggest problem was that there was no space for us to sit in the clinic, the clinic was cluttered with materials and the place was also dirty."

DISCUSSION

Most of the participants' narratives suggested that the first-rate performance of the work done by traditional healers encouraged them to choose those healers over Western-trained physicians.

Specifically, we learned of a better work ethic and a more intimate working relationship between the traditional care-givers and their clients. The low charges prompt answers given to patients' families about the causative agents of their diseases, excellent working relationships between the caregivers and their clients, and effective care at the traditional clinics was convincing of better treatment for the participants.

From their narratives, it was obvious that the traditional clinics were cluttered with the materials they used in their profession, thereby posing a hindrance or potential danger to easy patient movement and, consequently, making it difficult for patients and the healers to find much needed space. This also created unsanitary conditions in the clinics, according to participants narratives.

This study recommends improvements to achieve patient-friendly and hygienic environments in the form of better sanitation and de-cluttering of unwanted materials from the healing sites/clinics of the traditional healers in order to ensure optimal efficiency. This recommendation is motivated by the fact that participants believed that improvements in the environments of some of the traditional healers would ease their stress and improve their health when they are at these sites.

Limitations and future research

Although using twenty participants' experiences from five clinics for this study may appear limiting, it represents more than two-thirds of the traditional clinics in the research site. Also, we were aware of the dangerous possibility of our personal judgments intervening in their narratives. Being aware of these potential pitfalls helped, however, to mitigate them. Specifically, our awareness of this unique situation kept us on guard against intervening in the telling of participants' narratives. In the future, and based upon the fact that participants wanted improvement in the traditional clinic setting, a survey will be done to determine whether there have been improvements (structural and interactional) enacted by healers in order to enhance their profession.

REFERENCES

[1] Petti CA, Polage CR, Quinn TC, et al. Laboratory medicine in Africa: A barrier to effective health care. Clinical Infectious Diseases. 2006;42:377-82.

[2] Dacombe RJ, Squire SB, Ramsav ARC, Banda HT, Bates I. Essential medical Laboratory Services: their role in delivering equitable health care in Malawi. Malawi Med J 2006:18(2):77-9.

[3] Joint United Nations Programme on HIV/AIDS. 2011. Accessed 2012 Nov 01. URL: http://www.unaids.org/en/media/unaids/contentassets/documents/unaidspublication/2011/JC2216_WorldAIDSday_report_2011_en.pdf.

[4] World Malaria Report. 2011. Accessed 2012 Nov 01. URL: http://www.who.int/ malaria/world_malaria_ report_2011/WHOGMP_burden_estimates_qa.pdf.

[5] The World Health Organization. 2006. Accessed 2012 Nov 01. URL:who.int/gho/publications /world_health_statistics/whostat2006_10highlights.pdf.

[6] WHO/UNAIDS/PEPFAR. Task Shifting: Global Recommendations and Guidelines. Geneva. 2008. Accessed 2012 Nov 01. URL:http://www.who.int/healthsystems/task_ shifting/en/index.html.

[7] Health Poverty Action. Accessed 2012 Nov 01. URL: http://healthpovertyaction.org/ policy-and-resources/health-systems/the-global-shortage-of-health-workers/.

[8] Mullan F, Freyhwot S, Omaswa F, Wassermann T. Medical schools in sub-Saharan Africa. Lancet 2011;377:1113-21.

[9] Callaghan M, Ford N, Schneider H. A systematic review of task-shifting for HIV treatment and care in Africa. Hum Resources Health 2010;8:8.

[10] Maletnlema TN. Hunger and malnutrition: The determinant of development: the case for Africa and its food and nutrition workers. East Afr Med J 1992;69(8):424-7.

In: Child and Adolescent Health Yearbook 2013
Editor: Joav Merrick
ISBN: 978-1-63117-658-6

Chapter 29

PLUMMER'S NAIL (ONYCHOLYSIS) IN AN ADOLESCENT NIGERIAN GIRL WITH HYPERTHYROIDISM DUE TO GRAVES' DISEASE

Alphonsus N Onyiriuka*, Chinedu A Atamah and Louis C. Onyiriuka
Department of Child Health, University of Benin Teaching Hospital, Benin City, Nigeria

ABSTRACT

This is a case report of a 16-year-old Nigerian girl with Plummer's nail associated with hyperthyroidism (Graves' disease). The issue of excessive weight gain after therapy for the Graves' disease was also discussed. Following therapy, the patient gained 7 Kg over a period of 5 months. The diagnosis of hyperthyroidism due to Graves' disease was based on increased heart rate at rest, diffuse smooth goiter, mild ophthalmopathy, low TSH (thyroid stimulating hormone) level, elevated T3 (triiodothyronine) and T4 (tetraiodothyronine) levels. The case report emphasize the need for clinicians to be alert to the possibility of nail changes in adolescents with thyroid diseases and watch out for weight gain following successful therapy.

Keywords: Adolescence, hyperthyroidism, Graves' disease, Plummer's nail, onycholysis

INTRODUCTION

In patients with hyperthyroidism, onycholysis (separation of the nail plate from the nail bed) is referred to as "Plummer's nails" (1,2). Plummer's nail is unique for Graves' disease (1,3). In Plummer's nail, the nails often exhibit a concave shape ("scoop shovel" configuration)

*Corresponding author: Alphonsus N Onyiriuka, MD, Department of Child Health, University of Benin Teaching Hospital, PMB 1111, Benin City, Nigeria. Email: alpndiony@yahoo.com or didiruka@gmail.com.

and/or a distal onycholysis (2).Hyperthyroidism makes the nail brittle, leading to the separation of the plate from the nail bed (4).

In adults, nail changes are present in 5% of cases of hyperthyroidism (2). Reports of Plummer's nail in children and adolescents with hyperthyroidism are very scarce. A survey of standard textbooks of pediatrics as well as pediatric endocrinology revealed that there was no mention of nail changes in hyperthyroidism, indicating the need to raise awareness among clinicians of its association with hyperthyroidism in the pediatric age group (5,6). Given the assertion that Plummer's nail is unique to Graves' disease (3), its presence might be a useful clue to the diagnosis of Graves' disease, particularly in developing countries where availability of laboratory facilities for evaluation of endocrine disorders is grossly inadequate. Nail abnormalities are known to provide both subtle and obvious clues to common medical problems or severe systemic diseases (7). Indeed, it has been stated that the complete physician regardless of his field of specialty needs to be alert to the often significant manifestation of abnormal nail as a signal to important pathology (8). In this context, Nakat Sui and Lin (3) suggested that patients with unexplained onycholysis should be screened for asymptomatic thyroid disease.

This case report aims at stimulating the interest and raising awareness of the general paediatrician with regard to the association between abnormalities of the nail and hyperthyroidism in adolescence.

CASE REPORT

The patient was a 16-year old girl who was referred from a secondary healthcare facility in a neighbouring state. The presenting complaints were weight loss for 17 months, cessation of menses for 10 months and neck swelling for 8 months. The immediate symptoms that prompted seeking medical help were abdominal pain, vomiting and frequent watery stools all of 4 days duration. A review of the systems revealed a positive history of increased food intake, excessive sweating, palpitation, sweaty palms and a slight change in hand writing. She had emotional liability. No family history suggestive of thyroid disorder. There was no positive history of acute iodine exposure or ingestion of thyroid hormone. The patient does not practice pedicure. She attained menarche at the age of 12 years and her menstrual cycle had been fairly regular until the present illness. The patient is a secondary school graduate who has just secured admission into one of the Nigerian universities. The patient was the youngest of four children. Her mother is 53 years old. Her father died (from "Stroke") three years ago before the onset of her illness. Physical examination revealed an anxious-looking adolescent girl with fine finger tremor and mild ophthalmopathy. She weighed 44 Kg with a height of 162 cm (BMI=16.8 kg/m^2; 5th percentile). She had a diffuse, smooth, non-tender thyroid swelling measuring 4 x 6 cm. The goiter had no nodule, bruit or differential warmth. The Sexual Maturity Rating (SMR) was Tanner stage IV. The Plummer's nails (Onycholysis) and goiter are shown in Figures 1 and 2 respectively. She had tachycardia with bounding pulse (pulse rate 124/minute at rest). The blood pressure was 110/60 mmHg with the apex beat in the 5th left intercostals space mid-clavicular line. There was no cardiac murmur or finger clubbing. The abdomen was flat, soft with tenderness in the lower half. Bowel sound was normal.The urea and electrolyte profile were normal. Her haematocrit value was 34%.

The laboratory findings are displayed in table 1 and shows a low normal serum TSH and elevated T3 and T4 values.

Table 1. Laboratory findings in a 16-year-old girl with hyperthyroidism

Laboratory parameter	Normal serum values in UBTH	Observed serum values Initial	After 2 months
TSH	0.4-6.2 U/ml	0.6 U/ml	3.4 U/ml
T3	0.7-2.0 ng/ml	6.2 ng/ml	7.6 ng/ml
T4	4.8-10.8 μg/dl	35.2 μg/dl	19.8 μg/dl
Random blood glucose	4.7-6.7 mmol/L	6.2 mmol/L	-
Pelvic scan	Right ovarian cyst measuring 55.1 x 52.9 mm		
Neck scan	Thyroid lobes measure 36 x 17 mm (Right) and 36 x 15 mm (Left) with no focal or cystic mass lesion		
Abdominal scan	Normal		

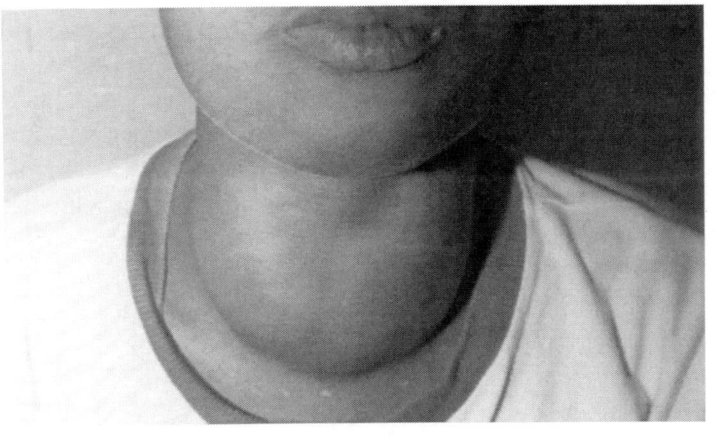

Figure 1.

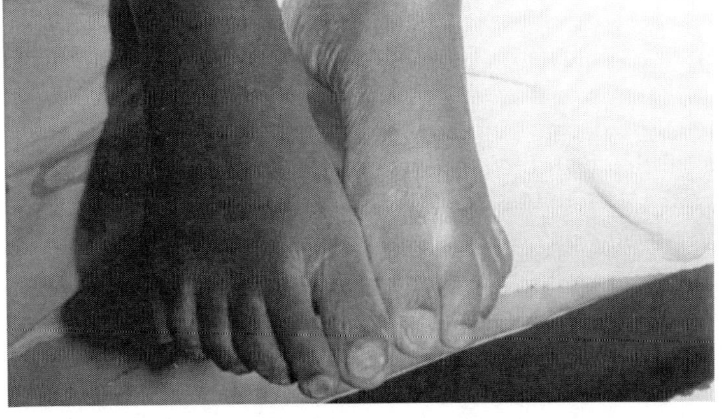

Figure 2.

A diagnosis of Hyperthyroidism due to Graves' disease was made. The gastroenteritis was also kept in view. She was rehydrated with intravenous fluid because of the gastroenteritis and attendant dehydration. Oral carbimazole and propanolol were commenced. The clinical condition improved as evidenced by the resting pulse rate which dropped to an average of 84/minute and she was less nervous. The patient was discharged from the hospital after 4 weeks and followed up in the Endocrine clinic. Her menses was restored and it was regular. She has since resumed her study in the University. Her weight rose to 51 Kg (BMI=19.4 kg/m^2) 5 month after discharge. However, she was lost to follow up.

DISCUSSION

In this patient, the diagnosis of hyperthyroidism due to Graves' disease was based on increased heart rate at rest, presence of diffuse goiter, low normal serum TSH (thyroid stimulating hormone) and elevated serum T3 (triiodothyronine) and T4 (tetraiodothyronine) values.This is in keeping with the criteria used for diagnosis of Graves' disease in a previous study (9). The finger tremor, mild ophthalmopathy and low Body Mass Index (BMI) were all consistent with the diagnosis of Graves' disease. Other causes of hyperthyroidism in childhood and adolescence include subacute thyroiditis, thyroid neoplasms, McCune-Albright syndrome, TSH hypersecretion, excess iodine or thyroid hormone ingestion. Epidemiologically, Graves' disease is by far the commonest cause of hyperthyroidism in the paediatric age group (5,6). The goiter in this patient was not tender as would be expected in thyroiditis. Thyroid cancer is rare in childhood (5,6). The child with thyroid cancer usually presents with a thyroid nodule or an asymptomatic asymmetrical neck mass (5,6). The goiter in the index patient was symmetrical, diffuse, smooth and non-tender, thereby making these other differentials less likely. In our patient, there was no history of acute exposure to iodine or ingestion of thyroid hormone. Hypermetabolic states such as severe anaemia, chronic infections, pheochromocytoma, and muscle-wasting disease may mimick hyperthyroidism clinically but results of thyroid function test are normal (5). In the index patient, the thyroid function tests were deranged.

The toe nails of the index patient was concave shaped, "scoop shovel" configuration, in keeping with the typical description of Plummer's nail in Graves disease (2). Most reports of Plummer's nail are in adults (3,4). Reports of its occurrence in children and adolescents with Graves' disease are scarce. In this context, the present report, hopefully, will contribute to raising the awareness of clinicians of the association of Plummer's nail with Graves' disease in the paediatric age group. This is even more relevant in developing countries where laboratory facilities for adequate investigation of endocrine disorders are often lacking. As proposed by Nakat Sui and Lin any patient (children and adolescents inclusive) with unexplained onycholysis should be screened for asymptomatic thyroid disease (3).

Following treatment and subsequent discharge, our patient gained weight with improvement in her BMI towards normal range. This is not surprising as previous studies have reported a similar finding among patients treated for Graves' disease (9-11). The index patient gained 7 kg five months after therapy and discharge from hospital. The mean weight gain six months after therapy was 5 Kg in the study by Brunova et al. (11). In one of the studies it was concluded that excessive weight gain within six months of treatment is seen in children with Graves disease and the gain in weight could persist (9). The risk of persistence of the weight gain makes it a challenge for the clinician, given the known adverse effects of overweight and obesity (12). The weight gain is believed to be due disappearance of hypermetabolism, linked to the hyperthyroid state (10).

In conclusion, it is our hope that the present report will contribute to raising the awareness of the general paeditrician concerning the association between nail changes (Plummer's nail) and Graves' disease. The issue of excessive weight gain following treatment for Graves' disease in adolescent patients is emphasized.

References

[1] Fawcett RS, Hart TM, Linford S, Stullberg DL. Nail abnormalities: clues to systemic disease. Am Fam Physician 2004;69(6):1417-24.

[2] Rosen T, Kleman GA. Thyroid and skin. In: Callen JP, Jorrizo JL, Greer KE, Pennys NS, Piette WW, Zone JJ, eds. Dermatological signs of internal disease, 2nd ed. Philadelphia, PA: WB Saunders, 1995:183-95.

[3] Nakat Sui T, Lin AN. Onycholysis and thyroid disease: a report of three cases. J Cutan Med Surg 1998;3(1):40-2.

[4] Atia A, Johnson BS, Aldelmalak HD, Sinnot B. Onycholysis (Plummer's nail) in a patient with hyperthyroidism. EndocrPract 2008;14(1):132.

[5] MorelliJG.In: Kliegman RM, Behrman RE, Jenson HB, Stanton BF, eds. Nelson textbook of pediatrics, 18th ed. Philadelphia, PA: Saunders Elsever, 2007:2731-4.

[6] Fisher DA, Grueters A. Thyroid disorders in childhood and adolescence. In: Sperling MA, ed. Pediatric endocrinology, 3rd ed. Philadelphia, PA: Saunders Elsevier, 2008:227-53.

[7] Noronha PA, Zubkov B. Nails and nail disorders in children and adults. Am Fam Physician 1997;55(6):2129-40.

[8] Scher RK. Toe nail disorders. ClinDermatol 1983;1(1):114-24.

[9] Van Veenendaal NR, Rivkees SA. Treatment of paediatric Graves' disease is associated with excessive weight gain. J ClinEndocrionolMetab 2011;96(10):3257-63.

[10] Portmann L, Glusti V. Weight changes in hyperthyroid patients: a challenge for clinicians? Rev Med Suisse 2007;3(105):854-8.

[11] Brunova J, Bruna J, Joubert G, Koninq M. Weight gain in patients after therapy for hyperthyroidism. S Afr Med J 2003;93(7):529-31.

[12] Han TS, Tijhuis MA, Lean ME, Seidell JC. Quality of life in relation to overweight and body fat distribution. Am J Public Health 1998;88: 1814-20.

[13] Visscher TL, Seidell JC. The public health impact of obesity. Annu Rev Public Health 2001;22:355-75.

In: Child and Adolescent Health Yearbook 2013
Editor: Joav Merrick
ISBN: 978-1-63117-658-6

Chapter 30

CHILD ABUSE AND ALCOHOL MISUSE IN A VICTIM: THE ROLE OF ETHNIC AND SOCIETAL FACTORS

Sergei V Jargin*
Peoples' Friendship University of Russia, Moscow, Russia

ABSTRACT

The association of child abuse with alcohol misuse in adolescent victims is known. A case report from the former Soviet Union (SU) is presented in this short communication, illustrating an immediate cause-effect relationship. An opportunity to stay away from the abusive atmosphere at home was provided by a drinking company of schoolmates including some older boys inspiring alcohol purchase and consumption. Ethnicity-related and other societal factors contributing to alcohol misuse and antisocial behavior in adolescents are discussed. Violence in families was a seldom theme in the professional literature of the former SU. Public organizations sometimes did not react to known cases of family violence. A part of the society appeared to be opposed to a broad discussion of family violence because it is to some extent accepted. There is no generally agreed policy with regard to child abuse; the matter being complicated by shortage of adequately trained personnel and limited access to foreign professional literature. The situation seems to be improving nonetheless: the growing Russian economy enables further development of the social welfare system, while broadening international cooperation must attract foreign expertise into the country.

Keywords: Child abuse, adolescents, alcoholism, antisocial behavior

INTRODUCTION

Associations of child abuse (CA) with alcohol misuse (1-3), mental disorders (4,5), poor social skills (6), antisocial behavior (7) and drug abuse (8) have been reported. CA sometimes

* Corresponding author: Sergei V Jargin, MD, Peoples' Friendship University of Russia, Clementovski per 6-82, 115184 Moscow, Russia. Email: sjargin@mail.ru.

persists in families from one generation to another (9,10); and there is a tendency of underreporting (11). Detection and reporting of CA, essential for its prevention and eradication, depend both on victims and perpetrators. It is easy to expose a socially unprotected abuser, for example, an alcoholic or mentally disordered individual. Otherwise, different tools can be applied to prevent the disclosure: distortion of facts and counter-accusations of libel; threats and intimidation of the former victim, acts against his financial or personal interests. Here is presented a case report from the former Soviet Union (SU), not associated with alcohol abuse in the perpetrators.

CASE REPORT

In the summer of 1959 Sergei (S) was three years old. His parents were divorcing and he was sent together with a nanny to a suburb village. They spent also the summers of 1960 and 1961, having little contact with other children; and the boy sat on a sofa or a bench days on end, which did not contribute to his physical development and social skills. In 1963 his mother remarried, the stepfather being 15 years older than S. The following risk factors of CA were present in this case: weak social support, a second younger child in the family, young age of the perpetrator and maltreatment history in his past (12). An ethnic factor obviously played a role: the stepfather was of Jewish descent, while S used to point out his Russian ethnicity. S was in a sense an ethnic misconception: his father and maternal grandfather were Russians, but maternal grandmother was at least partly of Jewish descent. Having a Jewish stepfather, who even worked for a short period at his school, S was, without understanding it, often treated by the social environment as a Jew, which was expressed by bullying. The bullying was sometimes visibly inspired by older persons including some teachers. The author does not intend to say that Jewish children were generally bullied in Soviet schools: it was different at various places; and especially at schools with diversified ethnic composition there were no visible signs of it. Many Jewish children were not bullied, because they behaved “adequately”: somewhat distanced, friendly, not denying their difference. On the contrary, S stressed his Russian ethnicity and behaved ambitiously, involuntarily provoking his social environment. S himself participated in bullying Jewish children, which cannot be morally justified, but is psychologically explicable in this particular case. Today Sergei regrets it and would like to ask all persons independently of ethnicity, towards whom he behaved inappropriately directly or indirectly as a result of his childhood trauma, to accept his sincere apologies. Fortunately, S managed to dispose of all ethnic prejudice in his later life. There is no other way in our age of globalization; and corresponding new ethics needs to be developed (13); which is however outside the scope of this paper. Probably, for the similar reason, the social environment was quite indifferent to the violence in their family. For example, S asked for help some of his companions, "hooligans" 2-4 years older than he; they discussed it but did not do anything. The maternal grandmother, who lived separately, wrote letters to the authorities about CA in the family, it had no effect either. Moreover, the ethnic factor obviously contributed to Sergei’s alcohol consumption: consciously and subconsciously he tried to appear as Russian as possible. This psychological mechanism, predisposing to alcohol consumption and antisocial behavior, seems to be active in some people of mixed descent; just to name the famous poet, actor and singer Vladimir Vysotsky, whose father was of Jewish origin. Vysotsky was immensely popular; he had an enduring effect on Russian mass culture (http://en.wikipedia.org/wiki/Vladimir_Vysotsky), avoided Jewish traits in his works and image, being at the same time prone to alcohol consumption.

The physical abuse was administered predominantly by slapping in the face and whipping with a belt. The first episode complicated by nasal bleeding happened when S was approximately 8 years old. Episodes of violence went along with intimidation and verbal abuse, in connection with physical abuse and out of it. There are statements in the literature that CA is heavily laden with emotions (14). In this case, it could have been so in the beginning, but later the scenes of abuse became more theatrical and less laden by true emotion on the part of the abuser. Battery and verbal abuse sometimes occurred before spectators: the mother, relatives and friends. Sometimes, the mother took part in battering, which has been described in the literature as a pattern where mothers participate in abuse of their children more often if their partners were stepfathers of victims rather than genetic fathers (15). A motive could have been subconscious revenge to the disloyal ex-spouse in the person of his son, probably on the background of dissociation, because maternal affection was visibly present, especially during early childhood, and spontaneously returned. As usual in such cases, everything associated with the physical abuse was laden with shame; and S rarely told anybody about it. Once he positively answered a question of a schoolteacher whether he had been physically punished; it had no consequences. Another teacher, puzzled by the nationalistic remarks made by S at school, came for a home visit. It was followed by a remission in violence of several months' duration, accompanied by success in his school studies; in agreement with reports that maltreated children are at risk of insufficient school functioning (16).

Apart from occasional participation in parties at home, where alcohol was not consumed in excess, and drinking up to a bottle of beer with a schoolmate, S had not consumed alcohol till the age of 13 years, when he drank a 750 ml bottle of fortified wine with an older boy. During the 1969-70 school year, his alcohol consumption increased up to 250 ml of vodka with beer or a 750 ml bottle of fortified wine at one session. An opportunity to stay away from the abusive atmosphere at home was provided by a drinking company of schoolmates including some older boys inspiring alcohol purchase and consumption. During the last two school years, S was repeatedly arrested by the militia (police) and spent several nights at a sobering-up station. Shortly after the start of his study at a university in 1973, a separate room was rented for S by his mother. One year later he was dismissed from the university due to drunkenness and truancy, served two years with the army and resumed university education after a 4-years' interruption. In 1979, on his mother's initiative, an intramuscular implantation of a disulphiram preparation Esperal® had been performed, which was followed by abstinence of about 8 months' duration. After a challenge from the environment, he resumed alcohol consumption; there were no signs of the disulphiram-ethanol reaction. S discontinued alcohol misuse at the age of approximately 35 years, working abroad in a non-challenging environment.

Discussion

The case should be classified as intimate partner violence (IPV), a common problem, affecting many children (17); it illustrates a cause-effect relationship between CA and early-onset alcohol consumption with antisocial behavior in an adolescent, facilitated by societal and ethnicity-related factors. Exogenous nature of the early-onset alcohol misuse is demonstrated by the fact that, in spite of considerable experience of alcohol consumption, S did not develop any physical dependence and discontinued alcohol misuse because of professional and familial reasons. He did not resume excessive alcohol consumption also later, having come back to Russia, in spite of the challenges from old buddies etc. It appears probable that, although family violence is associated with alcohol misuse during adolescence, a mentally healthy adult can overcome a psychological dependence on alcohol, developed as a consequence of CA. It is in agreement with the data showing no significant association between CA and alcohol abuse in male victims becoming adults (18,19) in contrast to adolescents (2,3). To finish the case report on an optimistic note, it should be mentioned that S made conscious efforts to achieve forgiveness of the perpetrators, and was obviously successful in it. It was reported that forgiveness is associated with improved alcohol-related outcomes (20). Moreover, his mother and the stepfather cooperated with the author of this paper in elucidation of the motives, of psychological, ethnic and social factors of CA. In particular, according to his mother's memory partly confirmed by those of S, behavioral and communication abnormalities noticed during his early childhood had probably been caused by partial isolation from other children and bullying by older boys, which was apparently in some cases inspired by adults and tolerated by his nanny. Later S overcame his communication difficulties, admittedly, not without help of alcohol. This is, in fact, another factor contributing to alcoholism, which can be ethnicity-related: to become "insider" through alcohol consumption. This mechanism was exploited: in workers', students' and intelligentsia companies, the ringleaders called zavodila could be observed, who manipulated others towards regular alcohol consumption, while non-drinkers were sometimes stigmatized (21).

Violence in families was seldom discussed in professional literature of the former SU (22). Existence of CA was sometimes plainly denied (23); many cases of CA remained therefore undisclosed (24). Public organizations sometimes did not react to known cases of family violence. The today's Russian-language professional literature on CA is still scarce and partly represented by compilations from foreign publications. A part of the society seems to be opposed to public discussion of family violence because it is to some extent accepted (22). There is no generally agreed policy with regard to the CA (25,26); the matter being complicated by shortage of adequately trained personnel and limited access to foreign professional literature (27). The situation seems to be improving nonetheless: a considerable part of CA has occurred in connection with excessive alcohol consumption and heavy binge drinking, which appears to be in decline in today's Russia (21,28,29). A conclusion is therefore optimistic: the growing Russian economy enables further development the social welfare system, while broadening international cooperation must attract foreign expertise into the country.

REFERENCES

[1] Makhija N, Sher L. Childhood abuse, adult alcohol use disorders and suicidal behaviour. QJM 2007;100(5):305-9.

[2] Caballero MA, Ramos L, González C, Saltijeral MT. Family violence and risk of substance use among Mexican adolescents. Child Abuse Negl 2010;34(8):576-84.

[3] Rothman EF, Bernstein J, Strunin L. Why might adverse childhood experiences lead to underage drinking among US youth? Findings from an emergency department-based qualitative pilot study. Subst Use Misuse 2010;45(13):2281-90.

[4] Larkin W, Read J. Childhood trauma and psychosis: evidence, pathways, and implications. J Postgrad Med 2008;54(4):287-93.

[5] Lown EA, Nayak MB, Korcha RA, Greenfield TK. Child physical and sexual abuse: a comprehensive look at alcohol consumption patterns, consequences, and dependence from the National Alcohol Survey. Alcohol Clin Exp Res 2011;35(2):317-25.

[6] Garbarino J. The consequences of child maltreatment: biosocial and ecological issues. In Gelles RJ, Lancaster JB (Editors). Child Abuse and Neglect. Biosocial Dimensions. New York: Aldine de Gruyter, 1987: 299–316.

[7] Jonson-Reid M, Presnall N, Drake B, Fox L, Bierut L, Reich W, Kane P, Todd RD, Constantino JN. Effects of child maltreatment and inherited liability on antisocial development: an official records study. J Am Acad Child Adolesc Psychiatry 2010;49(4):321-32.

[8] Gonzalez A, MacMillan HL. Preventing child maltreatment: an evidence-based update. J Postgrad Med 2008;54(4):280-6.

[9] Lancaster JB, Gelles RJ. Introduction. In: Gelles RJ, Lancaster JB (Editors). Child Abuse and Neglect. Biosocial Dimensions. New York: Aldine de Gruyter, 1987:3–14.

[10] Ney PG. Child mistreatment: possible reasons for its transgenerational transmission. Can J Psychiatry 1989;34(6):594-601.

[11] Rodriguez E, Lasch KE, Chandra P, Lee J. Family violence, employment status, welfare benefits, and alcohol drinking in the United States: what is the relation? J Epidemiol Community Health 2001;55(3):172-8.

[12] Hindley N, Ramchandani PG, Jones DP. Risk factors for recurrence of maltreatment: a systematic review. Arch Dis Child 2006;91(9):744-52.

[13] Jargin SV. Overpopulation and modern ethics. S Afr Med J 2009;99(8):572-3 continued in 2010;100(11):694 and 2011;101(8):494.

[14] Herbruck CC. Breaking the cycle of child abuse. Minneapolis: Winston Press, 1979.

[15] Alexandre GC, Nadanovsky P, Moraes CL, Reichenheim M. The presence of a stepfather and child physical abuse, as reported by a sample of Brazilian mothers in Rio de Janeiro. Child Abuse Negl 2010;34(12):959-66.

[16] Cicchetti D, Toth SL, Hennessy K. Child maltreatment and school adaptation: Problems and promises. In: Sigel IE, Cicchetti D, Toth SL (Editors). Advances in applied developmental psychology. Vol. 8. Child abuse, child development, and social policy. Norwood, NJ: Ablex, 1995:301–30.

[17] Zolotor AJ, Denham AC, Weil A. Intimate partner violence. Prim Care 2009;36(1):167-79.

[18] Widom CS, Hiller-Sturmhöfel S. Alcohol abuse as a risk factor for and consequence of child abuse. Alcohol Res Health 2001;25(1):52-7.

[19] Langeland W, Hartgers C. Child sexual and physical abuse and alcoholism: a review. J Stud Alcohol 1998;59(3):336-48.

[20] Webb JR, Robinson EA, Brower KJ. Mental health, not social support, mediates the forgiveness-alcohol outcome relationship. Psychol Addict Behav 2011;25(3):462-73.

[21] Jargin SV. On the causes of alcoholism in the former Soviet Union. Alcohol Alcohol 2010;45(1):104-5.

[22] Nikulina EA. Organizational and pedagogical prevention system of child abuse in families. Candidate Dissertation. Saratov: Saratov State University, 2006. [Russian]

[23] Kovac C. Paediatricians meet to tackle child abuse in former Soviet bloc. BMJ 2002;30;324(7340):756.

[24] Semenova IV. The problem of child abuse and the ways of its solution. In: Social pediatrics - problems, research, solutions. Proceedings of the Prof. N.G. Veselov 60 Years Anniversary Scientific and Practical Conference. Saint Petersburg, 28 November 2000:39–42. [Russian]

[25] Besschetnova OV. Social work with children - victims of abuse in families (analysis of domestic and foreign experience). Balashov: Niklolaev, 2003. [Russian]

[26] Smagina MV. Child abuse in family as a socio-cultural phenomenon in today's Russia. Candidate Dissertation. Stavropol: North Caucasus Social Institute, 2006. [Russian]

[27] Murphy J, Jargin S. International perspectives and initiatives: The state of medical libraries in the former Soviet Union. Health Info Libr J 2010;27(3):244-8.

[28] Jargin SV. Letter from Russia: child abuse and alcohol misuse in a victim. Alcohol Alcohol 2011;46(6):734-6.

[29] Jargin SV. Letter from Russia: minimal price for vodka established in Russia from 1 January 2010. Alcohol Alcohol 2010;45(6):586-8.

In: Child and Adolescent Health Yearbook 2013
Editor: Joav Merrick
ISBN: 978-1-63117-658-6

Chapter 31

UNDERNOURISHMENT AS UNDERLYING CAUSE OF A TEENAGER WITH EXTREME SHIFTS IN SERUM SODIUM

Eva MM Hoytema van Konijnenburg**, *Jaap W Groothoff*, *Tessa de Baat*, *Felix HK Kreier and Annemarie CM van Bellegem
Department of Paediatrics, Academic Medical Center/Emma Children's Hospital, Amsterdam, Netherlands

ABSTRACT

Undernourishment can be complicated with impaired kidney function and electrolyte disturbances. We hereby report the case of a 17-year-old girl with a history of brain surgery and epilepsy who was admitted to the hospital, because of generalized seizures. A hyponatraemia of 115 mmol/L, combined with a very low urine osmolality was present. In retrospect, the patient had a two-year history of progressive weight loss. Thereby, she started intentional vomiting and drinking excessive amounts of water. She was diagnosed with purging type anorexia nervosa with polydipsia. Over the following months, serum sodium shifted between 125 mmol/L and 150 mmol/L together with an increase in the frequency of seizures. The shifts in serum sodium are of multivariable cause: decreased protein intake combined with excessive water intake, partial nephrogenic diabetes insipidus and hypokalaemic tubulo-interstitial nephritis. Undernourishment plays a key role and a careful refeeding regimen should always be started.

Keywords: Renal insufficiency, nutritional status, water-electrolyte imbalance, eating disorders

* Corresponding author: Eva MM Hoytema van Konijnenburg, MD, Meibergdreef 9, 1105 AZ Amsterdam, The Netherlands. Email: eva.hoytema@gmail.com.

INTRODUCTION

Undernourishment is still a major health problem, mainly in developing countries, but also in the Western society. One of its possible consequences is impaired kidney function (1,2). An example of undernourishment in developed countries is anorexia nervosa. It is well known that anorexia nervosa patients may develop life-threatening electrolyte disorders, such as severe hypokalaemia and hypophosphataemia (3). These complications are either due to starvation, refeeding or purgative behaviour. Children and adolescents are especially at risk for these complications (3,4). However, it is less reported that undernourishment can also have serious adverse effects on osmoregulation. We present a case of anorexia nervosa with severe disturbances in serum sodium and discuss the pathophysiology.

CASE STORY

A 17-year-old girl was admitted to an intensive care unit because of generalized seizures. Serum electrolytes were low with sodium of 115 mmol/L (normal values 135-145 mmol/L) with a very low urine osmolality of 58 mOsm/kg H2O.

She had a medical history of therapy resistant epilepsy from the age of 6 years, caused by a benign cerebral tumour that was removed together with part of the frontal lobe at the age of 8. The epilepsy had relapsed six years after surgery. Furthermore, she had a two-year history of progressive weight loss with dieting and self-induced vomiting, an increased fluid intake and secondary amenorrhea, but she had not been evaluated for this. At presentation her weight was 44.1 kg (body mass index: 15.6 kg/m2).

During the subsequent admission at our paediatric clinic, she was diagnosed with purging type anorexia nervosa and polydipsia. She was put on a strict 2.5 litre fluid restriction. Her diet was gradually increased to 2000 kilocalories (84 g protein). Serum sodium was normal during this admission with a normal daily intake.

In the following months she was treated on an outpatient basis for her disorder and she was encouraged to eat according to her regimen and fluid restriction. However, she continued vomiting and drinking extreme amounts of water and was frequently admitted with seizures. The serum sodium levels showed shifts between 125 and 150 mmol/L in a few hours time. In order to test renal ability to concentrate urine, a fluid deprivation test was performed at an euvolemic state, followed by a DDAVP-test (intranasal administration of 5 μg 1-deamino-8D-arginine vasopressin, a vasopressin analogue). After 7 hours of fluid deprivation, the maximum urine osmolality was only 265 mOsm/kg (normal value >600 mOsm/kg). With DDAVP, the maximum urine osmolality inadequately increased to 695 mOsm/kg (normal value 900 mOsm/kg), thus indicating partial nephrogenic diabetes insipidus.

Today, a year later, despite intensive psychiatric and somatic therapy with a strict dietary regimen, unfortunately her weight has further decreased. She has been unable to stop vomiting, drinking excessive amounts of water and, in addition, has started to eat extra salt. Serum creatinine has been variably increased (maximum 117 umol/L), consistent with an eGFR (estimated Glomerular Filtration Rate) of 55 mL/min/1.73m2, based on the Cockcroft-Gault formula. However, it is difficult to accurately determine a GFR in severely underweight persons (5).

Discussion

In this case, anorexia nervosa, and thus undernourishment, presents with prolonged disturbances in serum sodium and seizures in a teenager with a history of epilepsy and brain surgery, complicated with recurrent episodes of excessive water intake.

There are several important pathophysiological factors that may lead to these shifts. First, overconsumption of (hypotonic) fluids in combination with a diminished protein intake leads to an increased risk for acute hyponatraemia. Under normal circumstances, a healthy person can drink at least 10 litres of water in 24 hours without developing hyponatraemia (6). However, the kidney cannot produce complete solute-free urine. This means that, even in the most diluted urine, a certain amount of osmoles have to be excreted. If the protein-intake is severely reduced, even 2 litres of water per 24 hours can induce hyponatraemia (7). In our patient, given the extremely low urine osmolality at admission, this is probably what happened first. Secondly, however, the reduced intake of solutes and massive intake of water also lowers the solute concentration in the renal medulla. This reduces the ability of the kidney to optimally concentrate the urine in demanding circumstances. Even after administration of DDAVP, urinary osmolality rises inadequately. In other words, the combination of massive water intake and decreased protein intake also induces a (partial) nephrogenic diabetes insipidus (8). This explains the rapid shifts from hypo- to hypernatraemia in this patient. Finally, a third condition may aggravate these problems. In undernourished children, prolonged extreme undernourishment can be accompanied by prolonged severe hypokalaemia. In eating disorders, this is often aggravated because of purgative behaviour. It is important to be aware that prolonged hypokalaemia can induce tubulo-interstitial nephritis and consequently lead to a decreased ability to regulate water and salt excretion. In that case, serum creatinine would be increased (despite decreased muscle mass) in the absence of dehydration (9).

Conclusion

The extreme shifts in serum sodium in this teenager are of multivariable cause and undernourishment plays a key role. It is therefore very important to always start a careful refeeding regimen in the case of severe hyponatraemia in an undernourished patient. If serum sodium has not recovered thereafter, it can be either because of a (surreptitiously) continuous inadequate diet or because of permanent kidney damage.

Acknowledgment

Competing interests: None. Funding: None.

REFERENCES

[1] Nations FAAOOTU. Global hunger declining, but still unacceptably high. 2010 Sep 10;1–2.

[2] Benabe JE, Martinez-Maldonado M. The impact of malnutrition on kidney function. Miner Electrolyte Metab 1998;24(1):20–6.

[3] Rosen DS, American Academy of Pediatrics Committee on Adolescence. Identification and management of eating disorders in children and adolescents. Pediatrics 2010;126(6):1240–53.

[4] Halperin ML, Bohn D. Clinical approach to disorders of salt and water balance. Emphasis on integrative physiology. Crit Care Clin 2002;18(2):249–72.

[5] Fabbian F, Pala M, Scanelli G, Manzato E, Longhini C, Portaluppi F. Estimation of renal function in patients with eating disorders. Int J Eat Disord 2011;44(3):233–7.

[6] De Wardener HE, Herxheimer A. The effect of a high water intake on the kidney's ability to concentrate the urine in man. J Physiol 1957;139(1):53-63.

[7] Thaler SM, Teitelbaum I, Berl T. "Beer potomania" in non-beer drinkers: effect of low dietary solute intake. Am J Kidney Dis 1998;31(6):1028–31.

[8] Evrard F, Da Cunha MP, Lambert M, Devuyst O. Impaired osmoregulation in anorexia nervosa: a case-control study. Nephrol Dial Transplant 2004;19(12):3034–9.

[9] Liang C-C, Yeh H-C. Hypokalemic nephropathy in anorexia nervosa. CMAJ 2011;183(11):E761.

SECTION FOUR – INTERNET ADDICTION

In: Child and Adolescent Health Yearbook 2013
Editor: Joav Merrick

ISBN: 978-1-63117-658-6

Chapter 32

CLINICAL SIGNS AND SYMPTOMS OF ADDICTIVE BEHAVIORS

Terpsichori N Korpa*, MD and Pinelopi V Papadopoulou, MSc
ADHD/LD Unit, Department of Child Psychiatry,
"P & A Kyriakou" Children's Hospital, Athens, Greece

ABSTRACT

Despite extensive research and clinical practice in the field of biological addictions, addictive behaviors associated with maladaptive patterns have not been sufficiently studied. As a result, adolescents, a clinical group with frequent referral to psychiatric units, are not adequately screened for behavioral addictions. The aim of this review is to supply the clinician with a guide containing the main clinical features of addictive behaviors and several ways to perform differential diagnosis and assess comorbidity. In the following text, the basic maladaptive behavior patterns connected to addiction are demonstrated: Pathological gambling, excessive internet use, eating addiction, sex addiction and compulsive buying disorder. It seems that addictive behaviors share common clinical signs such as preoccupation, loss of control and continuous use despite harmful consequences. Overlapping or coexisting with other psychiatric disorders is presented in the majority of the clinical cases. Early identification of the addiction type and related intervention can contribute to effective therapeutic management and lower odds for continuity in the adulthood. Mental health professionals should be educated in diagnosing and treating addiction. Implementing primary and/or secondary prevention programs is a matter of high importance. Clinical and diagnostic issues are discussed.

Keywords: Addictive behaviors, adolescents, clinical symptomatology, differential diagnosis, primary prevention

* Correspondence: Korpa N Terpsichori, Child and Adolescent Psychiatrist, ADHD/LD Unit, Department of Child Psychiatry, "P & A Kyriakou" Children's Hospital, Thivon & Levadeias Goudi 11527 Athens, Greece. E-mail: terpsikorpa@aglaiakyriakou.gr

INTRODUCTION

There exist a range of behavior patterns like pathological gambling, overeating, excessive Internet use, compulsive sex and buying, defined as addictive behaviors, which (including substance use-related addictive disorders) are associated with serious family, school/work and social problems. Many addicted individuals show clinical functional impairment as well. For this reason, addictive behaviors constitute major public health issues. Prevention, assessment and early intervention in this field are critical.

Clinical experts specialized in evaluating and treating addictive disorders support the view that patients, who give up alcohol or illicit drug use, usually transfer their addictive behavior to activities such as Internet, sex etc. Additionally, significant similarities can be recognized between biological and behavioral addictions. Adolescents exhibiting behavioral addictions often meet diagnostic criteria for substance use disorders (see table 1) (1).

Table 1. Diagnostic criteria for substance use disorders

Signs and symptoms of addictive disorders
Addictive disorders are diagnosed in case drug use/behavior pattern leads to clinically significant impairment or distress. Three or more of the following criteria are met since the last year.
1) *Tolerance.* The effects of the same amount of the drug/time spending on the activity are diminished over time.
2) *Withdrawal.* Psychological and physiological symptoms are observed when drug use/ behavior pattern is discontinued.
3) *Escalating use.* Greater drug use/display of behavior than intended.
4) *Continued drug use/engagement in the specific activity* despite adverse consequences.
5) *Desire and/or unsuccessful efforts to discontinue* drug use/display of behavior.
6) *Time and effort are spent* in order to acquire and use the substance/exhibit the specific behavior or recover from the effects of the drug use/addictive behavior.
7) *Significant social or occupational activities* are given up due to the drug abuse/ behavior pattern.

Behavioral addictions represent clinical entities, not classified in Diagnostic and Statistical Manual of Mental Disorders 4th ed. (DSM-IV) (2) (except pathological gambling), during which repetitive impulsive behaviors take place with a strong negative impact on the patient and his close environment.

Given the fact that the specific addictions are dangerous psychiatric conditions manifested in the developmental period of adolescence and that early onset of pathological gambling is connected to more psychiatric problems, family/social problems, substance use, cognitive problems and suicidal ideation, it is considered critical mental health professionals to be informed about the clinical symptomatology of these behaviors, so that they will able to identify the addiction and to manage it (3). In this review we will look at these main addictive behaviors.

PATHOLOGICAL GAMBLING

Nowadays, adolescents and young people are grown up in a society, where gambling, pathological or not, is an accessible and a socially acceptable activity. The mean age onset for pathological gambling is 11.5 years worldwide. According to international studies, the prevalence of the disorder is estimated to be 2-4 higher in adolescents compared to adults. It is noteworthy that 3.5-8% of adolescents aged 12-17 years are diagnosed as "pathological gamblers". Gambling in adolescence is associated with poor school performance, criminal behavior and family conflicts. Moreover, not only recreational but also pathological gambling are connected to psychiatric comorbidity in adults and high-risk behaviors in adolescents (4).

As mentioned above, pathological gambling is the only behavioral addiction described in this chapter, which is encoded in both international classification systems. More specifically, it is incorporated in the section "impulse control disorders" with other clinical disorders (pyromania, trichotillomania) in DSM-IV (see table 2), while in ICD-10 it is included in the category "personality and behavior disorders in adults". In February 2010, the DSM-V task force suggested that the "substance-related disorders" should be renamed "addiction and associated disorders" and pathological gambling should be introduced as the only behavioral addiction in the diagnostic textbook (5,6).

Table 2. Diagnostic criteria for pathological gambling

A)Persistent and repetitive maladaptive behavior pattern is displayed if the individual presents five or more of the following:
1) Is preoccupied with gambling.
2) Gambling with increasing amounts of money.
3) Has repeatedly unsuccessfully tried to control, diminish or discontinue gambling.
4) Restless or irritable when attempting to cut down or stop gambling.
5) Gambles as a way of escaping from problems or of relieving a dysphoric mood.
6) After losing its money, returns another day to get it back (i.e., "chasing one's losses").
7) Lies to gloze the extent of involvement with gambling.
8) Has committed illegal acts to stake gambling activities.
9) Has hazarded or lost an important relationship, job, or educational or career opportunity because of gambling.
10) Relies on others to obtain money to relieve a desperate financial situation provoked by gambling.
B) The gambling behavior is not better accounted for by a manic episode.

As far as the main clinical symptoms of the disorder are concerned, it could be argued that the addictive behavior, which accounts for the pathological involvement in the activity contains compulsive use, loss of control and continuous use despite adverse consequences (7). Finally, pathological gambling, as defined by DSM-IV, tends to be manifested along with further psychiatric disorders, including anxiety disorders, alcohol abuse and substance use disorders. Additionally, comorbid major depressive episode is relative common, as some researchers may claim that 2/3 of these patients could meet the diagnostic criteria for major depressive disorder (8). As a result, adolescents do represent a vulnerable social group, which is susceptible to present comorbid psychiatric disorders. For this reason, patients with pathological gambling should always be thoroughly assessed by a child psychiatrist in order to evaluate further psychological and psychiatric problems.

EXCESSIVE INTERNET USE

Nowadays, internet is widely used by adolescents in order to retrieve information, to entertain and to get socialized. However, it is possible Internet use to be transformed into abuse and to harm the individual's functioning. Several diagnostic terms have been used to describe the specific clinical condition, compulsive Internet use, pathological Internet use, problematic Internet use, Internet addiction etc. In fact, there are some studies, where excessive Internet use is classified in behavioral addictions or impulse control disorders (9). Regarding the disorder's prevalence in the general population, it is estimated that the 2-5.4% of adolescents in Europe and the 1-8.2% in Greece respectively does present this behavior pattern (10).

Young (11) initially introduced the diagnostic criteria for pathological internet use, subsequently Beard & Wolf (12), Shapira and colleagues (13) and Ko and colleagues (14) suggested their diagnostic framework by adapting Young's diagnostic pattern and trying to improve and enrich it. Tables 3 and 4 present Young's and Ko's diagnostic criteria (11,14). Summarizing, an adolescent should meet the following criteria, so that the Internet addiction disorder could be diagnosed: uncontrollable Internet use, significant distress, time spending, social, professional and financial difficulties and presence of the symptoms of abuse not only during manic or hypomanic episodes (15,16).

Table 3. Diagnostic scale for Internet Addiction (Young, 1996)

1)	Do you feel preoccupied with the Internet (think about previous online activity or anticipate next online session)?
2)	Do you feel the need to use the Internet for increasing amounts of time to achieve satisfaction?
3)	Have you repeatedly made unsuccessful efforts to control, cut back, or stop Internet use?
4)	Do you feel restless, moody, depressed, or irritable when attempting to cut down or stop Internet use?
5)	Do you stay online longer than originally intended?
6)	Have you jeopardized or risked the loss of significant relationship, job, educational or career opportunity because of the Internet?
7)	Have you lied to family members, therapist, or others to conceal the extent of involvement with the Internet?
8) 9)	Do you use the Internet as a way of escaping from problems or of relieving a dysphoric mood (e.g., feelings of helplessness, guilt, anxiety, depression)?

Excessive and problematic Internet use is connected to multiple adverse psychosocial conditions such as social isolation (17), aggressive behavior (18), ADHD (19,20), depression (19,20). Nevertheless, it is controversial whether Internet addiction is a primary or a secondary disorder resulting from the presence of other psychiatric disorders. Given the fact that adolescents often show higher odds for psychopathology, the adolescent exhibiting symptoms of Internet addiction is necessary to be assessed and treated with regard to a comorbid psychiatric disorder.

Table 4. Proposed diagnostic criteria for Internet addiction (adapted from Ko CH, Yen JY, Chen CC, Chen SH, Yen CF. Proposed diagnostic criteria of Internet addiction for adolescents. J Nerv Ment Dis 2005;193(11):728-33.)

A. Six or more of the following symptoms:	
1	Preoccupation with Internet activities.
2	Recurrent failure to resist the impulse to use the Internet.
3	Tolerance: a marked increase in Internet use needed to achieve satisfaction.
4	Withdrawal, as manifested by either of the following: a) symptoms of dysphoric mood, anxiety,irritability, and boredom after several days without Internet activity; b) use of Internet to relieveor avoid withdrawal symptoms.
5	Use of the Internet for a period of time longer than intended.
6	Persistent desire and/or unsuccessful attempts to cut down or reduce Internet use.
7	Excessive time spent on Internet activities.
8	Excessive effort spent on activities necessary to obtain access to the Internet.
9	Continued heavy Internet use despite knowledge of physical or psychological problem caused or exacerbated by Internet use.
B. Functional impairment. One or more of the following symptoms:	
1	Recurrent Internet use resulting in a failure to fulfill major obligations
2	Impairment in social relationships
3	Behavior violating school rules or laws due to Internet use
C. The Internet addictive disorder is not better accounted for by another disorder	

EATING ADDICTION

Excessive food intake in developed societies is associated with a high prevalence of overweight and obesity, which in turn contribute to insulin resistance, diabetes, hypertension and cardiovascular diseases. Binge eating dominating nowadays in the western world is attributed to the increased availability of food, sedentary lifestyle and financial cost that often results from the purchase of healthy food (21). Two assumptions have been proposed for eating addiction. According to the first, eating addiction is identified with eating disorders, as these patients often use drugs and exhibit low impulse control, overload with the substance abuse and serious symptoms with respect on eating when they are exposed to stressful events (22). According to the second hypothesis, it is speculated that foods with high concentration of sugar, carbohydrates, fat, salt and caffeine are addictive substances. Consequently, it is reasonable that many individuals are not able to control their impulse to eat them (21).

As far as the clinical symptoms of eating addiction are concerned, the main characteristics include the consumption of large quantities of food for prolonged periods, repetitive efforts to discontinue this behavior and continuous display of the maladaptive behavior pattern regardless of harmful consequences. Tolerance, time spent and effort are less common symptoms, while withdrawal and significant reduction of professional, social and recreational activities are rarely reported. The diagnosis of eating addiction is highly correlated to body mass index and therefore is particularly frequent in obese individuals and even more in obese patients with binge eating disorder (23).

The above mentioned are confirmed by findings from clinical studies. In a relevant study of Due et al. (24), 15.2% of overweight children stated that they “often”, “usually” or "always" feel addicted to food. Furthermore, not only the increased food intake, but also the emotional eating were significantly associated with the body mass index. In a recent qualitative study conducted in overweight and obese children and adolescents, it was concluded that the most common symptoms were the consumption of large quantities of food, the unsuccessful attempts to give up the excessive food intake and the continuous abuse despite adverse consequences. When participants were informed about the definition of "addiction", 29% indicated that they consider themselves addicted to the most of foods (25).

As a result, the clinical expert will be asked to assess adolescents who present symptoms of eating addiction such as strong desire for food and loss of control during the consumption of food. Assessment tools estimating eating addiction behavior patterns are the Eating Behaviors Questionnaire (EBQ) and the Yale Food Addiction Scale (YFAS), which are particularly valuable and can guide specialists to clarify the phenomenology of eating addiction disorders (23,26).

Sex Addiction

Sex addiction is defined as a pattern of sexual behavior that initially offers pleasure, but then becomes unfulfilling, self-destructive and uncontrollable. As a result, sex addiction refers to a person's disability to control its sexual thoughts and behavior, which provokes negative effects on personal, professional and social life (27).

Despite the fact that the term "sex addiction" is not included in the DSM-IV, the clinician can reclaim the diagnostic criteria for the substance use disorders and expand them by creating a framework for the diagnostic assessment of sex addiction behaviors. Any behavior characterized by loss of control, persistent display of the specific behavior, despite harmful effects and obsession or preoccupation, can potentially be named "addiction" (28). However, there are some categories of sex addiction that are acknowledged in DSM-IV as specific paraphilias. Moreover, sex addiction can be diagnosed under Paraphilia Not Otherwise Specified, Impulse Control Disorder NOS or Sexual Disorder NOS, depending on behavior that the individual shows (29). It has been suggested (28) that there are three levels of sex addictive behavior: a) The behaviors are perceived as normal and acceptable (masturbation, viewing pornography, prostitution, having multiple relationships), b) The individual exhibits illegal behaviors, which lead clearly to victimization but are considered nuisance crimes (exhibitionism, obscene phone calls) and c) The individual is engaged in illegal behaviors, which have serious consequences for the victim and legal effects for the offender (rape, incest, and child harassment) (28).

In addition, the sex addicted individual, moves through a four-step addiction vicious cycle, which includes four stages and becomes more intense each time it is repeated. In the first step, the person's mind is overwhelmed with thoughts about sex (preoccupation phase). In the second step, the addict's sexual routine leads to a respective sexual behavior (ritualization phase). At this stage, the preoccupation of the addict is intensified while feelings such as excitement and enthusiasm are strengthened. In the third stage (compulsive sexual behavior), the addict participates actively in a sexual behavior, which he/she is unable to control or discontinue. In the last stage (despair), the addict experiences a feeling of helplessness because of his/her behavior and his/her disability to impose on himself/herself (29).

The diagnostic assessment of sex addiction is a challenging process. Firstly, there are not few differences in sex addiction clinical symptoms between adolescents and adults. More specifically, occasional sexual behavior may not be considered pathological in adults, while in adolescents can or cannot be viewed as abnormal, as such behaviors influence the psycho-emotional development and the social adaptation of adolescents and can have a direct impact on the adult life. In any case, the risky sexual behavior pattern (absence of precaution, multiple affairs) is a condition that should be investigated by the clinician, but also generate suspicion for the presence of comorbid substance abuse disorder and other mental disorders (27).

Compulsive Buying Disorder

The specific disorder is relative common and can lead to serious personal and family functional impairment, as well as financial and legal problems (30). Not only clinical but also community studies show that 80-95% of persons with the disorder are women. The age of onset of compulsive buying disorder seems to be in the late teens or early twenties, though there are also some researchers reporting a mean age at onset of 30 years (31).

Individuals with compulsive buying disorder exhibit preoccupation with buying and strong desire to spend money. They devote significant time to these behaviors, while they often describe high levels of impulsivity and anxiety, which settle down only when a purchase is made.

According to Black (31), four phases of the disorder can be identified: a) anticipation, b) preparation, c) shopping, d) spending. During the first phase, the person with the disorder develops thoughts, impulses or preoccupations, which are related either to a specific object or to the action of shopping itself. In the second phase, the person prepares for shopping and spending money. This phase includes the decisions on when and where to shop, on what to wear and which credit cards to use. The third phase contains the actual shopping experience, which is described as extremely exciting. Finally, this process is completed with the payment and a feeling of frustration usually follows. The most frequently reported emotions prior to the act of buying are depression, anxiety, boredom, self-critical thoughts and anger, while relief from negative emotions and euphoria often follow (31).

As far as the comorbidity is concerned, clinical studies indicate that persons involved in compulsive buying often meet the diagnostic criteria for psychiatric disorders, which are coded in DSM-IV Axis I, mood disorders (21%-100%), anxiety disorders (41%-80%), substance use disorders (21%-46%) and eating disorders (8%-35%). Impulse control disorders are also relative common in these patients (21-40%). Furthermore, according to other studies, it is suggested that 33%-35% of persons with the disorder, presents obsessive compulsive disorder as well (30).

Discussion

It is now well-known that an addictive behavior does not necessarily imply a specific substance addiction (cannabis, marihuana, cocaine etc). On the contrary, the term "addiction" covers a set of multiple symptoms and behaviors, whose clinical "label" is differentiated depending on the activity that the patient is preoccupied.

First of all, the main symptoms of an addictive behavior do not differ significantly between the substance use-related disorders and the behavioral addictions. Moreover, it seems that the basic clinical signs remain the same among the addictive behavioral patterns and include compulsive use, loss of control and continuous use despite adverse consequences. It may be a little more complex for the clinician to diagnose behavioral addictions, since they do not contain biological symptoms and thus, they are not easy to recognize.

In specific, addictive behaviors such as pathological gambling (32), and excessive Internet use are commonly presented in adolescents and usually occur together with another psychiatric disorder. Furthermore, it is noteworthy that adolescence is a critical period, during which individuals often exhibit high-risk behaviors and are susceptible to manifest subclinical or clinical psychiatric symptoms. Screening for these disorders demands full child psychiatric assessment by a mental health professional with adequate clinical experience, as conducting differential diagnosis and evaluating comorbidity is not simple in this case. Addictive behaviors can either overlap with depressive disorders and impulse control disorders or coexist with other psychiatric disorders (substance dependence, depressive disorders etc.).

Primary care clinicians should be familiar with a range of addictive behaviors, so that they are able to screen adolescents and treat them. Early intervention may prevent the development of more severe morbidity and correlated psychiatric disorders among at-risk adolescents.

However, most of the advances in the primary prevention of addictive disorders have been in the field of drug abuse prevention. A series of studies have examined prevention strategies of drug abuse in adolescents, as during adolescence, young people begin to make independent decisions about their own behaviors.

Implementing evidence-based programs that have been shown to be effective and broadening and expanding them, particularly for the addictive disorders that have, until now, received less research attention, is a top priority.

Taken together, it is extremely significant to make prevention of addictive disorders a public health priority is extremely significant. Meanwhile, developing programs for a broader range of addictive behaviors will pave the way for effective management. Creating and evaluating public health policies on addictive disorders is of high importance.

All in all, this chapter offers a comprehensive review of various types of addictive behaviors and provides the clinician with informational material on the main clinical symptoms of the disorders in question. To which extent the specific disorders can extend across the lifespan? What are the subgroups of adolescents being at high risk? Should behavioral addictions be introduced in DSM-V? The above mentioned are critical issues to be clarified.

References

[1] Addictive behaviours, 2010. POSTNote. Accessed 2012 April 08. URL: http://www.parliament.uk/briefing-papers/POST-PN-356.

[2] American Psychiatric Association. Diagnostic and Statistical Manual of Mental Disorders (4th ed). Text Revision (DSM-IV-TR) Washington, DC: APA, 2000.

[3] Villella C, Cassano M, Martinotti G, La Torre G, Di Nicola M, Gliubizzi MD, et al. Behavioural addictions in adolescents and young adults: Results from a prevalence study. J Gambl Stud 2011;27:203–14.

[4] Caillon J, Grall-Bronnec M, Bouju G, Lagadec M, Venisse JL. Pathological gambling in adolescence. Arch Pediatrie 2012;19:173-9.

[5] Rantala V, Sulkunen P. Is pathological gambling just a big problem or also an addiction? Addict Res Theory 2012;20(1):1–10.

[6] Hodgins DC, Stea JN, Grant JE. Gambling disorders. Lancet 2011;378:1874–84.

[7] Chamberlain L. Understanding and diagnosing compulsive gambling. In: Coombs RH, ed. Handbook of addictive disorders. A practical guide to diagnosis and treatment. Chichster: John Wiley, 2004.

[8] Lloyd J, Doll H, Hawton K, Dutton WH, Geddes JR, Goodwin GM, et al. How psychological symptoms relate to different motivations for gambling: An online study of internet gamblers. Biol Psychiatry 2010;68:733-40.

[9] Tonioni F, D'Alessandris L, Lai C, Martinelli D, Corvino S, Vasale M, et al. Internet addiction: hours spent online, behaviors and psychological symptoms. Gen Hosp Psychiatr 2012;34:80-7.

[10] Kormas G, Critselis E, Janikian M, Kafetzis D, Tsitsika A. Risk factors and psychosocial characteristics of potential problematic internet use among adolescents: A cross-sectional study. BMC Public 2011;11:595.

[11] Young KS. Internet addiction: the emergence of a new clinical disorder. Cyberpsychol Behav 1998;1(3):237-44.

[12] Beard KW, Wolf EM. Modification in the proposed diagnostic criteria for Internet addiction. Cyberpsychol Behav 2001;4(3):377-83.

[13] Shapira NA, Lessig MC, Goldsmith TD, Szabo ST, Lazoritz M, Gold MS, et al. Problematic internet use: proposed classification and diagnostic criteria. Depress Anxiety 2003;17(4):207-16.

[14] Ko CH, Yen JY, Chen CC, Chen SH, Yen CF. Proposed diagnostic criteria of Internet addiction for adolescents. J Nerv Ment Dis 2005;193(11):728-33.

[15] Widyanto L, Griffiths M. Internet addiction: A critical review. Int J Ment Health Addict 2006;4:31–51.

[16] Aboujaoude E. Problematic Internet use: an overview. World Psychiatry 2010;9(2):85-90.

[17] Weiser EB. The functions of internet use and their social and psychological consequences. Cyberpsychol Behav 2004;4(6):723-43.

[18] Yen JY, Ko CH, Yen CF, Chen SH, Chung WL, Chen CC. Psychiatric symptoms in adolescents with internet addiction: Comparison with substance use. Psychiatr Clin Neurosci 2008;62(1):9-16.

[19] Ko CH, Yen JY, Chen CS, Chen CC, Yen CF. Psychiatric comorbidity of internet addiction in college students: An interview study. CNS Spectr 2008;13(2):147-53.

[20] Yen JY, Ko CH, Yen CF, Wu HY, Yang MJ. The comorbid psychiatric symptoms of internet addiction: Attention deficit and hyperactivity disorder (ADHD), depression, social phobia and hostility. J Adolesc Health 2007;41:93-8.

[21] Ifland JR, Preuss HG, Marcus MT, Rourke KM, Taylor WC, Burau K, et al. Refined food addiction: A classic substance use disorder. Med Hypotheses 2009;72:518-26.

[22] Garner DM, Gerborg A. Understanding and diagnosing eating disorders. In: Coombs RH, ed. Handbook of addictive disorders. A practical guide to diagnosis and treatment. Chichester: John Wiley, 2004.

[23] Meule A. How prevalent is "food addiction"? Front Psychiatr 2011;2:61.

[24] Due P, Damsgaard MT, Rasmussen M, Holstein BE, Wardle J, Merlo J, et al. Socioeconomic position, macroeconomic environment and overweight among adolescents in 35 countries. Int J Obes (Lond) 2009;33(10):1084-93.

[25] Pretlow RA. Addiction to highly pleasurable food as a cause of the childhood obesity epidemic: a qualitative Internet study. Eat Disord 2011;19(4):295-307.
[26] Corsica JA, Pelchat ML. Food addiction: true or false? Curr Opin Gastroenterol 2010;26(2):165-9.
[27] Sussman S. Sexual addiction among teens: A review. Sex Addict Compulsivity J Treat Prev 2007;14(4):257-78.
[28] Schneider JP. Understanding and diagnosing sex addiction. In: Coombs RH, ed. Handbook of addictive disorders. A practical guide to diagnosis and treatment. Chichester: John Wiley, 2004.
[29] Seegers JA. The prevalence of sexual addiction symptoms on the college campus. Sex Addict Compulsivity J Treat Prev 2003;10(4):247-58.
[30] Black DW. Compulsive buying disorder: A review of the evidence. CNS Spectr 2007;12(2):124-32.
[31] Black DW. A review of compulsive buying disorder. World Psychiatry 2007b;6:14-18.
[32] Derevensky JL, Shek DTL, Merrick J, eds. Youth gambling. The hidden addiction. Berlin: De Gruyter, 2011.

In: Child and Adolescent Health Yearbook 2013
Editor: Joav Merrick
ISBN: 978-1-63117-658-6

Chapter 33

Development of Internet Addictive Behaviors: Potential Pathophysiologic Mechanisms

Joseph Calles, MD, Donald E. Greydanus*, MD, DR HC (Athens) and Ahsan Nazeer, MD

Department of Child and Adolescent Psychiatry and Department of Pediatric and Adolescent Medicine, Western Michigan University Homer Stryker, M.D. School of Medicine, Kalamazoo, Michigan, United States of America

Abstract

In the near future, the accurate diagnosis and effective treatment of internet addictive disorders will rely on research-based knowledge of pathogenetic mechanisms. Progress in this area has been hampered by debates over whether internet addiction is a true addiction, and whether biophysiological (vs. behavioral) factors contribute to its development. This review provides a brief overview of the major areas of investigation into the etiology of internet addiction.

Keywords: Internet addiction, etiology, pathophysiology, comorbidity

Introduction

A certain proportion of adolescents will increase their time online to the point of interfering with certain obligatory functions, such as schoolwork, familial interactions, and even self-care.

---

* Correspondance: Donald E Greydanus, MD, Dr. HC (ATHENS), Professor and Chair, Department of Pediatric and Adolescent Medicine, Western Michigan University Homer Stryker MD School of Medicine, 1000 Oakland Drive, D48G, Kalamazoo, MI 49008-1284, United States. E-mail: Donald.greydanus@med.wmich.edu

As both clinicians and scientists, physicians always want to know why unhealthy behaviors occur, in order to develop effective therapeutic and preventative interventions. In the case of inappropriate time spent using the Internet, research into the cause of related "addictive" behaviors has been limited. What follows is an examination of some of the factors contributing to the relative paucity of research in this area. In addition, some speculations—derived from studies of addictive disorders—as to possible pathophysiologic mechanisms will be discussed.

Internet addiction: The argument over diagnosis

In order to accurately study any clinical entity, practitioners first must agree on how to define and diagnose the problem. The first proposed diagnostic criteria for Internet addiction (IA) were derived from the DSM-IV criteria for pathological gambling (1). In a commentary on this issue, Pies (2) argued against the inclusion of IA in the forthcoming DSM-V, based on the following points: the terms substance abuse and substance dependence—not addiction—appear in the DSM; dependence on a substance requires physiological tolerance and withdrawal, which have not been demonstrated with IA; and, given the high rate of comorbid psychiatric and behavioral problems associated with IA, the symptoms of IA would be better subsumed under well-established diagnostic categories. Even if IA were to qualify as an addiction, there would still be the need for a valid and reliable set of diagnostic criteria, especially for use in adolescents, the primary demographic group at risk for IA. Ko and colleagues have proposed such criteria (3), which, however, do not settle the debate over how IA should be diagnosed.

Internet addiction: The argument over categorization

If IA isn't an addiction, what is it? Pies also noted in his commentary (2) that IA actually describes behaviors that could be called compulsive or impulsive, i.e., the person feels compelled to be online excessively. The problem with categorizing excessive Internet use (EIU) as a compulsion is that, unlike the classic mental compulsions of obsessive-compulsive disorder (OCD), which are ego-dystonic (unwanted), the putative compulsions of IA/EIU are ego-syntonic (wanted). Describing the behaviors associated with IA as impulsive seems to be more relevant, as impulsivity implies emotionally based actions in the absence of awareness of, or concerns about, possible negative consequences. Cao, et al., explored the connection between impulsivity and IA in Chinese high school students (4). Using a well-validated questionnaire and a computer-based paradigm, the students with IA scored significantly higher on the measures of impulsivity than did controls without IA. Impulsivity is also known to be one of the core features of attention-deficit/hyperactivity disorder (ADHD). Yoo, et al., investigated the presence of IA in Korean elementary school students with or without ADHD (5). Using rating scales and checklists, the authors found "significant positive correlations" between ADHD scores and IA scores.

Internet addiction: Neurobiological features

Even if debates over how best to categorize and diagnose IA were resolved, the question of what causes IA would still be unanswered. In recent years researchers have looked at both brain structure and functions in an attempt to answer that question.

Zhou et al. (6) using voxel-based morphometry (VBM) analysis of magnetic resonance imaging (MRI), compared the brains of a small group of Chinese adolescents with IA to those of healthy, matched controls (6). They found that, compared to the healthy controls, adolescents with IA had lower gray matter density in the left anterior and posterior cingulate cortices, the left insula, and the left lingual gyrus. The researchers describe how the modulation of emotional behavior is the responsibility of the affected areas, and especially note that the insula "plays a crucial part in addiction." They conclude their article with the statement that the results "provide new insights into the pathogenesis of IA." In a similar study of Chinese college students, Yuan, et al. (7), found that on VBM analysis of brain MRI, subjects with IA showed atrophy in the bilateral dorsolateral prefrontal cortex (DLPFC), supplementary motor area (SMA), cerebellum, orbitofrontal cortex (OFC), and the left rostral anterior cingulate cortex (rACC). In addition, atrophy of the right DLPFC, the left rACC and the right SMA correlated with the duration of IA, which the study by Zhou, et al. (6), did not find. It is clear from these studies that there is an association between brain structure abnormalities and IA. It is not clear whether the brain changes cause behavioral symptoms, or whether the behaviors themselves cause the brain to change.

Some research has focused on the functional aspects of IA. Liu et al. (8) using functional MRI (fMRI), compared the brain regional homogeneity (ReHo) (representing nervous system activity) of Chinese young adults with and without IA (8). Compared to those without IA, the IA group demonstrated increased ReHo distributed over the cerebellum, brainstem, right cingulate gyrus, bilateral parahippocampus, right frontal lobe, left superior frontal gyrus, left precuneus, right postcentral gyrus, right middle occipital gyrus, right inferior temporal gyrus, left superior temporal gyrus and middle temporal gyrus. In their discussion, the authors speculate that the "enhancement of synchronization among the cerebellum, brainstem, limbic lobe, frontal lobe and apical lobe may be associated with reward pathways," i.e., the initiation and/or propagation of IA.

The psychophysiology of individuals with IA has also been studied too. Lu, et al., assessed the blood volume pulse (BVP), skin conductance (SC), peripheral temperature (PTEMP), and respiratory response (RESPR) in a group of high-risk IA abusers vs. a group of low-risk IA abusers while surfing the Internet (9). Risk status was determined using cutoff scores on the Chinese-language Chen Internet Addiction Scale (CIAS) (10). The analyzed data demonstrated that the BVP and RESPR values in the high-risk IA abusers were higher than for those in the low-risk group; conversely, the SC and PTEMP magnitudes were smaller in the high-risk than in the low-risk IA abusers. These results indicate that the sympathetic nervous system was highly activated in the high-risk IA subjects. Concurrently, the SC index revealed an activated parasympathetic nervous system in the high-risk IA group. Although the purpose of the study was related to improving the assessment of IA, the authors also discussed the relationships between addiction-related cues, autonomic nervous system activity, affective states, and behavior. They were careful to note that research data is unable to "make causal inferences regarding the etiological role of the nervous system in the prevention and treatment implications of IA (9)."

Researchers have also begun to explore the molecular biology of IA. Using positron emission tomography (PET) scans on Korean young adult males, with and without IA, Kim and colleagues (11) measured dopamine D2 receptor availability in the ventral striatum, dorsal caudate, and dorsal putamen. They found reduced D2 receptor availability in the bilateral caudate and left putamen in the IA group, the degree of dopamine receptor availability being inversely correlated with the severity of IA. The authors interpret the findings as suggestive of an association between IA and dysfunctions in dopaminergic brain systems, and note consistency with previous research showing reduced levels of D2 receptors in both substance-related and non-substance-related addictions. They also believe that their findings support the claim that IA may share similar neurobiological abnormalities with other addictive disorders.

Prompted by the apparent relationships between dopamine, ADHD and IA, Han et al. (12) conducted an open-label study of OROS methylphenidate HCl in Korean children with comorbid ADHD and IA for video games (12). After 8 weeks of treatment, there were significant reductions in both IA ratings and time spent on the Internet. The decreases in IA scores correlated with decreases in scores on measures of ADHD. Although the authors suggest that Internet video game play in their subjects might derive from the ADHD, both disorders involve abnormalities in the dopaminergic system. Given those similarities, they cautiously propose that methylphenidate be investigated as a potential treatment for IA, given its ability to increase brain levels of dopamine (13). In a different study, Han and colleagues (12) investigated the use of another dopaminergic agent, bupropion sustained release (SR), in a group of young adults with IA for a specific video game. When compared to healthy controls using fMRI data and clinical assessments, after 6 weeks of bupropion SR treatment the IA group demonstrated decreases in cravings for Internet video game play, total game play time, and cue-induced brain activity in the DLPFC. These studies speak to the involvement of the dopaminergic system in the symptomatology of IA. As in the structural studies previously noted, there is insufficient data to determine in which direction the cause-effect relationship operates between IA and dopaminergic dysfunction.

INTERNET ADDICTION: RELATIONSHIP TO OTHER ADDICTIONS

IA is neither the only, nor the most problematic, addictive behavioral problem in adolescents. However, since all addictions may share some common etiologic elements, the study of other addictions may shed light on the cause(s) of IA. One possible pathophysiologic factor to consider in adolescents with IA is adolescence itself. Although the majority of adolescent Internet users will not develop IA, for some individuals age-related neural changes may leave them more susceptible to developing IA and other addictions. In a review of the neurobiological connection between adolescent brain development and behavior, Casey and Jones (14) explain that in adolescents the signaling activity in the ventral striatal cortex (VSC) is relatively stronger than the activity in the prefrontal cortex (PFC). By adulthood, PFC activity predominates over activity in the VSC. The implication for addictions lies in the fact that the VSC is involved in "bottom up" control, which is associated with sensation-seeking and risk-taking behaviors, whereas the PFC is involved in "top down" control, which is associated with the ability to resist urges and delay gratification. The introduction of drugs, alcohol, and other strongly reinforcing sources of stimulation—such as the Internet—during adolescence, when VSC activity is higher than PFC activity, greatly increases the probability of developing addictive behaviors.

Volkow and colleagues (15) investigated how brain DA activity in various brain regions contributes to addiction. Their findings, in adults with addictions to various substances, demonstrated a reversal of the normal maturational ratio of frontal-to-striatal activity, meaning that in addicts the activity of frontal executive functions (e.g., emotional control and decision-making) is reduced, whereas the activity of the striatum is increased. Over time the relative increase of DA activity in the striatum is not related to the drug use itself, but to the anticipation of use. In other words, craving in response to drug-conditioned cues may be more reinforcing than the drug use itself. This is consistent with our experiences in working with youth with IA, where it is often easier for the adolescents to completely abstain from online activity than to have a limited amount of online access, which remains as a cue to increase online activity.

In addition to DA, other neurotransmitters/receptors seem to be involved in addictions, including serotonin, endogenous opioids and cannabinoids, GABA, and glutamate (16). Kirby et al. (17) specifically reviewed addiction vulnerability related to serotonergic mechanisms. As previously described, there is a connection between impulsivity and addiction, and the authors present data supporting that link, and also discuss potential avenues of research into serotonin and addictions. A specific form of IA is excessive online gambling, which in many respects is identical to regular pathological gambling. Treatment of a 36-year-old Korean male with gambling addiction, using the selective serotonin reuptake inhibitor (SSRI) fluvoxamine, yielded significant reductions in both self-reported symptoms of addiction and in frontal lobe and limbic area activation on fMRI (18). The authors could not say with certainty whether the fluvoxamine treated the pathological gambling directly, or indirectly through the treatment of comorbid depression. Another study investigated the effects of the SSRI escitalopram in adults with what the authors termed impulsive-compulsive Internet usage disorder (19). During the initial, open-label phase of active treatment there was a significant reduction in time spent on the Internet. However, in the subsequent double-blind, placebo-controlled discontinuation phase, there was no significant difference in time spent online between the escitalopram- and placebo–treated groups. It is clear that more research is needed regarding the relationship between serotonin and gambling, excessive online activities, and other addictions.

One of the criticisms of considering IA as an addiction is the absence of physical withdrawal symptoms in individuals with IA who have abruptly discontinued use of the Internet. It is important to remember that psychic withdrawal may actually be more debilitating than physical withdrawal to newly abstinent addicts—perhaps especially those with IA—as psychic withdrawal is related to craving, preoccupation, boredom, anxiety, sadness, and the desire to feel "normal" (16). Psychic withdrawal, as related to craving, can persist indefinitely in some individuals, and may play an important role in their eventual relapse.

Internet addiction: Research relevance to European adolescents

As can be readily perceived by examining the references for this review, the bulk of the research on IA is being conducted in Asia. One possible—and perhaps the most plausible—explanation is that the highest Internet connection speeds are available in several Asian countries. In fact, the countries with the fastest average connection speeds, ranked numbers 1, 2 and 3, are South Korea, Hong Kong and Japan, respectively (20). However, European countries may be closing the gap, as the seven countries that comprise the rest of the top 10 in Internet speed are in Europe (from number 4, the Netherlands, to number 10, Denmark). What remains to be seen is how Internet connection speed and IA may be related, and whether the neurobiological vulnerability toward developing IA differs between Asian and European youth.

Conclusion

Research into the pathophysiology of IA is in its infancy, and much of it is guided by research efforts in other areas of addiction science (21,22,23). The eventual adoption of consensus diagnostic and classification criteria for IA should contribute to an increase in the number of identified patients and to improvements in research study design. It is only a matter of time before consistent, verifiable causes of IA are discovered, which could lead to the development of effective pharmacotherapeutic agents.

References

[1] Young KS. Internet addiction: the emergence of a new clinical disorder. Cyberpsychol Behav 1998;1(3):237-44.

[2] Pies R. Should DSM-V designate "Internet Addiction" a mental disorder? Psychiatry (Edgmont) 2009;6(2):31-7.

[3] Ko CH, Yen JY, Chen CC, Chen SH, Yen CF. Proposed diagnostic criteria of Internet addiction for adolescents. J Nerv Ment Dis 2005;193(11):728-33.

[4] Cao F, Su L, Liu TQ, Gao X. The relationship between impulsivity and Internet addiction in a sample of Chinese adolescents. Eur Psychiatry 2007;22(7):466-71.

[5] Yoo HJ, Cho SC, Ha J, Yune SK, Kim SJ, Hwang J, et al. Attention deficit hyperactivity symptoms and internet addiction. Psychiatry Clin Neurosci 2004;58(5):487-94.

[6] Zhou Y, Lin FC, Du YS, Qin LD, Zhao ZM, Xu JR, et al. Gray matter abnormalities in Internet addiction: a voxel-based morphometry study. Eur J Radiol 2011;79(1):92-5.

[7] Yuan K, Qin W, Wang G, Zeng F, Zhao L, Yang X, et al. Microstructure abnormalities in adolescents with Internet addiction disorder. PLoS One 2011;6(6):e20708.

[8] Liu J, Gao XP, Osunde I, Li X, Zhou SK, Zheng HR, et al. Increased regional homogeneity in Internet addiction disorder: a resting state functional magnetic resonance imaging study. Chin Med J 2010;123(14):1904-8.

[9] Lu DW, Wang JW, Huang AC. Differentiation of Internet addiction risk level based on autonomic nervous responses: the Internet-addiction hypothesis of autonomic activity. Cyberpsychol Behav Soc Netw 2010;13(4):371-8.

[10] Chen SH, Weng LJ, Su YJ, Wu HM, Yang PF. Development of a hinese Internet addiction scale and its psychometric study. Chin J Psychol 2003;45:279-94.

[11] Kim SH, Baik SH, Park CS, Kim SJ, Choi SW, Kim SE. Reduced striatal dopamine D2 receptors in people with Internet addiction. Neuroreport 2011;22(8):407-11.

[12] Han DH, Lee YS, Na C, Ahn JY, Chung US, Daniels MA, et al. The effect of methylphenidate on Internet video game play in children with attention-deficit/hyperactivity disorder. Compr Psychiatry 2009;50(3):251-6.

[13] Volkow ND, Wang G, Fowler JS, Logan J, Gerasimov M, Maynard L, et al. Therapeutic doses of oral methylphenidate significantly increase extracellular dopamine in the human brain. J Neurosci 2001;21:RC121.

[14] Casey BJ, Jones RM. Neurobiology of the adolescent brain and behavior: Implications for substance use disorders. J Am Acad Child Adolesc Psychiatry 2010;49(12):1189-201.

[15] Volkow ND, Wang GJ, Fowler JS, Tomasi D, Telang F. Addiction: beyond dopamine reward circuitry. Proc Natl Acad Sci USA 2011;108(37):15037-42.

[16] Gardner EL. Addiction and brain reward and antireward pathways. Adv Psychosom Med 2011;30:22-60.

[17] Kirby LG, Zeeb FD, Winstanley CA. Contributions of serotonin in addiction vulnerability. Neuropharmacology 2011;61(3):421-32.

[18] Chung SK, You IH, Cho GH, Chung GH, Shin YC, Kim DJ, et al. Changes of functional MRI findings in a patient whose pathological gambling improved with fluvoxamine. Yonsei Med J 2009;50(3):441-4.

[19] Dell'Osso B, Hadley SJ, Allen A, Baker B, Chaplin WF, Hollander E. Escitalopram in the treatment of impulsive-compulsive internet usage disorder: an open-label trial followed by a double-blind discontinuation phase. J Clin Psychiatry 2008;69(3):452-6.

[20] Belson D, Möller R, Bergqvist S. Q2 2011 State of the Internet Webinar Akamai Technologies, Cambridge, MA, USA. Accessed 2013 Jan 6. URL: http://www.akamai.com/dl/akamai/Q2_2011_SotIPresentation.pdf

[21] Greydanus DE, Greydanus MM: Internet addiction in adolescents: The legacy of Dionysus versus Apollo in the 21st century. Asian J Paediatric Pract 2011.

[22] Greydanus DE, Greydanus MM: Internet use, misuse, and addiction in adolescents: Current issues and challenges. Int J Adolesc Med Health 2012;24: 22-30.

[23] Derevensky JL, Shek DTL, Merrick J, eds. Youth gambling. The hidden addiction. Berlin: De Gruyter, 2011.

In: Child and Adolescent Health Yearbook 2013
Editor: Joav Merrick

ISBN: 978-1-63117-658-6

Chapter 34

INTERNET ADDICTION AND PSYCHIATRIC COMORBIDITIES

Ahsan Nazeer, MD, Donald Greydanus**, MD, DR HC (Athens) and Joseph Calles, MD

Department of Child and Adolescent Psychiatry and Department of Pediatric and Adolescent Medicine, Western Michigan University, Homer Stryker MD School of Medicine, Kalamazoo, Michigan, United States of America

ABSTRACT

Internet addictive disorder is a term used to encompass numerous behaviors associated with Internet overuse. In academia, IAD continues to be a controversial concept and is currently not a part of Diagnostic and Statistical Manual-IV-TR. Recent research, mostly from Asian countries has played an increasingly important role in delineating the prevalence, diagnostic structure and associated medical and psychiatric comorbidities of this disorder. The following is a brief review of the current literature regarding IAD and psychiatric comorbidities.

Keywords: Internet addiction, Internet overuse, Internet use, Pathological internet use, Technology addiction

INTRODUCTION

Internet addictive disorder (IAD) is a relatively recent proposed addition to the ever-expanding list of addictive disorders (1). There is general consensus that this disorder consists

* Correspondance: Donald E Greydanus, MD, Dr. HC (ATHENS), Professor and Chair, Department of Pediatric and Adolescent Medicine, Western Michigan University Homer Stryker MD, School of Medicine, 1000 Oakland Drive, D48G, Kalamazoo, MI 49008-1284, United States. E-mail: Donald.greydanus@med.wmich.edu

of numerous sub-categories that include online shopping, gaming, web surfing, gambling and porn addiction.

Despite the fact that the Internet was initially conceptualized in the 1960's, it was not until the mid-nineties that personal computers started becoming a part of individual and family life. With the introduction of the World Wide Web, e-mail and websites such as MySpace, Facebook and Twitter, a gradual albeit steep paradigm shift occurred in the way individuals communicate and socialize. This phenomenon was more pronounced among individuals born during the early 1990's, also called Generation Z. Along with the innumerable benefits, this technology brought an addictive potential for a significant portion of the population that was hard to resist. This negative aspect reflected itself in persistent Internet use despite poor academic performance, chaotic family relationships and behavioral dyscontrol problems, detrimental to overall mental health. With the passage of time, the impact of this phenomenon has gained widespread recognition and in DSM-V, Internet Gaming Disorder is indentified in Section III as a disorder warrenting more research. Despite this growing tsunami of widespread impact, the published studies in western mainstream academic journals are scarce. Recently, with the collaboration of the Safer Internet Programme, southern and central European countries have started a project EU NET ADB. This project is designed to evaluate the prevalence, psychosocial correlates and comorbidities of Internet overuse in European minors (2).

In the meantime, most of the current state of knowledge is from studies published in Taiwan, South Korea and China. Few of them have addressed this issue in the adolescent population, although others have sought to include a broader sample of adolescent and adult individuals. Because of the global nature of this phenomenon and despite the cultural differences, research findings and outcomes are equally meaningful and applicable to the western and European societies.

INTERNET ADDICTIVE DISORDER AND DSM-V

American psychiatrist Ivan Goldberg first introduced the term "Internet addiction" (IA) in the mid-1990's. This was a parody effort on his behalf to draw attention to what he considered as an increasingly medicalized orientation of the recently published DSM-IV. Later, Young introduced this term into the mainstream literature to encompass numerous behaviors associated with Internet overuse including online gambling, cybersex and Internet relationships (3). Over the years, this term took on a life of its own, and now there are serious considerations as to whether this should be included in the future DSM editions as an identifiable and diagnosable mental disorder. As there is always a risk of over-inclusiveness, numerous mental health professionals continue to debate the true nature of this problem. Most of the debate has been focused on whether these behaviors can truly be labeled as an "addiction" versus whether a more neutral term such as "overuse" is warranted. Opponents in this debate propose that the Internet use in these cases is closely tied and secondary to underlying social and addictive behaviors including loneliness, pathological gambling and porn addiction, and that the Internet is simply a means to deal with those issues. They also point to the difficulty in accurately diagnosing and differentiating this disorder from loneliness, depression, self-medication and obsessions. Proponents of this disorder have been fascinated by the impact of this technology on the broader population and its psychological and emotional effects on individuals and the family (4). Researchers have noticed increased compulsive behaviors among non-addicted individuals, with more time being spent in online chat rooms, e-mail, online shopping, games and general web-surfing. This finding must be interpreted with caution as most of us have increased our use and dependence on computers and the Internet in everyday life due to its convenience, speed, comprehensiveness, and flexibility. During this social transition, use of institutions in our former society such as phone books, newspapers, music shops, bookstores, and postal (snail) mail have declined.

Sample variations, lack of consensus on the diagnostic criteria, and difficulties in finding a homogenous sample across studies have made it challenging to measure prevalence rates accurately. In a Finnish study published in 2004 of 12-18 year old youth, 1.4-1.7% reported Internet addiction (5). In a British study published in 2005, 18.3% of the college students were found to be addicted to online gaming (6). Current prevalence of IAD in the United States is not accurately known, but one estimate suggests it to be in the range of 0.3-0.7% while another suggests it is in the realm of 13.7% (7). Prevalence in Asia is estimated to be around 12%. Economic and cultural differences in self-disclosure and access to the Internet among societies are probably the main reasons for this variability. In Asia, Internet cafes abound, and there are more trained professionals who collect prevalence data during routine evaluations. In more affluent Western societies, the Internet is mostly being accessed from home, and social factors including shame and denial lead to minimized reporting of these behaviors to professionals (8).

PRE-EXISTING DISORDERS AND PRECURSORS OF INTERNET ADDICTIVE DISORDER

Internet use has a reinforcing component that is triggered by receiving immediate reward without the need for delayed gratification. Different personality characteristics including low self-esteem, shyness and impulsivity contribute to and collude with this reinforcing tendency to put certain individuals at higher risk for IA.

Clinical observations also suggest that individuals with IAD have a pre-existing personality and pathological dimension that perpetuate this risk, such as social isolation, compulsive personality, depression and loneliness. It is worth noting that despite the fact that some individuals have these pre-existing risk factors, it has proven to be quite challenging to make a causal association between pre-existing states or traits and the development of IAD (9). Depressive symptoms and attention deficit hyperactivity disorder (ADHD) are also said to be commonly associated with IAD, but most of the studies have been cross-sectional, without any conclusive results about the cause and effect of this disorder.

Only a few recent studies have attempted to focus on causality while providing further insights into the interactions of these complex variables. In an effort to identify traits that may trigger IA, researchers from China identified 59 university students who as freshmen were naïve to the Internet but after one year were diagnosed with IA. Pre- and post-Internet addiction psychopathology was measured with the Symptom CheckList-90 (SCL-90). Results showed increased obsessive behaviors before the diagnosis of IA, which were consistent with other studies looking at compulsive behaviors and addictive disorders. Scores on depression, anxiety and hostility scales were within the normal range before the diagnosis but were significantly elevated after 1 year of Internet use. This study failed to identify any predisposing pathological factors that could have triggered IA. On the other hand, this study clearly showed an increase in psychopathology after the onset of excessive Internet use. Despite these results, it is important to note that numerous other academic and psychosocial stressors could have caused emergence of psychopathology. These factors were not directly evaluated, making it harder to reach any conclusions about cause and effect (10).

In a Taiwanese prospective, population-based study, 517 adolescents from three different schools were randomly selected with goal of identifying predictors of IA. Participants completed the Brief Symptoms Inventory (BSI) along with IA and personality dimensional scales. The sample was followed for 1 year, and data points were collected at intervals. Results revealed low self-esteem, impaired family dynamics, online gaming, low reward tolerance and "high exploratory excitability" as predictors of the incidence of IA (11). The students who spent more than 20 hours per week on the Internet were at higher risk for this disorder. The same researchers later conducted a 2-year prospective study of 2162 adolescents. The goals were to identify the predictive value of the psychiatric symptoms and to see if there were gender differences among adolescents with Internet-addictive behaviors. Among the adolescents who completed the study questionnaire, 233 (10.8%) were found to fulfill the diagnostic criteria of IAD. Among general factors, being male and Internet use of greater than 20 hours per week were found to be associated with IA. Association of psychiatric symptoms showed some gender differences. ADHD, depression, hostility and social anxiety were found to be risk factors among females, while ADHD and hostility were risk factors for adolescent males. After controlling for age and race, ADHD was found to be the single most significant predictor of IAD in this study (12).

The results of the Taiwanese study can also be interpreted in light of the work done by Robert Cloninger who introduced a conceptual framework for the risk of alcoholism. In this seminal work from Denmark, he took report cards from 3rd graders and found predictive factors for two types of alcoholism. Type 1 alcoholics had been of high social reward dependence and harm avoidance in 3rd grade, while type 2 youth-onset alcoholics had in high in risk-taking and thrill-seeking groups in 3rd grade. The latter group also tended to be high as adolescents and adults in ADHD, delinquency, and other drug dependence, while the type 1 group only had legal problems related to driving under the influence and drug problems with sedatives. There appears to be a type 2 effect in the above mentioned studies on IAD.

Certain personality traits, including low self-esteem, sensation seeking, shyness, isolative tendencies and impulsivity appear to be common risk factors in individuals with IAD (13). A recent study from Greece accessed the psychological profile of 86 adolescents with a mean age of 15.3 years who already had become afflicted with IA. The sample was heavily skewed towards males (95.4%). Study findings suggest that impaired family dynamics, including dysfunctional relationships, problematic boundaries and family conflicts were the main predictors of IA in adolescents. Adolescents' perceptions of an unsupportive and confrontational parenting style also were associated with IA. These adolescents were also more prone to poor academic performance, including unexcused absences and dropping out of school, and with emotional problems including depressive symptoms (14).

There are numerous commonalities between the adolescents addicted to Internet use and the ones with addiction to illicit drugs, including alcohol and opioids. Both disorders are associated with, and at times preceded by, depression and ADHD. Impulsivity, novelty seeking, tendency for immediate gratification, familial discord and perceived perception of psychosocial difficulties have been found in both groups. Comparison among personality characteristics in adolescents with these addictive disorders was recently reviewed in a Taiwanese study. In this cross-sectional study, 3662 high school students were evaluated with the Tri-Dimensional Personality Questionnaire (TPQ) to assess the difference among personality characteristics between these two groups (15). The concept of tri-dimensional personality is based on Cloninger's model of personality characteristics that include: harm avoidance, novelty seeking and reward dependence (16). Researchers found high novelty seeking to be the most important predictor of IA and of substance use. Among other indicators, low harm avoidance was associated with substance use, whereas high harm avoidance was associated with IA (17). On a behavioral level, Internet addicts have shown tolerance, withdrawal and craving, which is also often found in other substance use disorders. The mesolimbic dopamine reward circuitry and abnormalities in this system have been reported among individuals with substance use disorders. Looking at that association, it is no surprise that neuroimaging studies have focused on this system in this population. One recent PET study of subjects with IAD has found decreased D2 receptor availability in the caudate and striatal areas of the brain. This finding is inversely related to the severity of IA and complements other studies that have found abnormalities in the dopaminergic system in individuals with substance use disorders (18). Table 1 summarizes the pre-existing factors that are found to be associated with IA.

Table 1. Pre-existing social, personality and psychiatric factors associated with internet addiction disorder

Interpersonal relations	Intrapersonal factors
Social impairment	Sensation seeking behaviors
Introversion	Borderline personality traits
Social anxiety	Narcissistic personality traits
Low self-disclosure	Compulsive personality
Hostility	Low self-esteem
Impaired family dynamics	Vocational impairment
Shyness	Poor academic performance

Comorbidities

Internet addiction disorder is associated with numerous psychiatric disorders and this association appears to be a rule rather than an exception. Comorbidity as a term usually refers to the existence of two or more distinct psychiatric or medical disorders. The professional literature has suggested that more than 40% of the DSM-IV psychiatric disorders are comorbid with each other. Studies have shown that IA is associated with more severe psychiatric symptoms, and numerous theories have been proposed ranging from shared etiological factors to reciprocal worsening of the symptoms when both disorders coexist (19). Some common psychiatric comorbid disorders found with IAD are: depression, substance use disorders, ADHD and numerous anxiety disorders including social phobia, generalized anxiety disorder and obsessive compulsive disorders. Despite the similarities among IAD, substance use disorders and compulsive disorders, the hierarchal classification of IA in DSM-V is still under debate. It is important to understand how the comorbid disorders interact with IAD to determine the best treatment strategy. Table 2 summarizes the comorbid factors associated with IA.

Table 2. Comorbid factors associated with Internet addiction disorder

Substance use disorders	Attention deficit hyperactivity disorder
Mood disorder-predominantly depression	Suicidal ideations
Anxiety disorders	Behavioral issues
Obsessive compulsive disorder	Impulse control disorders
Social anxiety disorder	Psychotic disorders-rare
Compulsive buying	Pyromania-rare
Gambling	

DEPRESSION, ALEXITHYMIA AND DISSOCIATION

Comorbid disorders are the major reason why individuals with IAD seek medical attention. As many as 86% of the individuals who struggle with Internet overuse/addiction have another DSM-IV psychiatric disorder (20). A recent Italian study reviewed the "first reason for psychiatric consultation" in their sample subgroup with IAD diagnosis. Results showed that 34% of the IAD sample initially sought clinical care for depression, 20% for attention/hyperactivity issues, 13% for sleep and anxiety problems and 1% for mood liability (20). In this study, Young's Internet Addiction Scale (IAS) was used to make a diagnosis of IAD. After further evaluation with SCID II, 15% of the sample met criteria for generalized and social anxiety disorder each, 14% each for ADHD and borderline personality disorder, 7% each for hypomania, binge eating disorder, dysthymia, and obsessive compulsive personality disorder. Interestingly, obsessive compulsive and dissociative symptoms were the only two psychiatric symptoms that were correlated with high IAS scores (20).

Another Italian study sought to identify the relationship between alexithymia, dissociation and IA among undergraduate students. Alexithymia is a personality trait that is characterized by difficulty in identification and expression of feelings. Results revealed that students with alexithymia had low self-esteem, were at higher risk of dissociative symptoms and were also more prone to IA (21). Other studies have also identified low self-esteem as an independent predictor of IA. In a recent Norwegian study that included youths and adults, 13% of the sample with IA was also positive for alcohol and substance abuse during the past year (22).

Depressive symptoms have been associated with IA. Researchers from Leeds used an online questionnaire to identify the individuals with IA. That group was then administered the Beck Depression Inventory (BDI). 1.2% of the 1319 respondents were categorized as IA and the results were compared with individuals classified as non-addicts (NA). Results showed more addictive tendencies in young males, and the IA group contrasted significantly with NA in their tendency to be moderately to severely depressed (23).

ATTENTION DEFICIT HYPERACTIVITY DISORDER

Attention deficit hyperactivity disorder is a disorder of attention, impulsivity and hyperactivity. It has been associated with IA in numerous studies (24). Individuals with this disorder have behavioral and neurobiological characteristics that make them more prone to the addictive potential of the Internet. They struggle with deficient working memory, impaired task flexibility and planning, and display behavioral dysregulation with preference for immediate reward. In a Taiwanese study of college students, ADHD was the most common (18.1%) comorbid disorder, with depression being the second (11.1%) on the list of comorbidities (25).

Gender differences appeared to be present, with the association of depression and IA being significantly stronger in males than in females. Other studies have tried to evaluate the particular symptoms of ADHD that are associated with IA.

In a study of college students from Taiwan, a sample of 2793 college students with an age range of 18-48 years were recruited from eight colleges. Symptoms of ADHD were evaluated by the Adult ADHD Self-Report Scale (ASRS). 12.9% of the sample was found positive for IA and 9.9% for adult ADHD. The association between the inattentive component of ADHD and IA was stronger in females than in males (26). The relationship between behavioral and personality trait of impulsivity and IA was evaluated in a Chinese study of 2620 high school students. The sample was evaluated with the Barratt Impulsiveness Scale-11 and by the GoStop Impulsivity Paradigm, a measure of behavioral impulsivity. Students with IA were found to be more behaviorally impulsive and also were found to have comorbid ADHD more often than the non-addicted group (27).

SUBSTANCE USE DISORDERS

The debate continues about whether to classify IA as an impulse control disorder or as a part of the substance use disorders (SUDs). Both IA and SUD share numerous common features, including being comorbid with ADHD and depressive symptoms. Psychological and psychosocial profiles of the individuals among both groups share the same characteristics, and both groups have more severe psychiatric symptoms than those without addictive disorders. Studies also have reported substance exposure among individuals with IA (15), but few studies have looked into the specifics of this association. Researchers from Taiwan evaluated 2114 students from senior high and vocational schools for IA and problematic alcohol use. Results showed an association between these two behaviors. Also, being male, parent-child conflicts, and having familial discord and friends with deviant behaviors were found to be risk factors for this association (28). This study was important in that it reviewed underlying psychosocial determinants in a methodological manner and found both of the disorders to share numerous factors. It is also worthwhile to note that Internet overuse can, by itself, facilitate substance use in susceptible adolescents by providing easy access to pro-drug websites and those from which one can order illicit or controlled prescription drugs. Studies have noted a significant number of adolescents going online to search health-related topics. Male adolescents who engage in high risk activities and are sensation seekers are more prone to visit the sites selling illicit drugs (29).

These individuals usually belong to lower socioeconomic class, have family discord, poor academic achievements, and a history of childhood abuse. These are the same characteristics that are also found in the group prone to IA (30). Understanding this and other common themes among these groups provides insights that can be used in establishing effective prevention and treatment programs in the community.

Table 3 summarizes the consequences of IA.

Table 3. Consequences of internet addiction

Problematic family relationships Legal troubles Academic failures High risk-taking behaviors Occupational difficulties	Loneliness Impaired frustration tolerance Fatigue Insomnia

Conclusion

Despite the fact that there are controversies about the labeling of this disorder, no one debates that Internet overuse remains a significant problem that is gradually blurring the boundaries of normal and pathological behavior. This appears to be more of a serious problem for adolescents growing up in this cyber age. Internet overuse also is a common denominator in numerous comorbid disorders including mood and substance use disorders. The reader is advised to be cautious in interpreting the results of the available studies, especially concerning etiological explanations. The triad of predisposing social factors, personality traits and comorbid psychiatric disorders can lead to a pathological condition that can be labeled as IA and for which treatment models used for substance abuse programs can be applied. In the meantime, understanding the nature of this disorder and screening for it in community clinics can identify at-risk individuals and can be a target for intensive interventions.

References

[1] Young KS. Psychology of computer use: addictive use of the Internet: a case that breaks the stereotype. Psychol Rep 1996;79:899-902.

[2] EU NET ADB. EU NET ADB: Research on the intensity and prevalence of the internet addictive behaviour risk among minors in Europe. Accessed 2012 Dec 30. URL: http://ec.europa.eu/information_society/apps/projects/factsheet/index.cfm?project_ref=SI-2010-KEP-4101007.

[3] Young KS. Internet addiction: the emergence of a new clinical disorder. Cyberpsychol Behav1996;3:237–44.

[4] Pallanti S, Bernardi S, Quercioli L. The Shorter PROMIS Questionnaire and the Internet Addiction Scale in the assessment of multiple addictions in a high-school population: prevalence and related disability. CNS Spectr 2006;11(12):966-74.

[5] Kaltiala-Heino R, Lintonen T, Rimpela A. Internet addiction? Potentially problematic use of the Internet in a population of 12–18 year-old adolescents. Addict Res Theory2004;12:89-96.

[6] Niemz K, Griffiths M, Banyard P. Prevalence of pathological internet use among university students and correlations with self-esteem, the General Health Questionnaire (GHQ), and disinhibition. Cyberpsychol Behav 2005;8:562-70.

[7] Aboujaoude E, Koran LM, Gamel N, Large MD, Serpe RT. Potential markers for problematic Internet use: a telephone survey of 2,513 adults. CNS Spectr 2006;11:750-55.

[8] Block JJ. Issues for DSM-V: internet addiction. Am J Psychiatry 2008;165:306-7.

[9] Morahan-Martin J. Internet abuse: Addiction? Disorder? Symptom? Alternative explanations? Soc Sci Comput 2005;23:39-48.

[10] Dong G, Lu Q, Zhou H, Zhao X. Precursor or sequela: pathological disorders in people with Internet addiction disorder.PLoS One 2011;6(2):e14703.

[11] Ko CH, Yen JY, Yen CF, Lin HC, Yang MJ. Factors predictive for incidence and remission of internet addiction in young adolescents: a prospective study. CyberpsycholBehav 2007;10(4):545-51.

[12] Ko CH, Yen JY, Chen CS, Yeh YC, Yen CF. Predictive values of psychiatric symptoms for internet addiction in adolescents: a 2-year prospective study. Arch PediatrAdolesc Med 2009;163(10):937-43.

[13] Xiuqin H, Huimin Z, Mengchen L, Jinan W, Ying Z, Ran T. Mental health, personality, and parental rearing styles of adolescents with Internet addiction disorder.CyberpsycholBehav 2010;13(4):401-6.

[14] Tsitsika A, Critselis E, Louizou A, Janikian M, Freskou A, Marangou E, Kormas G, Kafetzis DA. Determinants of Internet addiction among adolescents: a case-control study. ScientificWorldJournal 2011;19(11):866-74.

[15] Ko CH, Yen JY, Chen CC, Chen SH, Wu K, Yen CF. Tridimensional personality of adolescents with internet addiction and substance use experience. Can J Psychiatry 2006;51(14):887-94.

[16] Cloninger CR. A systematic method for clinical description and classification of personality variants: a proposal. Arch Gen Psychiatry 1987;44(6):573-88.

[17] Ahn DH. Korean policy on treatment and rehabilitation for adolescents' Internet addiction, in 2007 International Symposium on the Counseling and Treatment of Youth Internet Addiction. Seoul, Korea: National Youth Commission 2007: 497.

[18] Kim SH, Baik SH, Park CS, Kim SJ, Choi SW, Kim SE. Reduced striatal dopamine D2 receptors in people with Internet addiction. Neuroreport 2011;22(8):407-11.

[19] Yen JY, Ko CH, Yen CF, Chen SH, Chung WL, Chen CC. Psychiatric symptoms in adolescents with Internet addiction: comparison with substance use. Psychiatry ClinNeurosci 2008;62(1):9-16.

[20] Bernardi S, Pallanti S. Internet addiction: a descriptive clinical study focusing on comorbidities and dissociative symptoms. Compr Psychiatry 2009;50(6):510-16.

[21] De Berardis D, D'Albenzio A, Gambi F, et al. Alexithymia and its relationships with dissociative experiences and Internet addiction in a nonclinical sample. CyberpsycholBehav 2009;12(1):67-9.

[22] Bakken IJ, Wenzel HG, Gotestam KG, Johansson A, Oren A. Internet addiction among Norwegian adults: A stratified probability sample study. Scand J Psychol 2009;50(2):121-7.

[23] Morrison CM, Gore H. The relationship between excessive Internet use and depression: a questionnaire-based study of 1,319 young people and adults. Psychopathology 2010;43(2):121-26.

[24] Yen JY, Ko CH, Yen CF, Wu HY, Yang MJ. The comorbid psychiatric symptoms of Internet addiction: attention deficit and hyperactivity disorder (ADHD), depression, social phobia, and hostility. J Adolesc Health 2007;4:93-6.

[25] Ko CH, Yen JY, Chen CS, Chen CC, Yen CF. Psychiatric comorbidity of internet addiction in college students: an interview study. CNS Spectr 2008;13(2):147-53.

[26] Yen JY, Yen CF, Chen CS, Tang TC, Ko CH. The association between adult ADHD symptoms and internet addiction among college students: the gender difference. Cyberpsychol Behav 2009;12(2):187-91.

[27] Cao F, Su L, Liu T, Gao X. The relationship between impulsivity and Internet addiction in a sample of Chinese adolescents. Eur Psychiatry 2007;22:466-71.

[28] Ko CH, Yen JY, Yen CF, Chen CS, Weng CC, Chen CC. The association between internet addiction and problematic alcohol use in adolescents: the problem behavior model. Cyberpsychol Behav 2008;11(5):571-76.

[29] Westat and Annenberg School for Communication. Evaluation of the National Youth Anti-Drug Media Campaign: 2003 report of findings. Rockville, MD: Westat, 2003.

[30] Belenko S, Dugosh KL, Lynch K, Mericle AA, Pich M, Forman RF. Online illegal drug use information: an exploratory analysis of drug-related website viewing by adolescents. J Health Commun 2009;14(7):612-30.

In: Child and Adolescent Health Yearbook 2013
Editor: Joav Merrick
ISBN: 978-1-63117-658-6

Chapter 35

ASSESSMENT OF INTERNET ADDICTIVE BEHAVIOR

Mari Janikian, PhD*

Adolescent Health Unit, 2nd Department of Pediatrics "P & A Kyriakou" Children's Hospital, National and Kapodistrian University of Athens School of Medicine, The American College of Greece, Deree College, Graduate Program in Applied Psychology, Athens, Greece

ABSTRACT

A comprehensive assessment for the detection of internet addictive behaviors includes conducting a clinical interview usually in conjunction with a standardized assessment instrument, to examine several areas of functioning and to determine differential and co morbid conditions. This review provides a brief overview of the major instruments used to assess internet addictive behavior. Specifically, the chapter summarizes the general assessment process, the clinical interview as well as various tools measuring internet addictive behavior.

Keywords: Internet addictive behavior; assessment; instruments

INTRODUCTION

Assessment is a systematic process of obtaining information from psychological instruments and other sources used to draw inferences about characteristics of people. Assessment goals include screening, diagnosis and progress evaluation. A screening assessment is usually concise and is administered to identify individuals who have a disorder in need of remediation or may require further comprehensive evaluation. A diagnostic assessment targets one or more areas of functioning. It may address a specific diagnostic referral question (e.g., does the individual exhibit internet addictive behavior?) and it involves making suggestions for

* Correspondence: Mari Janikian, PhD, Psychologist, Assistant Professor of Psychology, The American College of Greece, Deree College, Graduate Program in Applied Psychology 6 Gravias Street, Aghia Paraskevi 15342 Athens, Greece. E-mail: mjanikian@acg.edu

intervention. A progress evaluation assessment focuses on the effectiveness of intervention procedures through time.

A comprehensive assessment for the detection of internet addictive behaviors includes conducting a clinical interview usually in conjunction with a standardized assessment instrument, to examine several areas of functioning and to determine differential and co morbid conditions. The purpose of this review is to summarize current information on the assessment of internet addictive behavior. Specifically, in this review we look at the general assessment process, the clinical interview as well as various measures of internet addictive behavior.

CLINICAL INTERVIEW

Detecting internet addictive behaviors upon clinical interview can be challenging (1). In the case of adolescents, obtaining reliable information from multiple sources is of critical importance. An interview should be conducted with an adolescent client first, prior to gathering data from the parents. Most of the interview techniques implemented with adults can be employed with adolescents, depending on their level of maturity. Individual interviews could be further followed-up with a family interview to gather information about interactions between family members.

The recommended format for the clinical interview includes history-taking (chief complaint, history of present illness, personal, family and social histories) and mental status examination in an age-appropriate manner (2). Questions about alcohol and drug use and about a family history of addiction need to be addressed. In the context of the initial interview, information regarding the extent and nature of internet use is collected. Particular attention should be given to chronologically trace the initiation of internet use, progress, maintenance factors and moderation efforts (2).

A semi-structured interview style is recommended, giving adolescents an opportunity to convey information in their own words, and also providing a comprehensive list of questions (e.g., 'How much time do you spend online daily or weekly?' 'What are your favorite applications or activities online?') In addition, symptoms of addiction need to be assessed, such as salience (craving), tolerance, preoccupation and persistence. The effect of internet use on one's academic and interpersonal contexts can be further examined, for example: 'Have you used the internet excessively to the extent of neglecting other activities?' Importantly, what adolescents do online needs to be assessed; creating personas, romantic relationships, and gaming can take on a variety of forms. As already indicated, it is important to corroborate obtained data from additional sources, such as the adolescent's parents or guardians, relatives, and teachers.

Internet addictive behaviors are seldom detected in isolation and thus psychological co morbidity needs to be further assessed. Commonly found co-occurring disorders in adolescence include both internalizing and externalizing problems (3 - 9). Notably prior to labeling an individual as presenting with internet addictive behavior, it should be evidenced that such behavior does not stem from an underlying condition, for example, a mood or psychotic disorder.

An adolescent's motivation to address their internet addictive behavior needs to be further assessed. The transtheoretical model of change (10) is useful in conceptualizing whether an adolescent is motivated to change. Specifically, an individual in the precontemplation stage is not thinking about making a change. In the contemplation stage, one is willing to examine a current behavior pattern and consider the risks involved. In the preparation stage, one contemplates specific plans of action towards particular behavior change and in the action stage implementation of these plans takes place. As individuals change, they usually alternate between the stages and cycle through them at various rates (11). Assessment of an adolescent's motivation for change is valuable for planning and tailoring interventions accordingly.

MEASURES OF INTERNET ADDICTIVE BEHAVIOR

Standardized instruments of internet addictive behaviors are limited. The ones that have been constructed mirror the variations in the diagnostic criteria for internet addictive behavior (12). The following section will review the main existing measures in the literature. It is important to note that these brief measures are not diagnostic, but responses that exceed established cut off scores could suggest a high likelihood of internet addictive behavior.

In earlier investigations, researchers attempted to create their own instruments in an effort to capture the main construct. In one of the first studies of internet addiction, Egger and Rauterberg (13) built a 46-item questionnaire that investigated patterns of use and experiences online. However, their categorization of addiction was based on a single item, asking participants (n=450) whether they felt they were addicted or not. A total of 10% identified themselves as internet addicts and reported high frequency of usage.

INTERNET ADDICTION DIAGNOSTIC QUESTIONNAIRE (IADQ) AND INTERNET ADDICTION TEST (IAT)

Young (9) conceptualized internet addiction in terms of pathological gambling (DSM-IV; 14). Young argued that many problematic internet users exhibited preoccupation with the internet, compulsive use and impairment in their functioning. She created the Internet Addiction Diagnostic Questionnaire (IADQ) or Young's Diagnostic Questionnaire (YDQ) as referred to in the literature, consisting of eight yes/no items (see table 1).

Individuals who endorsed five or more items on the IADQ over a period of six months were classified as internet dependent. In a self-selected sample (n=496), results indicated that the majority (60%) met criteria for internet addiction (9). However, while the IADQ provides a framework for defining addictive internet use, it is a one-cutoff-point instrument (15). Essentially, the IADQ does not allow for any measure of severity to account for the variation of internet addictive behavior symptoms (16). Conceptualizing internet addiction as a continuous construct from mild to severe presentation may provide flexibility in diagnosis and increased adequacy for both clinical and research practice.

Table 1. Internet Addiction Diagnostic Questionnaire (IADQ) / Young's Diagnostic Questionnaire (YDQ)

1	Do you feel preoccupied with the Internet (think about previous online activity or anticipate next online session)?
2	Do you feel the need to use the Internet with increasing amounts of time in order to achieve satisfaction?
3	Have you repeatedly made unsuccessful efforts to control, cut back, or stop Internet use?
4	Do you feel restless, moody, depressed, or irritable when attempting to cut down or stop Internet use?
5	Do you stay online longer than originally intended?
6	Have you jeopardized or risked the loss of a significant relationship, job, or educational or career opportunity because of the Internet?
7	Have you lied to family members, therapists, or others to conceal the extent of involvement with the Internet?
8	Do you use the Internet as a way of escaping from problems or of relieving a dysphoricmood (e.g., feelings of helplessness, guilt, anxiety, depression)?

In 1998 Young (9) devised an expanded version of the earlier IADQ, the 20-item Internet Addiction Test (IAT). The IAT measures the extent of an individual's involvement with the internet, the degree of preoccupation, loss of control, extent of lying about use, and general functioning (17). The questionnaire is based on a five-point Likert scale (0= n/a to 5=always) and contains 20 items (see table 2).

Table 2. Internet Addiction Test (IAT)

1	How often do you find that you stay online longer than you intended?
2	How often do you neglect household chores to spend more time online?
3	How often do you prefer the excitement of the Internet to intimacy with your partner?
4	How often do you form new relationships with fellow online users?
5	How often do others in your life complain to you about the amount of time you spend online?
6	How often do your grades or schoolwork suffer because of the amount of time you spend online?
7	How often do you check your e-mail before something else that you need to do?
8	How often does your job performance or productivity suffer because of the Internet?
9	How often do you become defensive or secretive when anyone asks you what you do online?
10	How often do you block out disturbing thoughts about your life with soothing thoughts of the Internet?
11	How often do you find yourself anticipating when you will go online again?
12	How often do you fear that life without the Internet would be boring, empty, and joyless?
13	How often do you snap, yell, or act annoyed if someone bothers you while you are online?
14	How often do you lose sleep due to late-night log-ins?
15	How often do you feel preoccupied with the Internet when offline, or fantasize about being online?
16	How often do you find yourself saying "Just a few more minutes" when online?
17	How often do you try to cut down the amount of time you spend online and fail?
18	How often do you try to hide how long you've been online?
19	How often do you choose to spend more time online over going out with others?
20	How often do you feel depressed, moody, or nervous when you are offline, which goes away once you are back online?

According to the IAT manual, the scale categorizes internet addictive behavior in terms of mild (31-49 points), moderate (59-79 points) and severe (80-100 points) impairment. A number of instruments, such as the Chinese Internet Addiction Inventory (CIAI; 15), are adaptations of the IAT. Validation studies have been conducted in France (18) and Italy (19).

The IAT has established acceptable psychometric properties (20). Using exploratory factor analysis, Widyanto and McMurran (20) identified six dimensions ("salience, excess use, neglecting work, anticipation, lack of self-control, and neglecting social life"), suggesting that the conceptualization of internet addiction needs to be multifactorial. Nevertheless this research sample was small (n= 86) and no cross-validation took place (15). More recently, recruiting a sample of 410 participants in a reevaluation of the IAT, researchers extracted three principle components from the test, including "withdrawal and social problems", "time management and performance" and "reality substitute" (21). This difference in factor structure may be the result of sampling and cultural variations. Chang and Law (21) conclude that examining the IAT dimensions stability, additional studies require being carried out on diverse populations. Overall, the IAT is an extensively used measure in the internet addiction literature (4).

INTERNET-RELATED ADDICTIVE BEHAVIOUR INVENTORY (IRABI)

Brenner (22) recruiting a sample of online survey respondents (n= 563) developed an instrument based on substance abuse criteria (DSM-IV; 14). The Internet- Related Addictive Behavior Inventory (IRABI) consists of 32 true/false items about excessive internet use. Brenner (22) reported satisfactory internal consistency for the scale (Cronbach's α=0.87). However, no further psychometric information was provided (23) and the specific instrument has never been used (24). The IRABI has been criticized about the extent to which its items measured behaviors indicating true signs of addiction (25).

PATHOLOGICAL INTERNET USE SCALE

Morahan-Martin and Schumaher (26) sampled university students (n= 277) to devise a scale using 13 true/false items assessing adverse outcomes of pathological internet use, including problems in academic, work and interpersonal contexts, withdrawal symptoms, distress and mood-altering usage. They considered any respondent answering favorably to four or more of the items as pathological internet users, without providing a rationale for the specific cutoff use (23). Morahan-Martin and Schumacher (26) did not report any psychometric properties of the PIU, with the exception of internal reliability (Cronbach's α= 0.8761).

GENERALIZED PROBLEMATIC INTERNET USE SCALE (GPIUS)

Caplan (27) created the 29-item Generalized Problematic Internet Use Scale (GPIUS) based on the cognitive-behavioral model (28) using a sample of 386 undergraduate students. The items were developed from three aspects: cognitions (e.g., 'I am treated better than others online than I am offline'); behavior (e.g., 'I use the net to make myself feel better when I'm down') and negative consequences (e.g., 'I have gotten into trouble with my employer or school because of being online'). An exploratory factor analysis revealed that the GPIUS consists of seven factors, including "mood change, perceived social benefits, negative outcomes related to internet use, compulsive use, excessive online time, withdrawal symptoms, and perceived social control" (27). Preliminary findings indicated that the scale has high internal consistency (Cronbach's α ranging from 0.78-0.85) and construct validity (27). The GPIUS has been further revised and updated (29).

ONLINE COGNITION SCALE (OCS)

A similar scale based on the cognitive-behavioral framework was developed by Davis, Flett, and Besser (30). The 36-item Online Cognition Scale (OCS) was created using a sample of undergraduate students (n= 211). Items were selected from instruments of pathological gambling, depression, impulsivity and procrastination. The scale is based on a seven-point Likert scale and contains items, such as, 'I often keep thinking about something I experienced online well after I have logged off;' 'I get more respect online than in real life;' and 'Using the internet is a way to forget about the things I must do but really don't want to do' (30). The confirmatory factor analysis resulted in a four-factor model: diminished impulsive control, loneliness/depression, social comfort and distraction. Davis et al. (30) reported high internal consistency of the scale as a total measure of problematic internet use (Chronbach's α = 0.94).

INTERNET ADDICTION SCALE FOR TAIWANESE HIGH SCHOOL STUDENTS (IAST)

Lin and Tsai (31-32) designed a 29-item scale for adolescents. The Internet Addiction Scale for Taiwanese High School Students (IAST) contains five dimensions: tolerance, compulsive use, withdrawal, related family, school, and health problems; and related interpersonal and financial problems. Scale items are rated on a four-point Likert scale of such statements as: "Although I plan to use the internet for a short time, I end up staying on-line longer than originally intended;" "When I tried to reduce my internet use, I felt anxious; "I have to search for more exciting information to achieve the original satisfaction that I found when I began using the internet;" "More than once, I cut classes to use the internet for something unrelated to school learning;" and "Communicating with on-line friends is more interesting than with people I meet in real life." Both the reliability and validity indeces of the IAST were reported to be satisfactory (33).

INTERNET ADDICTION SCALE (IAS)

The Internet Addiction Scale (IAS; 34) is another self-report measure consisting of 36 items. The IAS was developed based on the seven substance dependence criteria of the DSM-IV

(14) and two additional criteria (i.e., mood modification and salience) recommended by Griffiths (25). Respondents rate their agreeableness on a five-point Likert scale, with higher scores representing greater addiction rate on the internet. Preliminary results indicate that the IAS is a reliable measure with high internal consistency (Cronbach's α= .95) as reported by Nichols and Nicki (34). The IAS was found to consist of one factor relating to the negative consequences of excessive internet use. One criticism of the IAS is that using substance dependence diagnostic criteria to conceptualize internet addictive behaviors has been largely rejected in favor of behavioral addictions models (35).

PROBLEMATIC INTERNET USE QUESTIONNAIRE (PIUQ)

Thatcher and Goolam (23) created a 20-item questionnaire based on Young's (36) criteria for internet addiction. Items were further derived from a pathological gambling questionnaire and published literature on internet addiction symptoms. Respondents were asked to complete a five-point Likert scale, indicating the frequency of problematic internet behaviors (e.g., 'do you go online when you know there are more important things you should do?'; 'do you feel distressed when you cannot connect to the internet?'). The PIUQ was shown to have good internal reliability (Chronbach's α= 0.90) and a factor analysis suggested the following three-factor solution explaining 50% of the variance: online preoccupation, adverse effects, and social interactions. The questionnaire was shown to correlate with other predictors of problematic internet use, feelings of depression, isolation and loneliness, and Young's eight criteria of internet addiction (23).

PROBLEMATIC INTERNET USAGE SCALE (PIUS)

More recently, another multidimensional questionnaire is the 33-item Problematic Internet Usage Scale (PIUS; 37). Three factors were extracted, using principle component analysis, including negative consequences, social benefit/social comfort, and excessive use. The internal consistency coefficient of the scale was 0.94. Item total correlations ranged between 0.31 and 0.70. Test-re-test reliability was 0.81 and split half reliability coefficient was 0.83 (37). No inter-item or inter-factor correlation matrix was reported for the PIUS (38).

PROBLEMATIC INTERNET USE QUESTIONNAIRE (PIUQ)

Demetrovics and colleagues (39) published the Problematic Internet Use Questionnaire (PIUQ). The 18-item PIUQ was constructed by modifying Young's (9) Internet Addiction Test and including questions designed by the authors. Respondents provide a self-rating on a 5-point scale ranging from never (1) to always (5). Hungarian participants (n= 1037) were sampled online to establish the questionnaire's psychometric properties. A factor analysis yielded three subscales: Obsession, Neglect scale, and Control Disorder. A high internal consistency for each subscale was reported (Cronbach's α= .74-.87) and the correlation of every subscale with the total scale was above .80. The subscale test–retest reliability coefficients ranged between .76 and .90. Kelley and Gruber (24) further sampled American undergraduate students (n= 278) to conduct a confirmatory factor analysis of the PIUQ and examine its reliability and validity. Their results corroborated the problematic internet usage model suggested by Demetrovics et al. (39).

CONCLUSION

A number of important criticisms of the assessment instruments discussed need to be highlighted. First, there is disagreement regarding the underlying dimensions of the construct, as these scales are conceptualized using diverse theoretical models of internet addictive behaviors. Second, the assessment of problematic internet use via self-report measures is limiting given that respondents may not reply in a truthful manner or may not comprehend certain items. Third, most scales do not take into consideration all existing activities online such as social networking sites, pornography and others. Therefore an accurate evaluation of the extent and scope of internet use is not achieved. Fourth, there are concerns in terms of sampling. Respondents are commonly recruited from colleges and web sites without the use of a control group for comparison purposes. Very few studies have sampled adolescent populations for the development of their scales. Population biases may have been introduced to the preliminary results of the studies. Finally, no assessment measure discussed has been subjected to thorough testing of reliability and validity. Thus additional research is necessary to establish solid psychometric properties. Given the lack of a universally acceptable gold standard assessment or diagnostic tool, the use of clinical interviews within a comprehensive framework of clinical assessment becomes essential (12). Concluding, the continuing debate over the validity of internet addictive behavior as a diagnostic category has created obstacles in our current understanding of the etiology, assessment and treatment of the problem. As the internet continues to be an integral part of adolescents' life, the need for reliable and valid assessment procedures to measure problematic internet behaviors will continue to increase (40).

REFERENCES

[1] Young K, de Abreu C. Internet addiction: A handbook and guide to evaluation and treatment. Hoboken, NJ: John Wiley, 2011.

[2] Vijaya M, Sanju G. Lost online: An overview of internet addiction. Adv Psychiatr Treat 2007;13(1):24-30.

[3] Ghassemzadeh L, Shahraray M, Moradi A. Prevalence of internet addiction and comparison of Internet addicts and non-addicts in Iranian high schools. Cyberpsychol Behav 2008;11(6):731-33.

[4] Ha J, Yoo H, Cho I, Chin B, Shin D, Kim J. Psychiatric comorbidity assessed in Korean children and adolescents who screen positive for internet addiction. J Clin Psychiatry 2006;67(5):821-26.

[5] Kim EJ, Namkoong K, Ku T, Kim SJ. The relationship between online game addiction and aggression, self-control and narcissistic personality traits. Eur Psychiatry 2008;23(3):212-8.

[6] Kratzer S, Hegerl U. Is "internet addiction" a disorder of its own?A study on subjects with excessive internet use. Psychiatr Prax 2008;35(2):80-3.

[7] Nannan J, Haigen G. A study on college students' internet usage behavior, attitude and personality traits. Psychol Sci 2005;28(1):49-51.

[8] Petersen KU, Weymann N, Schelb Y, Thiel R, Thomasius R. Pathological internet use - epidemiology, diagnostics, co-occurring disorders and treatment. Fortschr Neurol Psychiatr 2009:77(5):263-71.

[9] Young K. Internet addiction: The emergence of a new clinical disorder. Cyberpsychol Behav 1998;1(3):237-244.

[10] Prochaska JO, DiClemente CC, Norcross JC. In search of how people change: Applications to addictive behaviors. In: Salovey P, Rothman AJ, Salovey P, Rothman AJ. Social psychology of health. New York: Psychology Press, 2003:63-77.

[11] DiClemente CC. Addiction and change: How addictions develop and addicted people recover New York: Guilford, 2003.

[12] Beard K. Internet Addiction: A review of current assessment techniques and potential assessment questions. Cyberpsychol Behav 2005;8(1):7-14.

[13] Egger O, Rauterberg M. Internet behavior and addiction. ETH Technical Report AP-01-96. Zurich: Swiss Federal Institute of Technology, 1996.

[14] American Psychiatric Association. Diagnostic and statistical manual of mental disorders, 4th ed. Washington, DC: APA, 1994.

[15] Huang Z, Wang M, Qian M, Zhong J, Tao R. Chinese Internet Addiction Inventory: Developing a measure of problematic Internet use for Chinese college students. Cyberpsychol Behav 2007;10(6):805-11.

[16] Dowling N, Quirk K. Screening for internet dependence: Do the proposed diagnostic criteria differentiate normal from dependent internet use? Cyberpsychol Behav 2009;12(1):21-7.

[17] Young K. Cognitive behavior therapy with internet addicts: Treatment outcomes and implications. Cyberpsychol Behav 2007;10(5):671-9.

[18] Khazaal Y, Billieux J, Thorens G, Khan R, Louati Y, Scarlatti E, et al. French validation of the Internet Addiction Test. Cyberpsychol Behav 2008;11(6):703-6.

[19] Ferraro G, Caci B, D'Amico A, Di Blasi M. Internet addiction disorder: An Italian study. Cyberpsychol Behav 2007;10(2):170-75.

[20] Widyanto L, McMurran M. The psychometric properties of the Internet Addiction Test. Cyberpsychol Behav 2004;7(4):443-50.

[21] Chang MK, Law SPM. Factor structure for Young's Internet addiction test: A confirmatory study. Comput Human Behav 2008;24:2597–619.

[22] Brenner V. Psychology of computer use: XLVII. Parameters of internet use, abuse and addiction: The first 90 days of the internet usage survey. Psychol Rep 1997;80:879–82.

[23] Thatcher A, Goolam S. Development and psychometric properties of the Problematic Internet Use Questionnaire.S Afr J Psychol 2005;35(4):793-809.

[24] Kelley K, Gruber E. Psychometric properties of the Problematic Internet Use Questionnaire. Comput Human Behav 2010;26(6):1838-45.

[25] Griffiths M. Internet addiction: Does it really exist? In: Gackenbach J. Psychology and the internet: Intrapersonal, interpersonal and transpersonal applications. New York, NY: Acad Press, 1998:61-75.

[26] Morahan-Martin JJ, Schumacher P. Incidence and correlates of pathological Internet use among college students. Comput Human Behav 2000;16(1):13-29.

[27] Caplan SE. Problematic Internet use and psychosocial well-being: Development of a theory-based cognitive-behavioral measurement instrument. Comput Human Behav 2002;18(5):553-75.

[28] Davis RA. A cognitive–behavioral model of pathological Internet use. Comput Human Behav 2001;17(2):187-95.

[29] Caplan SE. Theory and measurement of generalized problematic internet use: A two-step approach. Comput Human Behav 2010;26(5):1089-97.

[30] Davis RA, Flett GL, Besser A. Validation of a new scale for measuring problematic Internet use: Implications for pre-employment screening. Cyberpsychol Behav 2002;5(4):331-45.

[31] Lin SSJ, Tsai CC. Internet addiction among high schoolers in Taiwan. Boston, MA: 106th annual convention of the American Psychological Association, 1999.

[32] Tsai CC, Lin SSJ. Internet addiction of Taiwanese adolescents: an in-depth interview study. Washington, DC: 107th annual convention of the American Psychological Association, 2000.

[33] Tsai CC, Lin SSJ. Analysis of attitudes toward computer networks and Internet addiction of Taiwanese adolescents.Cyberpsychol Behav 2001;4:373–6.

[34] Nichols LA, Nicki R. Development of a psychometrically sound internet addiction scale: A preliminary step. Psychol Addict Behav 2004;18(4):381-4.

[35] Warden NL, Phillips JG, Ogloff JRF. Internet addiction. Psychiatr Psychol Law 2004;11:280–95.

[36] Young K. Caught in the net. New York, NY: John Wiley, 1996.

[37] Ceyhan E, Ceyhan AA, Gürcan A. The validity and reliability of the Problematic Internet Scale use. Educ Sci Theory Pract 2007;7:387–416.

[38] Jia A, Jia HH. Factorial validity of problematic internet use scales. Comput Human Behav 2009;25(6):1335–42.

[39] Demetrovics Z, Szeredi B, Rozsa S. The three-factor model of internet addiction: The development of the problematic internet use questionnaire. Behav Res Methods 2008;40(2):563–73.

[40] Beard K, Wolf E. Modification in the proposed diagnostic criteria for Internet addiction. Cyberpsychol Behav 2001;4(3):377-83.

In: Child and Adolescent Health Yearbook 2013
Editor: Joav Merrick

ISBN: 978-1-63117-658-6

Chapter 36

RISKS OF DEVELOPING INTERNET ADDICTIVE BEHAVIORS: SCOPE AND EXTENT OF INTERNET SITES USED

Kai W Müller**, Dipl-Psych., Klaus Wölfling, Dipl-Psych. and Michael Dreier, Dipl-Soz.

Outpatient Clinic for Computer Game and Internet Addictive Behaviour,
Mainz Clinic and Polyclinic for Psychosomatic Medicine and Psychotherapy,
University Medical Center, Johannes Gutenberg-University Mainz, Mainz, Germany

ABSTRACT

It is elucidated that the development of internet addiction includes three main factors. Those are 1) factors of the individual, 2) factors of the environment and 3) factors of the drug resp. behaviour. Those are related to a different kind of internet application use and motivational state such as (I) gaming, (II) social networking, (III) gambling, and (IV) distraction. These indicated aspects are going to be linked and this elaboration is especially focusing on the scope and extent of the internet applications that are used for each emphasis of use. Overall here the intersection of the indicated use of applications is tackled in relation to addictive factors. Media convergence and its advantages is discussed critically in context of internet applications and broader opportunities for activities such as streaming and playing games offered from platforms including enormous social components via smartphone. In this context the social networking component of online games is depicted, indicating that a successful gamer has the subliminal quest for socializing. The elaborated aspects are finally discussed and set into context to recent research and literature. The current lack of knowledge about different applications that lead to internet addictive behavior are circumscribed, relating to empirical evidence and solutions are discussed.

---

* Correspondence: Kai W. Müller, Dipl Psych, Research Associate, Outpatient Clinic for Bevahioral Addictions, Department for Psychosomatic Medicine and Psychotherapy at the University Medical Center of the Johannes Gutenberg-University Mainz (UMC-Mainz), Untere Zahlbacher Straße 8 55131 Mainz, Germany. E-mail: muellka@uni-mainz.de.

Keywords: Internet addiction, social belonging, media convergence, gaming, social networking, gambling, distraction, browser games

INTRODUCTION

Like in other addictions and addictive behaviours too, it is supposed that the addictive disorder originates from an interaction of different circumstances, pointing to a multi-factorial etiopathogenesis. Looking onto internet addiction, at present there is still a lack of knowledge concerning theoretical frameworks explaining its appearance. Moreover, most of those scarce approaches can't explain relevant mechanisms in the transition from a regular usage pattern to internet overuse, misuse, and finally addictive use.

From a theoretical point of view three closely interrelated factors are probable to play a role in developing internet addiction. Following early assumptions by Kielholz and Ladewig (1, addiction disorders – no matter whether substance-related or not – are fostered by:

- factors of the individual (e.g., personality, cognitive styles, the self)
- factors of the environment (e.g., family structure, social norms, socio-economic variables)
- factors of the drug resp. behaviour (e.g., contents, effects, availability, advertising) (1).

Up to now, there is considerable research concerning personal risk-factors potentially leading to an addictive use of the internet. It was shown that shyness (2), social insecurity (3), dysfunctional attachment styles (4), heightened vulnerability to stress (5) and certain personality factors like exaggerated neuroticism and diminished conscientiousness (6) are related to excessive and addictive use of both computer games and further internet applications. To a lesser extent, factors of the environment have been investigated. Still, it is plausible that general social acceptance of the internet as a potentially beneficial medium, as well as its broad availability is playing a role in developing addictive use.

Recent research has increasingly focused in identifying factors of the internet itself in explaining the attraction, as well as development of misuse and internet addiction. Professionals agree that it is not the internet itself that can be held responsible for addictive behaviours. Rather specific internet-related contents with unique characteristics are to be regarded as potentially addictive. As Young (7) stated in her early clinical contributions, five different types of internet addiction can be differentiated: gaming addiction (e.g., role-playing games, browser games), information overload (e.g., web surfing), "net compulsions" (e.g., online gambling or online shopping), cybersexual addiction (e.g., online sex), and cyber-relationship addiction (e.g., online relationships, chats, and social networks) (7). Indeed, recent studies confirm that there is considerable variation between the addictive potential of different internet applications. First of all, online games are seen as containing the most pronounced danger in developing Internet Addiction. For example, an Asian study revealed that about 90% of all internet-overusers were mainly playing online games (8). Epidemiologic surveys in Europe also show that gaming has to be regarded as the most prominent form of Internet Addiction (9). Likewise, a clinical investigation of a specialized outpatient clinic for the treatment of Internet Addiction confirmed that most of the treatment-seeking clients were preoccupied with online games, mostly Massive Multiplayer Online Role-Playing Games (MMORPG) (10). However, there is growing evidence that also communication-based applications might be regarded as comparably addictive (11). In a large-scale study by Morrison and Gore (2010) it was shown that apart from games, the use of social network sites (SNS) was closely related to Internet Addiction. It has been further demonstrated that overuse of SNS is also related to heightened depressive symptoms (9). A third critical application can be found in online gambling activities (12,13). Different professionals argue that internet-related gambling might be seen as more threatening than terrestrial gambling, because there are fewer limitations in using different gambling-sites, less age restrictions and accelerated dynamics of betting (14). However, at present there are no systematic investigations that relate to different important questions, like if there are specific risk factors (e.g., gender, personality) leading to one or another kind of Internet Addiction, or if there is comparable psychopathological strain among different types of internet addicts. Also, it is unclear if scope and kind of co-morbidity vary among those subtypes.

From a sociological perspective, the arrangement and presentation regarding different aspects of self strongly depend on certain relevant situations that social actors take part in (15). This is most important with regard to coherent in-group-communication and the coherent-communication-based group belonging (16). In the understanding of Strauss (1959) a social identity is assigned during the interactional process of negotiation (15). These thoughts are similar to Goffman´s view (1959) and his distinct presentation of an individual, which acts in different ways depending to be on the front or back stage (17). This interaction-based process of shifting, adjusting, and presenting strongly affects the social environment of social actors. The logic conclusion must be a detailed knowledge about the main leisure time activity of the individually chosen preferred peer-group. It is absolutely clear to the individual that certain knowledge is required to become part of special social areas. This phenomenon becomes evident in four different aspects: computer gaming, social networks, gambling, and use for distraction; this will be addressed later. The following paragraphs are also meant to shed some light on psychological effects and potential addictive characteristics of diverse popular internet applications like games, social networks, and online gambling. For that purpose, the different applications are depicted consecutively and discussed in terms of their sociological and psychological features. In conclusion, some thoughts about the internet itself and upcoming technological and content-based innovations, like the phenomenon of media convergence, are being addressed.

GAMING

Regarding computer gaming, knowledge is related to a minimum pool of internet sites or applications that have to be used to ensure the individual an increase of knowledge and granting access to other people that are also into gaming (16). This set of in-group-knowledge suggested pages and applications is enhancing the knowledge and thus the likelihood of integration into an in-group. Specific combinations of these significant symbols (16) are grouped up as a so called “Diderot set” (18). The arrangement of single Diderot unities is situation-guided, because it makes a difference if somebody plays Counter Strike 1.6 or

Counter Strike Source (CCS) (18). It is the difference of social localization (19). These two similar but at the same time differing games, which could be assigned to the same game genre first-person-shooter (FPS), require a minimum set of equipment to reach the target of successful long-term gaming. There have to be specific hardware conditions like a broadband internet connection, a headset, a gaming mouse, a huge gaming monitor with one of the lowest reaction times that are available on the market, and an excellent gaming computer to minimize lags which could affect the fun of gaming and the success of the player. So the gamer feels the challenge to own high-end gaming equipment to avoid disadvantages during the gaming experience. Beside those not absolutely necessary hardware demands, there are some software requirements which have to be met beside the game itself. To start simple there has to be a voice over IP-program (VoIP) which is used for communication and decision making. But there are additional important areas of usage that have to be covered. Gamers are members of clans or guilds; these gamer associations use specially manufactured homepages and forums for communication and gamer bonding. The ambitious gamer also needs to be up to date about the latest patches and game-related stories. Therefore well-known online magazines are used as well as highly specialized overall mod-community pages. The gamer has the urgent quest to update the personal knowledge about the game of choice. This update grants an in-group-position (16). If the gamer does not fulfill his community given quest, he will be excluded from the social areas that he has been part of so far. This exclusion from a social system depends on the specific learned knowledge that grants the inclusion into individually relevant subsystems of our society. The designed subsystem codes of gamers are highly professionalized, polarizing and coherent to be the insurance of being a social subsystem (20). In summary, the individually chosen target to be a valued part of a gamer community has to be achieved by using a specific set of internet applications, because if those are not used, exclusion impends.

SOCIAL NETWORKS

Since the appearance of the Web 2.0, the internet has become even more interactive and dynamic. Nowadays, when interacting with others, users are no longer restricted to simple chat surfaces typing in word after word and waiting for a reply. Social networks like Facebook®, MySpace® and Google+® have become an integral part of the World Wide Web. Thus, it doesn't surprise that SNS are one of the fastest growing and developing internet applications. Estimations on numbers of its users relate to approximately 500 million – which corresponds to one third of all regular internet users – with at least one profile in SNS (21). According to a recent study on internet behavior of 23420 minors aged between 9 to 16 years across Europe, a total of 57% confirmed having a personal profile on at least one social networking site (22). Also it has been shown that every second person registered in SNS is updating or cherishing his profile on a daily basis, pointing out high engagement concerning SNS-usage. Not surprisingly, between 2008 and 2009 an increase of about 566% in respect to time spent in SNS was recorded (21). Facing these high rates of people involved in social networking sites, the question arises: What makes these websites that interesting? First of all, SNS offer a quick and easy possibility to fulfill an evolutionary old desire: the desire of affiliation. Accordingly, research on adolescents has shown that 91% use SNS to stay in contact with friends they know personally (from real life contexts) and another 49% – interestingly, more often males – are motivated to find new friends via SNS (21). For human beings it is important to create social networks, to connect, and – of course – to compare with others. Social affiliation as a part of our evolutionary heritage (23) is one core desire and investigations emphasize its importance on health as well as psychosocial well-being, showing that there is a linkage between emotional and social loneliness and a poorer state of health, deterioration of job-performance, depressive symptoms and substance misuse (24).

In the year 2012 it is possible to gather a widespread community of friend-like kindred spirits in a totally different way compared to former times – one might state, that nowadays they are just one click away. Apart from this, it is now possible to draw a variety of social comparisons in an easy way, just by viewing the profiles of others and by observing how they change in the spade of time. However, the question arises in how far there are also dangers for psychosocial health embedded into these countless social comparisons. The huge amount of different profiles on SNS is turning the occurrence of upward social comparisons as inevitable. The more so because popular SNS like Facebook® are designed quite uniformly, making it easier to quickly recognize discrepancies and similarities between one's own and the other's profile. Frankly spoken, the user seems to be forced to draw social comparisons almost automatically (25). From social psychology it is known that being confronted with social objects that are recognized as highly discrepant (e.g., more attractive, more popular, more experienced, more active) from the self of the viewer can cause negative affective states and in turn decrease psychosocial well-being (25). Especially persons with lowered self-esteem might be particularly vulnerable to this effect. Indeed a preliminary study on this confirmed existence of that relationship experimentally (26). It was demonstrated that users of SNS who were confronted with highly discrepant profiles of (ideal) others were experiencing more negative feelings afterwards and developed a more negative view on themselves. These effects were more pronounced in women than in men as well as in persons with a weak self-esteem (26). However, deepened knowledge about the general effects of SNS-usage is lacking; especially concerning aspects of developmental psychology and psychosocial maturing. It is hard to say in how far social learning through SNS-mediated communication is affecting social competencies and social representations in children and adolescents. It is a matter of fact that computer-mediated communication has to be seen as a distinct, more reduced form of human communication; for example lacking nonverbal-information. From a theoretical point of view one can suppose that children primarily relating to connect with others through SNS might be at a disadvantage in respect to the development of a sound ability of understanding the complexity of (real life) social interaction, for example by having difficulties to encode non-verbal social cues. Indeed, a study by Mittal, Tessner and Walker (2007) demonstrated that adolescents with schizotypal tendencies, a personality disorder characterized by a need for social detachment and interpersonal problems, were both using more often SNS and online-games than healthy controls and the time spent with SNS was correlated negatively with the number of real-life friends (27). Certainly, more research is needed to appraise effects of SNS-use on social behaviour.

Apart from general negative effects that might occur, the addictive potential of SNS has been discussed recently, too. SNS have yielded attention by clinicians in Germany since Rumpf et al. (2011) published their final report of the PINTA study. The main focus of this large-scale epidemiological survey was to identify a representative prevalence of internet addictive behavior. A prevalence of 1% was measured among a total sample of 15,024 participants aged between 14 to 64 years. This overall prevalence was approximately divided equally between genders. There were 1.2% of male and 0.8% of female internet addicted users with a confidence interval of 1.0-1.6% (male) and 0.6-1.1% (female). The analyzed sub-sample of participants aged between 14 and 24 years displayed an increased overall prevalence of 2.4% with even more similar results regarding gender differences. 2.5% male and 2.4% female users had to be classified as internet addicted. This tendency increased again in adolescents of 14 to 16 years, where addicted behavior had to be assigned to 4% of the minors. Here the prevalence was shifted to a female dominance; meaning that prevalence for Internet Addiction among females was 4.9% compared to 3.9% of the male users (28).

These results prove that especially young female users are affected by internet addicted behavior. This conclusion is most interesting when it comes into consideration that social networks (77.1%) – followed by emailing (11.7%) – were the most relevant descriptive user referenced application of the internet for females. Males used social networks (64.8%) as well, (and) additionally online games (33.6%) (28). However, at present there are no representative investigations on the addictive potential of SNS and little is known about both, concrete prevalence rates and risk factors. Generally, addictive SNS-use has probably to be explained within frameworks of biopsychosocial models with phenomenological similarities to substance-related addictions and similar symptoms. Reasonably, core criteria of addictive SNS-use are to be expected concerning excessive use (time spent in SNS, updating one's own profile resp. surfing on other's profiles), tolerance (increasing use of SNS over time), salience resp. craving (i.e., behavioural, cognitive, and emotional preoccupation with the SNS usage; urge to check SNS), withdrawal symptoms (experiencing aversive physical and emotional symptoms when SNS-use is restricted) and loss of control resp. repeated use of SNS despite occurring negative consequences (poorer health, conflicts with family, neglect of partnership, and decreasing achievements in school or job). However, no systematic clinical investigations on this topic have been done so far, making it difficult to judge upon its clinical relevance.

GAMBLING

The pool of used gambling applications is low. When gambling starts, an information collecting research phase, which is used to improve the knowledge and gaming skills of the recipient begins. Until the gambler gets professional, the amount of used applications is cut down to a minimum. The main focus here is the used online gambling application. Inside this application, the gamer starts to boost confrontations with upcoming important events, using more than one game at the same time. Online poker gamblers use as much more tables simultaneously as they need to feel challenged and satisfy their perceived subjective amount of winning moments. Social and financial costs are increasing enormously while the gamer uses that huge amount of different gambling tables (29). Later on, some are doing internet research to find possibilities for financial revenue stream.

Across different studies, internet gambling behavior is seen as especially critical and hence associated with increased risk for loss of control and addictive use. It is still a matter of debate whether internet gambling addiction is a modern form of pathological gambling that just changed its environment from the terrestrial to the virtual or if it can be regarded as a further distinct subtype of Internet Addiction. In the end both perspectives have raison d'être and there is certainly consensus in regarding excessive internet-related gambling as a form of behavioral addiction, just like pathological gambling will be referred to in the upcoming revision of DSM (30). Moreover many researchers foresee increasing rates of people affected by internet gambling addiction, referring to proliferating gambling offers and variants in the internet. The possibility to engage in online gambling activities reaches from sports betting, virtual fruit machines, classic casino games like roulette and black jack and of course the vast amounts of poker sites.

Although it is unclear if internet gambling breeds new cases of pathological gamblers, clinical data show that there is a considerable overlap in pathological gamblers using terrestrial and online variants of gambling. An investigation of treatment seeking clients in a specialized outpatient clinic in Germany showed that about 42% of pathological gamblers admitted using online-gambling offers – apart from terrestrial ones – on a regular basis. Further epidemiologic data confirm that there is a remarkable overlap between addictive internet use and gambling in adolescents (12,13), possibly due to emerging convergence effects (31) that can be observed in the internet nowadays (e.g., playing poker within social network sites).

Apart from that, online gambling exhibits several features known to be addiction fostering in a special and sometimes enhanced manner. From research on the addictive potential of different games of chance it has become evident that frequency of single gambling-related events, diversity and range of betting possibilities, perceived winning odds, availability, payout intervals, occurrence of near-miss events and continuity can be regarded as markers indicating heightened addictive potential (32). Concerning internet gambling, all of those features have to be regarded as present. Not surprisingly, recent research in gambling German minors has shown that among gambling on slot-machines, participation in online gambling-activities was the strongest predictor for addictive use and psychopathological strain (13).

DISTRACTION

Distraction is highly related to an individual history of being reprimanded in everyday life and also on procrastination (33). One of the biggest and simultaneously most affective influences on the development of internet addictive behavior is given by an uncontrolled and non-focused use of internet applications or web pages. The danger of getting addicted in this case is not presented by interesting and immersing bounded internet applications. A distracting use is much more related to a missing applicable and appropriate alternative action, as well as (subjective) feelings of being overloaded by the everyday's demands, and resulting levels of stress. So here internet applications are used in a non-focused way and with a distracting manner. First empirical evidence leads to the assumption that in this case, internet use and misuse is strongly related to a certain kind of avoidant coping strategy that has been called "media-related coping" (34,35). Calming down arises in regards to internet areas that grant emotional highly protected reserves, since unpleasant persons could be blocked from communication lists and annoying thoughts of upcoming hassles and stressors that subjectively seem to overcharge the resources of the user can be suppressed for the moment of surfing. People are focused on the usage of joy-bringing applications, applications of their interest, applications that grant the updating of specific in-group knowledge (16). The user can get a very active and also very tough member of the internet which does not necessarily need to be similar to everyday life. So the user notices that a negative impact of the real life can be suffered easier when the focus of the own perception is shifted to the comforts of the internet world. The perceived self-efficacy is increased – at least in terms of the virtual environment – and the recipient notices that internet usage is not causing any harm. This subjective perspective supports a positive self-concept of the internet user. But adverse outcomes like loneliness and psychopathological symptomatology arise in the course of time and is significantly increased by the indication of an internet addictive behavior (36).

Table 1. Vicious cycle in internet addiction

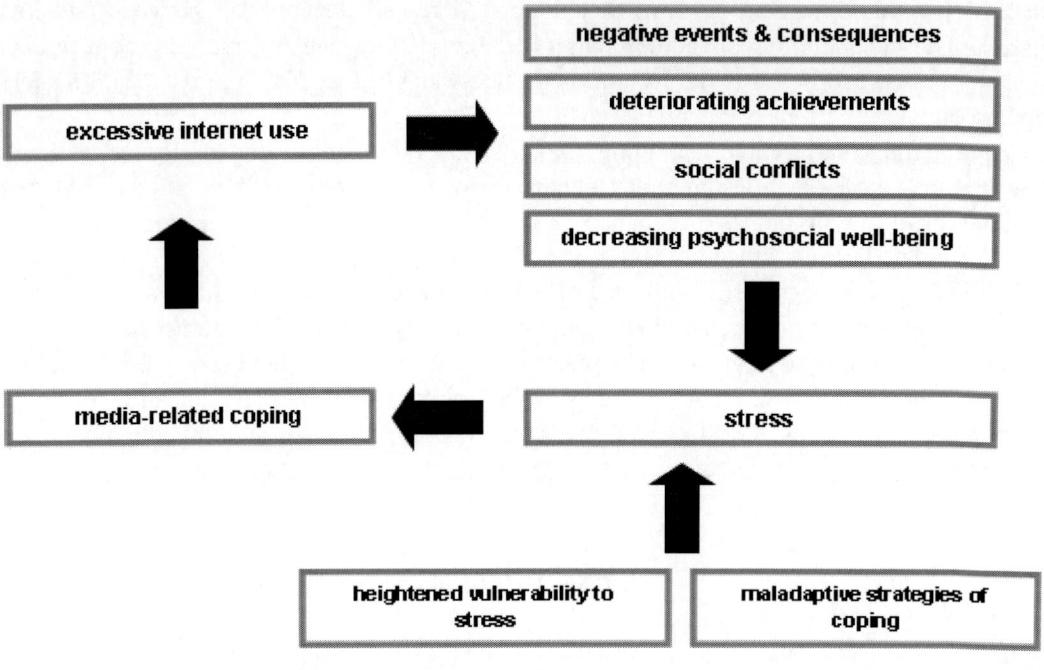

However, research reveals that one prominent risk factor for Internet Addiction has to be supposed in a heightened vulnerability to stress, combined with less effective and functional strategies of coping. Consequently, current etiopathological models of Internet Addiction are based on the tradition of diathesis-stress-models (37). Among the already mentioned media-related coping, further passive and avoidant ways of coping can be recognized in distracting, and suppression, as well as in tendencies to ruminate and in self-blaming (38). According to approaches of cognitive learning theories, the user at risk discovers the distracting infinity of the internet as a possibility to escape stressors and threats of daily life. Over the course of time he more and more (mis-) uses the internet as an external opportunity to regulate negative mood states and engages increasingly in that avoidant behavior. However, dysfunctional ways of coping do only have temporary relieving effects (39), soon resulting in the re-appearance of the stress-response that is encountered with a repeated increase of internet-related activities and time spent online. Out of this, even more negative events in the real world appear, potentially leading to further stressors like conflicts with friends or family members, bad grades or dissuasiveness. A vicious cycle arises, paralyzing the user at risk in a routine that can't be changed easily (see table 1).

MEDIA CONVERGENCE

In times of smartphones, which act as real-time linkage between the personal reality and the internet, virtuality becomes closer bounded to the individual way of life. The small and multifunctional devices are conquering the user market and applications are getting more open with no fixed focus at being used at one specific device. But this merging process is not only about smartphones; it is also about the general approaching process of different merely independently used media.

The most significant improvement of the gaming market started in United Kingdom in late 2011. A real time game streaming game provider was installed not as a game selling library like Steam®, but furthermore as an all in one solution. Onlive® is offering usual games combined with social network functions (40). They provide games on demand using common available devices like Mac®, PC, iPad®, Android™ or HDTV. Thus it becomes possible to play the most modern game in an appropriate graphic quality without the need for owning a new device for gaming. The minimum requirements are fulfilled by every modern netbook and a minimum wired or Wi-Fi connection of 2 Mbps. Social components have their benefit by using ShareBragClip™ videos linked to Facebook® or friend- and community functions. Because of technical restrictions – regarding pings – this offer is actually only available in Great Britain, but the startup was successful and other countries will follow. As one first example, this Onlive® business model stands for a new age of hardware and software merging and availability and thus represents media convergence in a very holistic and socially flavored way.

BROWSER GAMES INSIDE SOCIAL NETWORKS

Nowadays browser games are part of social networks. This has the advantage that social comparing and social bonding could be used by game developers and producers to increase the amount of money spent at the individually preferred game.

Browser games themselves do have a similarity in usage and approach with the Multi-User Dungeons (MUD) appearing in the 1970s (41). It was only possible to play one character per account, the battle system was simple, but there was an interactive component, which stimulated the gamers so that they got aware of the fun they had while playing with different gamers (42). Vanhatupa (2010) indicates that Earth 2025 was the first browser-based game released in October 1996. Later on everybody that had the ability to program browser games was able to offer his games using Facebook® as a platform for multiplication and selling (42). Especially the quality of graphics increased much more since Quake3 (1999) and later QuakeLive (2010) were developed and set new standards in the approach that should be used by game developing and game publishing companies (ID Soft, 2011), (43). This successful story of browser games based on their concept of direct comparing and interactional gaming has further increased, since Adobe Flash 11 was launched in 2011 including the relevant Software Developer Kit (SDK) to target Flash 11 and AIR3 to have the ability of 3D gaming as part of a browser game with an enormous increment of graphical quality and hardware saving at the same time (44).

Nowadays Minecraft proved that a successful game does not necessarily need high end graphic or interesting storyline. The most important thing about the Minecraft success is that gamers got the ability to create something totally new, something that was not foreseen or scripted by game designers. It is about something gorgeous like rebuilding Tolkien´s Middle-earth by an interested and organized group of gamers – it is the infinity of possibilities (45). Thus it has to be indicated that social communities and their potential of interaction are increased by technological development. The line of technological requirements has been crossed, so that games that are not presented in a highly polished dress, but armed with superior game design knowledge can reach areas of major selling and kudos.

One of the worldwide leaders of the browser game sector is Bigpoint. In 2011 they closed with over 228.800.000-registered gamers for their provided games (46). Another global player is Gameforge. They implemented a gamer comparison tool. Electing the top-star gamer of a day grants fame and honor to the game effort based player who becomes famous in the gaming and real life community, since the achievement is presented on the Gameforge homepage consecutively (47).

Lots of browser games try to enhance usability using a direct entry into the browser gaming world without creating an account. The gamer starts directly with the character-building screen and is not requested to enter personal data at the beginning. This step is presented later, when the gamer got in touch with the game. This familiarization is used to immerse the gamer and to bring him into the joining position. Nowadays intermittently reinforcing schedules are used in a similar way; game design focuses much more on subliminal accessing of monetization and a stepwise tender incensement of financial efforts.

WORLD OF WARCRAFT AS DISGUISED SOCIAL NETWORK

Having the ability of socializing with other gamers means assigning the biggest impact on the gamer that is using MMORPGS, since nearly every function or feature is presented in single player environments as well. But the social component of getting in touch with people who are interested in the same hobby like the recipient has conceivable impact. So the self-efficacy of the gamer is elevated since social reputation and honor is brought to him while others interact with the recipient (48). Gamers have the inevitable subliminal quest to group up to be able to finalize the upcoming quests or dungeons. Since the gamers are physically separated, but nevertheless interacting in a social way, it has to be indicated that they are part of "collective solitude". The final goal was the installation of the social norm sociability. And it is alarming that gamers have fairly sparse social reality connections (49).

From a clinical perspective, belonging to a seemingly stable social network that people affected by computer game addiction often refer to as their "virtual family" must be regarded as a crucial factor contributing to the maintenance of the addictive behavior. Early studies show that people at risk for problematic internet use over-interpret the depth and intimacy they experience while interacting with virtual others (50). At the same time, research has displayed that there is also a heightened expectancy in possibly meeting like-minded online (51). Clinically, it seems appropriate to refer in this context of an "online social-perception bias": People with high levels of introversion or even social insecurity feel attracted by the promises of interacting with others on a more detached and controlled level. So the internet with its endless pool of potential contacts and a maximum of anonymity and control over the user's impression management is attractive to them by nature. While virtually interacting with others via the internet, no matter if on social networking sites or as a member of a guild, the vulnerable user loses social inhibition, experiencing a formerly unknown feeling of social competency and thus regarding transient social encounters as exceptionally comforting, intimate, and lasting.

CONCLUSION

Social belonging was illustrated and embroidered as one of the essential indicators for the development of internet addicted behavior. Linkages were presented to computer gaming, gambling, and social networking. Gender aspects and the dominance of a prevalence dominated by female users in younger user groups were set into the context of social networking. However, there are still unresolved questions researchers have to take into consideration in further investigations on internet addictive behavior.

While there is remarkable progress in research on addictive computer gaming, knowledge is still partial about different forms of Internet Addiction. For instance, this is the case for the issue of addictive online gambling. Did the classic disorder of pathological gambling just shift its environment, expanding to the medium internet or are online gamblers to be seen differently concerning specific risk factors and symptomatology from terrestrial gamblers? First clinical impressions from specialized institutions for the treatment of pathological gambling suggest that there seems to be a subgroup of gamblers solely gambling online. These patients might be regarded as a distinct clinical population. However, further research is needed, especially concerning possible specific treatment programs of this subgroup.

Likewise, the question arises if there is distinct psychopathological strain within the different types of Internet Addictions. The question if addictive computer gaming is related to higher psychopathology than addictive use of social networking sites hasn't been addressed yet. Also specific etiological features have not been investigated systematically yet, although clinical case reports suggest that – like in the vast amount of substance-related addiction disorders – the existence of both, general risk factors and specific ones, seems to be reasonable.

Despite rapidly growing numbers of scientific publications on Internet Addiction there are still critical voices doubting the existence of this clinical phenomenon. Also there are still clinicians arguing that the internet must not be seen as potentially addictive to some users, but rather as a modern form of self-medication, helping socially inhibited people to carry out social connectedness through the World Wide Web. Undoubtedly, this might be true for some users. There might be introverted people profiting from the social contacts they establish in virtual worlds by generalizing this newly gained experience of social competency into the real world, turning them to address others out of a more confident position. But on the reverse, the opposite might be true as well. This could be the case in people avoiding essential learning experiences by hiding in social networking sites, chat fora or guilds, substituting real life friendships by online-contacts without being able to manage a transfer of their social experiences from the medium internet to the real world. It is improbable that these people take any advantages from the possibilities of the internet; rather it is probable that they get lost in a vicious circle, getting more and more disconnected in the real world because of their excessive internet use while compensating this disconnectedness by an even more intensified internet behavior. Simply stating that social interaction on the internet is a solution for the socially inhibited resembles proposing an agoraphobic to leave the house not until nightfall.

REFERENCES

[1] Kielholz P, Ladewig D. Die Abhängigkeit von Drogen. München: Deutscher Taschenbuch Verlag, 1973. [Gernman]

[2] Chak K, Leung L. Shyness and locus of control as predictors of internet addiction and internet use. Cyberpsychol Behav 2004;7:559-70.

[3] Wölfling K, Müller KW, Beutel ME. Reliability and validity of the Scale for the Assessment of Pathological Computer-Gaming (CSV-S). Psychother Psychosom Med Psychol 2011;61:216-24. [German]

[4] Ghassemzadeh L, Shahraray M, Moradi A. Prevalence of internet addiction and comparison of internet addicts and non-addicts in Iranian high schools. Cyberpsychol Behav 2008;11:731-3.

[5] Batthyány D, Müller K, Benker F, Wölfling K. Computer game Playing: Clinical characteristics of dependence and abuse among adolescents. Wiener Klin Wochenschrift 2009;121:502-9. [German]

[6] Müller KW. Clinical findings on computer game addiction: The role of personality, stress and coping. Eur Psychiatr 2010;25:1067.

[7] Young K. Internet addiction: Evaluation and treatment. Student BMJ 1999;7:351-352.

[8] Ko YS, Kim SJ, Kim BG. National research of internet addiction. Seoul: Korea Agency Digital Opportunity Promotion, 2007.

[9] Morrison CM, Gore H. The relationship between excessive internet use and depression: a questionnaire-based study of 1319 young people and adults. Psychopathol 2010;43:121-6.

[10] Beutel ME, Hoch C, Wölfling K, Müller KW. Clinical characteristics of computer game and internet addiction in persons seeking treatment in an outpatient clinic for computer game addiction. Zeitschrift Psychosom Med Psychother 2011;57:77-90. [German]

[11] Kuss DJ, Griffiths MD. Online social networking and addiction. A review of the psychological literature. Int J Environ Res Public Health 2011;8:3528-52.

[12] Tsitsika A, Critselis E, Janikian M, Kormas G. Association between internet gambling and problematic internet use among adolescents. J Gambl Stud 2010;27:389-400.

[13] Duven E, Giralt S, Müller KW, Wölfling K, Dreier M, Beutel ME. Problematisches Glücksspielverhalten bei Kindern und Jugendlichen in Rheinland-Pfalz. Universitätsmedizin Mainz, 2011. Accessed 2012 Nov 22. URL:http://www.unimedizinmainz.de/fileadmin/kliniken/verhalten/Dokumente/Broschuere_KIJU-RLP.pdf

[14] Griffiths MD. Gambling and gaming addictions in adolescence. Leicester: British Psychological Society, 2002.

[15] Strauss A. Mirrors and masks: The search for identity. Glencoe, IL: Free Press, 1959.

[16] Schütz A. Gesammelte Aufsätze II. Studien zur soziologischen Theorie. Den Haag: Martinus Nijhoff, 1972.

[17] Goffman E. The presentation of self in everyday life. New York: Anchor Books, 1959.

[18] Diderot D. Gründe, meinem alten Hausrock nachzutrauern. Über die Frauen. Zwei Essays. Berlin: Friedenauer Presse, 1992. [German]

[19] Bourdieu P. Distinction. A social critique of the judgement of taste. Harvard: Harvard University Press, 1984.

[20] Luhmann N. Die Gesellschaft der Gesellschaft. Frankfurt: Suhrkamp, 1997. [German]
[21] The Nielsen Company. Global Faces and Networked Places. 2009. Accessed 2013 Jan 06. URL:http://blog.nielsen.com/nielsenwire/wpcontent/uploads/ 2009/03/nielsen_globalfaces_mar09.pdf
[22] Livingstone S, Haddon L, Görzig A, Olafsson K. Risiks and Safety on the internet. The perspective of European children. Initial findings from the EU Kids Online survey of 9-16 year olds and their parents. 2010. Accessed 2012 Oct 30. URL: www.eukidsonline.de
[23] Regan PC. Functional features: An evolutionary perspective on inappropriate relationships. In: Goodwin R, Cramer D, eds. Inappropriate relationships: The unconventional, the disapproved, and the forbidden. Mahwah, NJ: Lawrence Erlbaum, 2002:25-42.
[24] Hawkley LC, Burleson MH, Berntson GG, Cacioppo JT. Loneliness in everyday life: Cardiovascular activity, psychosocial context and health behaviors. J Pers Soc Psychol 2003;85:105-20.
[25] Festinger L. A theory of social comparison processes. Hum Relat 1954;7:117-40.
[26] Haferkamp N, Krämer NC. Social Comparison 2.0: Examining the effects of online profiles on social-networking sites. Cyberpsychol Behav 2011;14:309-14.
[27] Mittal VA, Tessner KD, Walker EF. Elevated social Internet use and schizotypal personality disorder in adolescents. Schizophrenia Res 2007;94:50-7.
[28] Rumpf HJ, Meyer C, Kreuzer A, John U. Prävalenz der Internetabhängigkeit (PINTA). Bericht an das Bundesministerium für Gesundheit. Lübeck: Universitäten Greifswald Lübeck, 2011. [German]
[29] Fisher S. A Prevalence study of gambling and problem gambling in British adolescents. Addict Res 1999;7(6):509-38.
[30] Holden C. Behavioral addictions debut in proposed DSM-V. Science 2010;19:770-1.
[31] King D, Delfabbro P, Griffiths MD. The convergence of gambling and digital media: Implications for gambling in young people. J Gambl Stud 2010;26:175-87.
[32] Meyer G, Häfeli J, Mörsen C, Fiebig M. Die Einschätzung des Gefährdungspotenzials von Glücksspielen – Ergebnisse einer Delphi-Studie und empirische Validierung der Beurteilungsmerkmale. Sucht 2010;56(6):405-14. [German]
[33] Davis RA, Flett GL, Besser A. Validation of a new scale for measuring problematic internet use: Implications for pre-employment screening. Cyberpsychol Behav 2002;5(4):331-45.
[34] Davis R, Flett G, Besser A. Do people use the Internet to cope with stress? Chicago: 110th Annual Convention American Psychological Association, 2002.
[35] Wölfling K, Müller KW. Computerspielsucht. In: Batthyány D, Pritz A, eds. Rausch ohne Drogen. Substanzungebundene Süchte. Wien: Springer, 2009. [German]
[36] Gentile DA, Choo H, Liau A, Sim T, Li D, Fung D, Khoo A. Pathological video game use among youths: A two-year longitudinal study. Pediatrics 2011;127:318-30.
[37] Müller KW, Wölfling K. Computer game and internet addiction: Aspects of diagnostics, phenomenology, pathogenesis, and therapeutic intervention. Suchttherapie 2011;12:57-63.
[38] Wölfling K, Müller KW, Giralt S, Beutel ME. Emotionale Befindlichkeit und dysfunktionale Stressverarbeitung bei Personen mit Internetsucht. Sucht 2011;57(1):27-37.
[39] Lazarus RS. Psychological stress and the coping process. New York: McGraw-Hill, 1966.
[40] Onlive. 2011. Accessed 2012 Oct 30. URL: http://www.onlive.com/
[41] Barton M. Dungeons and desktops. The history of computer role playing games. Wellesley: AK Peters, 2008.
[42] Vanhatupa JM. Browser games for online communities. Int J Wireless Mobile Networks 2010;2(3):39-47.
[43] QuakeLive. 2011. Accessed 2012 Oct 30. URL: http://www.quakelive.com/
[44] Adobe. 2011. Accessed 2012 Oct 30. URL: http://labs.adobe.com/
[45] Wölfling K, Müller KW. Computerspiel- und Internetsucht: Klinische Betrachtungen und psychologische Effekte. In: Kommission für Jugendmedienschutz der Landesmedienanstalten, ed. KJM-Schriftenreihen Band 2: Umstritten und Umworben – Computerspiele – Eine Herausforderung für die Gesellschaft. Berlin: Vistas, 2010:158-73. [German]
[46] Bigpoint. 2011. Accessed 2012 Oct 30. URL: http://de.bigpoint.com/
[47] Gameforge. 2011. Accessed 2012 Oct 30. URL: http://en.gameforge.com/

[48] Yee N. Ariadne - Understanding MMORPG addiction. 2002. Accessed 2012 Oct 30. URL: http://www.nickyee.com/hub/addiction/home.html

[49] Ducheneaut N, Yee N. Collective solitude and social networks in world of warcraft. In: C. Romm Livermore C, Setzekorn K, eds. Social networking communities and e-dating services: Concepts and implications. Hershey: IGI Global, 2009:78-100.

[50] Greenfield DN. The nature of internet addiction: Psychological factors in compulsive internet use. Boston, MA: Meeting American Psychological Association, 1999. Accessed 2012 Oct 03. URL: http://virtual-addiction.com/internetaddiction.html

[51] Hahn A, Jerusalem M. Internetsucht: Jugendliche gefangen im Netz. In: Raithel J, ed. Risikoverhaltensweisen Jugendlicher. Erklärungen, Formen und Prävention. Opladen: Leske Budrich, 2001. [German]

In: Child and Adolescent Health Yearbook 2013
Editor: Joav Merrick
ISBN: 978-1-63117-658-6

Chapter 37

ONLINE SOCIAL NETWORKING USE: ASSOCIATIONS WITH ADOLESCENT WELL-BEING AND INTERNET ADDICTIVE BEHAVIORS

Eleni C Tzavela*, MSc and
Foteini M Mavromati, MSc/Post-MSc Dip
Adolescent Health Unit, 2nd Department of Pediatrics "P & A Kyriakou" Children's Hospital, National and Kapodistrian University of Athens School of Medicine, Athens, Greece

ABSTRACT

In the last decade social networking sites (SNSs) have gained immense popularity and have become an integral part of youth daily social practice. The popularity of SNS is intuitively linked to the multiplicity of the features and opportunities afforded therein; including, profile making, "friending", commenting, and communication. Some of these online opportunities are closely linked to adolescent developmental needs. There is good evidence that SNS offer fertile ground for identity development by providing training for exercising independence and social skills and for experimenting with one's identity. Peer acceptance, self-worth and identity exploration are today expressed and negotiated online on SNS. Social platforms have re-defined the ways by which adolescent daily communication and developmental struggles are expressed, and as such constitute a new context for development. Nonetheless, for some adolescents SNS use may be a way to compensate for offline personal difficulties, at times turning into an excessive or "addictive" behavior. SNS may be addictive and "SNS addiction" may be seen as a subtype of internet addictive behaviors, namely within the range of the cyber-relationship addictions. To date there is only limited empirical evidence supporting the addictive "potential" of SNS use and as such it is not possible to draw clear and robust linkages and conclusions.

---

* Correspondence: Eleni C Tzavela, Developmental Psychology, MSc., , Adolescent Health Unit, 2nd Department of Pediatrics "P & A Kyriakou" Children's Hospital, National and Kapodistrian University of Athens School of Medicine, 24 Mesogeion Avenue, Goudi 11527, Athens, Greece. E-mail: etzavela@med.uoa.gr

Keywords: Adolescence, development, internet addictive behaviors, social networking sites (SNS), well-being

INTRODUCTION

Social network sites (SNSs) are internet-based social platforms, which allow people to interact online. Structurally, SNS are a cross between a yearbook and a community website (1). The first notable SNSs that introduced user profiles and featured friends' lists were launched in the mid-1990s (Classmates.com in 1995; Sixdegrees.com in 1997). Few would have guessed that within 15 years, SNSs would gain immense popularity and prominence, would attract over half a billion users, and ultimately become an integral part of youth culture. Sites such as Facebook and MySpace have penetrated the adolescent social scene by re-organizing and re-defining daily social practice, including the formation and maintenance of peer relations. For most adolescents SNS are a continuation of their offline sociability and routine, often seamlessly integrating their offline and online reality; while for others, SNS use may be a way to negotiate difficulties or fill offline 'gaps', and may turn into an excessive or "addictive" habit. It has been suggested that SNS may be addictive and that "SNS addiction" maybe be seen as a subtype of internet addiction, namely within the range of cyber-relationships addictions (2).

This review aims to define and review SNS use and practices in adolescence, with focus on the psychological underpinnings of use on adolescent development, and on associations with internet addictive behaviors.

DEFINING SNS

Social network sites are part of a new wave of technology often collectively referred to as Web2.0 tools or social media.

In a more complete definition, provided by Boyd and Ellison (3), SNSs are described as web-based services that allow individuals to (a) construct a public or semi-public profile within a bounded system; (b) articulate a list of other users with whom they share a connection; and (c) view and traverse their list of connections and those made by others within the system (3). SNS are virtual communities (such as Google Groups) yet bear few differences from the latter; in virtual communities, the emphasis is on the content created whereas in SNSs the emphasis is on the user and his or her network (4). SNSs are about people and relationships. Content is created in SNSs - and this is often elaborate and embellished for adolescent users- but content is social and typically personal.

In sum, SNSs are online platforms that afford technology-mediated communication and a way to share information and content with a network of individuals.

Trends in SNS use

The popularity of social media across ages and countries is undeniable. Data from 2010 reveal that 75% of Internet users worldwide visit a social network or blog when they go online — which represents a 24% increase over the same period the year before. The average user (internationally) spends 66% more time using SNS than a year ago (from 3 ½ hours in 2009 to 6 hours in April 2010) (5). Both in Europe and in the USA social networking represents the fastest growing content category. While in 2010 in the USA social networking constituted the most preferred online activity, in Europe social networking comes second in preferences, following search/navigation (which represents 84% of online users). Europeans spend the equivalent of one day a month online (24:20 hours) with important variability noted across countries (6). Overall, the world now spends 22.7 percent of all online time on social networking.

Adolescents: The lion's share in SNS use

The profile of social networking users in Europe reveals that that 15-24 year olds represent 25% of users and the most significant of all age groups (6). One quarter of MySpace users are adolescents (7). For adolescents SNS use has displaced other online social media, snatching time from e-mailing and instant messaging (5). Social networking is not part of adolescent communication; it *is* adolescent communication (8). Data from the EU Kids Online Survey collected in 2010 revealed that in Europe 93% of children 9-16 are online (at least weekly) and of these about 60% have their own social network profile (9). American data from the 2009 Pew Internet & American Life Project suggests similar internet use across the Atlantic, (93% of American adolescents 12-15 years are online and) 73% of online teens between the ages of 12 and 17 use SNSs. (10), an increase from 58% in 2007 (11). Adolescents and young adults undoubtedly maintain the lion's share in SNS use.

Age trends and restrictions

It appears that the popularity of social networking increases with age, since at 13-14 years of age 73% report having a social networking profile, while in middle adolescence (15-16 years) figures rise to 82%/ (9). Moreover, in Europe significant variability was shown across countries, with Greece being in the lower end of SNS use, where54% of children 9-16 years report having a profile, while on the highest end is the Netherlands where 80% have a profile.

With regard to pre-teen use of social networks, a lot of public attention has been drawn on age restrictions for registration in SNSs. Some sites require 13, 16, or 18 years as the minimum age of registration It appears that age-restrictions are frequently violated since one quarter of European preadolescents 9-11 years old and half of 11-12 years old, have their own social networking profiles (9). Facebook has introduced in a Statement of Rights and Responsibilities an age restriction of 13 years for use.

Gender trends in SNS use

Social networking is equally popular among boys and girls in Europe, with 60% of girls and 58% of boys 9-16 years having a profile (9). Similar gender trends were shown among American teens (10). Notably, a gender discrepancy is revealed in middle adolescence in the U.S.A.: 70% of online girls 15-17 years have created a profile, while only 57% of boys of the same age have done the same (11).

Friends' SNS and Facebook

The largest SNS category used in adolescence is friends' SNS with greatest popularity enjoyed by Facebook, MySpace, Friendster and Twitter. Facebook was launched in 2004 and was originally available only for college students until 2005, when it opened up to the public. Facebook has an educational orientation and is said to cater (or initially did) to youth of higher educational and socio-economic status. Data from 2010 reveal that adolescents and young adults account for 27% of Facebook users. (6). Facebook is the leading social networking site in 15 out of 18 countries assessed in the comScore report, representing 63% of social networking penetration. Only in Poland and in the Netherlands have other social networks reached audiences larger than Facebook, with Nasza-klasa.pl and Hyves obtaining first place respectively. The 15-24 year olds represent 25.3 percent of SNS users and this age group shows preference for Facebook and Twitter. Boyd (2007) offers an interpretation of adolescents' site preferences, suggesting that each site has an orientation towards a social issue (3).

Features, affordances and concerns

The popularity of SNS among youth is linked to the multiplicity of its features and to the consequent opportunities afforded therein. The core features of SNS include: profile making, friending (organizing and managing "friends" lists), commenting, and sending messages (giving and receiving feedback). Additionally, users can download music and videos, upload music, update personal profiles and information, upload and tag photos, blog, as well as create and share virtual objects.

Profile-making

SNSs are also referred to as *profile sites* because registered members place on their profile personal information that they want to share, thus creating a personalized online representation. SNS profiles are entirely user-generated, which empowers users with creativity and control over content. Personal interests are combined with embellishments, songs or video-clips, making up the user's digital representation. Online profiles are comparable to interactive scrapbooks or photo-albums (12).

The profile photo is one of most important means of self-presentation because it represents, in whole or in part, the user's physical identity. It appears in search results and alongside every turn of online interaction. Profile choices are subject to personal taste and peer norms, and are often updated.

As suggested by Livingston, adolescents' profile design is not solely a matter of individual choices but rather is guided by assumptions on what their friends would enjoy viewing (13).

Profile privacy settings

The visibility of a profile is specified by the users. Particularly for adolescents visibility control is a widely discussed topic and a case of public concern. Of European adolescents using SNS, 43% report that they keep their profile private (accessed only their friends) and another 28% report that their profile is partially private, enabling friends of friends and networks to see their profile (9). Following public campaigns, adolescents are becoming more cautious about their privacy setting. One study conducted in 2010 comparing adolescents online social behaviors and assessing the privacy setting of almost 10,000 MySpace profiles, found that between 2006 and 2009 a significant change was evidenced in the nature of personal content made publicly available (7).

Friending

Most SNS link their members through the creation of personal networks. A user can either initiate or receive "friend" requests, and this process (*friending*) collectively generates a "friend" list, which is publicly displayed on the profile. SNS friending can for some adolescents, become a chase of numbers, and proof of popularity. SNS friending practices do not share many common features with offline befriending. It is common for adolescents to undertake intense friending, adding on users they barely know and as a result opening up their profile and information to a wide group of users. Pursuing large numbers of friends, even thousands, is a common activity in Facebook (14). It is a widespread belief among youth that a large number of friends reveals social desirability and thus marks an appealing feature of one's profile. This notion was tested in an empirical study and it was revealed that the relationship between the number of friends a profile owner has and observers' perceptions of social attractiveness is curvilinear (inverted U-shape) (15). Both a very low (<100) and a very large number of friends (>300) were associated with low social attractiveness. Social attractiveness ratings were shown to be highest for profiles displaying about 300 friends.

European findings from 2010 suggest that half of children 9-16 years have fewer than 50 contacts in their preferred SNS, and only one in five had 100-300 contacts (9). Considerable country-specific variability was shown with 20% of Greek adolescent and pre-adolescents reporting more than 300 contacts, and another 18% reporting 100-300 contacts respectively. Thus, almost 40% of Greek children 9-16 years report over 100 contacts (9).

Commenting and communication

The primary reason teens use social network sites is to stay in touch with friends (16). As many as 83% of teenage users have added comments to pictures that their friends have posted; 77% have posted public messages to friends' pages and about half send instant messages or chat through these sites (11). Social networking sites provide numerous communication features. While email is still used to communicate with adults and authorities, MySpace has become the primary asynchronous communication tool for teens (1). For users daily "tasks" include checking personal messages, friend additions, bulletin board posts, event announcements and new blog posts.

Psychological and developmental underpinnings of SNS use

Adolescent development

Adolescence is a period marked by major physical, cognitive, and emotional changes. As adolescents struggle to make the transition from protected childhood to independent adulthood, the peer group "becomes the vehicle of that transition" (17). Peer relationships become of primary importance to adolescent's well-being and friendship quality significantly correlates to adjustment. Conformity to the peer group peaks at 13-15 years. Adolescence is a time of juggling conformity and independence, gradually developing one's individual identity. Erikson described the task of identity formation as a normative struggle between the adolescent's perception of self and others' view of self As Harter suggested, there is no developmental period in which evaluations regarding the self are as likely to affect self-esteem and well-being, as in adolescence (18).

A new context for adolescent development

A lot of the transitional struggles negotiated by today's adolescents are similar to those of adolescents of previous generations'; conformity to peers, conflict with adults and the need for gradual independence prevails across time. What has changed is *the ways* that youth communicates; expressions, language, and habits have changed trailing technological advancements. Youth has always had the need and the habit to congregate, to form cliques and crowds. What was previously done on the corner store or in the mall is today done online on social networking sites. SNSs are often compared to hangout places of previous generations (12). Similarly, peer conflict and problematic behaviors have moved online. Some of the problems have been confronted and addressed in the past, while others are new-maybe byproducts of the new era- such as in the case of cyber-bullying. Children have always been bullied but this was taking place in the schoolyard. Now these same conflicts have moved online and have become more salient and visible to a wider public. The internet has re-defined the ways in which adolescent daily communication and developmental struggles are expressed. Peer acceptance, self-worth and identity negotiation are now expressed in a new social environment: online social media. Social media have attained such a prominent position in the lives of adolescents that by all accounts constitute the forum where daily social practice plays out - a new context for development.

SNS attractions to adolescents and needs met

People use the media based on their needs and motives, and media use is reinforced by gratifications obtained (19). Undoubtedly, the web makes it easier to engage in social interaction. Social interaction has been identified as a primary motive for social media adoption. In adolescence the need to connect to peers is pivotal and the peer context has been shown to influence achievement of developmental tasks (19). Social media diminish communication barriers– both practical (i.e., cost, distance) and inter-personal (introversion, shyness), thus facilitating fulfillment of the fundamental need to connect. The need to belong (i.e., be part of a group), is yet another fundamental human motivation associated to today's youth's involvement in virtual communities. It has been empirically shown that the need to belong is a predictor of SNS adoption for females (4). Another appealing feature of SNSs is profile creation and this preferred activity may be associated with the adolescent need for identity exploration. Profile creation allows for self-experimentation via the process of generating of one's self-representation. This activity is also linked to the development of independence (12). Finally, the absence of authority and lack of parental control in the context of SNS use is an additional feature that appeals to adolescents. Adolescents enthusiastically adopt the online realm because it represents their space- visible by the peer group more than by adults, and enjoy a relatively safe opportunity to conduct their social psychological tasks (13). As the same author suggests, for today's adolescents self-actualization includes a negotiation between online opportunities (identity, intimacy and sociability) and risks (privacy, abuse) afforded by internet mediated communication.

What is the influence of online communications on adolescent well being?

The effect of internet use and social media in particular, on social relationships is still a matter of intense debate. One dominant hypothesis, the *displacement hypothesis*, posits that time spent on social media displaces offline interaction (with friends and family), amplifying social isolation and adversely affecting social development. One of the very first studies suggesting this type of effect was carried out at Carnegie-Mellon University in the late nineties, only a few years after the appearance of first social networks (20). This study's authors suggested that internet use was associated with declines in social involvement and psychological well-being, and that people may be substituting offline ties with online ones. Similarly, Green and Block have suggested that online communication is a distracting alternative to deeper interactions (21). Along the same lines, Mesch (2006) examined Israeli adolescents' social ties and found - in support of the displacement hypothesis- that internet use was negatively related to family closeness and positively related to family conflict (22).

The opposing, and more positive view, is the *stimulation or increase hypothesis*, which argues that online communication can increase social interaction, thus enhancing well-being. Valkenburg and Peter (23) suggest that online communication is facilitative in connecting with old friends and making new ones, and that time with friends as well as quality of friendships is enhanced (23). Notably, a significant association has been suggested between well-being and feedback received from other SNS users; namely, positive feedback enhanced adolescents' self-esteem while negative feedback decreased self-esteem (24).

It appears that the relationship between SNS use and well-being may be mediated by personality traits (i.e., sociability), or pre-existing competences. SNS participation benefits may be more prevalent in some personality types, such as socially anxious individuals, a position also referred to as the *social compensation hypothesis*. Extroversion has been associated with larger social networks in SNS, suggesting that typically SNS friends are first made offline (23). Correa et al. (25) recently found that extroversion is the most significant personality trait predicting social media usage for emerging adults. Similarly, in their most recent research Kraut and colleagues (26) proposed that internet use was associated with better outcomes for extroverts than for introverts (27). In 2009, Lee concluded a longitudinal investigation and found that adolescents who had strong social ties at earlier ages (i.e., middle childhood) were more likely to use online communications, which in turn predicted more cohesive friendships (27). The same author suggested that the motives of socially competent individuals may entail the maintenance of existing relationships, while socially isolated individuals may be primarily motivated to initiate new relationships online (27). Moreover, Facebook usage was found to interact with measures of self-esteem to predict psychological well-being, suggesting that SNSs might provide greater benefits for users experiencing low self-esteem and low life satisfaction (14). A recent American Pew national survey (28) researched how social network site use by adults is related to overall social networks (offline included). Their findings suggest that there may be little validity to concerns that SNS users have smaller offline social networks, or less closeness, or are exposed to less diverse experiences. It was shown that people with large offline social networks (and with more education) gravitate to specific SNS platforms, such as LinkedIn and Twitter. Finally, and most interestingly, the authors found that frequent use of Facebook is associated with having closer social ties. It could therefore be the case that Facebook use supports intimacy, rather than undermines it (28). Similar results were shown in a longitudinal study which followed adolescents into young adulthood (29). The authors suggest that in SNS youth enact their long-standing patterns of face-to-face interactions, and that better adjusted adolescents were more likely to be using SNSs in early adulthood. This view postulates that the internet is merely a medium in which pre-existing behavioral patterns are expressed.

PUBLIC CONCERN AND PUBLIC POLICY

Since the explosion of social networking, and in particular after 2006, there has been growing concern among parents, teachers' and policy makers with regard to adolescents' safety on these sites. Some adolescents use SNSs in ways which compromise their safety, such as sharing personal information publicly. Some problems associated with safety online stem from adolescents' ability to fully control their profile content and privacy setting, which are typically not subjected to parental control. Adolescents' relative immaturity and their need to be voiced can be problematic when they are expressed online. Social networking use has been vilified with primary focus on the ways privacy and safety are compromised exposing children and adolescent to harassment, cyber-bullying, substance abuse and even hate crimes. Public attention has also been awarded on the new social conventions, which SNS have introduced: the notion of "friendship", privacy and intimacy management, the permanence of what is uploaded and the associated risks such as harassment (30).

In Europe, in the last five years, multiple organizations have launched public campaigns aiming to safeguard online children and adolescents. One such notable effort has been made by the European Commission's *Safer Internet Programme,* which aims at empowering and protecting children and young people online by awareness-raising initiatives and by fighting illegal and harmful online content and conduct. In the USA an important step was taken in 2006 when the House of Representatives passed the Deleting Online Predators Act of 2006, a bill that explicitly restricted the use of SNSs and chat rooms in schools and libraries. These bills offer a promise of protection through containment. Such legal actions localize the problem onto the children themselves, instead of regulating SNS content or implementing age restrictions for access.

THE ADDICTIVE "POTENTIAL" OF SNS

Although online activity and communication can widen and strengthen the social networks of adolescents, excessive SNS-use also incorporates the risk of developing a dependent or addictive behavior towards the specific online activity. According to Young, there are four types of internet addiction: a) computer addiction; b) information overload; c) cybersexual addiction; and d) cyber-relationship addiction (2). "SNS addiction" would accordingly fall under the fourth category since the main motive for using SNSs is the establishment and maintenance of both online and off-line relationships (31).

To date, empirical evidence addressing the addictive potential of SNS is limited, and there is no standardized definition of "SNS addiction". On a theoretical level, if seen from a bio-psychosocial perspective, "SNS addiction" includes the standard addiction symptoms met in other behavioral and substance-related addictions, including: mood modification (i.e., use of SNSs resulting in a positive change in emotional state), salience (i.e., cognitive, behavioral and emotional preoccupation with SNS engagement), tolerance (i.e., continuous increase of SNS use over time), withdrawal symptoms (i.e., experiencing unpleasant emotional or physical symptoms in cases of non-use or restricted use), conflict (i.e., SNSs use resulting in interpersonal or intrapsychic problems), and relapse (i.e., reverting back in excessive SNSs engagement after a brief period of abstinence) (32). Seen from an alternative perspective, "SNS addiction" can be defined as a "syndrome at the centre of which is impaired control over behaviors, and this loss of control is leading to significant harm" (33). Within this definition, both psychological and physical symptoms are presumed but social networking is not equated to a substance. The later perspective is consistent with Young's conceptualization of internet addiction, linking it to pathological gambling- an impulse control disorder (34). Therefore, in the examination of SNS's addictive potential any "impaired control" leading "to cravings and a complete preoccupation with a habit" is to be considered psychological in nature (35), and such symptoms could suggest problematic SNS use.

Spending excessive amounts of time on SNS has been associated with reporting symptoms of internet addictive behaviors. In a study conducted in Greece, a significant association was shown between SNS frequent use in adolescence and all IAT (Internet Addiction Test) (34) domains. Specifically, frequent SNS users scored higher on Salience, Excessive Use, Neglect Work, Anticipation, Lack of Control and Neglect Social Life domains as compared to adolescents who used SNS rarely or never (36).

Moreover, as previously mentioned, the relationship between SNS use and well-being may be mediated by personality traits (i.e., sociability), or by pre-existing competences. Empirical evidence addressing the addictive potential of SNSs-use, though limited, appears to be in line with the proposition of mediated effects. For instance, in 2009 Pelling and White

(37) surveyed 233 undergraduate university students and found that addictive tendencies for SNS-use were significantly predicted by measures of self-identity and belongingness. The authors suggested that participants who identified themselves as SNS users or who sought a sense of belongingness through SNSs engagement, appeared to be at risk for developing SNS addiction.

Empirical findings also suggest that young people's preference for online communication and consequent excessive SNS-use is related to specific personal characteristics such as self-esteem and self-efficacy. For instance, Morahan-Martin and Schumacher found that lonely, anxious or depressed individuals used the internet primarily as a means for seeking emotional support, interacting with pre-existing or new contacts, and as a chance to behave online in less inhibited ways (38). The compensation for weak offline social skills may constitute an underlying reason why some individuals engage in increased SNS use, which in turn makes them more prone to addictive online behavior (39). Moreover, Wilson et al., (40) found that in a university student sample of 201 participants (aged 17 to 24 years old), the personality and self-esteem factor significantly predicted level of SNS-use and addictive SNS tendency. In particular, the results indicated that individuals who were characterized by high extroversion or low conscientiousness were the ones who engaged more frequently in SNS use and displayed higher levels of addictive tendency.

Finally, Kuss and Griffiths (31) conducted a review of the relevant psychological literature in an effort to investigate the addictive potential of online social networking. According to this review, negative influences of SNS usage include decrease in real life social community participation, deterioration in academic performance, as well as the experience of relationship problems. Each of these negative effects may in turn act as an indicator of potential SNS addiction. Moreover, the authors suggested that certain personality traits and particularly extroversion and introversion constitute predictors of higher levels of SNS use, which in turn may be associated with the potential of SNS addiction. What differs is the underlying motivation of SNS use: extroverts may be involved in excessive use in order to enhance their social networks, while introverts in order to compensate for the lack real life social networks (27, 31).

Conclusion

Social media are an integral part of adolescent life. Most adolescents, having grown up online, have fully embraced the daily use of SNS and have been exposed to both opportunities and risks (13). There is substantive evidence that SNS offer fertile ground for identity development by providing a training ground for exercising independence, for developing social skills and for experimenting with one's identity – all of which constitute core adolescent developmental tasks. Adolescents need education and guidance to use SNS with safety and respect for self and others. Proper awareness raising programs are essential and have been found to be effective in modifying adolescent online behaviors. Parental online mediation needs to be embedded in family routines, as well as the setting proper boundaries and developmentally appropriate limitations. Parents need to become as digitalized as it takes to follow their adolescent children online.

As far as the addictive potential of SNS use is concerned, there is only limited empirical evidence supporting it and therefore it is not possible to draw clearcut and robust linkages and conclusions. Different scholars, however (41), have noted that the excessive use of new technologies, and especially SNSs, may be particularly addictive to young people and adolescents. Therefore it is essential for future research to investigate SNS addiction with a focus on this specific and often more vulnerable age group. Finally, as noted by Kuss and Griffiths (31), future studies need also to draw particular attention on the issue of possible co-addiction and co-morbidity in relation to SNS addiction. A significant number of mental disorders coexist with additional clinical problems and specification of such comorbid conditions is essential in order for clinical practice and treatment outcomes to be improved.

ACKNOWLEDGMENT

The authors thank Dr. Spiros Gangas for assisting in the final editing of the manuscript.

REFERENCES

[1] Boyd D, Jenkins H. MySpace and deleting online predators act (DOPA). MIT Tech Talk 2006. Accessed 2012 Dec 30. URL: http://www.danah.org/papers/MySpaceDOPA.html

[2] Young K. Internet addiction: Evaluation and treatment. Student BMJ 1999;7:351-2.

[3] Boyd D, Ellison NB. Social network sites: Definition, history, and scholarship. J Comput-Mediated Commun 2007;13(1):11.

[4] Gangadharbatla H. Individual differences in social networking site adoption. In: Romm-Livermore C, Setzekorn K, eds. Social networking communities and e-dating services. London: Information Science Reference, 2009.

[5] Blog Nielsen. What Americans do online: social media and games dominate activity 2010. Accessed 2012 Dec 30. URL: http://blog.nielsen.com/nielsenwire/online_mobile/what- americans-do-online-social-media-and-games-dominate-activity/

[6] Aquino C, McCarthy C. 2010 Europe digital year in review. comSCORE, 2011. Accessed 2011 August 24, URL:

[7] http://www.comscoredatamine.com/2011/02/2010-europe-digital-year-in-review/

[8] Patchin JW. Changes in adolescent online social networking behaviors from 2006 to 2009. Comput Hum Behav 2010;26:1818-21.

[9] Wandel TL. Student use of social media. In: Romm-Livermore C, Setzekorn K, eds. Social networking communities and e-dating services. London: Information Science Reference, 2009.

[10] Livingstone S, Ólafsson K, Staksrud E. Social networking, age and privacy. EU KIDS Online 2011. Accessed 2012 Dec 30. URL: http://www2.lse.ac.uk/media@lse/research/EUKidsOnline/ShortSNS.pdf

[11] Lenhart A, Purcell K, Smith A, Zickuhr K. Social media & mobile internet use among teens and young adults. Washington DC: Pew Internet American Life Project, 2010.

[12] Lenhart A, Madden M, Macgill AR, Smith A. Teens and social media: The use of social media gains a greater foothold in teen life as they embrace the conversational nature of interactive online media. Washington, DC: Pew Internet American Life Project, 2007.

[13] Muri M. Teen and social networking services: an overview. In: Romm-Livermore C, Setzekorn K. Social networking communities and e-dating services. London: Information Science Reference, 2009.

[14] Livingstone S. Taking risky opportunities in youthful content creation: teenagers' use of social networking sites for intimacy, privacy and self-expression. New Media Society 2008;10:393.

[15] Ellison NB, Steinfield C, Lampe C. The benefits of Facebook "friends": Social capital and college students' use of online social network sites. J Comput-Mediated Commun 2007;12(4).

[16] Tong S, Van Der Heide B, Langwell L, Walther JB. Too much of a good thing? The relationship between number of friends and interpersonal impressions on facebook. J Comput-Mediated Commun 2008;13(3):531-49.

[17] Lenhart A, Madden M. Teen content creators and consumers. Washington, DC: Pew Internet American Life Project, 2005.

[18] Bee H, Boyd D. The developing child. Boston: Allyn Bacon, 2007.

[19] Harter S. The construction of the self: a developmental perspective. New York: Guilford, 1999.

[20] McQuail D. Mass communication theory: An introduction, 2nd ed. London: Sage, 1987.

[21] Kraut R, Patterson M, Lundmark V, Kiesler S, Mukophadhyay T, Scherlis W. Internet paradox: A social technology that reduces social involvement and psychological well-being? Am Psychol 1998;53(9):1017-31.

[22] Green MC, Block TC. Antecedents and civic consequences of choosing real versus social activities. Media Psychol 2008;11(4):566-92.

[23] Mesch G. Family relations and the Internet: Exploring a family boundaries approach. J Fam Commun 2006;6(2):119–38.

[24] Valkenburg PM, Peter J. Online communication and adolescent well-being: testing the stimulation versus the displacement hypothesis. J Comput-Mediated Commun 2007;12(4).

[25] Valkenburg PM, Peter J, Schouten AP. Friend networking sites and the relationship to adolescents' well-being and social self-esteem. Cyberpsychol Behav 2006;9:585-90.

[26] Correa T, Hinsley AW, De Zuniga HG. Who interacts on the web? The intersection of users' personality and social media use. Comput Hum Behav 2010;26:247-53.

[27] Kraut R, Kiesler S, Boneva B, Cummings J, Helgeson V, Crawford A. Internet paradox revisited. J Soc Sci 2002;58(1):49-74.

[28] Lee S. Online Communication and adolescent social ties: Who benefits more from Internet use? J Comput-Mediated Commun 2009;14(3).

[29] Hampton KN, Goulet LS, Rainie L, Rurcell K. How people's trust, personal relationships, and civic and political involvement are connected to their use of social networking sites and other technologies. Washington, DC: Pew Internet American Life Project, 2011.

[30] Mikami AY, Szwedo DE, Allen JP, Evans MA, Hare AL. Adolescent peer relationships and behavior problems predict young adults' communication on social networking websites. Dev Psychol 2010;46(1):46-56.

[31] Livingstone S, Haddon L, Görzig A, Ólafsson K. Risks and safety on the internet: The perspective of European children. Full Findings. London: EU KIDS Online, 2011.

[32] Kuss DJ, Griffiths MD. Online social networking and addiction: A review of the psychological literature. Int J Environ Res Public Health 2011;8:3525-52.

[33] Griffiths MD. A "components" model of addiction within a biopsychosocial framework. J Subst Use 2005;10:191-7.

[34] West R. Theory of addiction. Oxford: Wiley-Blackwell, 2006.

[35] Young KS. Internet addiction: The emergence of a new clinical disorder. Cyber Psych & Behav 1998; 1: 237-244.

[36] Phillips H. Hooked: Why your brain is primed for addiction. New Scientist 2006. Accessed 2012 Dec 30. URL: http://www.newscientist.com/article/mg19125661.200-hooked-why-your-brain-is-primed-for-addiction.html?full=true

[37] Tsitsika A, Tzavela, E, Janikian M, Critselis E, Tzavara H, Kormas, G, Sakou I, Bakoula C. Is social networking (SN) in adolescence associated with internet addictive behaviors (ADB)? Poster presented at the 17th European Annual Meeting of the International Association of Adolescent Health (IAAH) 2012, Antalya, Turkey.

[38] Pelling EL, White KM. The theory of planned behavior applied to young people's use of social networking web sites. Cyber Psychol Behav 2009;12:755-9.

[39] Morahan-Martin J, Schumacher P. Loneliness and social uses of the Internet. Comput Hum Behav 2003;19:659–71.

[40] Davis RA. A cognitive-behavioral model of pathological Internet use. Comput Hum Behav 2001;17:187–95.

[41] Wilson K, Fornasier S, White KM. Psychological predictors of young adults' use of social networking sites. Cyberpsychol Behav 2010;13(2):173-7.

[42] Echeburua E, De Corral P Addiction to new technologies and to online social networking in young people: A new challenge. Adicciones 2010;22:91-5.

In: Child and Adolescent Health Yearbook 2013
Editor: Joav Merrick
ISBN: 978-1-63117-658-6

Chapter 38

PSYCHOLOGICAL RESEARCH AND A SOCIOLOGICAL PERSPECTIVE ON PROBLEMATIC AND ADDICTIVE COMPUTER GAME USE IN ADOLESCENCE

Michael Dreier*[*], Dipl.-Soz., Klaus Wölfling, Dr. Dipl.-Psych. and Kai W. Müller, Dipl.-Psych.
Outpatient Clinic for Behavioral Addictions Mainz,
Department of Psychosomatic Medicine and Psychotherapy,
University Medical Center, Johannes Gutenberg-University Mainz, Mainz, Germany

ABSTRACT

Psychological, sociological and neurobiological factors are introduced and each component describes its relevance to the development of excessive and addicted computer gaming. The psychological argumentation discusses diagnostic criteria, the relation to substance related disorders, and predictors. The sociological approach focuses cultural aspects and describes the negotiating-process of social in- or exclusion using consumption-sociological theories. Above neurobiological aspects got elaborated in regard to the mesolimbic dopaminergic reward system. Strong evidence was gained in EEG-methodology based paradigms. Beyond each sub-discipline it is not only argued within the relevant discipline, furthermore the argumentation is combined to create a multi-disciplinary etiopathogenetic model.

Keywords: Computer game addiction, etiopathogenetic model, psychological factors, sociological factors, neurobiological factors, vulnerability

* Correspondence: Michael Dreier, Dipl.-Soz. Research Associate, Outpatient Clinic for Behavioral Addictions Mainz,, Department of Psychosomatic Medicine and Psychotherapy, University Medical Center of the Johannes Gutenberg-University Mainz (UMC-Mainz), Untere Zahlbacher Straße 8 55131 Mainz, Germany. E-mail: michael.dreier@uni-mainz.de

INTRODUCTION

There is no question at all: Computer games are meant to be fun and therefore they are designed primarily to be attractive. Inducing enjoyment is one key feature of every commercially successful game. Since its beginning the market of video and computer games has developed rapidly. Thinking of "prehistoric" games of the 80ies like Pac Man® nowadays causes associations of rough pixels, coarse movements and squeaky sounds. At best, it makes one feel nostalgic and it might make one feel puzzled (and) contemplating how these ancient games could ever have brought joy and distraction to the gamer. Thinking ahead, this might be one cause for the fact that addictive computer gaming has not been widely discussed in the 1980ies, but nowadays is. Like Internet Addiction, which must be seen as a broader label for a bunch of different internet-related subtypes of behavioral addictions, Computer Game Addiction (CGA), mostly related to games that can be played online, like Massively Multiplayer Online Role-Playing Games (MMORPGs), can cause similarly severe psychosocial and health-related problems in a limited number of vulnerable individuals – having nothing to do with a mere recreational activity.

Although it is evident that the number of publications on Internet Addiction has grown over the past years, specific studies on CGA as a major subtype of Internet Addiction are comparatively rare. Generally, research on the topic of Internet Addiction must be considered carefully, because there are still no studies focusing on a comparison of its different subtypes. Following Young (1998), Internet Addiction has to be understood as a major, rather unspecific category containing a number of different online-activities that can become addictive (1). It might be puzzling that despite many epidemiologic surveys on Internet Addiction, there is still no clear evidence for the question, how frequency and specific prevalences of different subtypes among Internet Addiction are distributed. However, some surveys investigated which online activities contribute significantly to an addictive use of the internet. Although varying in detail, a majority of studies came to the conclusion that playing online games has to be regarded as a major predictor for Internet Addiction (2,3). Apart from epidemiological surveys, results of investigations in clinical samples also suggest the unique role of online-games. Analyses of clients seeking treatment because of Internet Addiction in a specialized Outpatient Clinic for Behavioral Addictions in Germany illustrate that more than half of the clinical sample was using internet applications like chats and social networks in a non-pathological way, whilst solely playing online games excessively (4). A further investigation on the general rehabilitation system of Germany found that 4.2% of the included patients with main diagnoses of alcohol and marijuana addiction met criteria for a comorbid Internet Addiction. Among them, playing online games was identified as the strongest predictor for addictive internet use (5). So, many factors point out that CGA has to be recognized as an outstanding subtype of Internet Addiction. According to that, this chapter aims at focusing on the phenomenology of Computer Game Addiction, its potential origins, epidemiology, and clinical features. In the very beginning, a short summary on relevant features of modern computer games and their relation to addictive gaming will be depicted. At the end of the deliberations, a biopsychosocial model explaining the development of addictive gaming will be introduced.

FUN OF GAMING VS. NEED FOR GAMING

Most of research on addictive gaming concludes that especially using online games is related to CGA. Both, epidemiological as well as clinical studies identified online-games as predictors for addiction (6,4). Interestingly, there are further differences between different types of online-games. While addictive potential in so called casual games seems to be negligible, experiences of excessive and uncontrolled use in respect to browser games and - to a higher extent – MMORPGs seem to be more common. So it is reasonable that there are unique features of MMORPGs turning them to be addiction fostering to some of its users. Yet it has to be stated unambiguously that it is the minority of users developing addictive use.

General psychological research on the experiences of joy while playing video games has identified three major aspects, turning video games as enjoyable, namely exploration, feeling challenged by the competition, and experiencing success (7).

Most of MMORPGs offer the opportunity to the gamer to nearly get lost into seemingly endless virtual landscapes. Owning a so-called Avatar means starting a journey through the generously programmed widths of mostly fantastic surroundings, without having the feeling to reach the world's end at last. In fact, with most of these games having add-ons being traded out frequently, this feeling isn´t wrong at all: The virtual world of the games theoretically is meant to touch infinity. The player can spent hours, even days wandering through those fantastic scenes without making it to the final frontier of the programmed end of the world. Accordingly, the gamer´s perception of the virtual world is described best with attributes like endlessness, freedom and unrestrictedness. The design of this endless space is mostly made of sophisticated graphics and a high degree of diversion. The player passes castles and ruins, roams through deep canyons, icy mountains, passes dry deserts and enchanted forests, sails shoreless oceans to get into unknown towns and villages.

In contrast to former single-player video or console games, MMORPGs are played via the internet. Thus, it is secured that the player won't experience the above depicted virtual worlds on his own, but instead with a large number of other like-minded owners of different Avatars. So on his way through the mystics of the world, the player will encounter other players, exploring the environment on their own, pursuing their own goals and motives. Leagues but also rivalry might arise, leading to competitions and battles the player has to sew in order to strengthen his position. This obligation to struggle with others becomes all the more exciting for the player because he knows that he doesn't compete with an anonymous artificial intelligence, but with real humans from all over the world. Success in these challenging conflicts grants the player more power, better equipment and a heightened prestige. The amended equipment can be used to conquer more difficult or hidden places in the virtual world. Gaming success is directly addressed in specific high score rankings posted in game-related fora, ensuring interested others will take notice from the player´s impressive gaming career.

Apart from fun factors, there are also first research results on potentially addictive elements implemented into games. In the study on adolescent MMORPG-users, five features were identified as predictors for addicted gaming, which are 1) curiosity, 2) reward, 3) role playing, 4) belonging and 5) commitment (8). Curiosity can be seen as related to graphical effects and sound elements attracting the gamer´s attention and elevating him into a feeling of tension (sensoric curiosity). Additionally, the endless and mystical widths of MMORPGs are stimulating cognitive components of the curiosity motive. The gamer constantly is getting the idea that soon something could happen. Possessing a powerful and successful avatar is rendering the game to a source of reinforcement. In addition, MMORPGs seem to make use of schedules of intermittent reinforcement that is known to create behavioral responses particularly resistant to extinction. Being able to explore and to experience success underneath an anonymous shield that the avatar can be regarded as, and this way acting out fantasies and attitudes that are impaired in the real world is a further point of addictive attraction. Finally, being an integral part of a virtual society with clear structures and roles, rights and duties is interacting with the gamer´s desire for social affiliation that might not be fulfilled sufficiently in real world societies or families. In general, it becomes clear that those game features can´t be sufficient to cause addictive gaming on their own. Further responsible aspects must be taken into consideration, like neurobiology, personality and sociological variables that will be discussed later on.

The Phenomenon of Gaming: A Sociological Perspective

Research on computer game addiction is a primarily psychological dominated field. Nevertheless it is helpful to implement paradigms and theoretical background of other society-relevant sciences with a broader perspective. From a sociological point of view there are two comprehending ways of deepening consideration. The first is a macro-sociological approach, which treats computer gaming as a social mass phenomenon based on developments in the gaming industry as well as commercials and society's development. The second is a micro-sociological view illustrating explanatory approaches. The upcoming sociological essay will include a micro-sociological perception, but will also be linked to macro-sociological aspects using meso-sociological understandings. Thus the social phenomenon computer gaming will be presented in a media convergence environment, which includes psychological research as well as sociological aspects of changes within post-modern societies. The framework, which leads to individual situations that are supportive of a development of computer gaming addictive behavior, will be elucidated by the use of the model of man RREEMM, consumption sociological approaches, consumption styles as well as group affiliation.

Introducing the RREEMM Model as a Consumption Sociological Approach

One of the most important sociological fundamentals is the question, which model of man should be referred to. Since the focus is on gaming, the Homo Ludens has been used often in this context. The argumentations of the Homo Ludens followers are comprehensible, but Huizinga argues that the aim of the game is directly located inside the played game itself (9).

A defined game ending time is not given in modern games like Massive Multiplayer Online Role-Playing Games (MMORPGs) or even Facebook games. Other gamers can continue gaming and thereby go for an intention to obtain their advantages, which directly reduce the value of the gamer's avatar or account. Since others are solving quests, gathering experience points or find excellent war gear, this disadvantage has to be whitewashed by extended gaming periods of the gamer.

The modern view on computer gaming allows to implement the RREEMM model (Resourceful, Restricted, Expecting, Evaluating and Maximizing Man) (10) as a versatile model of a consuming social actor. This model combines five essential characteristics of a social actor. This individual is classified as a resourceful, restricted, expecting, evaluating and maximizing man. It contains three systematically related elements. Those are environment (restriction, evaluation and expectation), change or continuity (resourcefulness) and choice (maximization of utility). The resulting framework is highly dynamic (10). The roots of this approach were initiated by the thoughts of Meckling (1976). He provided a model of man called REMM, composed of the parts resourceful, evaluating and a maximizing man (11). To improve the model and bring it onto a higher level of meaning and scientific explanatory power, Lindenberg (1985) added restrictions and expectations (10). Thus the RREEMM social actor approach combines the advantages of the Homo Sociologicus and the advantages of the Homo Economicus and is adding the component resourceful (12) (see table 1).

The trench warfare between the proponents of the Homo Economicus and those of the Homo Sociologicus can be brought to a constructive end by the use of this approach. Simultaneously it enhances the range of sociological validity without losing the eye for details and it is primarily used in consumption sociology.

Table 1. RREEMM merging the models of man (Adapted from Esser H. Soziologie. Allgemeine Grundlagen. Frankfurt am Main: Campus, 1993).

	homo oeconomicus	homo sociologicus	REMM-model	RREEMM-model
Resourceful			✓	✓
Restricted	✓			✓
Evaluating		✓	✓	✓
Expecting		✓		✓
Maximizing	✓		✓	✓

To embark upon a deeper description of this model of man the acronym itself will be chronologically divided into its individual parts. The first is the opportunity of being able to learn in social situations and being equipped with an inventive mind. Lindenberg calls this resourceful (10). The social actor is also restricted by the environment and since he is a part of society he is regimented by the law as well as by common norms and values. Subjective probabilities are attached to future events by the social actor, turning the social actor to an expecting individual.

There is a unique ranking order used to evaluate upcoming events. Finally man is maximizing regarding his utility in decision making (10). Flinn and Alexander (1982) described those maximizing behavioral patterns (13):

> ''1. Imitating those who appear successful 2. Behaving oppositely or differently from those who appear unsuccessful (anti-imitation) 3. Accepting advice and instructions from those with an interest in one's own success. These will include: (a) genetic relatives; (b) investors in reciprocity; (c) others who share the same interests (e.g., any group member, in some circumstances) 4. Viewing skeptically advice and instructions given by an individual with interests that conflict with one's own in regard to the topic being instructed'' (13).

THE RREEMM MODEL AND ITS PERSPECTIVE ON COMPUTER GAMING

This model of man was presented to describe an ordinary human inhabitant of our planet. It has been implied that this model is a consumption sociological one.

To bridge the gap this model is describing a consuming actor. One of the parts that could be consumed are the offers and promises of the internet or computer games. Hereafter the characteristics of the RREEMM model of man will be applied to an ordinary inhabitant of a digitalized virtual world. The presentation will be done in the same chronological order as the characteristics for ordinary humans were presented.

Resourcefulness is given to a gamer, since he learns during interaction, which social conditions are established as social norms. Those rules can defer from ordinary social norms. The reason for this is that the in-game reality is restricted by specific game-focused rules.

Those restrictions affect the gamer, since they give a framework that includes the gamer's abilities. If the avatar is not permitted to jump by the developer, the gamer has no in-game opportunity to do so. Beside this small restriction the gamer is restricted by available time. He is not able to have one minute more than the everyday available 24 hours neither inside nor outside the game. The social actor is expecting, since he has an imagination about upcoming events. Thus the gamer will expect special loot or rewards for killing a final boss in any kind of game, because he learned in other games or in the game he is actually playing that those hard quests or dungeons will be rewarded in an appropriate way. Based on his inventive mind the gamer is able to evaluate new situations on the base of prior experiences.

Finally the gamer tries to maximize his use of restricted gaming time by re-grouping in adequate parties and consuming his joy using this computer game.

COMPUTER GAMERS AND THEIR INTERACTING CONSUMPTION BASED GROUPING

To understand why consumption is focused that strongly in this disquisition, a definition of a consumer is required. A consumer is a person who gains enjoyment by the use of goods and objects. Even thoughts about those goods or objects evoke the stimulus for fantasies or dream worlds, without requiring the process of buying or owning those stimulating goods. Thus it is also possible to enjoy and consume feelings or even locations (14). This accommodates the fact of a socially loaded environment. On the one hand goods or objects are evaluated due to the personal preference order, but on the other hand those mostly as individual perceived preferences are regarded as social norms and values which were communicated and socialized in primary and secondary socialization (15). Although an interaction with such described goods does not appear to be social in an original-sociological way, but it has to be notified that it is absolutely social in the way that has also been described by Latour (14,16). Consumption-focused social acting is the leading social behavioral pattern of our society. Particularly with regards to non-physical goods of consumption, society has experienced an extension of consumable goods. This extension is based on the change of awareness (17,18). Secondary socialization is not brought to somebody through family; it is furthermore oriented by peer group and other significant people (15). Expressive goods as well as social-emotional components are mainly adjusted to ones peer group (24). Empirical consumption preferences based on group belongings in relation to a certain peer group could be identified (19).

DEALING WITH STATUS SYMBOLS

If a good is deemed to be rare, it is requested and it is simultaneously noticed and understood by others, then this good becomes a status symbol (20). These goods are requested due to their shortage as well as a subjective increment in perceived importance. The value of a good gets reliable, if adequate conditions of exchange are set. Social systems differ particularly in regard to the resources that are defined as rare (21). The framework of shortage is set by game designers in the developing process of a computer game. The interaction inside the game is establishing rules, while the game is proceeding. Usually the most occasional items or achievements are special items, which drop from final bosses or achievements, which are granted after the user invested lots of play time. In all likelihood it will take several runs to find the targeted item. In all cases, time and not necessarily gaming skill is demanded of the gamer. If one sacrifices enough time, he will find the targeted joy-bringer. The gamer has to provide some kind of time and social pre-financing in order to reach the targeted good (22). Shortage increases the need for individualization, because the unregulated competition is cut down to specific entities (23). Especially due to this shortage, social distinction and systemic borders cannot be crossed by arbitrary access to consumption goods (23). So decisions are not made in an individual way on a meta-level. Thus a woman that is going to buy a fashionable up-to-date summer hat is anticipating the reaction and the suspected applause, which her peer group members will give to her (18). In computer games decision-making is similar to the focused group. This leads to social recognition and to a membership in a special social group. Recognition is negotiated in a social process and so affirmed or undermined. Of course consumption goods are socially impregnated, so the social assignment of group memberships is based on the information, which has a disposition and is communicated due to significant symbolic content (24). This society relevant additional benefit is increasing in modern societies (25). Because of a world that is growing more anonymous, status symbols are gaining importance, since they give the opportunity to create a communicable identity. Especially those goods are socially impregnated, which signalize dysfunction in a common way. This is based on historic development, stating that individuals that do not have to work physically have a worthwhile social position (24). The relation is particularly evident in clothes, nutrition, accommodation, leisure time, and the use of media (26). Status symbols are loaded with an expressive-communicative function, comparable with the crown of a king. The crown shows the desire to occupy certain social areas. Especially consumption-oriented actors are highly social-linked to their peer group (27). Therefore the original function of goods becomes irrelevant and the use of social objectives is enhanced (28). So nowadays dysfunction changes into a social function. For instance an armour that is characterized by maximum stats is not necessarily wanted. It depends on the effort that has been spent obtaining this specific item and not its perfect stats. That's why a comparison between two avatars leads to privileging the avatar that is wearing the more desirable armour and not the stats-identic common one. The fact that is on the basis of this decision is that the preferred gamer spent days or months getting this armour and thus signalizes his or her knowledge about the game as well as a high in-game degree of self-expectation. Party slots are always limited and social territories are claimed, understood and reproduced in everyday computer gaming interaction. If only on slot is left and there is one inquirer that is perfectly equipped regarding the look and origin and not only regarding his stats, this gamer would be highly likely part of the party, if no social obligations are affecting the decision. Perceiving goods as socially impregnated is the premise giving social actors the opportunity to use them as a communicator (29). The assessment of status is characterized as a social process, which is marked by the occupation and taking of social positions, thus social status is distributed (30).

GAINING AN IDENTITY VIA COMPUTER GAMING

By observing the use of these consumption goods it is feasible to get an imagination of the individual self-concept, causing identity and interaction to intertwine (31). Thus consumption affects the individual in an identity creating way. This culminates in the development of two different identities, such as an individual and a collective identity (14). Heraldic goods (32) support the individual in creating an imaginary, fictive self, armed with the ability to communicate this fictive self to its social environment (27). One result is the social tendency of trying to get individual. This individualization is structural-generating (33). For example media, which enhances individualization, is a way of standardization (33). Paradoxically individualization can also be described as equal heterogeneity (33). Thus the individually and perfectly equipped avatar of a computer gamer is reducing his individualization. Social facts are reduced in their complexity by using significant symbols to make social status comprehensible. The used consumption goods tell others a lot about the values and norms of the consumer. Though, cheap clothes make cheap people (28). Virtual clothes fulfill the same function. In the virtual world of MMORPGs, the social actor can be defined as prosumer (34). In this context visible imbalances are considered as motivating factors. Social feedback motivates the social actor adjusting its individual image to the present situation and to the interaction partner (35). Satisfaction is not reached until the psychologically felt social distance to the situational relevant group is reduced, thus the actor has the ability to use specific behaviors to achieve the aimed group affiliation (18). If a social actor does not reach his personal or other-districted aims, he starts to compensate by using consumption goods. Compensation can get out of hand leading to excessive purchasing, material fixation or extreme experience-orientation. This compensation will not be sufficient to cover the real-world social wounds sufficiently or even heal them (27). But consumption based on a high effort or price is speaking a clear language. It is speaking the language of social distinction and also the language of compensation (25).

In conclusion status symbols are readable in a significant way. Social actors have an exact imagination of consumption goods used by others. In a MMORPG environment it is thus possible to identify special achievements or legendary items, since avatars are promenading like advertising pillars (21). The knowledge about valuable and desirable items or achievements is well spread and is getting reproduced during the process of social interaction until the acting framework is modified by the game providing company or modding community.

Since the need to distinguish and to search for social confirmation is one of the biggest acting motivations of man, social imitation of successful gamers representing promenading advertising pillars provokes interplay of distinction and imitation (27). For the regular gamer it is obvious that if he wants to reach social reputation, he has to decorate his avatar with socially recognized or even socially desirable items or achievements. Since cheap people are represented by cheap clothes or in a gaming environment with bad war gear, which are subjectively correlated with the expected abilities of the relevant gamer (28). So items once perceived as valuable and satisfying become inflationary and worthless, when a new add-on is launched. Thus the gamer feels the informal pressuring quest to reproduce the original social distance to other gamers, since he or she does not feel individual, special and unique anymore (36). Bourdieu (1987) described this social phenomenon as reciprocal refusing refusal (37). The effect is enhanced by the use of gatekeeper goods, whose ownership actively include or exclude social actors from specific social groups and consequently assign reputation inside the gaming clan or guild or even inside the game (36). Naturally social actors need the acknowledgement of their fellow man, but the modern extrinsically guided man is raising this acknowledgment to his control source and to the center of his compliance and reception ability (17). One of the most important keys to group belonging and collective identity is the knowledge of the specific group internals. This knowledge is mostly incoherent, inconsistent, and only partially clear, but in a relationship to an in-group member it has the appearance of being coherent, clear, and consistent. Group belonging is engrained with the different facets of socially passed knowledge and gaming is a specific one (33).

ABOUT THE QUESTIONS OF PREVALENCE AND NOSOLOGICAL CLASSIFICATION

In the meantime several studies on the prevalence of CGA exist across different countries. While quite patchy prevalence rates were reported in early studies, more recent ones estimate its appearance much more realistic and consistent. This is probably due to the fact that there is more and more consensus about diagnostic criteria for CGA, resembling those of substance-related addiction disorders and pathological gambling, as it is also the case for the broader clinical concept of Internet Addiction. Accordingly, core criteria for CGA can be seen in the excessive use (time and frequency of playing), tolerance (increasing amount of time spending playing), craving (recurrent thoughts on the game, strong urge to use the game), withdrawal symptoms (aversive physical and emotional events in case of impairment), loss of control (losing the sense of time while playing), and continued gaming behavior despite facing negative consequences (conflicts with others, social isolation, lack of sleep, deteriorating achievements). Like other forms of internet addictive behaviors, CGA can be conceptualized as a non-substance-related kind of addiction (behavioral addiction). Concerning Internet Addiction, CGA can be understood as one major part under the umbrella of this broader concept, similar to the addicted use of social networking sites or chats. However, most of prevalence studies on CGA suffer from different methodological shortcomings, like relying on convenience samples, being selective because by focusing only on adolescents or solely relying on online-surveys. So there is still a lack of solid knowledge on its prevalence in community-based representative samples.

In Germany, a large-scale epidemiologic survey on 15,168 15-years old adolescents revealed that 1.7% had to be classified as computer game addicted, with boys (3.0%) being much more often affected than girls (0.3%). Compared to non-addicted regular gamers this clinical group showed significant shortcomings concerning school performance and reported more frequent quarrels with friends and family members (38). In an Austrian sample of 1,068 adolescents between 12 and 18 years a prevalence of 2.7% was found (39). The clinical group displayed elevated levels of psychosomatic problems (pain symptoms), experienced higher pressure because of bad grades in school, reported of being less able to concentrate, and had increased scores in school phobia. Moreover, minors with CGA reported playing favourably when feeling depressed, stressed or anxious than regular gamers. In addition, CGA correlated significantly with dysfunctional ways of coping and was part of a coping strategy by itself (media-related coping). Most of the studies that were conducted in Asia reported higher prevalence rates (e.g., 8.7%) (40), but in general, boys seem to be more prone to CGA than girls.

Recently, one of the first longitudinal studies was published. In their analysis Gentile et al. (2011) were using three measure points in an adolescent sample with respect of stability of CGA and co-occurring psychopathological strain. Results showed that depression, anxiety, and social phobia were reduced in case of a remission of an addictive gaming behavior, whereas signs of depression, anxiety, and social phobia increased while an addictive gaming behavior developed. The most striking result of this investigation was the finding that the remission rate among addicted adolescents was restricted to only 14% of them. The authors concluded that addictive gaming must not be reduced to a mere phenomenon of a developmental crisis due to an overload of psychosocial adaptation processes (41). Rather, addictive gaming resembles a stable psychopathological phenomenon, inter-correlating with heightened psychopathological strain.

About the Role of the Brain

Perceiving CGA as one form of addiction makes it reasonable to think of the mesolimbic dopaminergic reward system as one key structure being involved in its development and maintenance. This functional brain structure, including circuits of the ventral tegmental area, nucleus accumbens, and the limbic system has been shown to play a crucial part in all kinds of addcition disorders (42). Here the key assumption is that the reward system is activated whenever unexpected positive events are caused by a certain behavior, following principles of the operant conditioning. Behaviors leading to a reinforcement (e.g., satisfaction, positive emotional arousal), are associated with the release of extracellular dopamine in the nucleus accumbens. The link between the antecedent behavior and the expected outcome is something the individual learns by mechanisms of neuroadaptive strengthening of the synaptic transmission. In consequence, potentially rewarding behaviors have a higher probability of being repeated by the individual. Research has shown that drug ingestion has the same effects as natural reinforcers, with the peculiarity that most of psychoactive substances have the potential to maximize the neurotransmissions described above, potentially leading to overuse, misuse and addiction in the vulnerable individual.

There are some studies focusing on neurobiological dynamics in computer game addicted individuals. One study by Thalemann, Wölfling, and Grüsser (2007) was using an EEG-methodology based on the paradigm of specific cue-reactivity (43). Persons fulfilling criteria for CGA were compared to regular computer gamers and different pictures consisting of neutral, positive, negative, and drug-related ones were presented. In addition, screenshots of different computer games completed the set of stimuli. The results of the study showed that in contrast to regular gamers, addicted subjects displayed a heightened amplitude in the so called Late Positive Complex that is regarded as an indicator of deepened emotional processing of perceived objects. The authors concluded that this enhanced emotional responsivity indicates a higher emotional arousability by critical cues in addicted gamers, leading to a heightened craving for playing computer games and in turn might predict an increased probability for relapse (43). In a further study, relying on the same paradigm, but using functional magnetic resonance imaging, similar differences between addicted and regular gamers were found (44). Subjects suffering from CGA showed specific activation of right dorso-lateral prefrontal and right orbifrontal regions. Moreover, these activation patterns were correlated with reported craving by the subjects. These results are important because of two aspects: First, similar brain activations were found in persons with cocaine-dependence and in pathological gamblers, illustrating neurobiological proximity of CGA with further addictions (45). Secondly, the results allow for a deepened understanding of CGA. The dorso-lateral prefrontal cortex is involved in processes of working memory, linking present perceptions to former experiences (46). The right orbifrontal cortex is involved in evaluating motivational values of stimuli (47). Moreover it has projections to the limbic system, indicating an integration of motivational drive and emotional expectations. This makes it plausible, that being confronted with specific cues (e.g., gaming commercials) is causing an elevated level of arousal in the computer game addicted, leading to re-activation of memory based emotional contents promising reward by using the game, increase the motivation to use the game and evoke craving, a process that is well known from other forms of addiction.

Definately, more research is needed concerning the complexity of addicted computer gaming and involved brain regions. But up to now it has to be stated that research has given first insights in an altered neurobiological functioning in addicted gamers that shows conspicuous parallels with different forms of addiction disorders.

Thoughts about Origins and Maintaining Factors of Addicted Gaming

First of all it has to be noticed that systematic research on CGA is scarce, especially concerning longitudinal studies, which could clarify causal relationships between addicted gaming and predisposing factors. So, most of the ideas on risk factors for CGA are derived from clinical observations or from investigations on general Internet Addiction. However, sound models on the etiopathology of CGA are of substantial interest concerning both the development of specific prevention strategies and psychotherapeutic interventions as well. As in other addictions it is reasonable, that CGA originates from the interlude of three global aspects, according to the trias model by Kielholz and Ladewig (1973), namely features of the person, features of the illicit drug (in this case, of the computer game), and social circumstances (48). However, there is justified assumption that a further distinction has to be drawn between different stages of gaming intensity, like excessive and addictive gaming, and of course being interested in computer games at all. So development of mere gaming habits has to be part of a sound etiopathologic model, too. While addictive gaming fulfills full clinical appearance of a psychopathological disorder, excessive gaming might be regarded as a pre-stage of addictive use, mainly being characterized by a large amount of time spent gaming and an upcoming retreat from activities and social contacts. So it seems appropriate to assume different risk factors, influencing being solely attracted by games, developing an excessive pattern of gaming, and getting addicted eventually. Figure 1 is depicting a selection of possible variables effecting the development of gaming habits. Following an etiopathological model of CGA, developed by Müller and Wölfling (2011), that is called vulnerability-process-model of CGA (VPMC), the depicted model adds several hypotheses to the VPMC by postulating that there are two types of risk factors on the gamer´s personality, that affect excessive and addictive gaming differently (49) (see figure 1). Moreover, according to biopsychosocial assumptions, circuits of different variables (e.g., dysregulations within neurotransmission, cognitive biases, dysfunctions within the family) are believed to act as dynamics maintaining the addicted gaming behavior. Basic assumptions of this model have been profed empirically, like an unique manifestation of the Big-Five. Primarily in CGA increased neuroticism, as well as decreased conscientiousness and extraversion have to be regarded as global risk constellations within personality (50). Also, deficits in coping and heightened proneness to stress were found in epidemiological and clinical investigations (51).

Before pathological use is arising, general characteristics of the game (availability, popularity) play a role in attracting the gamer. And of course, also gaming habits of important in-group members like the peer-group are playing a role in getting engaged in a certain game. However, research has shown that being attracted by computer games is partially predicted by several personality characteristics, like self-transcendence and novelty seeking (52) and it is reasonable that also boredom susceptibility and impulsivity can be regarded as further variables, leading to a pronounced consumption of the game. These personality constellations have different contributions on gaming intensely, like heightening the sense of presence, a phenomenon that makes the gamer feel like being part of virtuality that is crucial for later reinforcing effects like the experience of flow. Also, as stated by recent findings (8), factors introduced in this essay like competition and being able to explore an appealing virtual environment are in-game features getting the gamer bound to the game, potentially leading to high levels of immersions (that is getting lost into the game) and in progress, excessive use.

This transition from mere interested to excessive gaming potentially is fostered by further vulnerabilities of the gamer, like neuroticism, heightened vulnerability to stress, dysfunctional coping strategies and a negative self-concept. Further crucial factors for the development of addictive gaming can be seen in particular motivational states raising the importance to stay in the game. Discovering the game as a substitute for real life experiences and misusing the game as a possibility to compensate real-life shortcomings (like feeling unattractive or weak, missing social acceptance or success) leads to an increase of the meaning of the game, transferring it to a major source of reward, pleasure, and the external regulation of emotions. The pathogene dynamics increase as the gamer spends more and more hours exploring virtual worlds while neglecting real life issues.

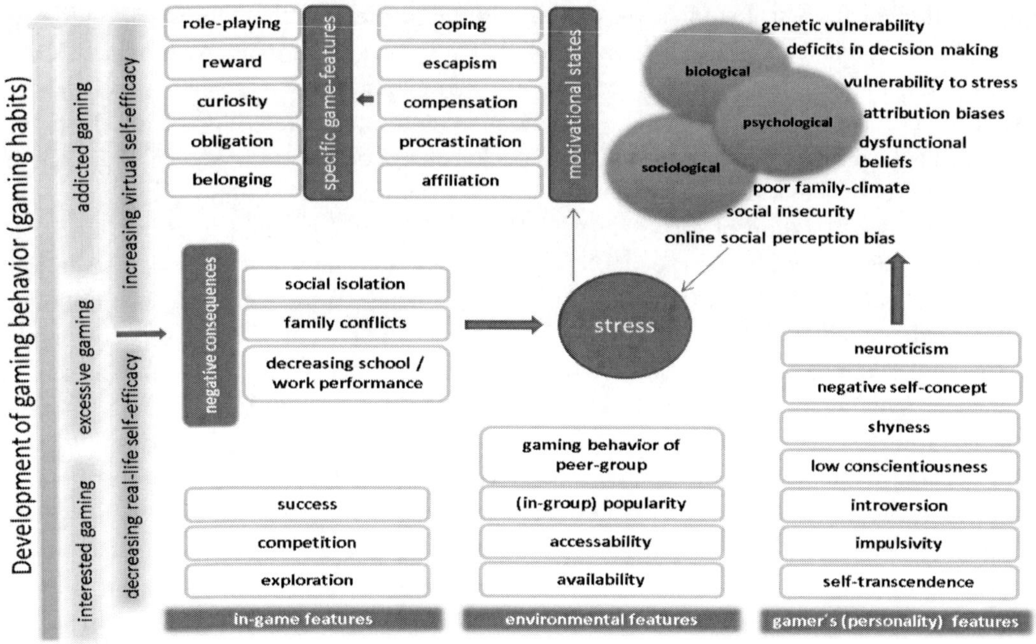

Figure 1. Variables effecting the development of gaming habits.

First occurring repercussions because of the growing intensity of gaming can be expected in terms of family conflicts, social withdrawal, and decreasing school or job performance.

All of these consequences have been proofed empirically (3,4). As the game undergoes a change in meaning for the gamer in the meantime, rendering virtual worlds to seem more comforting and secure, occurring stressors are responded to be even heightened retreat into virtuality. Thus, a vicious circle is implemented.

Neurobiologically, the reward system of the excessive gamer is affected by getting more and more sensible to the game as a potentially rewarding stimulus, while natural reinforcers lose their rewarding potential stepwise.

Accompanied by phenomena like loss of control, craving and symptoms of withdrawal, tolerance is leading to even more excessive gaming behavior. At this stage, addictive use of the game is established and the gamer´s former (intended) wanting to be engaged playing is replaced by having to be engaged in the game.

About Psychological Strain and the Need for Treatment

There are first clinical studies on CGA pointing out psychopathological burden, high rates of co-morbidity, and significant decreases in the level of functioning of the affected. Analyses of psychopathological symptoms of addictive gamers emphasize that there is considerable psychological strain associated with addictive surfing and gaming (53). Main motivations for getting psychotherapeutic treatment can be found in becoming an active part of daily life again, getting re-integrated in social systems, and being able to manage one´s life again (4).

Similar to the treatment of Internet Addiction, there are only few publications on psychotherapeutical approaches in CGA due to this disorder´s novelty. Although there are no randomized clinical control studies yet, possible strategies for psychotherapy can be derived from general experience with addiction disorders. From that point of view, treating CGA or Internet Addiction in general, requires comparable therapeutic efforts.

For the purpose of an exact planning of the intervention, detailed diagnostic efforts have to be realized. Knowing about the client´s background, personality, social situation and associated psychopathological symptoms resp. co-morbidities is essential for an expedient treatment. Also exploration of the client´s gaming history, gaming habits (genres used), and potential risky use of further internet applications is inevitable since it is the basis for defining concrete aims of the intervention (e.g., gaining abstinence from MMORPGs). Following cognitive-behavioral approaches that have been demonstrated empirically of being highly effective in the treatment of addictions (54), systematic analyses of situational factors leading to enhanced craving is crucial for the therapeutical process. Identifying related emotions, physical responses, and cognitions, especially dysfunctional automatic cognitions is the first step in changing the problematic behavior successively. Strategies of cognitive restructuring seem to be appropriate for that reason. Psychoeducative elements, addressing possible origins of the disordered gaming and associated neurobiological mechanisms are supportive strategies, helping the client to better understand the disorder and facilitate processes of destigamtization. Of course, specific circumstances responsible for maintenance of the addictive gaming behavior that mark possible risk factors for relapse should be thematized, too. Trainings of social competence and stress management can contribute to a successful intervention. Therapeutic supervised exposition to critical gaming contents is expected to be a further utterly helpful strategy. The technique of exposition, that has turned out to be highly effective in the treatment of alcohol (55) serves two therapeutic purposes: Firstly, it can help the patient to understand, that being confronted with addictive contents (e.g., the client´s avatar) has effects on the level of arousal experienced by the client and still can cause enhanced craving despite a phase of abstinence from the game. In this context, this strategy is an elaborated kind of psychoeducation. Secondly, by getting prepared to start the game, but impairing the "last click", the strength of automatic stimulus-response dynamics is weakened and, in the long-term, processes of extinction are initiated.

Up to now, there are no studies questioning long-term effects of psychotherapy in CGA. So it remains unclear if similar high rates of relapse have to be expected like in other addictions. However, research on this topic has just begun and one might hope for a further dissemination of studies. Current discussions on including Internet Addiction into the upcoming DSM-V (56) certainly would contribute to the acceleration of that necessary process, for knowing CGA and Internet Addiction means being able to encounter this new kind of psychic disorder.

CONCLUSION

It was stated that an understanding of Computer Game Addiction requires several aspects like neurobiological, personal and sociological ones. Thus this chapter is presenting a fruitful combination of neurobiological aspects, sociological perspectives and psychological understanding of CGA. It was clearly emphasized that the importance of a holistic understanding needs to be taken into consideration if one thinks about the development of computer game addiction.

The sociological view included the consumption sociological RREEMM model, which has been described with a special focus on gaming. The strong influence of the social environment that affects the human being was elucidated as well. Aspects of group belonging and gained joy were set into the context of gaming and elaborated on a strong base of sociological theories. Therefore it was inevitable to define and describe sociological fundamentals to offer the opportunity of enhanced sociological understanding to the reader. Society's effects on the individual development of social actors were set into the context of gaming as a cultural aspect. The environment leads human beings into situations that can improve the likelihood of getting addicted. These were presented in a macro-sociological level as a part of society's development. The focus was set on micro-sociological situations of interacting with peers and the special development of values and norms, which may lead to group affiliation and thus to an increased social empowering self. The important linkage between macro- and micro-sociology was also presented in situations that require individual decisions based on a socially defined and created (virtual) world. It was indicated that the need for social reputation has to be realized during social interaction while the individual perceived preference order has to be negotiated.

From a psychological point of view diagnostic criteria and the relationship to non-substance related disorders were presented. The criteria have been elaborated on detail. Gender allocation of CGA was also described and it was stated that boys seem to be more prone to CGA than girls. Especially individual life situations that are related to depression, anxiety, and social phobia show close associations to the development of CGA. On a psychological level playing online was identified as the most prominent predictor for CGA. This is most precarious since online gaming can happen from a very secure and hidden place, where social phobia or anxiety is not tackled. The need for treatment is very clear, since it was stated that there is a need for re-integration into the social system.

On a neurobiological level, the mesolimbic dopaminergic reward system was indicated as one key structure that is involved in the development of CGA, since the reward system is triggered when certain individually positive perceived stimuli are presented – such as gaming. These results were stressed by EEG-methodology based paradigms.

The variables that effect the development of gaming habits were presented and the impact regarding specific combinations of neurobiological, psychological and sociological aspects was described within a framework of in-game-, environmental and personality features. The strict nexus of neurobiology with its brain developmental information, personality factors that has been discussed in the context of the development of a computer game additive behaviour and the embedding in a sociological framing, leads to an enhanced and stronger understanding of the discussed social phenomenon. Thus this essay culminates in the combined understanding of neurobiological, sociological and psychological perspectives on CGA and is presenting ideas and aspects that have not been part of CGA research so fare.

REFERENCES

[1] Young KS. Internet addiction: The emergence of a new clinical disorder. Cyberpsychol Behav 1998;1:237-44.

[2] Tsitsika A, Critselis E, Kormas G, Filippopoulou A, Tounissidou D, Freskou A, et al. Internet use and misuse: a multivariate regression analysis of the predictive factors of internet use among Greek adolescents. Eur J Pediatr 2009;6:655-65.

[3] Beutel ME, Brähler E, Glaesmer H, Kuss DJ, Wölfling K, Müller KW. Regular and problematic leisure time internet use in the community. Results from a German population-based survey. Cyberpsychol Behav Soc Network 2011;14:291-6.

[4] Beutel ME, Hoch C, Wölfling K, Müller KW. Clinical characteristics of computer game and internet addiction in persons seeking treatment in an outpatient clinic for computer game addiction. Zeitschrift Psychosom Med Psychother 2011;57:77-90. [German]

[5] Müller KW, Koch A, Beutel ME, Dickenhorst U, Medenwaldt J, Wölfling K. Komorbide Internetsucht unter Patienten der stationären Suchtrehabilitation: Eine explorative Erhebung zur klinischen Prävalenz. Psychiatr Praxis, Submitted. [German]

[6] Morrison CM, Gore H. The relationship between excessive internet use and depression: a questionnaire-based study of 1319 young people and adults. Psychopathol 2010;43:121-6.

[7] Klimmt C. Dimensions and determinants of the enjoyment of playing digital games: A three-level model. In: Copier M, Raessens J, eds. Level up: Digital Games Research Conference. Utrecht: Faculty of Arts, Utrecht University, 2003:246-57.

[8] Hsu SH, Wen MH, Wu MC. Exploring user experience as predictors of MMORPG addiction. Comput Educ 2009;53:990-9.

[9] Huizinga J. Homo ludens: a study of the play-element in culture. Boston: Beacon Press, 1995.

[10] Lindenberg S. An assessment of the new political economy: Its potential for the social sciences and for sociology in particular. Sociol Theory 1985;3(1):99-114.

[11] Meckling W. Values and the choice of the model of the individual in the social sciences. Schweizerische Zeitschrift Volkswirtschaft Statistik 1976;4(1):545-59. [German]

[12] Esser H. Soziologie. Allgemeine Grundlagen. Frankfurt am Main: Campus, 1993. [German]

[13] Flinn MV, Alexander R. Culture theory. The developing synthesis from biology. Hum Ecology 1982;10(3):383-400.

[14] Brewer J. Was können wir aus der Geschichte der frühen Neuzeit für die moderne Konsumgeschichte lernen?. In: Diegrist H, Kaelble H, Kocka J, eds. Europäische Konsumgeschichte. Frankfurt am Main: Campus, 1998:51-74. [German]

[15] Berger P, Luckmann T. The social construction of reality. A treatise in the sociology of knowledge. New York: Anchor Books, 2004.

[16] Latour B. A new sociology for a new society. Introduction to the participant network theory. Frankfurt am Main: Suhrkamp, 2007.

[17] Riesman D, Denney R, Glazer N. The lonley crowd. New Haven, CT: Yale University Press, 2001.

[18] Wiswede G. Soziologie des Verbraucherverhaltens. Stuttgart: Enke, 1972. [German]

[19] Wiswede G. Konsumsoziologie – eine vergessene Disziplin. In: Rosenkranz D, Schneider N, eds. Konsum. Soziologische, ökonomische und psychologische Perspektiven. Opladen: Leske Budrich, 2000:23-72. [German]

[20] Stihler A. Die Entstehung des modernen Konsums. Berlin: Duncker Humblot, 1998. [German]

[21] Hahn A. Soziologische Aspekte der Knappheit. In: Heinemann K, ed. Soziologie wirtschaftlichen Handelns. Sonderheft 28. Opladen: Westdeutscher Verlag, 1987:119-132. [German]

[22] Fisher S. A prevalence study of gambling and problem gambling in British adolescents. Addict Res 1999;7(6):509-38.

[23] Luhmann N. Funktion der Religion. Frankfurt am Main: Suhrkamp, 1977. [German]

[24] Bosch A. Konsum und Exklusion. Eine Kultursoziologie der Dinge. Bielefeld: Transcript, 2010. [German]

[25] Haseloff OW. Personale und soziale Funktion des privaten Verbrauchs. In: Rosenberger G, ed. Konsum 2000. Veränderung im Verbraucheralltag. Frankfurt am Main: Campus, 1992:141-56. [German]

[26] Lüdtke H. Expressive Ungleichheit. Zur Soziologie der Lebensstile. Opladen: Leske Budrich, 1989. [German]

[27] Stihler A. Ausgewählte Konzepte der Sozialpsychologie zur Erklärung des modernen Konsumverhaltens. In: Rosenkranz D, Schneider N, eds. Konsum. Soziologische, ökonomische und psychologische Perspektiven. Opladen: Leske Budrich, 2000:169-86. [German]

[28] Veblen T. The Theory of the leisure class. An economic study of institutions. New York: Dover, 1994.

[29] Featherstone M. Consumer Culture and Postmodernism. London: Sage, 1991.

[30] Siegrist J. Soziale Krise und Gesundheit. Eine Theorie der Gesundheitsförderung am Beispiel von Herz-Kreislauf-Risiken im Erwerbsleben. In: Krohne HW, Netter P, Schmidt L, Schwarzer R. eds. Gesundheitspsychologie. Band 5. Göttingen: Hogrefe, 1996. [German]

[31] Abels H. Interaktion, Identität, Präsentation. Kleine Einführung in interpretative Theorien der Soziologie. 3. durchgesehene Auflage. Wiesbaden: Verlag für Sozialwissenschaften, 2004. [German]

[32] Heubach FW. Produkte als Bedeutungsträger: Die heraldische Funktion von Waren. Psychologische Bemerkungen über den kommunikativen und imaginativen Gebrauchswert industrieller Produkte. In: Eisendle R, Miklautz E, eds. Produktkulturen. Dynamik und Bedeutungswandel des Konsums. Frankfurt am Main: Campus, 1992:177-197. [German]

[33] Schulze G. Die Erlebnisgesellschaft. Kultursoziologie der Gegenwart. 2. Auflage. Frankfurt am Main: Campus, 2005. [German]

[34] Kempf M. Die internationale Computer und Videospieleindustrie. Structure, Conduct und Performance vor dem Hintergrund zunehmender Medienkonvergenz. Hamburg: Igel, 2010. [German]

[35] Jäckel M. Soziologie. Eine Orientierung. Wiesbaden: Verlag für Sozialwissenschaften, 2010. [German]

[36] Simmel G. Fashion. Am J Sociol 1957;62:541-58.

[37] Bourdieu P. Distinction. A social critique of the judgement of taste. Harvard: Harvard University Press, 1987.

[38] Rehbein F, Kleinmann M, Mößle T. Prevalence and risk factors of video game dependency in adolescence: Results of a German nationwide survey. Cyberpsychol Behav Social Network 2010;13:269-77.

[39] Batthyány D, Müller KW, Benker F, Wölfling K. Computerspielverhalten – Klinische Merkmale von Abhängigkeit und Missbrauch bei Jugendlichen. Wiener Klin Wochenschrift 2009;121:502-9. [German]

[40] Choo H, Gentile DA, Sim T, Li D, Khoo A, Liau AK. Pathological video-gaming among Singaporean youth. Ann Acad Med Singapore 2010;39:822-9.

[41] Gentile DA, Choo H, Liau A, Sim T, Li D, Fung D, et al. Pathological video game use among youths: A two-year longitudinal study. Pediatrics 2011;127:318-30.

[42] Robbins TW, Everitt BJ. Limbic-striatal memory systems and drug addiction. Neurobiol Learning Memory 2002;78:625-36.

[43] Thalemann R, Wölfling K, Güsser SM. Specific cue-reactivity on computer game related cues in excessive gamers. Behav Neurosci 2007;121(3):614-8.

[44] Ko CH, Liu GC, Hsiao S, Yen JY, Yang MJ, Lin WC, et al. Brain activities associated with gaming urge of online gaming addiction. J Psychiatr Res 2009;43:739-47.

[45] Crockford DN, Goodyear B, Edwards J, Quickfall J, el-Guebaly N. Cue-induced brain activity in pathological gamblers. Biol Psychiatr 2005;58(10):787-95.

[46] Goldman-Rakic P, Leung HC. Functional architecture of the dorsolateral prefrontal cortex in monkeys and humans. In: Stuss D, Knight R, eds. Principles of Frontal Lobe Function. Oxford: Oxford University Press, 2002:85-95.

[47] Rolls ET. The orbitofrontal cortex and reward. Cerebral Cortex 2000;10(3):284-94.

[48] Kielholz P, Ladewig D. Die Abhängigkeit von Drogen. München: Deutscher Taschenbuch Verlag, 1973. [German]

[49] Müller KW, Wölfling K. Computer game and internet addiction: Aspects of phenomenology, pathogenesis, diagnostics and therapeutic intervention. Suchttherapie 2011;12:57-63.

[50] Montag C, Jurkiewicz M, Reuter M. Low self-directedness is a better predictor for problematic internet use than high neuroticism. Comput Hum Behav 2010;26:1531-5.

[51] Wölfling K, Müller KW, Beutel ME. Reliability and validity of the scale for the assessment of pathological computer-gaming (CSV-S). Psychother Psychosom Med Psychol 2011;61:216-24. [German]

[52] Ravaja N, Saari T, Salminen M, Laarni J, Holopainen J, Järvinen A. Emotional response patterns and sense of presence during video games: Potential criterion variables for game design. In: Hyrskykari A, ed. Proceedings of the NordiCHI. New York: ACM Press, 2004:339-347.

[53] Jang KS, Hwang SY, Choi JY. Internet addiction and psychiatric symptoms among Korean Adolescents. J Sch Health 2008;78(3):165-71.

[54] Toumbourou JW, Stockwell T, Neighbors C, Marlatt GA, Sturge J, Rehm J. Interventions to reduce harm associated with adolescent substance use. Lancet 2007;369:1391-1401.

[55] Marlatt GA. Cue exposure and relapse prevention in the treatment of addictive behaviors. Addict Behav 1990;15:395-9.

[56] Holden C. Behavioral addictions debut in proposed DSM-V. Science 2010;19:770-1.

In: Child and Adolescent Health Yearbook 2013
Editor: Joav Merrick
ISBN: 978-1-63117-658-6

Chapter 39

REAL WORLD HIGH-RISK PATTERNS ASSOCIATED WITH INTERNET ADDICTIVE BEHAVIORS

Efi Barlou, MD*
Adolescent Health Unit,
2nd Department of Pediatrics "P & A Kyriakou" Children's Hospital,
National and Kapodistrian University of Athens School of Medicine,
Athens, Greece

ABSTRACT

Internet addiction is a newly emerged behavior problem in adolescents and it is proposed to be included to previously defined behavioral problems. According to problem behavior theory, use of alcohol, smoking, and illicit substance use, have been grouped as problem behaviors, which have the same psychosocial proneness including the variables of social environment, perceived environment, personality, and behavior. This review underlines the importance of addressing internet addiction as problem behaviour of adolescence in order to design prevention and intervention programmes. Adolescents who manifest one high risk, problem behaviour should be evaluated for comorbidity of Internet addiction and vice versa.

Keywords: Internet addiction, problem behaviors, comorbidity

INTRODUCTION

The use of the concept of risk has been primarily biomedical, reflecting a concern for adverse outcomes related to morbidity and mortality. The epidemiological research has concentrated to locate agents or conditions that are associated with an increased probability of outcomes

* Correspondence: Efi Barlou, MD, Child Psychiatrist, Scientific collaborator, Adolescent Health Unit, 2nd Department of Pediatrics "P & A Kyriakou" Children's Hospital, National and Kapodistrian University of Athens School of Medicine, 24 Mesogeion Avenue, Goudi 11527, Athens, Greece, E-mail: info@youth-health.gr

that compromise health, quality of life, or life itself. More recently the concept has expanded into the domain of behavior, underlying the importance of high-risk behavior patterns in the development or deterioration of clinical disorders and illnesses.

Overall the empirical evidence supports the existence of organized patterns of adolescent risk behaviors. These patterns taken together probably reflect an adolescent's way of "being in the world". Their organization raises questions about the origin or source of the covariation and patterning. The answer probably lies part in the social ecology of adolescent life, an ecology that provides socially organized opportunities to learn risk behavior together and normative expectations and part in the fact that different risk behaviors can serve the same functions. Considerable research has shown that adolescent risk behaviors are functional, purposive, instrumental and goal- directed and that these goals are often central to normal adolescent development. Smocking, drinking, illicit drug use, risky driving or early sexual activity can be instrumental in gaining peer acceptance and respect; in establishing autonomy from parents; in repudiating the norms and values of conventional authority; in coping with anxiety, frustration and anticipation of failure or in affirming maturity and marking a transition out of childhood and toward a more adult status (1).

Internet addiction is a newly emerged behavior problem in adolescents and it is proposed to be included to previously defined behavioral problems. According to problem behavior theory1, use of alcohol, smoking, and illicit substance use, have been grouped as problem behaviors, which have the same psychosocial proneness including the variables of social environment, perceived environment, personality, and behavior. These variables serve either as instigations for engaging in problem behavior or controls against involvement on problem behaviour. It is suggested that the balance between instigations and controls determines the degree of proneness for problem behaviour. The overall level of proneness reflects the degree of psychosocial conventionality- unconventionality characterised each adolescent.

The concepts that constitute the perceived-environment system include social controls, models, and support. Problem behavior proneness in the perceived environment system includes low parental disapproval of problem behavior, high peer approval of problem behavior, high peer models for problem behavior, low parental controls and support, low peer controls, low compatibility between parent and peer expectations, and low parent (relative to peer) influence.

The concepts that constitute the personality system include a patterned and interrelated set of relatively enduring, sociocognitive variables—values, expectations, beliefs, attitudes, and orientations toward self and society—that reflect social learning and developmental experience. Problem behavior proneness in the personality system includes lower value on academic achievement, higher value on independence, greater social criticism, higher alienation, lower self-esteem, greater attitudinal tolerance of deviance, and lower religiosity.

The concepts that constitute the behavior system include both problem behaviors and conventional behaviors. Problem behaviors include alcohol use, problem drinking, cigarette smoking, marijuana use, other illicit drug use, general deviant behavior (delinquent behaviors and other norm-violative acts), risky driving, and precocious sexual intercourse. Involvement in any one problem behavior increases the likelihood of involvement in other problem behaviors due to their linkages in the social ecology of youth—with socially organized opportunities to learn and to practice them together—and to the similar psychological meanings and functions the behaviors may have.

Eysenck (2) has suggested that certain personality traits are prominent vulnerability factors for addiction, regardless of the type of addiction. According to this theory there are three major dimensions of personality, P (psychoticism), E (extraversion) and N (neuroticism); these are uncorrelated with each other, and cover different areas of personality. Personalities characterised by high P are aggressive, cold, egocentric, impersonal, impulsive, antisocial, unempathetic, creative and tough- minded. The majority of studies are linking P personality traits with addiction.

According to Gray's Reinforcement Sensitivity Theory, the behavior inhibition system (BIS) responds to punishment and results in behavior withdrawal and arousal, while the behavior activation system (BAS) responds to reward and results in behavior approach and arousal (3). High BAS-sensitive persons are more prone to engage in approach behavior for stimuli with reward. Thus, high-level BAS subjects should be more engaged in addictive behaviors. Besides, lower self esteem, attitudinal tolerance or deviance, lower life satisfaction, poor family function, peer influence and family history of addiction, seem to create an underlying causal mechanism that Internet addiction shares with the others addictive behaviors and disorders.

Numerous studies have underlined the role of dopamine in reward, signaling and addiction (4). Measurement of the levels of released endogenous dopamine in healthy people during a video game (goal-directed motor task) showed increased release and binding of dopamine to its receptors in the striatum (5). Playing a video game is one of many examples of anticipatory or motivated behavior where dopamine is involved in the learning of predicted reward. In particular, the nigro-mesolimbic dopaminergic pathway has been implicated in the addictive properties of many drugs of abuse, including: cocaine, heroin, amphetamine, alcohol and nicotine. These agents are known to increase extracellular dopamine levels in the nucleus accumbens, partly via blockade of the specific dopamine reuptake channels. It has been suggested that the dopamine D3 receptor, which is highly enriched in nucleus accumbens, plays an important role in reinforcement and reward.

In the cases that these risk behaviors turn into addictive disorders, the psychosocial risk that emerges, compromise the entire range of personal development and social adaptation in adolescence. It can delay or block the accomplishment of normal developmental tasks, the adoption of expected social roles, the acquisition of essential skills, the achievement of the sense of adequacy and competence, and the appropriate preparation for transition in the next stage of life trajectory, young adulthood.

INTERNET ADDICTION AND ILLICIT DRUG USE

Even though there is a great amount of research data focusing on substance addiction in adolescence and a growing literature on the Internet addiction, the link between these two addictive behaviors has not yet been established. Nevertheless, there are few recent studies demonstrate a strong correlation between these addictive disorders. These studies are focusing primarily at the common personality characteristics that these two disorders share.

Personality is reported to play an important role in the predisposition, precipitation and perpetuation of substance use disorder. Many studies have highlighted the characteristics of an "addictive personality' which include impulsivity, sensation seeking, psychotism and a tendency towards social deviance. These studies have used several personality questionnaires, to ascertain whether users of addictive drugs share some common characteristics. The oldest model is the Eysenck's PEN model (2). Studies involving hallucinogenic drugs and addictive substances with the use of the Eysenck's Personality Questionnaire (EPQ) have consistently demonstrated a pattern of high scoring on the psychoticism factor of the PEN model, that includes individuals who would be readily addicted to those types of behavior that are reinforcing, and will continue to indulge in these behaviors even after the circumstances giving rise to them have changed. Those individuals would be grouped as "addictive personalities.

A number of studies have suggested that certain personality traits correlate with online addictive behaviors. A study of adult online game users found that aggression and narcissistic personality traits were positively correlated with online game addiction (6). In another study of Taiwanese high school students, Internet dependents scored significantly higher on overall sensation seeking and disinhibition than the Internet nondependents (7). A study of Taiwanese high school students found that adolescents with Internet addiction were more likely to have substance use experience (8). High novelty seeking (NS), high harm avoidance (HA), and low reward dependence (RD) predicted a higher proportion of adolescents with Internet addiction, while high NS, low HA, and low RD predicted a higher proportion of adolescents with substance use experience. A survey of Chinese high school students examining a possible connection of chemical substance abuse and online addiction revealed that the Internet addiction group had significantly higher scores on the EPQ subscales of neuroticism, psychoticism, and lie than the control group (9).

In a recent study among the Greek adolescents, it is found that the PEN personality profile of an Internet user, presents distinct differences as the level of pathological use increases, from moderate to heavy and on to addictive use (10). Likewise, subjects with lifetime or recent experience of illicit substance use had different PEN personality profiles than those with no such experience. Seeking online pornography was the sole Internet activity that tended to be more frequent among adolescents who had a recent experience of illicit substance use. In the same study, had been detected increased levels of Internet abuse both among adolescents who had a recent experience of illicit substance use and among those adolescents who have had a similar experience anytime during their lifetime.

INTERNET ADDICTION AND PROBLEMATIC ALCOHOL USE

Problematic alcohol use is a substance addiction, which leads to negative impact for adolescents. It is also a typical problem behavior as defined by problem-behavior theory (11). High BAS-sensitive persons are more prone to engage in approach behavior for stimuli with reward, such as alcohol use. Besides, lower self esteem, attitudinal tolerance of deviance, lower life satisfaction, poor family function, peer influence, and family history of alcoholism have been reported to be associated with problem alcohol use of adolescents based on problem behavior theory.

One study had assessed whether these proved associated factors of alcohol use also correlate with Internet addiction (12). Possessing the following psychosocial factors: being male, having friends with deviant behavior or alcohol use, having high parental–adolescent or intra-parental conflict, having family regular alcohol use or lower family function, having lower self-esteem or lower life satisfaction, and positive attitude toward alcohol were all associated with problematic alcohol use. This result corresponded to problem behavior theory. In addition, these psychosocial factors, which were defined in problem behaviour theory, were also associated with Internet addiction. These results suggested that Internet addiction shares the same psychosocial proneness with problematic alcohol use.

This study demonstrated that adolescents with problem behavior had lower resources and perceived limited life chances (12). Thus, problematic alcohol use may serve as a coping mechanism for dealing with stress, frustration, inadequacy, and failure—or the anticipation of failure. It also functions to express solidarity with peers to demonstrate identification with the youth culture. Results demonstrate that the psychosocial proneness was also associated with Internet addiction and it was associated with problematic alcohol use. Since Internet is cheap, it could provide adolescents with a value-poor resource to get information and friendship with others.

Several characteristics of Internet use could explain its function on adolescents with problem behaviors. Such characteristics are: a) the anonymity and fluidity of identity of the Internet that relieves adolescents of their original identity with anticipation of limited future, b) the sense of control experienced online that serves as a coping mechanism for the helplessness in real life, c) the chance to get success in the virtual world while playing games online that helps cope with lower self-esteem and poor life satisfaction in the real world, d) the freedom to make a lot of friends by playing online games and participate in chat rooms and social networks that could provide compensation for their real-life poor support resources. Finally, Internet provides an environment free from traditional culture. In it, problem behaviors may be recognized, rationalized, and mutually encouraged by others. The lack of monitoring in the Internet provides them with a subjective sense of autonomy and maturity.

CONCLUSION

Internet addiction when viewed as problem behaviour of adolescence gives us the opportunity to design prevention and intervention programmes. Adolescents who manifest one high risk, problem behaviour should be evaluated for comorbidity of Internet addiction and vice versa. Besides, Internet addiction should be prevented and intervened with and grouped with other problem behaviors based on problem behavior theory.

REFERENCES

[1] Jessor R. Risk behavior in adolescence: A psychosocial framework for understanding and action. J Adolesc Health 1991;12:597–605.

[2] Eysenck HJ. Addiction, personality and motivation. Hum Psychopharmacol 1997;12(2):79–87.

[3] Gray JA. Neural systems of motivation, emotion and affect. In J. Madden (Ed.), Neurobiology of learning, emotion and affect. New York: Raven Press, 1991:273-306.

[4] Spanagel R, Heilig M. Addiction and its brain science. Addiction 2005;100(12):1813–22.

[5] Koepp MJ, Gunn RN, Lawrence AD, Cunningham VJ, Dagher A, Jones T, et al. Evidence for striatal dopamine release during a video game. Nature 1998;393:266–8.

[6] Kim E, Namkoong K, Ku T, Kim S. The relationship between online game addiction and aggression, self-control and narcissistic personality traits. Eur Psychiatry 2008;23:212–8.

[7] Lin S, Tsai C. Sensation seeking and internet dependence of Taiwanese high school adolescents. Comput Hum Behav 2002;18:411–26.

[8] Ko C, Yen J, Chen C, Chen S, Wu K, Yen C. Tridimensional personality of adolescents with internet addiction and substance use experience. Can J Psych 2006;51:887.

[9] Cao F, Su L. Internet addiction among Chinese adolescents: prevalence and psychological features. Child Care Health Dev 2007;33:275–81.

[10] Fisoun V, Floros G, Siomos K, Geroukalis D, Navridis K. Internet addiction as an important predictor in early detection of adolescent drug use experience-implications for research and practice. J Addict Med 2012;6(1):77-84.

[11] Hays RD, Stacy AW, DiMatteo MR. Problem behavior theory and adolescent alcohol use. Addict Behav 1987;12:189–93.

[12] Ko CH, Yen JY, Yen CF, Chen CS, Weng CC, Chen CC. The association between Internet addiction and problematic alcohol use in adolescents: the problem behavior model. Cyberpsychol Behav 2008;11(5): 571-6.

Submitted: December 01, 2012. *Revised:* December 27, 2012. *Accepted:* January 01, 2013

In: Child and Adolescent Health Yearbook 2013
Editor: Joav Merrick

ISBN: 978-1-63117-658-6

Chapter 40

MANAGEMENT OF INTERNET ADDICTIVE BEHAVIORS IN ADOLESCENTS

Gabriela Elena Chele*, PhD, George Macarie, PhD and Cristinel Stefanescu, PhD
University of Medicine and Pharmacy "Gr T Popa",
Iasi and Clinical Hospital of Psychiatry "Socola", Iasi, Romania

ABSTRACT

The pathological addiction is a disease subject to rather simple criteria: losing control on the amounts consumed, spending a lot of time for consuming or recovering from the effects caused by consumption, the obsessive wish to relapse and the impossibility of giving up this behavior, despite the negative consequences. In the international classification of diseases (ICD 10), the expression addiction syndrome is often used, and clinic diagnosis criteria are provided. The typical wrong attitude is present in the future addict much before the disease appears. It is not the substance or the computer (which are, basically, available to everyone) which is decisive for acquiring an addiction. What is decisive is a person's decision to use this substance in order to obtain certain effects. The change of the behavioral pattern requires specialized intervention. The therapeutic management include the cognitive-behavioral therapy combined with the motivational interview, where the purpose is to normalize the deviant behavior.

Keywords: Addiction, internet, management, therapy

INTRODUCTION

The new addictions of modern man raise the question whether these gambling, shopping, sports, work, Internet addictions are indeed as dangerous as those caused by the use various

* Correspondence: Gabriela Elena Chele, PhD, Assistant Professor, University of Medicine and Pharmacy "Gr T Popa", Iasi and Psychiatrist, Clinical Hospital of Psychiatry "Socola", Str.Universitatii nr.16 700115, Iasi, Romania. E-mail: gabrielachele@yahoo.com

substances? With a view to explaining this perspective on a relatively new phenomenon, Michel Lejoyeux, the head of the Department on Addiction of the Bichat Hospital in France, points out that nowadays, society encourages excess and finding pleasure in hyper-consumption. "All of the sudden, he explains, the persons who try too hard to adapt to the dominant social model – finding unlimited pleasure – become addicted. It is the case of Freud's patients, who became hysterical because they suppressed their desires in order to conform to the dominant model, the reserve" (1). Moreover, Marc Valleur, a chief physician at the Marmottan Medical Centre in France noted: "Our society is ambivalent: it favours hyperconsumption and stigmatizes it at the same time. It is precisely this ambivalence which amplifies the addiction phenomenon" (2). It is rather difficult to imagine that someone could ask for a consult because he/she works too much or does too much sport. We are all dependent on many things, and it is not considered a disease. In this context, how do we know if certain behavioral addictions are similar in nature to ones of the drug addicts and therefore potentially just as dangerous? When it is pathological, addiction invades the subject's existence to the detriment of any other affective and social commitments. The pathological addiction is a disease subject to rather simple criteria: losing control on the amounts consumed, spending a lot of time for consuming or recovering from the effects caused by consumption, the obsessive wish to relapse and the impossibility of giving up this behavior, despite the negative consequences. Nevertheless, it is generally considered that only two behavioral additions can be compared to hard drugs: gambling and shopping. These are the sole behavioral addictions causing so much harm that the patient seeks treatment on his/her own initiative.

Alan Leshner stated, "addictions can be defined as mental diseases with behavioral manifestations in the social context" (3). Many specialists point out that an atypical response to stress can contribute to acquiring, maintaining or relapsing into an excessive use of the computer. Emotional, social or physical stress can trigger or strengthen the computer addiction. Recent data show that the corticotrophin (CRF) released into the amygdaline nucleus can be a critical neuroadaptive mechanism responsible for developing addictions and consecutive compulsive behavior. In a person, the risk of relapse involves multiple factors, which probably interact in synergy. In context, stress acts as a motivation for relapse, together with other factors such as behavioral habits resulting from long and excessive computer use or prolonged break syndrome (3,4).

In the United States, excessive gambling is subject to debate, i.e., whether it can be considered or not as an addiction to a product. Since 1980, this disorder appeared in DMS IV TR, comprising classifications of mental diseases. Excessive gambling is entered in the category ''disorders of impulse control", next to pyromania, kleptomania, and not in the category ''disorders caused by a substance" (5,6).

From a social point of view, excessive gambling acts as a drug. Clinically, excessive gambling is close to drug addiction. First, the person seeks pleasure, and then pleasure brings about negative consequences. One has to do it again to feel pleasure and ease the suffering. The effect of the game is closer to stimulants, such as cocaine and amphetamines, rather than to the opium category. Gambling does not cause physical addiction, like the substances from the opium class, but a psychological addiction, similar to that caused by stimulants. From the moment the gambler stops, he/she is tortured by the irresistible desire to start again. Moreover, the pathological gambler is often an alcohol and/or nicotine consumer (7,9).

At a certain point, the addict becomes aware of his/her addictive behavior as a problem, which is getting more and more serious for himself/herself and the people around him/her, however, he/she will not give it up. From this perspective, there is a similarity to other obsessive behaviors, which can reach the point of transgressing human dignity. Some personality traits also modify, but this change is insidious and can go unnoticed for a long time. For instance, the addictive behavior pushes the person to self-delusion and lie, as he/she needs a complicated explanation system in order not to lose self-respect, but also the others' respect. As long as a person complies with the values of the society, freedom, self-determination and self-control, fulfilling social functions and health, there is no pathologic behavior (9).

The term is used only if the person has transgressed these values, if the person's range of interests has narrowed and if the addictive behavior occurs more and more often, but provides less satisfaction. Finally, an alcoholic will notice that drinking didn't bring any satisfaction, and a workaholic will lose interest in the results of his work, so his behavior is no longer influenced by success or by the results of his work. In the end, this self-dynamics of addiction leads to the progressive incapacity to feel pleasure (10,11).

In the international classification of diseases (ICD 10), the expression addiction or dependence syndrome is often used, and clinic diagnosis criteria are provided. If at least three of the following six criteria apply, the addiction syndrome is present (12):

- A strong desire or sense of compulsion to take the substance;
- Difficulties in controlling substance-taking behaviour in terms of its onset, termination, or levels of use;
- A physiological withdrawal state when substance use has ceased or have been reduced, as evidenced by: the characteristic withdrawal syndrome for the substance; or use of the same (or closely related) substance with the intention of relieving or avoiding withdrawal symptoms;
- Evidence of tolerance, such that increased doses of the psychoactive substance are required in order to achieve effects originally produced by lower doses (clear examples of this are found in alcohol- and opiate-dependent individuals who may take daily doses sufficient to incapacitate or kill nontolerant users);
- Progressive neglect of alternative pleasures or interests because of psychoactive substance use, increased amount of time necessary to obtain or take the substance or to recover from its effects;
- Persisting with substance use despite clear evidence of overtly harmful consequences, such as harm to the liver through excessive drinking, depressive mood states consequent to periods of heavy substance use, or drug-related impairment of cognitive functioning; efforts should be made to determine that the user was actually, or could be expected to be, aware of the nature and extent of the harm.

Two criteria refer to signs of the interruption syndrome and of tolerance. Therefore, four of the six criteria refer to the compulsive nature. It remains the essential component of the addiction syndrome (12).

So for internet addiction the following four criteria would be relevant:

1. The persistence of the intense desire to use the computer;
2. The difficulty to control one's behavior;
3. Function disorders, including the neglect of pleasures and interests;
4. Danger to oneself.

The DSM IV TR uses the term "substance dependence" instead of addiction. A series of American professional organizations (American Pain Society, American Academy of Family Physicians, American Society of Addiction Medicine and Federation of State Medical Boards) prefer the term addiction to dependence, in order to make a clear distinction between compulsive use and physical dependence (13).

In 1957, the WHO experts introduced the expressions ''physical dependence" and ''mental dependence". The latter is reflected in the abstinence syndrome. The "physical dependence" manifests as pathological states consisting in the organic need to use alcohol/drugs in order to avoid the effects occurring when use stops. It does not occur for all types of drugs, but it is often caused by alcohol and especially by the consumption of heroine and morphine. The addict suffers a series of unpleasant physical phenomena, called withdrawal symptoms.

"Psychic dependence" or "psychological dependence" manifests through behavioral change and a particular mental state consisting in the imperative mental need to consume alcohol (or drugs) periodically or permanently, in order to feel pleasure or to eliminate mental distress. This dependence is caused by all types of drugs, including alcohol, but also by the computer. Computer addicts use the computer to feel pleasure or to avoid nervousness, anxiety, irritability, insomnia, depression, which are characteristic to the withdrawal state (10,11,13). The typical wrong attitude is present in the future addict much before the disease appears. It is not the substance or the computer (which are, basically, available to everyone), which is decisive for acquiring an addiction. What is decisive is a person's decision to use this substance in order to obtain certain effects.

THERAPEUTIC MANAGEMENT

The therapeutic management is similar to the one for eating disorders, where the purpose is to normalize the deviant behavior. The cognitive-behavioral therapy is combined with the motivational interview. The motivational interview (MI) is a direct communication method, which focuses on the client and aims at increasing the intrinsic motivation for change by exploring and solving the ambivalence. It is an intervention style, a particular means of interacting with the client, oriented towards a well-established objective, for instance, reducing or giving up the risk behavior.

It is carried out in an empathic, positive atmosphere, which facilitates the change of the client's behavior and life style. This makes it easier to overcome resistance, solve the ambivalence, commit to change and persevere.

The MI intends to increase the awareness of the problem and the need to act, in the context of the increase of the self-efficiency feeling (14).

MOTIVATION AND THE DECISION TO CHANGE

Our existence is determined by the decisions we make at different points in life. Some are insignificant, and we seem to make them automatically, while some others influence substantially our existence and are associated with a high level of stress. Similarly, an addict makes a series of decisions, which, at a behavioral level, translate into actions such as starting to use the computer, maintaining this activity or ending it.

In adolescence, the brain systems dealing with motivation are in full development process. Motivation is based on a complex of biological, psychological, family and social factors. These factors determine the probability that a person may choose to enter, maintain and adopt on the long run a certain strategy aiming at a change, in other words, that person's motivation (15). However, in the enormous mass of the persons who use the computer, there is a group displaying a behavior that could become problematic, and within this group, there are the future computer abusers and addicts. In their case, the change of the behavioral pattern requires specialized intervention.

AMBIVALENCE AND RESISTANCE

The persons suffering from computer-use disorders are, most of the times, aware of the dangers and negative effects of computer addiction in the short-run and long run. However, they persist in the abuse, and this is, in fact, a diagnosis criterion of the disorder. Often, users find themselves torn between wishing to change or not to change. This is the case of the patients who go to a specialist only to explain that their problems aren't serious. This hesitation between the desire to change and the desire to maintain the addictive behavior, accompanied by feelings of guilt, shame, sadness and anger, defines the consumer's ambivalence towards the addictive behavior. All along the cycle of change, ambivalence is part of the recovery process and an important issue the therapist must take into account. The therapist:

- should accept and normalize the client's ambivalence
- should help the client to openly express and clarify his/her ambivalence
- should not mistake ambivalence for resistance or denial of problems and should not ignore the role of the computer as a coping mechanism in the client's life.

If the client's ambivalence is not accepted and clarified, there will be tensions in the relationship with the therapist, especially when there is pressure for change. These tensions can take different forms, illustrating the resistance to change. There are four types of resistance:

- the conflict with the therapist
- the interruption of the communication
- the denial of the problem
- the disregard of the therapist.

Therefore, the motivation, the ambivalence towards change and the resistance to change are factors characterizing the change process, which influence the relationship with the therapist and are influenced by this relationship (16, 17).

THE CYCLE OF CHANGE

Prochaska and Di Clemente created a transtheoretical model (founded on 18 distinct theories on change), called the cycle of change. It refers to the change that occurs both in the absence and in the presence of a therapist (18). The stages of the cycle of change:

- Pre-contemplation defines the stage in which the person does not consider changing or does not want to change his/her behavior; it is the "honeymoon" of the addiction, when only the pleasurable effects of the behavior are visible, while the negative consequences are completely ignored. For instance, in this stage, the person realizes only that the long hours spent in front of the computer give him/her a pleasant state of relaxation or help him/her avoid certain situations he/she couldn't face in the past (18,19).
- Contemplation is the stage in which the person becomes aware of the negative, unpleasant consequences of the behavior, too, starts to worry and to consider the possibility of change; he/she is ambivalent and doubtful of the need to change (18,19).
- Decision/Preparation. The change starts to be seen as a necessity, as the consumer experiences more and more painfully the unpleasant effects. He/she plans to make a change in the near future, but is not sure of what he/she has to do next (18,19).
- Action is the stage in which the person takes actual steps for achieving change, but they are still hesitating. For instance, he/she joins a specialized therapy programme, but then quits and goes back to the computer abuse; later, he/she will seek again specialty treatment (18,19).
- Maintenance. The client achieved his/her objective – for example, ceasing the undesirable behavior – and focuses on maintaining the new behavior acquired (18,19).
- Relapse. The client experiences the recurrence of the symptoms and, confronted with their consequences, decides what he/she will do next. The options are: resuming treatment and rejoining the recovery programme or, on the contrary, returning to the previous addictive behavior (18,19).

PSYCHOTHERAPY

The persons who fulfil the DSM IV TR diagnosis criteria for pathological gambling can be included in a psychotherapeutic program (13).

Retrospective studies show that the adults addicted on pathological gambling admit having started gambling early, at ages between 10 and 19. Just as the beginning of sexual relations and using alcohol and drugs, gambling can be a way in which adolescents try to discover their own identity. Most teenagers who gamble do it for fun or as a means of socializing. However, just like adults, more and more adolescents have a gambling problem. The pathological gambling usually starts in adolescence and it mainly affects boys. For most of them, the evolution is insidious. There can be years in a row when he/she plays with his/her friends for a limited amount of time, with acceptable preset losses (social gambling) and then, there is a sudden onset of the addiction, which can be caused by a larger exposure to games or by a stressor. The gambling pattern can be regular or episodic, and the evolution is usually chronic. These behavioral fixations, by their impulsivity and stringency, make the transition towards the clear pathology of the impulse control disorder and allow connecting the psychological pathology to the socio-cultural context. Premorbid personality has several characteristics: the person is unstable, he/she is easily bored and always seeks for a new source of pleasure, he/she is optimistic, uninhibited and unscrupulous, he/she desperately wants money, not to save it, but to spend it. By repetition, the pleasure gradually strengthens, followed by need and fixation. The younger the gambler, the more vulnerable he/she is and the deeper the algorithm of pleasure is incorporated. While family, professional and social relationships deteriorate, he/she engages in financial problems, he/she lies, at first out of shame, and then he/she can become anti-social (lies, steals, extorts) (20).

Recent approaches debate the conceptualization of gambling as a non-pharmacological addiction and as an obsessive-compulsive disorder (21). The former is supported by the co-morbidity of gambling with various pharmacological addictions, as well as by the genetic alterations and the modifications of the central neuro-mediators, which are connected with pathological gambling and other types of addiction, within the system of reward deficiency. Research has showed that monoamine neurotransmission may be disrupted in pathological gamblers (21). There is a reduction in the dopamine level and an increase in the 3,4-dihydroxyphenyl acetic acid and homovanillic acid values. The noradrenalin and the 3-metoxy-4-hydroxyfhenyl glycol levels were also high, but the 5-hydroxytryptamine and the 5-hidroxyindol acetic acid levels do not change. Other preliminary studies incriminate the dysfunction of serotonin (21). Griffiths (2004) stated, "the psycho-social and biological characteristics of the acquisition, development and persistence of the gambling behavior require a biological, psychological and socio-demographic analysis" (22). Pathological gambling in adolescents is associated with increasing juvenile delinquency and crime, with altered relations and with negative effects on academic performance and activity. Teenagers involved in gambling give up school, family and friends for it. Contrary to the general opinion, research shows that money is not the main reason why they take up this behavior. Money, in fact, is just a means to keep playing. They develop a number of dissociative behaviors: they break out into another world, in which, most often, their ego changes too. Teenagers addicted on gambling say that, when they are gambling, all their problems disappear and nothing else matters (22).

Adolescents dependent on gambling have a low self-esteem, a high depression rate and an increased risk of developing addiction or poly-addiction. The research on personality traits shows that they are much more irritable, extrovert, anxious, they generally have difficulties in conforming to social norms and a low self-discipline (23).

For such an adolescent, a good day means entering the virtual gambling room with 20$, gambling all day long and losing all the money. A bad day means losing the 20$ in less than 10 minutes. In children and adolescents with gambling problems, this is a social problem with serious psychological, social and economic implications. There are certain signs for identifying addiction in children and teenagers; however, as compared to the addiction on alcohol and other substances, this problem is not always discovered. Considering the devastating effect on the family when a family member is addicted on gambling, we should be very careful when treating such a child. In recent years, e-gambling, including both Internet gambling and mobile gambling, has become important on this market, opening new territories and opportunities, such as mobile services offered by casinos, electronic lotteries or sport bets. Thus, children have access to gambling outside the parents' control. Age doesn't represent an exclusion criterion anymore (24).

The cognitive therapy was developed to treat adults with depression and anxiety disorders. It is based on the theory according to which behavior is secondary to the way persons think about themselves and their roles in the world. The therapy uses an active, direct approach, limited in time, based on the techniques that attempt to change the person's cognitive process by changing his/her behavior and feelings. It is a short-term therapy, comprising generally 15-20 sessions in 12 weeks. It borrows its structural characteristics from behavioral therapies: organizing therapy sessions based on an agenda, working on problems in collaboration with the patient, introducing certain tasks that need to be carried out, a limited number of sessions, validating results by controlled exercises. Without denying the importance of the conditioning mechanisms, the cognitive theory contributes to the scientific model by taking into consideration conscious and unconscious thinking as a moderator of behaviors. In other words, the cognitive theory strengthens the meaning of the behavioral therapy (25,26,27).

The problem solving techniques provide various alternate solutions for solving problem-situations and increase the probability of selecting the most adequate answer:

- analyzing alternate solutions: the ability to find various possibilities of problem solving in interpersonal situations;
- analyzing the route to take for achieving the goal: becoming aware of the intermediate steps necessary for achieving the desired goal;
- analyzing consequences: the ability to identify the potential results of a certain act or of a certain solution;
- analyzing causes: the ability to connect a fact to another fact in time or to understand why a certain fact triggers actions taken by other persons;
- sensitivity for interpersonal problems: the ability to identity a problem, the intensification of its personal aspects and the prevention of a possible confrontation (26,27).

From a cognitive-behavioral perspective, pathological gambling is described as a behavior triggered by external or internal stimuli (1). The first winnings strengthen the behavior. Once the addiction is set in, the gambling behavior can be triggered by simply entering a casino. The gambler hates being interrupted and he/she avoids at all costs the consequences of ending the game. Irrational beliefs play a major role in triggering and maintaining the pathological state. Most players are prisoners of the fate metrication and control illusion. This belief takes many forms, from the rule of series, according to which each game depends on the others, to the adoption of superstitions, fetishes, rituals. The gamblers draw up complex, but ridiculous statistics, hoping to anticipate the winning numbers on the basis of the previous ones. This magical thinking gives them the certainty that they can master the hazard and the game. Repeated failures and great losses of any kind do not shake their faith in these irrational beliefs.

Freud's psychoanalytical approach of gambling emphasizes the self-destructive nature of the game. In his view, the gambling behavior results from the wish to lose and from a masochist tendency combined with the fight against the guilt feeling. (28).

Another method for treating computer/internet addiction is the model of the 12 steps, based on a model for the anonymous alcoholics, or combining the various interventions of the cognitive behavioral therapy with the interpersonal therapy for moderate computer users; this can address other disorders associated with this addiction, too, such as social phobia, affective disorders, marital dysfunctions, professional failure, sexual abuse in children.

It is important to understand internet compulsive behavior in order to establish also the acquisition of other types of addiction (alcohol, drugs, etc.) or other psychiatric conditions (19).

TREATMENT STRATEGIES FOR COMPUTER ADDICTION

Time management

The aim is to interrupt this routine by introducing new activities. For instance, the patient wakes up in the morning and checks his/her e-mail. We ask him/her to take a shower first and then check his/her e-mail.

The external alert

Is a simple technique, in which the patient sets an alarm clock to ring after a certain period of time, letting him/her know that it is time to shut down the computer.

The activity plan

The patient plans all his/her activities for a certain amount of time.

The abstinence

The therapist and the patient establish which are the most addictive activities and the therapist asks the patient to stop doing them, but allows him/her to use applications less used previously. This does not mean that the patient cannot do other on-line activities that the therapist considers less attractive for his client and which have been less used in the past.

The card

The patient writes on a card five major problems caused by Internet addiction and on another card five major benefits resulting from giving up the Internet use. The purpose is to motivate him/her in the moments when he/she is tempted to transgress the treatment strategy.

The inventory of activities

The patient writes down the activities he/she gave up in order to spend more time online (fishing, golf, meeting his/her friends). Then they should be organized on an importance scale: 1. very important, up to 5. the least important.

Support group

The support group is created and functions according to the same principles as the one for alcoholics and drug addicts. Some patients become Internet addicts because they have no social life. Young discovered that the support group successfully contributed to the treatment of the Internet addiction developed by lonely, disabled and retired persons. This study revealed that people who spend most of their time alone at home use online interactive applications, such as chat rooms, in order to compensate for the lack of social life. The persons who faced stressful situations, such as the loss of a loved person, a divorce, the loss of their job, can end up using the Internet in excess in order to forget about the problems they have in real life. In these situations, the treatment should focus on improving social life.

The therapist must help the patient to find the support group that is the most suited for his/her problems. These groups are made up according to the patients' needs and help them come into contact with persons dealing with the same kind of problems (29,30).

Family therapy

The family therapy focuses on (31,32):

- instructing the family on the manner in which Internet can become addictive
- reducing the critical attitude towards the Internet addiction
- improving relations and communication within the family, which may become a risk factor
- encouraging the family to help the addict participate in other activities and to listen to his/her needs and feelings.

With the help of his/her family, the patient can recognize the symptoms of the addiction and fight them.

In recent years, the studies on Internet addiction became more numerous and the research aimed especially at recognizing the Internet addiction as a disturbance of habits and impulse in the future DSM. Future research should focus on proving the way in which mental disorders, such as depression and obsessive-compulsive disorder, play an important role in developing the Internet addiction. Longitudinal studies should demonstrate how personality traits, family dynamics and communication abilities can influence people in becoming addicted. Moreover, studies should illustrate the efficiency of the various types of therapies.

Counselling in the Treatment of Addictions

Counselling is one of the essential elements of a therapeutic intervention programme in addictions. It starts from the premise that the person suffering from an addiction or at risk of becoming addicted needs external support in order to be able to solve the multiple problems caused by the addictive behavior or pre-existent to it. Counselling is a general therapeutic intervention based on the creation of a therapeutic relationship – the therapeutic alliance that generates the trust environment that allows to give advice or to elaborate strategies for overcoming the negative situation caused by excess consumption.

The results of the counselling programmes depend, among others, on learning new approaches for solving old problems, possibly by implementing more counselling and encouragement techniques, by constantly rewarding the patient for his efforts, by the therapist's positive, supportive emotional involvement in overcoming the helplessness feelings and other similar feelings, expressed in moderate, realistic interpretations of typical deviance or relapse situations, by patience and lack of ambition.

Many things depend on the patient's resources, health, simultaneous mental illnesses, social and family support (29,30,33).

Pharmacological Therapy

The pharmacological therapy is recommended for each manifestation of co-morbidity associated to addiction: depression and anxiety, obsessive compulsive disorder, social phobia, eating disorders, hyperkinetic disorders with attention deficit. Shapira (34) obtained very good results on the patients suffering from depression and anxiety by using inhibitors of the serotonin receptors or other antidepressants.

Electroconvulsive Therapy

While many experts in the United States still try to decide if the Internet addiction is a real disease, China has taken very seriously this disorder. Many clinics and camps for Internet addicts were created in order to treat hundreds of Chinese children and teenagers who spend many hours a day online. They are included in games and socialization programmes with other children in the real worlds instead of staying for hours at the computer, where they live in a virtual world. In extreme cases, they take medication and are even submitted to the electroconvulsive therapy in order to solve their problems. About 70% of the children who go to these camps are cured by the time they leave (35).

The famous Chinese television CCTV broadcasted, within the show "The Economic half-hour", coverage on "Young Internet addicts", which focused on young people suffering from Internet addiction under treatment. The show emphasized that this addiction results from the lack of supervision, and the causes are mainly sociological and psychological, and now many institutions and parents seek a treatment for the children's addiction. Electroconvulsive therapy, medication and violence have been used and they already caused physical and mental harm in many Chinese teenagers. Recently, the incident regarding a teenager with Internet addiction who was beaten to death in a treatment clinic of the Guangxi province got to the public's attention. While people keep debating on the Internet addiction in teenagers, there are more than 300 institutions for Internet addiction treatment. The rehabilitation treatment for Internet addiction has become an industry of billions of yuan in China. At the same time, all kinds of non-standard treatment methods were invented and caused physical and mental prejudice to many of the children undergoing treatment. The electroconvulsive therapy was used in 12 sessions within 4 months. Many people who were treated by this method suffer from severe headaches and are frightened of this therapy. The therapist claims that "these experiences must cause discomfort for the treatment to be effective". As a result of this TV coverage, on the basis of the data presented, this method of treatment has been banned.

During the investigation, the reporter noticed that the centre was using a DX-2A electroshock device for the therapy, and this kind of device had been created for the treatment of manic psychosis. Some experts who studied the device reported that, due to the severity of the treatment this device inflicts, there are serious health risks for patients suffering from cardiac and pulmonary disorders, from hepatic and renal diseases, for elderly persons and children and for people suffering from troubles of the central nervous systems. Therefore, it should be used very carefully, or else it may cause serious cognitive disorders. According to the national certification authority, the device DX-2A is an illegal product (35).

On the other hand, even if the Chinese Ministry of Health banned the use of the controversial electroconvulsive therapy for the Internet addiction due to its unsure safety and to the doubtful treatment efficiency, the newspaper Oriental Morning Post reported that many parents of Internet-addicted adolescents still support this harmful therapy. It is estimated that 13-16 million Chinese young people suffer from Internet addiction. Hundreds of therapy groups for Internet addicts emerged throughout China. Radical methods are widely used, varying from medication to military-type education for discipline and self-control, to electric shock and violent punishments. Most of these methods are not only inhuman, but also unscientific and inefficient. However, due to the parents' ignorance and despair, many of these non-professional organisations made fortunes.

The treatment of the manifestations of co-morbidity associated with pathological gambling reveal frequent cases of alcoholism (52%), major depression (28%), bipolar disorder (24%), and anxiety disorder (28%). Depression can be caused by gambling or can be the triggering factor for gambling.

REFERENCES

[1] Lejoyeux M. A chacun son type d'addiction, LeParisiene. Accessed 2012 Nov 12. URL: http://www.leparisien.fr/societe/a-chacun-son-type-d-addiction-28-10-2009-690637.php

[2] Valleur M. Les nouvelles formes d'addiction: l'amour, le sexe, le jeux video. Paris: Champs Flammarion, 2004. [French]
[3] Leshner A. Addiction is a brain disease, Issues in science and technology. Accessed 2012 Nov 12. URL: http://www.issues.org/17.3/leshner.htm
[4] Bramer MA. Computer game-playing. New York: Ellis Horwood, 1983.
[5] Young K, Pistner M, O'Mara J, Buchanan J. Cyber-disorders: The mental health concern for the new millennium: Cyber Psychol Behav 1999;2(5);475-9.
[6] Ward Gailey C. Mediated messages: Gender, class, and cosmos in home video games. J Popular Culture 1993;27(1):81-97.
[7] Block JM. Issues for DSM-V: Internet addiction. Am J Psychiatry 2008;165:306-7.
[8] Tanner L. Is video-game addiction a mental disorder? Accessed 2012 Nov 12. URL: http://www.msnbc.msn.com/id/19354827/
[9] Derevensky JL, Shek DTL, Merrick J, eds. Youth gambling. The hidden addiction. Berlin: De Gruyter, 2011.
[10] Jackson LA, Alexander von Eye, Biocca F. Children and internet use: Social, psychological and academic consequences for low-income children, 2006. Accessed 2012 Nov 13. URL: http://www.apa.org/science/psa/sb-jackson.html
[11] Lieber CS. To drink (moderaly) or not to drink. N Engl J Med 1984;310(13):864-8.
[12] World Health Organization. Classification of mental and behaviourral disorders: Clinical descriptions and diagnostic guidelines. Geneva: World Health Organization, 1992.
[13] American Psychiatric Association. Diagnostic and statistical manual of mental disorders, 4th ed), text rev. Washington, DC: APA, 2000.
[14] Miller WR. Enhancing motivation for change in substance abuse treatment. Rockville, MD: Substance Abuse Mental Health Services Administration, Treatment Improvment Protocol (TIP) series, 1999.
[15] Shaffer D, Gould MS, Rutter M, Sturge C. Reability and validity of a psychosocial axis in patients with psychiatric disorders. J Am Acad Child Adolesc Psychiatr 1991;30(1):109-15.
[16] Jones SG. Doing Internet research: Critical issues and methods for examining the Net. Thousand Oaks, CA: Sage, 1999.
[17] McKim WA. Drugs and behavior, 6th ed. Upper Saddle, NJ: Prentice Hall, 1997.
[18] Prochaska JO, DiClemente, CC, Norcross JC. In search of how people change: Applications to addictive behaviors. Am Psychol 1992;47(9):1102-14.
[19] Prelipceanu D, Ezechil D. Management of case. In: Textbook of treatment in abuse of substance, edition a II-a. Bucureşti: Editura Infomedica, 2002.
[20] Anderson Craig A. şi Brad J. Bushman. Effects of violent video games on aggressive behavior, aggressive cognition, aggressive affect, psychological arousal and prosocial behavior: A meta-analytic review of the scientific literature. Psychology 2001;12:353-9.
[21] Chambers RA, Taylor JR, Potenza MN. Developmental neurocircuity of motivation in adolescence: A critical period of addiction vulnerability. Am J Psychiatry 2003;160:1041-52.
[22] Griffiths M. Technological addictions. Clin Psychol J 2004;71:14-9.
[23] Shead NW, Derevensky JL, Gupta R. Risk and protective factors associated with youth problem gambling. Int J Adolesc Med Health 2012;22(1):39-58.
[24] Volberg RA, Gupta R, Griffiths MA, Olason DT, Delfabbro P. An International perspective on youth gambling prevalence studies. Int J Adolesc Med Health 2012;22(1):3-38.
[25] Almqvist F, Kumpulainen K, Ikäheimo K, Linna SL, Henttonen I, Huikko E, et al. Behavioural and emotional symptoms in 8-9 year-old children. Eur Child Adolesc Psychiatr 1998;4(4):7.
[26] Beck JS. Therapy basics and beyond. New York: Guilford, 1995.
[27] Beck AT. Cognitive therapy and the emotional disorders. New York: International Universities Press, 1976.
[28] Freud S. Introduction in psychoanalysis. Hertfordshire: Wordsworth Editions Classic World Literature edition, 2012.
[29] Young KS. Internet addiction: The emergence of a new clinical disorder. Internet Addict 1996;2:12-5.
[30] Young KS. Caught in the net: How to recognize the signs of internet addiction and a winning strategy for recovery. New York: John Wiley, 1998.

[31] Van Heusen A, van den Eerenbeemt E. Therapie familiale et generation, France: Pressed Universitaire de France, 1994. [French]

[32] Shaffer HJ, Hall MN, Vander Bilt J. Computer addiction: a critical consideration, Am J Orthopsychiatry 2000;70(2):162-8.

[33] Wieland DM. Computer addiction: Implications for nursing psychotherapy practice. Perspect Psychiatr Care 2005;41(4):153-61.

[34] Shapira NA. Problematic internet use. Toronto: 151st annual meeting of the American Psychiatric Association, 1998.

[35] Cohen D, Flament M, Taieb O, Thompson C, Basquin M. Electroconvulsive therapy in adolescence. Eur Child Adolesc Psychiatry 2000;9(1):1.

Submitted: December 05, 2012. *Revised:* December 28, 2012. *Accepted:* January 05, 2013

In: Child and Adolescent Health Yearbook 2013
Editor: Joav Merrick

ISBN: 978-1-63117-658-6

Chapter 41

EUROPEAN PUBLIC HEALTH POLICIES AND INTERVENTIONS FOR DETECTING AND DETERRING INTERNET ADDICTIVE BEHAVIORS IN ADOLESCENTS

Artemis Tsitsika**, MD, PhD, Mari Janikian, PhD and Vasiliki Dimitrakopoulou
Adolescent Health Unit,
2nd Department of Pediatrics "P & A Kyriakou" Children's Hospital,
National and Kapodistrian University of Athens School of Medicine,
Athens, Greece

ABSTRACT

As the phenomenon of Internet addictive behavior constitutes a growing European public health issue, it is important to consider a number of policies for addressing it. This review briefly outlines basic recommendations for parental, educational and state levels. Implications for future research are further addressed.

Keywords: Internet addictive behaviors, policy implications, future research

INTRODUCTION

Internet addictive behavior is considered to be an ever-growing European public health issue. Research studies have indicated that Internet addictive behavior rates among minors seem to differ from country to country depending on the age group, cultural differences, and

---

* Correspondence: Artemis Tsitsika, MD, PhD, Assistant Professor in Pediatrics and Adolescent Medicine, Head of the Adolescent Health Unit, 2nd Department of Pediatrics "P & A Kyriakou" Children's Hospital, National and Kapodistrian University of Athens School of Medicine, 24 Mesogeion Avenue, Goudi 11527, Athens, Greece. E-mail: info@youth-health.gr

technological tools used. Specifically, different countries have indicated different internet addictive behaviors prevalence rates.

In its most recent study in 25 European countries, the EU Kids Online project (1) estimated to what extent European adolescents aged 11 to 16 might be at risk of suffering from internet addictive behavior. The study found that 12% said that they had very often or fairly often 'tried unsuccessfully to spend less time on the Internet'. Some 13% said that they had 'spent less time' than they should with either family or friends or doing schoolwork because of the time spent on the Internet. About 16% said that they had very or fairly often 'caught themselves surfing when they were not really interested'. Some 12% said that they had very or fairly often 'felt bothered when they could not be on the Internet', and finally some 5% said that they had gone without eating or sleeping because of the internet. Looking at those who said that one or more of these things had happened to them very or fairly often puts a total of 30% of European adolescents aged 11-16 that has to some extent experienced problems with excessive internet use, ranging from 14% in Italy to 50% in Estonia. It is important however to differentiate between excessive use and internet addictive behavior.

IMPLICATIONS FOR PUBLIC HEALTH POLICIES

During adolescence young people attain increased independence over their online behaviors. Public health policies and interventions for detecting and deterring internet addictive behaviors need to be sensitive to the interaction between the specific adolescent developmental stage and contextual influences. The following recommendations need to be addressed:

Recommendations for parents

Raising awareness among parents also represents a challenge, as on the one hand they are primary caregivers who are able to prevent and react in case of abuse, but on the other hand they are often not aware of the specifics of online behaviors. Specific recommendation includes:

- Participation in the education of the child to ensure safety on the internet from an early age
- Enhancement of adolescents' resiliency and skills from an early age so that they do not resort to the Internet as a means of combating loneliness and boredom
- Nourishing the personality of the adolescents and their socialization
- Highlighting the dangers of non-controlled Internet use of adolescents from an early age
- Strengthening the role of play in the development of the child and parental involvement in a creative manner with adolescents
- Reasonable use of the Internet by parents to provide appropriate role-modeling.

Recommendations for education

School curricula need to reflect current online practices and the age of adolescents' initiation online. A trend of continuously initiation at younger ages, should guide the shift of e-safety, i.e., to early primary school. Moreover, adolescents' online preferences need to be considered in the context of local educational systems and the way they serve this new generation of technologically savvy youth. There is a need to integrate new technologies in order to enhance learning and motivate young people through their preferred applications. Educational practices and tools must be updated for this new generation of learners (2).

The internet is a means through which educators can approach adolescents, and it can be a powerful educational tool. SNS platforms can be used as classroom resources and educational tools to support learning. Good practice guidelines of social media use can be integrated into school curricula, thereby empowering adolescents to maximize communication benefits while minimizing online contact risks. Specific recommendations include:

- Inclusion of modules in the educational process on the safe and judicious use of the internet
- Inclusion of activities through the Internet to enhance effective uses of internet
- Enhancing self-esteem of adolescents and group work to serve as deterrent factors of isolation of adolescents online
- Enhancing the talents of adolescents and strengthening social sensitivity
- Training teachers in preventing the phenomenon of Internet addictive behavior and in ways to reintegrate adolescents in the school system.

Recommendations for the state

The EU Safer Internet Programme is committed to initiatives such as the Safer Social Networking Principles for the EU (3) with a common goal to which include seven principles signed originally by 14 SNS providers in 2009, subsequent monitoring by the EU (4,5). In regards to addictive behaviour industry, future versions of such initiatives could include campains of internet addictive behavior risks. Local governments and public bodies need to be informed and guided by current challenges in adolescents use of online technologies and in the associated implications on a state level. Specific recommendations include:

- Assisting in the education curriculum development and lifelong education of teachers
- Creating school competitions, exhibitions and other events to celebrate the safe and moderate internet usage
- Strengthening the role of parental associations and fostering alliances between schools and parents
- Training health care professionals on Internet addictive behavior issues
- Activating prevention centers on information for adolescents suffering from internet addictive behavior

- Planning to protect adolescents from the dangers of the internet (harassment, gambling, child pornography, fraud, etc.)
- Proposing legislative measures in the context of countries aiming to protect adolescents (Internet cafés, dangerous toys, cyber crime, etc.)
- Strengthening the team spirit of stakeholders to meet the needs of adolescents
- Organizing campaigns for safe internet use emphasizing events that promote team spirit and online creativity
- Creating initiatives that support social services to families affected by internet addictive behavior.

FUTURE DIRECTIONS

Further research on a European level is required to give specific answers about the size of the problem, the factors that lead adolescents to develop addictive behavior whether the conduct is harmful to adolescents, the existence of co-morbidities, stage of development of addiction to the Internet, strengthening the factors that can contribute to discouraging adolescents' expressions of addictive behaviors, their awareness on this issue and provide finally, the basis for further action and study.

Research findings will constitute a useful tool for planning major initiatives in social institutions to moderate usage by adolescents yet will help to inform parents and raising educational institutions and health care professionals in preventing the symptoms of internet addiction. The accumulated knowledge on both the status of internet addictive behavior among young people and possible prevention mechanisms in European member states, will serve as an essential tool for stakeholders and policy makers. Finally, the American Psychiatric Association in reviewing the 5th edition of the Diagnostic and Statistical Manual of Mental Disorders (DSM-V) mandated the necessity of additional research in the field on internet addictive behavior. Future findings will perform a crucial role in providing additional data to the global scientific community regarding this novel behavioral pattern.

Concluding, in order to gain a clear understanding on the phenomenon of internet addictive behavior and to help on European scale, it is highly important to tackle the issue beyond national borders, both as a holistic approach for all participating countries, and through cross-national comparisons, which will lead to proper and targeted awareness raising and policy making in the future.

REFERENCES

[1] Livingstone S, Haddon L, Görzig A, Ólafsson K. EU Kids online final report. London: EU Kids Online, LSE, 2011.

[2] Oblinger DG, Oblinger JL. Educating the net generation. Educause 2005. Accessed 2013 Dec 01. URL: www.educause.ed/educatingthe netgen/

[3] European Commission. Safer social networking principles for the EU. Luxembourg: European Commission, Safer internet programme, Luxembourg, 2009. Accessed 2013 Dec 01. URL: http://ec.europa.eu/information_society/activities/social_networking/ docs/sn_principles.pdf

[4] Staksrud E, Lobe B. Evaluation of the implementation of the safer social networking principles for the EU Part 1: General report. Luxembourg: European Commission Safer Internet Programme, 2010.
[5] Donoso V. Results of the assessment of the implementation of the safer social networking principles for the EU on 14 websites: Individual reports of testing of 14 social networking sites. Luxembourg: European Commission, 2011.

Submitted: December 10, 2012. *Revised:* January 02, 2012. *Accepted:* January 12, 2013

In: Child and Adolescent Health Yearbook 2013
Editor: Joav Merrick
ISBN: 978-1-63117-658-6

Chapter 42

INTERNET ADDICTION, MEDIA USE AND DIFFICULTIES ASSOCIATED WITH SLEEPING IN ADOLESCENTS

Stephanie J Stockburger, MD, FAAP and Hatim A Omar, MD, FAAP*

Division of Adolescent Medicine, Department of Pediatrics, University of Kentucky, Lexington, Kentucky, United States of America

ABSTRACT

The objective of this review article is to summarize the current literature regarding internet addiction; media use, and sleep disruption in adolescents. Design: Systematic review of current literature. Methods: The data was obtained through literature review of articles published in the last 10 years. Conclusion: Internet addiction and media use have the power to have great influence over the sleep of children and adolescents and it is important to take advantage of the positive effects of media while minimizing the potentially negative, but severe, consequence of sleep disruption.

Keywords: Internet addiction, media, mobile phone, cellular phone, computer, television, sleep, insomnia

INTRODUCTION

Media use including the internet, cellular phones, and smart phonesis becoming increasingly common. According the American Academy of Pediatrics, today's children are spending an average of seven hours a day on entertainment media (1). Worldwide, as of June 30, 2012 there were 2,405,518,376 internet users (2). Asia is the largest internet user in the world

* Correspondence: Professor Hatim A Omar, MD, Division of Adolescent Medicine, UK Healthcare, Department of Pediatrics, KY Clinic Room J422, Lexington, KY 40536-0284, United States. E-mail: haomar2@uky.edu

(44.8% of total world use), with Europe coming in second (21.5%) and North America coming in third (11.4%) (2). Social media is also increasingly popular. As of September 30, 2012 there was estimated to be 937,407,180 Facebook users (3). Other types of electronic device use, including cell phone use, are also considerably high. A Pew Research Report from 2012 found that 88% of US adults own a cell phone of some kind as of April 2012 and of these cell phone owners, more than half (55%) use their cell phone to go online (4). In Japan, the number as of cell phone users is similarly high. In 2009, 74.8% of the general population and 84.0% of the adolescent population (ages 13-19) own a cell phone (5).

Internet addiction is a growing and newly recognized concern along with the ever-increasing consumption of electronic media. Internet addiction is based on the DSM-IV definition for substance dependence and pathological gambling (6). It is "problematic internet use, wherein an individual's inability to control his or her use of the internet causes marked distress and/or functional impairment" (6). Internet dependents have been found to lose sleep due to late-night logons, feel life would be boring without the internet, and delay other work to spend time online (7). People with internet addiction tend to spend many hours online avoiding interpersonal relationships with real and known people (8). Internet addicts may have comorbid psychiatric disorders such as higher levels of depression and suicidal ideation as well dysthymia, ADHD, OCD, social phobia, and schizophrenia (9,10).

There is a growing body of evidence supporting the relationship of internet addiction, media use, and sleep disturbance. With the number of internet, electronic media, and cell phone users growing daily the scientific community is gaining awareness of the potential problems media use may cause in relation to sleep. Several studies have shown that the use of electronic media is associated with sleep disorders (5). It is known that media use affects children's dreams, sleep-wake transitions, and can cause overall sleep disturbances (11,12). This has the potential to greatly affect children and adolescents as they are also commonly users of electronic media but are also growing and developing and tend to have increased sleep requirements.

Children's bedrooms are now connected to "global networks" through the use of cell phones and internet (13). Sleep is vitally important to the growth, behavior, emotional development, and cognitive functioning of children and adolescents (14). Children may develop behavior problems due to sleep deficiencies which may interfere with learning (15). Changes in sleep quality or duration may also have a significant impact on hormone release, cardiovascular activity and glucose regulation and may have an overall impact on morbidity (16). Therefore, due to the ever-expanding use of electronic media, and the vital importance of sleep, it is important to examine the relationship between the two for the health of our children, adolescents, and society.

Methods

Literature search was conducted using PudMed and included terms such as "internet", "internet addiction", "media", "sleep", "sleep difficulty", "sleep disturbance", and "insomnia." Of the articles found, the references were reviewed which revealed further relevant literature.

Through the synopsis of articles below, this review investigates the role of media use (including internet addiction, internet use, mobile phones, and computers) on sleep, particularly as a cause of sleep disturbances. It specifically focuses on media use and the subsequent sleep disturbance in children and adolescents.

DISCUSSION

Internet addicts face difficulties with sleep disturbance as well as excessive daytime sleepiness according to multiple studies. Internet addicts often stay up late into the night using the internet. In a questionnaire study of 4,318 incoming university students at a university in Taiwan internet addiction was found to be a significant predictor of poor sleep ($p=0.002$) (16). Another questionnaire study of 2,336 high school students in South Korea found that the prevalence of insomnia, witnessed snoring, apnea, teeth grinding, and nightmares was highest in internet addicts. In addition, internet-addicted students had 5.2-fold more excessive daytime sleepiness than non-addicted students (17). A study of 719 Chinese adolescents in Hong Kong who participated in a school-based cross-sectional study revealed that 17.2% qualified as having internet addiction and 51.7% of those students were also identified as insomniacs. After internet use time and gender were adjusted for, internet addiction ($p<0.001$) and insomnia ($p<0.001$) demonstrated a significant association with depression (18).

It appears that circadian rhythm sleep disorder, delayed sleep phase type is reinforced by the time spent on the internet during the night. These individuals have a recurrent pattern of sleep disruption which leads to excessive sleepiness and insomnia. This is thought to be due to a mismatch between the sleep-wake schedule which is required by the environment and the ongoing sleep-wake pattern (19). This type of sleep disturbance may cause significant distress and impairment in social and occupational functioning (19). A study of 448 adult online gamers who were mainly young university graduates showed high rates of internet addiction (44.2% for Goldbert Internet Addiction Disorder Scale and 32.66% for the quantitative Orman Internet Stress Scale). The gamers also self-reported significantly higher rates (3 times more) of daytime sleepiness, sleep deprivation due to play, irritability, low mood and emotional changes since online gaming onset (20). Thus, in accordance with the circadian rhythm sleep disorder, the disturbance is causing significant distress and impairment in functioning.

Computer games and television, in addition to online gaming, may cause sleep impairment. In a study of seven healthy males (average age 24.7 +/- 5.6 years) played computer games (specifically shooting games) and were then evaluated in a sleep laboratory were found to have significantly shorter REM sleep after playing the games than after the control conditions. They were also found to have significantly longer sleep latency and higher heart rate after playing the games (21).

The content of electronic media has also been shown to appear in the dreams of children. A study which consisted of 2,546 children in a random sample of 15 secondary schools in Flanders, Belgium who completed a questionnaire about their television viewing habits, computer game playing, and pleasant dreams and nightmares found that media content frequently showed up in dreams. For 33% of the children, TV content showed up frequently in nightmares. Computer games were associated with nightmares in 5% of girls and 10% of boys. Influences were not always negative however. In 60% of 13 year olds and 50% of 16 year olds reported having pleasant dreams related to television (12).

Television exposure has been shown to be associated with sleep disturbances in 5 to 6 year old children. A randomized population-based survey was administered to 321 parents of children ages 5-6 years. The survey evaluated TV viewing, sleep disturbances and psychiatric symptoms. It was found that active television viewing and passive television exposure were related to sleeping difficulties. Specifically, passive television exposure ($p<0.01$) and viewing adult-targeted television programs ($p<0.01$) were strongly related to sleep disturbance (11).

Media use after lights out, especially cell phone use is increasingly common and may be related to being involved in bullying and being a bully victim. A study of 1656 school children in Flanders, Belgium (average age 13.7 years in youngest group and 16.9 years in oldest group) completed questions on the use of the mobile phone for receiving and transmitting text messages or calls via a questionnaire. Only 38% of the subjects never used their mobile phone after lights out. Those who used it more than once a week after lights out were 5.1 times more likely to be very tired (95% CI 2.5-10.4). The study concluded that mobile phone use after lights out is very prevalent among adolescents and is related to increased levels of tiredness (13). Another study which examined data from the cross-sectional survey of psychopathologies conducted for 19,436 Japanese students found that bullying status was significantly associated with irregular bedtime (OR = 1.23 and 1.41 for pure bullies and bully-victims, respectively). This study concluded that school-based interventions for sleep pattern and cellular phone usage may reduce bullying (22).

The presence of a television, computer, or cell phone in a child's or adolescent's bedroom also impacts sleep behaviors. In a cross-sectional survey of 40 students in 8th and 9th grade (mean age 14 +/- 0.8) in Israel who completed the modified School Sleep Habits Survey and the modified Electronic Media and Fatigue Questionnaire, the presence of electronic media inside the bedroom was associated with later bedtime, increased exposure ($p=0.004$), increased sleep latency (p,0.001), and decreased sleep duration.

This article concluded that electronic media exposure during unstructured and unmonitored leisure time contributes to altered sleep patterns (23). Another study of 19,299 elementary-school children in China who completed a parent-administered questionnaire found that media presence in the bedroom and media use were positively correlated with later bedtimes and awakening times. They also found a shorter duration of sleep during weekdays and weekends (14). This study shared the conclusion of the previous study that media in a child's bedroom has a negative effect on children's sleep patterns (14).

The effect of media exposure may not only temporarily impair sleep patterns but the effects may be cumulative. A prospective cohort study with self-reports and a follow up questionnaire after one year which evaluated adolescents in Flanders, Belgium and consisted of 1,656 school children found that even moderate use (use about once a week) of the mobile phone after lights out doubles the risk of long term tiredness ($P<0.0001$) (13).

In another study, already discussed, which examined computer game playing and internet use in addition to television viewing and time to bed and time out of bed found that media use lead to a delayed time in bed but did not seem to lead to a compensatory behavior of sleeping later on the weekends. Therefore, the study hypothesized in the concluding remarks that the effects of lack of sleep may be cumulative (24). These sleep problems may lead to daytime sleepiness, behavior problems, and even accidents (24).

Limitations of these studies exist. Many studies have been completed in Belgium, South Korea, and China. More studies need to be done in other parts of the world. Also, many studies obtain data by using questionnaires (retrospective subjective reports). More information may be gleaned from prospective diaries and the use of more objective measures such as actinography or more studies using polysomnography (23). Future directions of investigation may focus on content of electronic media, daytime cognitive functioning, academic achievement, and reasons for screen use (23).

A growing body of evidence demonstrates the negative effect that media may play on the sleep, and consequentially the lives, of children and adolescents. Along with evaluating the problem comes finding solutions. In 2009 the journal Ergonomics published principles for the wise use of computers by children which includes ensuring personal safety and privacy, encouraging appropriate social development, and facilitating appropriate physical development (25).

The American Academy of Pediatrics recommends limiting screen time and offering educational media and non-electronic formats including books, newspapers and board games. Parents should watch television with their children. There should also be "screen-free" zones at home by making sure there are no televisions, computers, or video games in children's bedrooms. Children and teenagers should have no more than one or two hours a day of media exposure. It is important for kids to spend time on outdoor play, hobbies, reading, and using their imaginations in free play. No television is recommended until the age of 2 years. A child's brain is rapidly developing during the first few years.

Young children learn by interacting with people, not screens (1). Following these guidelines will enable children and adolescents to continue to take advantage of the positive effects of media while minimizing the potentially negative, but severe, consequence of sleep disruption.

REFERENCES

[1] Media and Children. American Academy of Pediatrics. Accessed 2013 Jan 10. URL: http://www.aap.org/en-us/advocacy-and-policy/aap-health-initiatives/Pages/Media-and-Children.aspx

[2] Internet users in the world. Internet World Stats 2012. Accessed 2013 Jan 10. URL: http://www.internetworldstats.com/stats.htm

[3] Facebook users in the world. Internet World Stats 2012. Accessed 2013 Jan 10. URL: http://www.internetworldstats.com/facebook.htm

[4] Smith A. 17% of cell phone owners do most of their online browsing on their phone, rather than a computer or other device. Pew Research Center 2012. Accessed 2013 Jan 10. URL: http://pewinternet.org/Reports/2012/Cell-Intenet-Use-2012.aspx

[5] Munezawa T, Kaneita Y, Osaki Y, Kanda H, Minowa M, Suzuki K, et al. The association between use of mobile phones after lights out and sleep disturbances among Japanese adolescents: a nationwide cross-sectional survey. Sleep 2011;34(8):1013-20.

[6] Shapira NA, Goldsmith TB, Keck PE, Khosla UM, McElroy SL. Psychiatric features of individuals with problematic internet use. J Affect Disord 2000;57:267-72.

[7] Nalwa K, Anand AP. Internet addiction in students: a cause of concern. Cyberpsychol Behav 2003:6:6:653-6.

[8] Tonioni F, Alessandris LD, Lai C, Martinelli D, Corvino S, Vasale M. Internet addiction: hours spent online, behaviors, and psychological symptoms. Gen Hosp Psychiatry 2012;34:80-7.

[9] Ha JH, Yoo HJ, Cho IN, Chin B, Shin D, Kim JH. Psychiatric comorbidity assessed in Korean children and adolescents who screen positive for internet addiction. J Clin Psychiatry 2006;67:821-6.

[10] Kim K, Ryu E, Chon MY, Yeun EJ, Choi SY, Seo JS, et al. Internet addiction in Korean adolescents and its relation to depression and suicidal ideation: a questionnaire survey. Int J Nurs Stud 2006;43:185-92.

[11] Paavonen EJ, Pennonen M, Roine M, Valkonen S, Lahikainen AR. TV exposure associated with sleep disturbances in 5- to 6-year-old children. J Sleep Res 2006;15:154-61.

[12] Bulck JV. Media use and dreaming: the relationship among television viewing, computer game play, and nightmares or pleasant dreams. Dreaming 2004;14(1):43-9.

[13] Bulck JV. Adolescent use of mobile phones for calling and for sending text messages after lights out: results from a prospective cohort study with a one-year follow up. Sleep 2007;30(9):1220-3.

[14] Li S, Jin X, Wu S, Jiang F, Yah C, Shen X. The impact of media use on sleep patterns and sleep disorders among school-aged children in China. Sleep 2007:30(3):361-7.

[15] Aronen ET, Paavonen EJ, Fjallberg M, Soininen M, Torronen J. Sleep and psychiatric symptoms in school-age children. J Am Acad Child Adolesc Psychiatry 2000;39(4):502-8.

[16] Cheng SH, Shih CC, Lee IH, Hou YW, Chen KC, Chen KT, et al. A study on the sleep quality of incoming university students. Psychiatry Res 2012;197:270-4.

[17] Choi K, Son H, Park M, Han J, Kim K, Lee B, et al. Internet overuse and excessive daytime sleepiness in adolescents. Psychiatr Clin Neurosci 2009;63:455-62.

[18] Cheung LM, Wong WS. The effects of insomnia and internet addiction on depression in Hong Kong Chinese adolescents: an exploratory cross-sectional analysis. J Sleep Res 2011;20:311-7.

[19] Rotunda RJ, Kaas SJ, Sutton MA, Leon DT. Internet use and misuse: preliminary findings from a new assessment instrument. Behav Modif 2003;27:484-504.

[20] Achab S, Nicolier M, Monnin J, Trojak B, Vandel P, Sechter D, et al. Massively multiplayer online role-playing games: Comparing characteristics of addict vs. non-addict online recruited gamers in a French adult population. BMC Psychiatry 2011:11:144.

[21] Higuchi S, Motohashi Y, Liu Y, Maeda A. Effects of playing a computer game using a bright display on presleep physiological variables, sleep latency, slow wave sleep and REM sleep. J Sleep Res 2005;14:267-73.

[22] Tochigi M, Nishida A, Shimodera S, Oshima N, Inoue K, Okazaki Y, et al. Irregular bedtime and nocturnal cellular phone usage as risk factors for being involved in bullying: a cross-sectional survey of Japanese adolescents. PLoS ONE 2012;7(9):1-7.

[23] Shochat T, Flint-Bretler O, Tzischinsky O. Sleep patterns, electronic media exposure and daytime sleep-related behaviours among Israeli adolescents. Acta Paediatr Taiwan 2010;99:1396-1400.

[24] Bulck JV. Television viewing, computer game playing, and internet use and self-reported time to bed and time out of bed in secondary-school children. Sleep 2004;27(1):101-4.

[25] Straker L, Pollock C, Maslen B. Principles for the wise use of computers by children. Ergonomics 2009;52(11):1386-1401.

Submitted: December 16, 2012. *Revised:* January 10, 2013. *Accepted:* January 22, 2013.

In: Child and Adolescent Health Yearbook 2013
Editor: Joav Merrick

ISBN: 978-1-63117-658-6

Chapter 43

CYBERBULLYING: A BRIEF REVIEW

Amy L Burnett, John A Yozwiak and Hatim A Omar*
Division of Adolescent Medicine, Department of Pediatrics, University of Kentucky College of Medicine, Lexington, Kentucky, United States of America

ABSTRACT

The objective of this review is to summarize the prevalence of internet use among the adolescent population and the growing threat of cyberbullying. This manuscript also addresses the difference between cyberbullying and traditional bullying and the negative psychological effects that result from cyberbullying. Important intervention and prevention strategies for parents and school officials are noted as well.

Keywords: Cyberbullying, internet addiction, traditional bullying, electronic

INTRODUCTION

In a world of Internet dependency and constantly evolving technology, today's youth are becoming more comfortable with having endless information and instant communication at their fingertips. It is estimated that 93% of adolescents, ages 12 to 17 years, use the internet and 75% of this population have their own cell phone (1). Twenty-five percent of those having a cell phone uses it for social media (2). This group averages 3,364 text messages a month, with girls sending and receiving 2.5 times as many texts as boys on a daily basis (1). Adolescents spend an average of 10 hours a day using various forms of media (3). Even though this access allows an increase in media skills and constant social interaction, there are also negatives to this type of access, one being cyberbullying.

---

* Corresponding author: Professor Hatim A Omar, MD, Division of Adolescent Medicine, UK Healthcare, Department of Pediatrics, KY Clinic Room J422, Lexington, KY 40536-0284, United States. Email: haomar2@uky.edu.

Cyberbullying

Cyberbullying has been defined as "willful and repeated harm inflicted through the medium of electronic text" (4). The concept of cyberbullying has become more popular over the past decade as teens continue to use various forms of media to harm others. In the United States, 16.2% of students reported being electronically bullied, either through email, text messages, chats rooms, or social media (5). Surveys have shown that females are twice as likely than boys to be the victim of cyberbullying (5). Conversely, 10% to 20% of adolescents across the world admit to bullying others (3). Studies have shown that somewhere between 33% and 75% of those victims of cyberbulling are also bullied at school (6).

Cyberbullying and traditional bullying are similar in many aspects, seeing as both involve an exchange of hurtful words and or threats from a bully to a victim. The main differences in the two forms of bullying are that cyberbullying allows the bully to remain anonymous, lacks supervision from adults, and victims are extremely accessible at all times, which ultimately results in decreased inhibitions and overall more hurtful exchanges (7). Cyberbullying is somewhat more concerning than traditional bullying because the victims are unable to find a feeling of safety when going home, seeing as media is available at all times and can reach them wherever they go. It is thought that the victims of cyberbullying actually suffer more and have more negative effects due to the lack of escape (8). This form of bullying is rarely punished, seeing as most of the aggressors are anonymous online and law enforcement does not typically intervene in such situations unless there is immediate concern for one's safety (8).

Even though all victims of bullying may experience negative outcomes, research suggests that the effects of cyberbullying may be more severe and have a much greater impact on its victims (3). Overall, self esteem is lower in these victims compared to non-victims (9). These individuals display many negative psychological issues, including depression, anxiety, anger, and worry (7). Cyberbullying victims typically obtain less sleep and eat less than non-victims (3). Studies show that school performance declines in these students, resulting in a drop in grades, increased absences, poorer concentration, and increased behavior issues while at school (7). Those who are being bullied through electronic means are eight times more likely to carry a weapon to school than those students who experience no bullying (1). Many studies have shown that the discussed negative effects had a more profound presentation in those students who did not know the identity of their attacker (10). Even though the psychological effects are significant in these victims, there is no physical harm with cyberbullying (11).

Intervention and Prevention

With the growing numbers of cyberbullying victims, much attention has been given to intervention and prevention of this problem. Participation in social media sites and willingness to give personal information online are two risk factors for these attacks (12). Studies have suggested that, to prevent children from becoming victims of cyberbullying, parents need to be educated about the types of technologies that are being used by their children, have open discussions with their children about what they do when online, have privacy settings that monitor/shield what their children are able to access, and actually supervise their children while online (3).

Parents are able to do a great deal from home in terms of supervision, but it is important for school officials to get on board with intervention and prevention efforts as well. There is sometimes hesitancy from school officials to get involved in attacks that happen away from school, which only worsens the outcome for the victims (9). Most states now require school officials to intervene when such threats are made aware, as they now have added cyberbullying into anti-bullying policies (6). More research is needed regarding the schools' role in this form of abuse and to clarify the legal responsibility to act in certain situations (10).

Internet addiction is a topic that is currently being studied since the explosion of the Internet and the ease and portability of Internet accessing devices. This controversial addiction, generally defined as spending an excessive amount of time online that results in an interference with daily activities, jobs, and relationships, is a concern for today's youth (13). It is estimated that nearly 9 million Americans fall into the category of Internet addicts, which has become detrimental to one or more aspects of their life (14). Internet addiction is concerning for the overall state of the country due to a decrease in productivity, a decrease in interpersonal relations, and an increase in negative health effects related to this issue (15).

Research suggests that there may be a relationship between cyberbullying and excessive use of the internet. For instance, computer proficiency and time spent on-line were related to cyberbullying victimization and offending in an on-line survey of over 1,300 adolescents (8). Raya, Casas, Del Ray, and Ortega examined the connection between cyberbullying and excessive use of the Internet among almost 900 students, and found that excessive internet use predicated cyberbully victimization (17). In a survey that included 177 seventh graders, the students who used computers more frequently were more likely to bully others on-line. However, no relationship was found between the frequency of using computers and being a victim of cyberbullying in this sample (16). Features that are associated with Narcissistic Personality Disorder have been suggested to underlie these maladaptive behaviors (18).

Another potential underlying variable is depressive symptomatology. Youth who report depressive symptomatology are more likely to be the victim of harassment on the internet than their counterparts with mild or no symptomatology (19). In addition, mood disorders are related to excessive Internet use (20). Symptoms of depression may increase the vulnerability to excessive use of the internet and involvement in cyberbullying victimization and/or perpetration. Alternatively, cyberbullying victimization and/or perpetration and excessive use of the Internet may result in depressive symptomatology. Additional research is needed to identify the direction of casualty, and further explore these and other possible mechanisms underlying these constructs.

CONCLUSION

Cyberbullying is a growing problem among adolescents due to their exposure and access to the Internet and cell phones. The negative effects that result in such bullying can result in severe psychological distress, increasing the rates of depression, substance abuse, legal trouble, and suicide among the adolescent population. It is important for parents, school officials, and health care providers to develop better ways of educating students about safe electronic interactions and activities, detecting the threat/risk of cyberbullying, and helping those at risk combat such attacks.

Our access to constantly evolving technology is a great benefit to all aspects of today's world, but much more emphasis is needed in using this plethora of information and instant access to benefit one's overall self and to become more productive members of society. The internet provides adolescents with many opportunities and benefits. The internet's popularity and ubiquitous nature may also lead to pitfalls, such as cyberbullying and excessive use of the Internet. These drawbacks present researchers, clinicians, and policymakers with unique challenges. Whereas the results of research thus far have provided valuable information about these issues, additional research is needed to further describe and explain them, their relationship with each other, as well as their unique correlates, predictors, and features. Ideally, the product of these investigations will yield additional information about the extent to which these constructs are related, which in turn may lead to the development of effective interventions.

REFERENCES

[1] Strasburger VC, Jordan AB,Donnerstein E. Children, adolescents, and the media: health effects. Pediatr Clin North Am 2012;59:533-87.

[2] O'Keeffe GS. Overview: new media. Pediatr Clin North Am 2012;59:589-600.

[3] Donnerstein E. Internet bullying. Pediatr Clin North Am 2012;59:623-33.

[4] Patchin JW,Hinduja S. Bullies move beyond the schoolyard: A preliminary look at cyberbullying. Youth Violence Juv Justice 2006;4:148-69.

[5] Eaton DK, Kann L, Kinchen S, Shanklin S, Flint KH, Hawkins J, et al. Youth risk behavior surveillance - United States, 2011. MMWR Surveill Summ 2012;61:1-162.

[6] Schneider SK, O'Donnell L, Stueve A,Coulter RWS. Cyberbullying, school bullying, and psychological distress: A regional census of high school students. Am J Public Health 2012;102:171-7.

[7] Tokunaga RA. Following you home from school: A critical review and synthesis of research on cyberbullying victimization. Comput Hum Behav 2010;26:277-87.

[8] Hinduja S,Patchin JW. Cyberbullying: An exploratory analysis of factors related to offending and victimization. Deviant Behav 2008;29:129-56.

[9] Patchin JW,Hinduja S. Cyberbullying and self-esteem. J Sch Health 2010;80:614-24.

[10] Hoff DL,Mitchell SN. Cyberbullying: causes, effects, and remedies. J Educ Admin 2009;47:652-65.

[11] Sourander A, Brunstein Klomek A, Ikonen M, Lindroos J, Luntamo T, Koskelainen M, et al. Psychosocial risk factors associated with cyberbullying among adolescents: a population-based study. Arch Gen Psychiatry 2010;67:720-8.

[12] Mesch GS. Parental mediation, online activities, and cyberbullying. Cyberpsychol Behav 2009;12:387-93.

[13] Guan S-S, A.,Subrahmanyam K. Youth internet use: Risks and opportunities. Curr Opin Psychiatry 2009;22:351-6.

[14] Byun S, Ruffini C, Mills JE, Douglas AC, Niang M, Stepchenkova S, et al. Internet addiction: metasynthesis of 1996-2006 quantitative research. Cyberpsychol Behav 2009;12:203-7.

[15] Moreno MA, Jelenchick L, Cox E, Young H,Christakis DA. Problematic internet use among US youth: a systematic review. Arch Pediatr Adolesc Med 2011;165:797-805.

[16] Li Q. New bottle but old wine: A research of cyberbullying in schools. Comput Human Behav 2007;23:1777-91.

[17] Raya L, Casas JA, Del Ray R,Ortega R. Bullying, addiction to Internet and control of information: A prediction model of cyberbullying. 2008. Accessed 2013 Jan 01. URL: http://www.bullyingandcyber .net/media/cms_page_media/50/D.5..pdf

[18] EKŞİ F. Examination of Narcissistic Personality Traits' predicting level of Internet addiction and cyber bullying through path analysis. Educ Sci Theor Pract 2012;12:1694-706.

[19] Ybarra ML. Linkages between depressive symptomatology and Internet harassment among young regular Internet users. Cyberpsychol Behav 2004;7:247-57.

[20] Park S, Hong KE, Park EJ, Ha KS,Yoo HJ. The association between problematic internet use and depression, suicidal ideation and bipolar disorder symptoms in Korean adolescents. Aust NZ J Psychiatry 2012 Oct 9. [Epub ahead of print]

In: Child and Adolescent Health Yearbook 2013
Editor: Joav Merrick
ISBN: 978-1-63117-658-6

Chapter 44

THE IMPACT OF THE INTERNET ON THE SEXUAL HEALTH OF ADOLESCENTS: A BRIEF REVIEW

Julia Springate and Hatim A Omar*
Division of Adolescent Medicine, Department of Pediatrics, University of Kentucky, Lexington, Kentucky, United States of America

ABSTRACT

The object of this review is to summarize the impact of the Internet on the sexual health of adolescents. This article examines the use of websites, blogs and chat rooms as sources for sexual health information for adolescents. The influence of Internet pornography on sexual behaviors and attitudes is addressed. The use of the Internet as a place to find sexual partners is also assessed. During a time of great physical, emotional and sexual change, the Internet is playing a huge role in the decisions adolescents are making, both positive and negative.

Keywords: Adolescent, sexual health, internet, pornography, relationships

INTRODUCTION

Media has always played a large role in the lives of adolescents. In recent years, the rise of new media has increased this role. New media includes the Internet—blogs, chatrooms, social networking sites and other websites (1). Approximately 75% of households and most schools have Internet access. This means that 93% of 9-17 year olds are online. 30% of these adolescents have internet access in their bedrooms, meaning that they are most likely unmonitored. These teens use the internet at least four days per week for an average of two hours at a time (1).

* Corresponding author: Professor Hatim A Omar, MD, Division of Adolescent Medicine, UK Healthcare, Department of Pediatrics, KY Clinic Room J422, Lexington, KY 40536-0284, United States. Email: haomar2@uky.edu.

All of this time on the internet begs the question, what are adolescents doing online? Studies indicate that the most popular uses are looking up health information, school research, news information and information about movies, music and television (2). Adolescence is a time of much curiosity, especially regarding health and 75% of youth, as of 2004 had used the internet to look up health information (2). Two of the three most frequently researched topics on the Internet regarding health are sexual health (such as sexual activities, pregnancy and contraception) and sexually transmitted diseases. Sexual health is an important area of interest to adolescents, and the internet is providing information to them.

Young people turn to the internet for information regarding sexual health for many reasons. One of the most important reasons is the anonymity that is given by the internet. Many adolescents feel embarrassed and ashamed of sexual questions and do not want to approach their health care provider (3). It is also easy to access, free of charge and very interactive—aspects that are very important to adolescents (4).

Because of the large availability of information, interaction and media, the internet is playing a huge role in the lives of adolescents—especially in their sexual health.

Internet as a Source for Sexual Health Information

Adolescents are undergoing physical, cognitive and social changes (4). These changes stimulate questions regarding health, relationships and sexuality. Because teens want a confidential source of information regarding these sensitive topics, the internet is perfect. Adolescents turn to the internet because of its safety, anonymity, constant availability and transcendence from adult control (1). Sources of information include web pages, bulletin boards, newsgroups, forums and chartrooms, to name a few (4). According to a study conducted concerning a popular health bulletin board, posts concerning questions about sexual technique, contraception and pregnancy garnered the most questions as well as views and therefore the most interest from adolescents (4). The fact that adolescents seek out important information online has proven to be both positive and negative.

On one hand, the internet provides a place for adolescents to ask questions that they may not ask otherwise. Studies have shown that 41% of young adults changed their behavior, because of health information they found online, and almost half had contacted their physician as a result of the information (1).

Although the internet can provide much needed health advice, it can also be negative. There is always the possibility that the information is inaccurate or misleading. In the realm of sexual health—especially sexually transmitted diseases and contraception—mistakes can be very costly, causing pregnancy or serious infections such as HIV (1). Many websites promote condom use and abstinence, but few share other safe strategies such as decreasing number of partners or delaying first intercourse (1). Also, teens with low health literacy are more likely to use slang terms when looking for sexual health information, which may expose them to less credible websites (1). While 57% of adolescents trust the advice they come across, there are no standards for what qualifies as credible in the world of the Internet (2).

While the internet may provide information for teens regarding sexual health that information may not always be reliable. For this reason, it is important that adolescents check the reliability of the source as well as talk to their health care professional.

Internet as a Source for Pornography

While finding health information on the Internet can be positive and negative in the lives of adolescents, seeking pornography online is almost always detrimental. 42% of youth between the ages of 10 and 17 years have been exposed to online pornography in the past year (5). Out of these youth, 66% said that the exposure was accidental or unwanted (5). Compared with adolescents that have not been exposed to online pornography, those that had been exposed were more likely to have early coitarche, have higher numbers of partners, use alcohol during sexual encounters and participate in anal sex (5). These behaviors are high-risk and put adolescents in danger regarding their sexual health.

Not only does pornography affect the behavior of adolescents, it also influences their attitudes and ideas. Adolescents who view online pornography are more likely to have less progressive gender role attitudes, condone extramarital sex and exhibit sexually permissive attitudes (6). Increased sexual permissiveness indicates that these adolescents believe that casual sex is acceptable, relationships with multiple partners are normal, andone-night stands are acceptable (6). Teens who view online pornography are generally not concerned with the social consequences of their actions and have a skewed view of societal norms regarding sex (5). Because of this influence, these adolescents often participate in more high-risk sexual activities (6).

Internet as a Source for Relationships

High-risk sexual behaviors can impact an adolescent's entire life. Throughout adolescence and beyond, youth develop an interest in sex and relationships. While they show curiosity, they are often too shy to pursue it (7). The internet allows adolescents to keep their sexual activities hidden. As was the case with sexual health questions, the internet provides anonymity, perceived safety and ease of access when searching for sexual partners (8).

Unfortunately, the perception of safety is displaced. Studies show that young adults who seek sex partners online are at a greater risk for sexually transmitted diseases than their peers who do not seek sex partners online (8). Adolescents who seek sexual partners online are more likely to have early coitarche, more partners, and more anal sex than peers who did not have internet partners. These outcomes are similar to the adolescents that viewed online pornography. However, the same adolescents were also more likely to use condoms during vaginal and anal sex, discuss STDs with their partner, and visit prevention oriented chatrooms (8,9).While high-risk behaviors were more prevalent with internet partners, these adolescents were also practicing some safety measures.

Conclusion

Overall, the internet is a catch-22 when it comes to the sexual health of adolescents. It provides adolescents with a confidential place to seek health information. However, it opens the door for adolescents to find incorrect health information, pornography and high-risk partners. It is clear that both benefits and detriments are present. It will be of great importance in future years to find a way to use the Internet to improve the sexual health of adolescents, rather than damage it.

REFERENCES

[1] Brown JD, Keller S, Stern S. Sex, sexuality, sexting and sexed: adolescents and the media. Prev Res 2009; 16(4):12-6.

[2] Kanuga M, Rosenfeld WD. Adolescent sexuality and the internet: The good, the bad, and the URL. J Pediatr Adolesc Gynecol 2004; 17(2):117-24.

[3] Harvey JH, Brown B, Crawford P, Macfarlane A, McPherson A. Am I normal? Teenagers, sexual health and the internet. Soc Sci Med 2007; 65(4):771-81.

[4] Suzuki LK, Calzo JP. The search for peer advice in cyberspace: An exampination of online teen bulletin boards about health and sexuality. J Appl Devel Psychol 2004; 25(6):685-98.

[5] Braun-Courville DK, Rojas M. Exposure to sexually explicit web sites and adolescent sexual attitudes and behaviors. J Adolesc Health 2009; 45(2):156-62.

[6] Lo V, Wei R. Exposure to internet pornography and Taiwanese adolescents' sexual attitudes and behaviors. J Broad Elec Media 2005; 49(2):221-37.

[7] Subrahmanyam K, Greenfield PM, Tynes B. Constructing sexuality and identity in ana online teen chat room. J Appl Devel Psychol 2004; 25(6)651-66.

[8] McFarlane M, Bull SS, Rietmeijer CA. Young adults on the internet:risk behaviors for sexually transmitted diseases and HIV. J Adolesc Health 2002; 31(1):11-6.

[9] Doring NM. The internet's impact of sexuality: A critical review of 15 years of research. Comp Hum Behav 2009; 25(5):1089-1101.

In: Child and Adolescent Health Yearbook 2013
Editor: Joav Merrick ISBN: 978-1-63117-658-6

Chapter 45

DEVELOPMENT OF AN INTEGRATED INTERVENTION MODEL FOR INTERNET ADDICTION IN HONG KONG

Daniel TL Shek, PhD, FHKPS, BBS, JP [*,1,2,3,4,5]
and Hildie Leung [1]
[1]Department of Applied Social Sciences,
The Hong Kong Polytechnic University, Hong Kong, PRC,
[2]Centre for Innovative Programmes for Adolescents and Families,
The Hong Kong Polytechnic University, Hong Kong, PRC,
[3]Kiang Wu Nursing College of Macau, Macau, PRC,
[4]Department of Social Work, East China Normal University, Shanghai, PRC
[5]Division of Adolescent Medicine, Department of Pediatrics, Kentucky Children's Hospital, University of Kentucky College of Medicine, Lexington, Kentucky, United States of America

ABSTRACT

In response to the severe lack of indigenously developed preventive and counseling services for young people displaying Internet addiction problem, the Community Chest of Hong Kong funded a pioneering project entitled "Youngster Internet addiction prevention and counseling service". Besides provision of preventive services at the community, school, family and individual levels, individual-based and family-based counseling services were developed for young people displaying Internet addiction problem. In this paper, the major features of the counseling model are outlined, including emphases on controlled and healthy use of the Internet, understanding the change process in adolescents with Internet addiction problem, use of motivational interview methods, adoption of a family perspective, multi-level counseling at the individual, peer and family levels, and the use of both case and group approaches. The process of intervention in this counseling model is also described. Evaluation findings provide support for this integrated intervention model.

* Correspondence: Professor Daniel TL Shek, PhD, FHKPS, BBS, JP, Chair Professor of Applied Social Sciences, Faculty of Health and Social Sciences, Department of Applied Social Sciences, The Hong Kong Polytechnic University, Room HJ407, Core H, Hunghom, Hong Kong. E-mail: daniel.shek@ polyu.edu.hk

Keywords: Internet addiction; family intervention; individual counseling; motivational interviewing

INTRODUCTION

Despite potential educational and entertainment value of the Internet, its attractive nature may create addiction in young people. In fact, there are research findings showing that problematic or pathological use of the Internet adversely affects the physical, psychological, social, and spiritual health of adolescents (1,2). There are also research findings showing that problem use of the Internet is quite prevalent in young people in the West (3,4) and the Asian contexts (5,6). For instance, according to a report on youth Internet addiction disorder published in 2009, approximately 14.3% of adolescents in China aged between 13-17 years and 15.6% of those aged between 18-23 years who had access to computers suffered from Internet addiction (7). Studies conducted in Taiwan found that 18.8% of high school students (8) and 17.9% of senior high school students (9) were classified as being addicted to the Internet.

With specific reference to Hong Kong, Leung (10) concluded that 37.9% of the respondents were identified as Internet addicts. In another study (11), it was estimated that roughly 20% of the respondents could be classified as Internet addicted. In a longitudinal study of Internet addiction in students in Hong Kong, findings showed that Internet addiction is a common risk behavior in secondary school students. Using Young's 10-item Internet Addiction Test, roughly one-fourth of Secondary 1 and Secondary 2 students could be classified as having Internet addiction. Besides, both psychosocial and familial factors have been associated with Internet addiction among youths (12-14).

Specifically, Shek and Lu (12) found that the possession of positive and clear identity and general positive youth development predicted a lower probability of Internet addiction. Furthermore, adolescents with divorced parents were more likely to engage in pathological use of the Internet; perceived parental rearing behaviors that were lacking emotional warmth, rejecting, and punitive, were also associated with Internet addiction in adolescents (15).

In contrast to the growing Internet addiction in the global contexts, related work on intervention is scattered and was conducted in unsystematic manners (16,17). Furthermore, there is very little published work on successful intervention models in the Chinese contexts. Intervention models in the Chinese contexts are important because there is evidence showing that Chinese people displayed more pathological gambling behavior than did non-Chinese people (18,19). The widespread use of opium in China before the Opium War also suggests that we need Chinese models on addiction.

With the funding from the Community Chest of Hong Kong, a pilot project entitled "Youngster Internet addiction prevention and counseling service" was launched by the Jockey Club Wah Ming Lutheran Integrated Service Centre, Hong Kong Lutheran Social Service, and Lutheran Church-Hong Kong Synod (LC-HKS).

The major objectives of this pilot project were: a) to provide preventive education programs at the community, school, family, and individual levels; and b) to conduct a pilot project on individual- and family-based counseling services for young people who have displayed Internet addictive behavior. In this paper, the basic features of the intervention model and the process of intervention are outlined.

FEATURES OF THE INTERVENTION MODEL

As there are few validated intervention models for Internet addiction in the global and local contexts, the Research Team attempted to pull intervention strategies and techniques together in the fields of substance abuse, family counseling, and peer support group. Essentially, the intervention model adopted in this pilot project has the following features:

1. Emphasis on controlled and healthy use of the Internet: Instead of proposing complete abstinence of Internet use, it is argued that Internet use is intrinsically neutral. As such, controlled and healthy use was regarded as the desired outcome. This principle can also facilitate the involvement of the adolescent client in the counseling process.

2. Understanding the change process in adolescents with Internet addiction behavior: In the stages of change model (20, 21), there are several stages in the process of change, including pre-contemplation, contemplation, determination, action, maintenance, and relapse. In the pre-contemplation stage, the client may not think that his/her Internet use behavior is problematic and he/she does not consider changing his/her Internet use behavior. In the contemplation stage, the person starts to realize that his/her Internet use behavior is problematic and considers the possibility of changing. However, the consideration is ambivalent in nature. In the determination stage, the person decides to change his/her Internet use behavior. In the action stage, the person starts to decrease his/her online time. The person is successful in changing if he/she can maintain the changed Internet use behavior. Otherwise, relapse occurs and he/she might go through the stages of change again.

This model was used in the present context to understand the needs of adolescents with Internet addiction problem and their family members. In the intervention model, counseling tasks in relation to these different stages of change were devised. The details are described in Table 1 and Table 2.

3. Utilization of motivational interviewing model: Motivational interviewing is a directive, client-centered counseling style for eliciting behavior change by helping clients to explore and resolve ambivalence (22-24). It assumes that the responsibility and capability for change are within the client. Five basic principles are intrinsic to motivational interviewing. These include: a) expression of empathy via reflective listening to convey understanding of the client's thinking and feeling; b) pointing out discrepancy between the client's current behavior and future goals; c) avoid unnecessary arguments which evoke resistance to change; d) resistance and ambivalence are viewed as normal and are explored openly; e) support self-efficacy by building the client's confidence that he/ she can make a change. There are research findings supporting the effectiveness of motivational interviewing in the context of addiction (reference?).

4. Adoption of the family perspective: Instead of simply blaming adolescents for addictive behavior, it is noteworthy that such behavior may be a result of different ecological factors, particularly family factors (25,26). According to the family perspective, an adolescent with Internet addictive behavior represents a symptom of a dysfunction within a family rather than the individual's maladjustment. For example, the child's Internet addictive behavior might be a symptom of the marital and parenting conflicts amongst the parents. Furthermore, it is proposed that change in an individual member of the family system would cause change in other family members as well as the whole family system. For example, a father changing his way in dealing with the son's Internet addictive behavior can improve his relation and communication with the son, and the son might react by becoming more willing to cooperate when the father disciplines his Internet use behavior. Indeed studies have found Internet-specific parenting practices, such as the increase in quality of parent-child communication on the use of Internet (27), and the maintenance of appropriate parental norms regarding Internet use (28), to be negatively associated with pathological Internet use among adolescents.

Table 1. Individual-Based and Family-Based Counseling Tasks in the First Few Stages of the Change Process

Stages of Change	Individual-Based Counseling	Family-Based Counseling
Pre-Contemplation	• Making connection by expressing empathy. • Understanding the daily functioning, thinking, and feeling with respect to different areas such as school, peer and family contexts. • Understanding the needs and concerns of the client. • Understanding the positive and negative aspects of Internet use. • Developing discrepancy between what one wants and the current Internet use behavior.	• Helping parents to handle emotions aroused by their children's Internet addictive behavior. • Helping parents to understand their children's needs and other problems behind the Internet addictive behavior. • Identifying the interaction patterns which maintain the Internet addictive behavior.
Contemplation	• Constructing decisional balance about change and no change which is in favor of changing current Internet use behavior. • Strengthening self-efficacy so as to enhance the possibility of change.	
Determination	• Developing plans for changing Internet use behavior, not just an Internet use time table, but also a short-term plan about study or career. Different resources, such as the Youth Pre-Employment Training Program might be introduced whenever appropriate. • Engaging the client to join peer support groups, interest classes, or voluntary services.	• Facilitating direct and congruent parent-child communication, thus improving their mutual understanding and relationships. • Breaking the circular interaction patterns which maintain the Internet addictive behavior. • Developing and strengthening interaction patterns of dealing with the conflict about Internet use, which in turn promote healthy Internet use habits.
Action	• Strengthening problem solving skills for handling the difficulties in carrying out the action plan. • Providing support to develop self-efficacy. • Expressing empathy for those facing difficulties during the changing process.	

Table 2. Individual-Based and Family-Based Counseling Tasks in the Maintenance and Relapse Stages

Stages of Change	Individual-Based Counseling	Family-Based Counseling
Maintenance	• Identifying and handling the factors associated with the risk of relapse. • Strengthening social support network.	• Maintaining support and encouragement for developing healthy Internet use habits.
Relapse	• Providing supportive environment for learning from relapse and motivating to re-cycle through the stages of change.	• Helping parents to handle emotions caused by relapse. • Identifying the improved interaction patterns and those still needing to be improved. • Helping parents to maintain supportive family environment and motivating them not to give up.

In short, Internet addiction often occurs in the family context which results in serious conflicts between the adolescents and their parents. As there are family theories and research suggesting that family factors are etiological as well as therapeutic factors underlying addiction problems, family-based counseling is considered important in this pilot project. The systemic view, which is the foundation of different family therapies, was employed as the theoretical backdrop of family-based counseling utilized in this project.

5. Multi-level counseling model: Based on the preceding discussion, an intervention model incorporating the following elements was developed:

- *Individual counseling component:* The intervention model is an integration of the process of change model and motivation interviewing techniques. It is proposed that different counseling elements are intrinsic to different stages of change (see Table 1 and Table 2). The techniques intrinsic to the individual-based counseling model can be seen in Table 3.
- *Family counseling component:* Based on the systemic and family perspectives, it is argued that intervention at the family level such as enhancement of family functioning and improvement of parenting skills are important. The related family counseling tasks in relation to different stages can be seen in Table 1 and Table 2. The techniques intrinsic to the family-based counseling model can be seen in Table 4.
- *Peer support component:* Besides intervention at the individual and family levels, peer relation is also important for adolescents. In the context of addiction, peer influence has been found to be an important factor for substance abuse (29). At the same time, peer support is also very important for the maintenance of healthy Internet use habit. As such, different supportive activities including volunteer groups and interest classes were organized in this pilot project. The objectives of these activities included the improvement of social skills, establishment of supportive social network, realization of one's strengths and potentials, and promotion of healthy social engagement amongst the program participants.

Table 3. Summary of Individual-Based Counseling Techniques

Motivational Interviewing
Elicitation of Self-Motivational Statements ■ Self-motivational statements regarding adolescent clients' talk of concerns about online behavior, desire, reasons, ability and commitment for change were elicited. ■ Such statements should be elicited from the adolescent clients rather than being told or imposed.
Handling Resistance ■ Avoided argumentation which elicited resistance. ■ Reflection which exaggerated the adolescent clients' resistance of changing the Internet addictive behavior might induce the adolescent clients to say the opposite. ■ Double-sided reflection highlighted the ambivalence experienced, with the emphasis that the adolescent clients had the responsibility to choose whether they wanted to change.
Good Things and Less Good Things ■ Good things about going online were explored together with the adolescent clients, followed by the less good things about going online. ■ Adolescent clients tended to be more willing to discuss the "less good things" after the "good things". Both sides had been discussed thoroughly and summarized appropriately.
Decisional Balance ■ The discussion was similar to "good things" and "less good things" except that it focused on future behavior. ■ The pros and cons of changing the Internet addictive behavior were identified and compared with the pros and cons of not changing the behavior. ■ Emphasized that adolescent clients could make differences and they could choose to live in the way they really wanted.
Values Exploration ■ Encouraged the adolescent clients to rank different value statements. ■ The meaning of value statements, discrepancies between values and their current online behavior, and perceived barriers and opportunities of decreasing discrepancies were discussed. ■ This process helped the adolescent clients to evaluate whether their behavior fulfilled their short-term needs while violated the values they treasured in the long run.
Discussion of the Stages of Change ■ The stages of change were explained and the adolescent clients were asked to determine their current stage. ■ The adolescent clients were also helped to review whether they experienced different stages of change in the past and what would cause them to move between different stages.
OARS (Open-end questions, Affirmations, Reflective listening, and Summarization) ■ Basic techniques of motivational interviewing summarized by the acronym OARS (Open-end questions, Affirmations, Reflective listening, and Summarization) were also applied.
Other Individual-Based Counseling Techniques
Feedback on Online Behavior ■ Objective assessment on Internet addiction was conducted and the results were discussed.
Construction of Personal Inventory ■ A list of activities that had been neglected after the adolescent clients' establishment of Internet addictive behavior was constructed. ■ This technique helped the adolescent clients to evaluate the negative impacts of deterring the engagement in interesting or important activities due to the Internet addiction behavior.
Construction of Behavioral Contract ■ Set time limit on using the Internet. ■ Explored alternatives which could occupy the free time after spending less time online. ■ Difficulties of implementation and the related solutions were discussed.
Development of Career Plan ■ Developed career plan and related action plan such as taking courses or applying jobs. ■ This aspect was essential for those who had left school and were unemployed, as they had a lot of free time to stay online if the non-engaged situation persisted.

Note: Techniques are based on Miller (1995)

Table 4. Summary of Family-Based Counseling Techniques

Family-Based Counseling
Reframing the Symptoms of Internet Addiction ■ The mutual influences of family members' interactions were emphasized in the counseling process. The interaction patterns regarding the adolescent clients' Internet addictive behavior (such as inconsistent parenting) were examined to help the parents identify their influences. ■ To broaden parents' understanding of their children's online behaviors, Internet addictive behavior could also be reframed as their children's attempt to fulfill their interpersonal needs through online activities.
Dealing with Unbalanced Power ■ In some cases, the family power structure was upside down as children's superior computer knowledge might cause their parents to feel powerless in disciplining their children's Internet use behavior. Support was given to the parents for performing appropriate parenting roles. ■ External stoppers such as parent-child service plan provided by some Internet service providers, which enabled the parents to control their children's online time, could be introduced as a way to empower the parents.
Resolution of Conflicts ■ As there were continuous daily conflicts related to the Internet use behavior of the adolescent clients, such as when to go offline and the adolescent clients staying online during meal time, helping the parents and the adolescent clients to resolve the conflicts was a very important task. ■ Skills for handling the emotions aroused by the conflicts were introduced and discussed with the parents and the adolescent clients. ■ Facilitation of congruent communication which considered the self, others, and the context in parent-child interaction was important. This process attempted to find the solution which was accepted by both the parents and the adolescent clients.
Discussion of the Stages of Change ■ The stages of change were explained and the parents were asked to identify which stage of change best described their children's current situation. ■ The model helped to reframe the idea of "my child did not want to change" into "my child was in the pre-contemplation stage, which was the first step of change". It helped the parents to understand that change was a progressive process instead of simplifying it as a dichotomy of "change" or "not change". ■ Parents were helped to identify appropriate actions to motivate their children in the different stages of change.

Note: Techniques are based on Hanna and Brown (1995).

6. Utilization of case work and group work: As peer relations are very important in adolescent development, peer support group approach was used as a supplement to the casework approach. With the use of group dynamics, mutual support, and modeling opportunities, group members can learn from each other. With group atmosphere characterized by empathy, sincerity, and respect, group members serve not only to help them establish positive self-image, but also act as role models for others. Peer support group can also help group members establish social support network, which would help them maintain healthy Internet use habits.

In short, through the use of case work and group work, the proposed intervention focused on enhancing adolescents' motivation to change, changing the adolescents' cognitions and Internet addictive behavior, changing the dysfunctional familial interactive patterns, and eventually helping the adolescents to develop healthy Internet use habits.

CLIENTS IN THE INTERVENTION PROGRAM

A total of 59 cases participated in the project. Generally speaking, cases that were identified as Internet addicts by one of the assessment tools described in the evaluation report (30,31) were eligible for receiving the service. However, there was one case that did not meet the above assessment criteria. As he almost met the diagnostic criteria of Young's 10-item questionnaire (i.e., he responded "Yes" to 3 of the questions) and he desperately wanted to be helped, service was provided to him. Regarding the gender of the program participants, 58 were males and 1 was female. Most of them were early adolescents (aged 11-15 years; N=29) and late adolescents (aged 16-18 years; N=27), with 3 program participants aged over 18 years. The educational background of the program participants was as follows: primary education (N=7); Secondary 1 to Secondary 3 (N=33); Secondary 4 to Secondary 5 (N=18); Secondary 6 or above (N=1). Different sources of referral for the cases were identified, including school social workers (N=27), parents (N=22), teachers (N=5), non-school social workers (N=4), and siblings (N=1).

THE INTERVENTION PROCESS

Stage 1 (Initial Contact and Establishment of Relationship)

For the cases referred by social workers and teachers, relevant information including adolescent clients' Internet use habits, impacts of their Internet use habits on adolescent clients' daily social functioning, methods that had been used to help adolescent clients, and the effects of those methods was collected. The referrers were also informed that we would intake the cases only if the adolescents met the assessment criteria.

For most of the cases, it was the parents who sought help (either by themselves or via school social workers) for their children's Internet addiction problem. They usually felt helpless and wanted to depend on the worker. In the initial contact, their involvements in the counseling process were emphasized and the stages of change were also explained to them, such that they would be aware that change was a process that needed time to take place. In addition, the parents were asked about how they dealt with the problem and how the parents and their children reacted to each other's reactions.

In the initial contacts with the adolescents, information in different areas, including which online games the adolescent clients played, time spent on the Internet, adolescent clients' interests and hobbies, and initial impression about the referral was collected. Other relevant information was also collected so as to determine where (e.g., school or home), when (e.g., weekday after school or Sunday afternoon), and how (e.g., individual interview, joint interview together with parents or phone contact) to render the service to them in the later stage of the counseling process. As the adolescent clients were often at the stage of pre-contemplation or contemplation, they were not really motivated to see the worker. As such, acceptance and empathy were crucial. It was important to make connections with the adolescent clients by showing the interest in "understanding" their thinking and feelings rather than "solving" the Internet addiction problem.

Stage 2 (Intervention involving individual-based counseling, family-based counseling and peer support group)

After establishing working relationships with the adolescent client, the evaluation questionnaire containing the Internet addiction assessment tools was administered. Except the one case mentioned above, if the adolescent client met the criteria in one of the assessment tools, he/she would receive both individual-based counseling and family-based counseling and he/she would be invited to join the peer support group. The major goal of the intervention would be to help the adolescent client to develop healthy Internet use habit (i.e., a decrease in Internet addiction symptoms).

Individual-based counselling

The adolescent clients were often at the stage of pre-contemplation or contemplation and they were unmotivated to see the worker. Based on the implementation experiences, three categories of adolescent clients with Internet addiction problems were identified.

- For the first category, the adolescent clients did not have specific goals and they felt their lives were boring. They spent a lot of time online as they could not find other interesting things for them to kill time. It was very difficult to motivate them to change their Internet use habits as they did not see that there would be any serious negative consequences. It was very difficult to motivate them to move from the pre-contemplation stage to contemplation and determination stages by finding out their needs and desire so as to narrow the discrepancy between what they wanted and what they had to do. It was a good way to strengthen relationships with them through activities and helped them to establish meaningful connections with peers. At the same time, it was crucial to facilitate the adolescent clients and their parents to improve the communication and mutual understanding so that they could handle the conflicts due to the adolescent clients' Internet addictive behavior in a better way.
- The second category included adolescent clients with emotional problems who used Internet as a way to escape from the depressive mood. As long as they could better handle their emotions, they would less depend on the Internet and were motivated to change. They could also develop their own action plans and reduced the time on the Internet. Thus, it was also essential for the parents to understand that their children concealed the emotional problems under the Internet addictive behavior. This did not only remove the stress which might intensify the children's emotional problems and drove them to increase the Internet use for escaping, but also provided a supportive environment for the adolescent clients to handle their emotional problems. It should also be noted that in some cases, psychiatric intervention might be necessary.
- The last category included adolescent clients characterized by poor self-image. Basically, the lack of successful experience in daily life made them turn to seek gratification from the Internet by being absorbed in playing one or a few online games. They would spend a lot of time on the same online game or even buy some powerful weapons of the game, so that they could maintain a high status in the online

game. They were trying to build successful and competent images in the online games. Thus, it was essential to help them establish positive self-images through doing voluntary works, which could provide the opportunity for them to gain successful experience and realize their own strengths. Parental support and compliments were also important for creating a positive cycle for the adolescent clients to start establishing healthy Internet use habits.

Family-based counseling

Where appropriate, conjoint family interviews and family counseling sessions were carried out to facilitate the parents and their adolescent children to understand their mutual expectations, to improve the parent-adolescent relationships, and to foster healthy parent-adolescent interactions.

Peer support group

Originally, it was planned to organize groups for both the adolescent clients and their parents separately. However, a lot of difficulties were encountered. First, as the adolescent clients lived in different districts, such as Tseung Kwan O, Shatin, and Sheung Shui, they were not motivated to travel a long distance to join the group. Second, as many parents had very long working hours, it was very difficult to arrange suitable time schedules for forming groups with enough number of group members. As a result, only a support group for adolescent clients was organized. For adolescent clients who had not joined the support group, the workers would motivate them to be volunteers or join the interest classes so as to promote healthy social engagement, and to realize their strengths and potentials. Eventually, nine adolescents became volunteers or joined the interest classes.

Because adolescents with Internet addictive behavior displayed problems of loneliness and weak social networks, supportive networks for them were important. As such, peer support group was designed with the following objectives:

1. To help group members to recognize their own strengths and establish positive self-images.
2. To help group members to experience how to honestly face themselves and other people, so as to establish friendship with others.
3. To help group members to establish mutual respect, support, and caring relationships.

To avoid labeling effect, the support group took the form of a volunteer group. To ensure homogeneity of the group, members were at the determination stage (i.e., they had decided to improve their Internet using behaviors) and the group size was small with no more than eight members. However, as it was difficult to recruit suitable participants who would commit to the group and were at the similar stage of change when the group was scheduled to start, the group size turned out to be smaller with five members only.

Besides, strong emphases on interaction amongst members and mutual sharing and caring were made. The worker was expected to act as a role model and demonstrate congruence, respect, and care in running the group. On the other hand, members were expected to have strong commitment and positive expectations about themselves. Broadly speaking, the objectives of each session in the peer support group are as follows:

- First session: Knowing each other; establishing group norms; sharing individuals' expectations;
- Second and third sessions: Team building; recognizing one's strengths;
- Fourth and fifth sessions: Self-exploration; sharing with others;
- Sixth session: Expressing mutual support and encouragement; consolidation of the group experience.

The main themes and activities for each session in the peer support group are listed in Table 5.

Table 5. Main themes and activities for each session in the peer support group

Session	Main Themes and Activities
1	Brief introduction: The worker welcomed group members, introduced the group's objectives, and highlighted the importance of keeping the commitment to join the group. Ice breaking: Played 2 ice breaking games. Knowing each other: The worker and members drew an icon, and wrote down 3 characteristics of the icon which could represent them, and then shared. Establishing group norms: Forming pairs. Each pairs brainstormed 3 group norms, which they thought were most important, and represented those norms in actions. Other members guessed the meanings of those actions. Sharing expectations: Members re-drew and shared their icons by adding some changes to the icons to represent their expected changes when the group ended.
2 & 3	Team building: Played 2 team building games. In debriefing, the worker facilitated members to recognize others' contribution in completing the tasks. Finally, the worker summarized the contribution with the following "contribution cards": The picture of a brain: having some creative ideas. The picture of eyes: having insight on formulating workable action plans. The picture of ears: willing to listen and accept different opinions. The picture of a mouth: willing to discuss and share opinions with others. The picture of a heart: caring about others feelings and safety. The picture of hands: actively taking part in the tasks and trying different methods. The picture of legs: being supportive and encouraging when facing difficulties. Recognizing own strengths: Assigned 4 team tasks. After completing each team task, two members were selected. Other members chose "contribution cards" to represent those two members and explained the reasons for their choices. Besides, the worker secretly placed the "contribution cards" in the individual envelopes for all members to recognize their contribution in the task. After completing all the four team tasks, the worker displayed the "contribution cards" in each envelope openly for the members to discuss who should get which set of "contribution cards". It was common for the members to have different opinions with the worker, and it was demonstrated that they observed something not noticed by the worker. Finally, members chose one "contribution card" for themselves and shared an experience during which they demonstrated similar performance in their daily life.

Table 5. (Continued)

Session	Main Themes & Activities
4 & 5	Self-exploration and Sharing with others: Members took four instant photos for facial expressions which represented the feelings of "happy", "angry", "afraid", and "sad". Then they pasted their photos on an A3 worksheet, which was divided into four parts. In each part, they pasted one photo and then wrote down the most unforgettable event related to the particular feeling. After completion of the four parts, members shared with others about those events related to the feelings of "happy", "angry", "afraid" and "sad", why those events were so unforgettable, and why those events elicited those feelings.
6	Expressing mutual support and encouragement: A birthday party was organized for members whose birthdays were near. They were encouraged to organize birthday parties for other members in the future. Information facilitating future contact (i.e., MSN or email accounts) among members was exchanged for maintaining support after the group ended. Consolidation of the group experience: Members' feelings and thoughts about the group were discussed. The changes among members were explored. Based on the group experience, future development of the group, such as the possibility of continuing the group, commitment of members, and the major goal of the group that should be continued, was also discussed. Evaluation: Members filled in the evaluation form, commented and discussed what they liked and disliked about the group.

Stage 3 (Termination and Follow Up)

When the adolescent clients successfully established healthy Internet use habits or the families agreed that they were able to handle the children's Internet use problem by themselves, changes in the adolescent clients' Internet use habits and the family relationships were systematically evaluated.

Table 6. Condensed case illustration of individual-based and family-based counseling

Case Background
Yan was a Secondary 4 student of a Band 1 secondary school. Her parents divorced when she was in Primary 6. She was the only daughter and currently living with her mother. During her primary school education, she always obtained the first place in examinations. However, she started spending a lot of time online during her summer holiday in Secondary 1. Her school performance deteriorated and she barely got promoted to Secondary 4 in the same school. In addition, there were a lot of conflicts with her mother regarding her Internet use behavior.
The Intervention Process
Initial Contact and Assessment (About three months, with interviews every two weeks) A. Individual-based counseling with Yan and her mother while focusing on Yan ■ Expressing empathy and setting goal. ■ Understanding Yan's daily functioning, thinking, and feeling in different areas. ■ Understanding the needs and concerns of Yan. ■ Helping Yan to understand the positive and relatively less positive facts about the Internet. ■ Helping Yan's mother to handle emotions aroused by Yan's Internet addictive behavior. B. After gathering the basic information and preparing Yan and her mother, family-based counseling via joint interviews was conducted ● Facilitating Yan's mother to understand Yan's needs, as well as other problems behind the Internet addictive behavior. ● Identifying the interaction patterns which might maintain the addictive behavior of Yan.

Intervention (About nine months, with interviews every month as stable working relationships had been established)
A. Enhancement of parent-child interaction through joint interviews
● Facilitating direct and congruent parent-child communication.
● Breaking the circular interaction patterns which maintained the Internet addictive behavior.
● Developing and strengthening interaction patterns for dealing with the conflicts about Internet use.
B. Enhancement of Yan's motivation to change
■ Developing discrepancy between what was wanted and the current Internet use behavior.
■ Strengthening self-efficacy so as to increase the possibility of change.
■ Developing plans for changing Internet use behavior, not just an Internet use timetable, but also a short-term plan about her study or career.
■ Engaging her to join peer support groups, interest classes, or voluntary services.
■ Identifying and handling the factors associated with the risk of relapse.
■ Examining her social support network.
C. Promotion of effective resolution of conflict
● Encouraging use of "I" message and time out methods for avoiding over-emotional reactions.
● Maintaining support and encouragement for healthy Internet use habits.
● Helping Yan's mother to handle emotions caused by relapse.
● Identifying the improved interaction patterns and those still needing to be improved.
Termination and Follow Up (About six months)
As Yan's Internet use behavior and the parent-child relationship stabilized, the case was systematically evaluated and terminated with the agreement of Yan and her mother. The worker then followed up by making phone contacts with Yan and her mother every month to keep track of Yan's Internet use behavior and their relationship; this lasted for six months.

The cases would then be terminated and followed up for six months. A summary of the intervention process and the intervention goals through a case illustration is shown in Table 6.

EVALUATION OF THE INTERVENTION MODEL

Several evaluation mechanisms were used to evaluate the effectiveness of the program. As far as objective outcome evaluation is concerned, a one-group pretest-posttest design with different outcome indicators (Internet addiction behavior, attitude to Internet addiction, parenting and psychological well-being) was employed (30). Results showed that Internet addiction behavior of the program participants significantly dropped after they joined the program and there were some changes in parenting after the intervention.

Regarding the findings based on subjective outcome evaluation, several observations can be highlighted from the study. First, all program participants agreed that the objectives of the program had been achieved via counseling and they felt much better as compared with the first time they received counseling. Second, all participants regarded the counseling as helpful. Third, most of the respondents (92.5%) agreed that they had learned how to deal with their own problems through counseling. Fourth, most of them agreed that they were more able to solve their own problems as compared with the first time they received counseling.

Qualitative analyses based on seven adolescents and three parent cases showed several observations. First, the impression about the program was basically positive. Second, the impression about the workers was also basically positive. Third, there were positive changes in Internet use amongst adolescent clients after receiving the service. Fourth, there were positive changes in family relationships after receiving the service. Fifth, there were positive interpersonal relationship and cognitive changes in the informants after receiving the service. Sixth, several causes of change in the informants were identified (31).

Taken as a whole, the initial evaluation findings are very positive and they suggest the clinical utility of the integrated counseling model for young people with Internet addiction problem. Of course, the limitations of the existing evaluation of the integrated model should be realized. In future, randomized clinical trials and longitudinal evaluation studies should be conducted to examine the sustained effects of the program. In view of the lack of evidence-based addiction intervention programs in Hong Kong (32), the present study can be regarded as an interesting addition to the literature.

REFERENCES

[1] Hur MH. Demographic, habitual, and socioeconomic determinants of Internet addiction disorder: an empirical study of Korean teenagers. Cyberpsychol Behav 2006;9(5):514-25.

[2] Young K. Internet addiction: symptoms, evaluation, and treatment. In: VandeCreek L, Jackson T, editors. Innovations in clinical practice: a source book. Sarasota, FL: Professional Resource Press; 1999. p.19-31.

[3] Johansson A, Götestam KG. Internet addiction: characteristic of a questionnaire and prevalence in Norwegian youth (12-18 years). Scan J Psychol 2004;45:223-9.

[4] Bayraktar F, Gün Z. Incidence and correlates of Internet usage among adolescents in North Cyprus. Cyberpsychol Behav 2007;10(2):191-7.

[5] Ko CH, Yen JY, Yen CF, Lin HC, Yang MJ. Factors predictive for incidence and remission of Internet addiction in young adolescents: a prospective study. Cyberpsychol Behav 2007;10(4):545-51.

[6] Yang SC, Tung CJ. Comparison of Internet addicts and non-addicts in Taiwanese high school. Comput Hum Behav 2004;23:79-96.

[7] China Youth Internet Association. 2009 Report on youth Internet addiction disorder, 2010 [Internet]. Available from: http://mat1.gtimg.com/edu/pdf/wangyinbaogao.pdf

[8] Ko CH, Yen JY, Liu SC, Huang CF, Yen CF. The associations between aggressive behaviors and Internet addiction and online activities in adolescents. J Adolesc Health 2009;44(6):598-605.

[9] Yen JY, Ko CH, Yen CF, Wu HY, Yang MJ. The comorbid psychiatric symptoms of Internet addiction: attention deficit and hyperactivity disorder (ADHD), depression, social phobia, and hostility. J Adolesc Health 2007;41(1):93-8.

[10] Leung L. Net-generation attributes and seductive properties of the Internet as predictors of online activities and Internet addiction. Cyberpsychol Behav 2004;7(3): 333-48.

[11] Working Group of @er.com, Tang MY, Shek DTL. Internet addiction among Chinese young people: a report on youth characteristics. Hong Kong: Hong Kong Jockey Club Wah Ming Integrated Youth Services Centre, Hong Kong Lutheran Social Service, LC-HKS, 2006.

[12] Shek DTL, Yu L. Internet addiction in Hong Kong adolescents: profiles and psychosocial correlates. Int J Disabil Hum Dev 2012;11(2):133-42.

[13] Shek DTL, Yu L. Internet addiction phenomenon in early adolescents in Hong Kong. ScientificWorldJournal 2012. doi:10.1100/2012/104304.

[14] Shek DTL, Yu L. Internet addiction in Hong Kong adolescents: a three-year longitudinal study. J Pediatr Adolesc Gynecol 2013;26(3 Suppl):S10-7.

[15] Huang XQ, Zhang HM, Li MC, Wang JN, Zhang Y, Tao R. Mental health, personality, and parental rearing styles of adolescents with Internet addiction disorder. Cyberpsychol Behav Soc Netw 2010;13(4):401-6.

[16] Orzack MH, Voluse AC, Wolf D, Hennen J. An ongoing study of group treatment for men involved in problematic Internet-enabled sexual behavior. Cyberpsychol Behav 2006;9(3):348-60.

[17] Shek DTL, Sun RCF, Yu L. Internet addiction. In: Pfaff DW, editor. Neuroscience in the 21st century. Berlin: Springer, 2013:2775-811.

[18] Shek DTL, Chan EML, Wong RHY. Comorbid mood and adjustment disorders among pathological gamblers seeking treatment in Hong Kong. Int Gamb Stud 2012. doi: 10.1080/14459795.2012.6890000.

[19] Shek DTL, Chan EML, Wong RHY. Associations between pathological gambling and psychiatric comorbidity among help-seeking populations in Hong Kong. ScientificWorldJournal 2012. doi: 10.1100/2012/571434.

[20] Prochaska JO, DiClemente CC. The transtheoretical approach: crossing traditional boundaries of theory. Homewook, IL: Dow Jones/Irwin, 1984.

[21] Prochaska JO, DiClemente CC. Toward a comprehensive model of change. In: Miller WR, Heather N, editors. Treating addictive behaviors: processes of change. New York: Plenum, 1986:3-27.

[22] Miller WR. Motivational enhancement therapy with drug abusers. Albuquerque, NM: Department of Psychology and Centre on Alcoholism, Substance Abuse, and Addictions (CASAA), University New Mexico, 1995.

[23] Miller WR, Rollnick S. Motivational interviewing: preparing people for change. New York: Guilford, 1991.

[24] Rollnick S, Miller WR. What is motivational interviewing? Behav Cogn Psychother 1995;23:325-34.

[25] Hanna SM, Brown JH. The practice of family therapy: key elements across models. Pacific Grove, CA: Brooks/Cole, 1995.

[26] Shek DTL. Family functioning and psychological well-being, school adjustment and substance abuse in Chinese adolescents: are findings based on multiple studies consistent? In: Prester TA, editor. Psychology of adolescents. New York, NY: Nova Science, 2003:15-37.

[27] Van Den Eijnden RJ, Spijkerman R, Vermulst AA, Van Rooij TJ, Engels RC. Compulsive Internet use among adolescents: bidirectional parent–child relationships. J Abnorm Child Psych 2010;38(1):77-89.

[28] Liu QX, Fang XY, Deng LY, Zhang JT. Parent–adolescent communication, parental Internet use and Internet-specific norms and pathological Internet use among Chinese adolescents. Comput Hum Behav 2012;28(4):1269-75.

[29] Shek DTL. Tackling adolescent substance abuse in Hong Kong: where we should and should not go. ScientificWorldJournal 2007;7:2021-30.

[30] Shek DTL, Tang MY, Lo CY. Evaluation of an Internet addiction treatment program for Chinese adolescents in Hong Kong. Adolescence 2009;44(174):359-73.

[31] Shek DTL, Tang MY, Working Group of @er.com. Youngster Internet addiction prevention and counseling service: an evaluation study. Hong Kong: Hong Kong Jockey Club Wah Ming Integrated Youth Services Centre, Hong Kong Lutheran Social Service, LC-HKS,2008.

[32] Shek DTL, Lam MC, Tsoi KW. Evidence-based social work practice in Hong Kong. In: Thyer B, Kazi M, editors. International perspectives on evidence-based practice in social work. London: Venture Press, 2004:213-22.

Submitted: December 15, 2012. *Revised:* January 02, 2013. *Accepted:* January 24, 2013.

SECTION FIVE – ACKNOWLEDGEMENTS

In: Child and Adolescent Health Yearbook 2013
Editor: Joav Merrick
ISBN: 978-1-63117-658-6

Chapter 46

ABOUT THE EDITOR

Joav Merrick, MD, MMedSci, DMSc, is professor of pediatrics, child health and human development affiliated with Kentucky Children's Hospital, University of Kentucky, Lexington, United States and the Division of Pediatrics, Hadassah Hebrew University Medical Centers, Mt Scopus Campus, Jerusalem, Israel, the medical director of the Health Services, Division for Intellectual and Developmental Disabilities, Ministry of Social Affairs and Social Services, Jerusalem, the founder and director of the National Institute of Child Health and Human Development. Numerous publications in the field of pediatrics, child health and human development, rehabilitation, intellectual disability, disability, health, welfare, abuse, advocacy, quality of life and prevention. Received the Peter Sabroe Child Award for outstanding work on behalf of Danish Children in 1985, while still living in Denmark and the International LEGO-Prize ("The Children's Nobel Prize") for an extraordinary contribution towards improvement in child welfare and well-being in 1987.

Contact

Office of the Medical Director, Health Services, Division for Intellectual and Developmental Disabilities, Ministry of Social Affairs ans Social Services, POBox 1260, IL-91012 Jerusalem, Israel. E-mail: jmerrick@zahav.net.il

In: Child and Adolescent Health Yearbook 2013
Editor: Joav Merrick

ISBN: 978-1-63117-658-6

Chapter 47

About the National Institute of Child Health and Human Development in Israel

The National Institute of Child Health and Human Development (NICHD) in Israel was established in 1998 as a virtual institute under the auspicies of the Medical Director, Ministry of Social Affairs and Social Services in order to function as the research arm for the Office of the Medical Director. In 1998 the National Council for Child Health and Pediatrics, Ministry of Health and in 1999 the Director General and Deputy Director General of the Ministry of Health endorsed the establishment of the NICHD.

Mission

The mission of a National Institute for Child Health and Human Development in Israel is to provide an academic focal point for the scholarly interdisciplinary study of child life, health, public health, welfare, disability, rehabilitation, intellectual disability and related aspects of human development. This mission includes research, teaching, clinical work, information and public service activities in the field of child health and human development.

Service and academic activities

Over the years many activities became focused in the south of Israel due to collaboration with various professionals at the Faculty of Health Sciences (FOHS) at the Ben Gurion University of the Negev (BGU). Since 2000 an affiliation with the Zusman Child Development Center at the Pediatric Division of Soroka University Medical Center has resulted in collaboration around the establishment of the Down Syndrome Clinic at that center. In 2002 a full course on "Disability" was established at the Recanati School for Allied Professions in the Community, FOHS, BGU and in 2005 collaboration was started with the Primary Care Unit of the faculty and disability became part of the master of public health course on "Children and society". In the academic year 2005-2006 a one semester course on "Aging with disability" was started as part of the master of science program in gerontology in our collaboration with the Center for Multidisciplinary Research in Aging. In 2010 collaborations with the Division of Pediatrics, Hadassah Medical Centers, Hebrew University, Jerusalem, Israel.

Research activities

The affiliated staff have over the years published work from projects and research activities in this national and international collaboration. In the year 2000 the International Journal of Adolescent Medicine and Health and in 2005 the International Journal on Disability and Human development of De Gruyter Publishing House (Berlin and New York), in the year 2003 the TSW-Child Health and Human Development and in 2006 the TSW-Holistic Health and Medicine of the Scientific World Journal (New York and Kirkkonummi, Finland), all peer-reviewed international journals were affiliated with the National Institute of Child Health and Human Development. From 2008 also the International Journal of Child Health and Human Development (Nova Science, New York), the International Journal of Child and Adolescent Health (Nova Science) and the Journal of Pain Management (Nova Science) affiliated and from 2009 the International Public Health Journal (Nova Science) and Journal of Alternative Medicine Research (Nova Science).

National collaborations

Nationally the NICHD works in collaboration with the Faculty of Health Sciences, Ben Gurion University of the Negev; Department of Physical Therapy, Sackler School of Medicine, Tel Aviv University; Autism Center, Assaf HaRofeh Medical Center; National Rett and PKU Centers at Chaim Sheba Medical Center, Tel HaShomer; Department of Physiotherapy, Haifa University; Department of Education, Bar Ilan University, Ramat Gan, Faculty of Social Sciences and Health Sciences; College of Judea and Samaria in Ariel and in 2011 affiliation with Center for Pediatric Chronic Diseases and Center for Down Syndrome, Department of Pediatrics, Hadassah-Hebrew University Medical Center, Mount Scopus Campus, Jerusalem.

International collaborations

Internationally with the Department of Disability and Human Development, College of Applied Health Sciences, University of Illinois at Chicago; Strong Center for Developmental Disabilities, Golisano Children's Hospital at Strong, University of Rochester School of Medicine and Dentistry, New York; Centre on Intellectual Disabilities, University of Albany, New York; Centre for Chronic Disease Prevention and Control, Health Canada, Ottawa; Chandler Medical Center and Children’s Hospital, Kentucky Children’s Hospital, Section of Adolescent Medicine, University of Kentucky, Lexington; Chronic Disease Prevention and Control Research Center, Baylor College of Medicine, Houston, Texas; Division of Neuroscience, Department of Psychiatry, Columbia University, New York; Institute for the Study of Disadvantage and Disability, Atlanta; Center for Autism and Related Disorders,

Department Psychiatry, Children's Hospital Boston, Boston; Department of Paediatrics, Child Health and Adolescent Medicine, Children's Hospital at Westmead, Westmead, Australia; International Centre for the Study of Occupational and Mental Health, Düsseldorf, Germany; Centre for Advanced Studies in Nursing, Department of General Practice and Primary Care, University of Aberdeen, Aberdeen, United Kingdom; Quality of Life Research Center, Copenhagen, Denmark; Nordic School of Public Health, Gottenburg, Sweden, Scandinavian Institute of Quality of Working Life, Oslo, Norway; Centre for Quality of Life of the Hong Kong Institute of Asia-Pacific Studies and School of Social Work, Chinese University, Hong Kong.

Targets

Our focus is on research, international collaborations, clinical work, teaching and policy in health, disability and human development and to establish the NICHD as a permanent institute at one of the residential care centers for persons with intellectual disability in Israel in order to conduct model research and together with the four university schools of public health/medicine in Israel establish a national master and doctoral program in disability and human development at the institute to secure the next generation of professionals working in this often non-prestigious/low-status field of work.

Contact

Joav Merrick, MD, MMedSci, DMSc
Professor of Pediatrics, Child Health and Human Development
Medical Director, Health Services, Division for Intellectual and Developmental Disabilities, Ministry of Social Affairs and Social Services, POB 1260, IL-91012 Jerusalem, Israel.
E-mail: jmerrick@zahav.net.il

SECTION SIX – INDEX

INDEX

#

A

B

C

D

E

F

G

H

I

J

K

L

M

N

O

P

Q

R

S

T

U

V

W

X

Y

Z